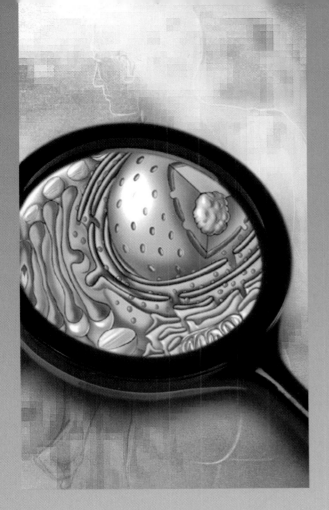

The Human Body in Health and Illness

Barbara Herlihy, PhD, RN
Professor
University of the Incarnate Word
School of Nursing
San Antonio, Texas

Nancy K. Maebius, PhD, RN
Instructor
The Health Institute of San Antonio
San Antonio, Texas

Illustrations by **Caitlin H. Duckwall**
Duckwall Productions
Baltimore, Maryland

W.B. SAUNDERS COMPANY
A Harcourt Health Sciences Company
Philadelphia • London • New York • St. Louis • Sydney • Toronto

W.B. SAUNDERS COMPANY
A Harcourt Health Sciences Company

The Curtis Center
Independence Square West
Philadelphia, Pennsylvania 19106

Library of Congress Cataloging-in-Publication Data

Herlihy, Barbara L.

The human body in health and illness / Barbara Herlihy,
Nancy K. Maebius.—1st ed.

p.   cm.

Includes index.

ISBN 0–7216–6107–6

1. Human physiology.   2. Physiology, Pathological.   I. Maebius,
  Nancy K.   II. Title.
  [DNLM: 1. Physiology.   2. Pathology.   QT 104 H549h 2000]

QP34.5.H46 2000   612—dc21

DNLM/DLC   99-26386

THE HUMAN BODY IN HEALTH AND ILLNESS   ISBN 0–7216–6107–6

Printed in the United States of America

Last digit is the print number: 9   8   7   6   5   4   3   2

To my family:
    my husband, Jeremiah
    my children, Joseph and Kellie
    my sister, Jean
    my furry friend, Pretzyl
BH

To my family:
    my father, Robert C. Kingsland
    my husband, Jed
    my children, Stephen, Maria, Elizabeth, Tom, Brian, Andrew
    my grandchildren, Allison and Sarah
NKM

To the Instructor

Yes! Another textbook on anatomy and physiology . . . but this one is different—very, very different. For one thing, it is interesting and sometimes amusing. *The Human Body in Health and Illness* tells the story of the human body, with all its parts and the way these parts work together. It is a story that we have told many times in our classes. It is also a story that gets better with each telling, because the body continues to reveal its mysteries and how marvelously it has been created. It is our hope that you enjoy telling the story as much as we do. This book has been a labor of love; it is the fruit of a lifetime of teaching anatomy and physiology and loving every minute of it.

The Human Body in Health and Illness is a basic anatomy and physiology text that is addressed to the student who is preparing for a career in the health professions. The text is written for students with minimal preparation in the sciences; no prior knowledge of biology, chemistry, or physics is required. The text provides all the background science information needed for the understanding of anatomy and physiology. The basic principles of chemistry are presented in two chapters and set the stage for an understanding of cellular function, fluid and electrolyte balance, and digestion. Microbiology basics are included in Appendix A.

The anatomy and physiology content is presented in a traditional order, from simple to complex. The text begins with the description of a single cell and progresses through the various organ systems. There are two key themes that run through the text. The first theme is the relationship between structure and function—the student must understand that an organ is anatomically designed to perform a specific physiologic task. The second major theme is homeostasis—the role that each organ system plays in sustaining life, and what happens when that delicate balance is disturbed.

Textbook Strengths

We believe that the text has many strengths:

- The anatomy and physiology are clearly and simply explained. A beautiful set of illustrations, complete with cartoons, supports the text. In fact, the story of the body is told as much through the art as through the written word. A promise: You will be delighted with the reaction of your students to this art program!

- This text truly integrates pathophysiology; it is not merely boxed or tacked on at the end. The integrated pathophysiology is used primarily to amplify the normal anatomy and physiology. For example, the text describes the role of the bone marrow in the production of blood cells. The integrated pathophysiology describes the effects of bone marrow depression in relation to anemia, infection, and bleeding. The pathophysiology of bone marrow depression amplifies the role of the bone marrow and helps the student make the transition to clinical applications.

- In addition to the pathophysiology, other topics are liberally integrated throughout the text. These include common diagnostic procedures such as blood count, lumbar puncture, urinalysis, and electrocardiogram. Pharmacologic agents are also introduced and, like the pathophysiology, are used to amplify the anatomy and physiology. For instance, the discussion of the neuromuscular junction is enhanced by a description of the effects of neuromuscular blocking agents. Because of the effort to make clinical correlations, this text sets the stage for the more advanced health science courses, including pharmacology, medical and surgical nursing, and maternity nursing.

- Medical terminology is introduced, defined, and used throughout the text. Common clinical terms, such as hypokalemia, vasodilation, hypertension, and diagnosis are defined and re-used so that the student gradually builds a substantial medical vocabulary. Appendix B is a concise list of medical and eponymous terms.

- The text incorporates many amusing anecdotes from the history of medicine. Although the human body is perfectly logical and predictable, we humans think, do, and say some strange things. Tales from the crypt provide some good laughs and much humility.

Features

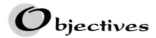
Objectives

The objectives identify the goals of the chapter.

••• Key Terms

The key terms are pronounced, thoroughly explained in the chapter, and defined in the glossary.

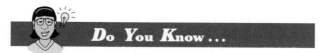
Do You Know...

Most of these boxed vignettes refer to clinical situations; others relate interesting historical events.

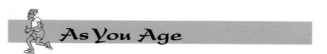
As You Age

These identify the major physiologic changes that occur with aging.

Summary Outlines

At the end of each chapter is a detailed summary outline. The outline serves as an excellent review of the chapter and helps the student pull the content together.

Review Your Knowledge

These "short-answer" questions review the major points of the chapter and ask the students to integrate key concepts.

✳ SUM IT UP!

Sum it up paragraphs appear regularly throughout the chapters and help the student to pull together key concepts.

Disorders of . . .

These tables describe specific disorders related to individual body systems.

Appendices. The three appendices provide supplemental information in microbiology, medical terminology, and laboratory values.

Appendix A includes the basics of microbiology. Key microbiologic terms, such as pathogen, nosocomial infection, opportunistic infection, and normal flora, are defined. An inclusive list of key terms is summarized in a table. The types, characteristics, and laboratory identification of microorganisms, such as bacteria, viruses, rickettsia, and fungi, are briefly described. The pathogens and the diseases caused by these pathogens are summarized in an extensive table. The information provided in this Appendix provides the basic information necessary for topics such as asepsis and the pharmacology of antimicrobial therapy.

Appendix B includes an introduction to medical terminology and a listing of eponymous terms. A table of prefixes, suffixes, and word roots provides ample information for a beginning course in medical terminology.

Appendix C is a section on laboratory values. Laboratory values for common blood tests, such as hemoglobin, WBC differential count, and blood electrolytes, are listed. Also included is a table of laboratory values for routine urinalysis.

Glossary. The extensive glossary includes a pronunciation guide and a brief definition of all key terms and many other words in the text.

Ancillary Package

Study Guide. The Study Guide for *The Human Body in Health and Illness* is thorough and designed to help the student integrate the information presented in the text. The Study Guide is divided into three parts: Part I, *Mastering the Basics,* contains matching, labeling, and coloring exercises for each content area in the corresponding textbook chapter. *Putting It All Together,* the second part, contains multiple-choice practice quizzes, completion exercises, and case studies that integrate the chapter content. Part III, *Challenge Yourself!,* contains critical thinking questions.

Instructor's Manual. The Instructor's Manual is composed of five parts: Part I, Introduction; Part II, Chapter Summary Outlines with corresponding Learning Activities; Part III, Test Bank of over 565 multiple-choice questions; Part IV, Answers to the Review Your Knowledge questions in the textbook; and Part V, the Study Guide answers.

The Learning Activities in Part II help convert the passive student into an active learner. For example, there are numerous clinical case studies, directions for the use of modeling clay, suggestions for the construction of collages, and an emphasis on creating a print-rich environment by the use of word walls and word sorts. Our students use, enjoy, and learn from these activities.

Color Transparencies. A set of 55 full-color transparencies of the major illustrations is available.

ExaMaster. A test bank of over 565 NCLEX-style questions is available. The computerized format allows the instructor to modify or add to the basic list of questions.

The Instructor's Manual, transparencies, and computerized test bank are free to adopters of the textbook. Contact your W.B. Saunders Company sales representative for information.

••• TO THE STUDENT

This book will take you on a cycle from the simplest to the most complex structure in the anatomy and physiology of a human being. You will also learn about what happens when human beings become ill with disorders of those structures. To help make learning this enjoyable and fun, we've spotlighted the following special features for you:

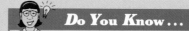

••• Key Terms

Action potential (ăk′shən pə-tĕn′shəl)
Brain stem (brān′ stĕm)
Cerebellum (sĕr″ə-bĕl′əm)

● **Key Terms** with **Pronunciation Guides** open each chapter. They are in bold type in the book and are defined in the Glossary

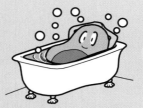

Do You Know...

What is meant by a blood clot on the brain?

Although the brain is well protected, a head injury may cause bleeding. Boxers, for instance, are often hit in the head. As the head snaps in response to the blow, blood vessels rupture, and bleeding

● **Do You Know?** boxes, often illustrated, pique your interest with novel background information related to A&P.

*O*bjectives

1. Define the two divisions of the nervous system.
2. List three general functions of the nervous system.
3. Compare the structure and functions of the neur

● **Objectives** for learning at the beginning of each chapter give you goals to keep in mind while you read.

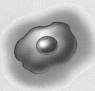

● Full-color **Cartoons** bring anatomy and physiology closer to you with humor, clarity, and insight.

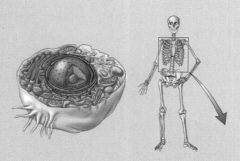

● **Original, full-color illustrations** help you make sense of anatomy and physiology structure, function, and concepts.

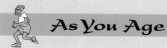

As You Age

1. Beginning at the age of 30, the number of neurons decreases. The number lost, however, is only a small percentage of the total number of brain cells and does not

● **As You Age** contains bulleted lists describing how human A&P is affected by the aging process.

Disorders of the Nervous Tissue . . .

Alcohol-induced neurotoxicity	Chronic and excessive ingestion of alcohol cau nervous system. The result is mental deterioratio concentrate, irritability, and uncoordinated mo syndrome is an alcohol-related type of encepha
Alzheimer's disease	A degenerative disease of the brain usually Alzheimer's disease is characterized by progro paired intellectual function. Evidence suggests the frontal and temporal lobes.

- **Disorders of the . . .** are pathophysiology tables that describe disorders related to specific body systems.

✳ **SUM IT UP!** The CNS, especially the brain, performs eloquently as a conductor. It coordinates the various organ systems of the body efficiently, with fine precision. The brain makes us hu-

- **SUM IT UP!** paragraphs throughout each chapter help you to quickly scan and review the key concepts.

Glossary

Adrenalin (ə-drĕn′ə-lĭn) See epinephrine.
Adrenergic fiber (ăd″rə-nŭ ′jĭk fī′bər) A fiber that secretes norepinephrine at the axon terminal; postganglionic fibers of the sympathetic nervous system are adrenergic fibers.
Adrenocorticotropic hormone (ACTH) (ə-drē″no-kôr″tĭ-kō-trŏp′ĭk hōr′mōn) A hormone secreted by the anterior pituitary gland; it stimulates the adrenal cortex to secrete steroids, particularly cortisol.

Appendixes

*Microbiology Basics
*Medical Terminology and Eponymous Terms
*Laboratory Values

Summary Outline

The purpose of the nervous system is to bring information to the central nervous system, interpret the information, and enable the body to respond to the information.
I. The Nervous System: Overview
  A. Divisions of the Nervous System
    1. The central nervous system (CNS) includes the brain and the spinal cord.

- The **Summary Outline** at the end of each chapter serves as a study tool. Use them to review your reading and prepare for exams.

Review Your Knowledge

1. How is the central nervous system different from the peripheral nervous system?
2. What is the difference between neuroglia and neurons? Name the functions of astrocytes and ependymal cells.

- **Review Your Knowledge** questions are at the end of each chapter.

Enhance your learning of the textbook content with the accompanying **Study Guide for The Human Body in Health and Illness.** The Study Guide has something to offer students at all levels of learning, from labeling and coloring exercises to multiple choice practice tests and case studies.

Acknowledgments

Writing, editing, illustrating, publishing, and marketing a new anatomy and physiology book has involved the combined efforts of many outstanding individuals. Grateful thanks to the staff at W.B. Saunders, especially

- Robin Levin Richman, Senior Developmental Editor, for her terrific efforts to coordinate it all. No words can express our gratitude for her kindness, patience, persistence, openness of thought, and good humor;
- Terri Wood, Editor, Nursing Books, for her great effort in seeing this book through to completion;
- Debra Osnowitz, Developmental Editor, for her editing and encouragement;
- Caitlin Duckwall, of Duckwall Productions, for the beautiful illustrations. Her cartoons, created with the help of her husband Rob, put the finishing touches on an outstanding art program;
- Annette Ferran, Copy Editor;
- Jonel Sofian, Designer; and
- Pete Faber, Senior Production Manager.

In addition, we would like to thank Ilze Rader, former Senior Editor, Nursing Books, who got this project off the ground, and Marie Thomas, Senior Editorial Assistant, who was a wonderful support.

We thank the many reviewers who offered many valuable suggestions:

Cynthia Amerson, MS, BSN, RN, Northeast Texas Community College, Mt. Pleasant, Texas; **Mary Snipes Armstead, MA, BSN, RN,** New Horizons Regional Education Center, Hampton, Virginia; **L. Adrienne Bowlus, MSN, RN,** Apollo Career Center, Lima, Ohio; **Reitha Cabaniss, MSN, RN,** Bevill State Community College, Sumiton, Alabama; **Cynthia D. Casey, BSN, RN,** Hinds Community College, Jackson, Mississippi; **Anne M. Comiskey, BSN, RN,** Nassau BOCES, Westbury, New York; **Justine Ann Coppinger, MS, CGC,** Genetic Counselor, Division of Reproductive Genetics, The University of Utah, Salt Lake City, Utah; **Monica G. DeCarlo, MSN, RN,C,** Indiana County Area Vocational-Technical School, Indiana, Pennsylvania; **Julia C. Dent, MEd, EdS, BSN, RN,** Coastal Georgia Community College, Brunswick, Georgia; **Kathleen Dolin, BSN, RN,** Monroe County Area Vocational-Technical School, Bartonsville, Pennsylvania; **Delores L. Garner, MS, BSN, RN,** Hinds Community College, Jackson, Mississippi; **Lois Harrion, MS, RN,** Simi Valley Adult School, Simi Valley, California; **M. Rita Hejtmanek, MS, RN,** Tulsa Technology Center, Tulsa, Oklahoma; **Phyllis S. Howard, BSN, RN,** Kentucky Technical Institute, Ashland Campus, Ashland, Kentucky; **Donna Leach Kane, BS, RN,** Louisiana Technical College, South Louisiana Campus, Houma, Louisiana; **Janice M. Kilgallon, MSN, RN,C,** Passaic County Technical Institute, Wayne, New Jersey; **Patricia Laing-Arie, RN,** Meridian Technology Center, Stillwater, Oklahoma; **Valerie I. Blickos Leek, MS, RN,C,** Cumberland County Technical Education Center, Bridgeton, New Jersey; **Carolyn Morrison Maybee, PHN, BSN, RN,** Citrus College, Glendora, California; **Marion Elizabeth Monahan, MAEd, RN,** Jefferson County Vocational-Technical School, Reynoldsville, Pennsylvania; **Sally J. O'Neil, MSEd, BS, RN,** W.F. Kaynor Regional Vocational-Technical School, Waterbury, Connecticut; **Donna N. Roddy, MSN, RN,** Chattanooga State Technical Community College, Chattanooga, Tennessee; **Ruth A. Speakman, MEd, BSN, RN,** Apollo School of Practical Nursing, Lima, Ohio; **Kathleen G. Stilling, MS, RN,C,** Johnston School of Practical Nursing, Baltimore, Maryland; **Donna Welty Stoner, BSN, RN,** Amarillo

College, Amarillo, Texas; **Barbara Gayle Talik, MEd, BSN, RN,** Northwest Technical Institute, Springdale, Arkansas; **Kiska H. Varela, MSN, RN, ANP,** Texas Careers, San Antonio, Texas; and **Loretta Lucille White, MSN, RN,** IVY Technical State College, Greencastle, Indiana.

Barbara Herlihy thanks her students and friends at the University of the Incarnate Word. For three years they have been asking the same question, "Have you finished the book yet?" Yes! And thank you. Thanks to Jerry Herlihy for typing tables and putting up with messy paper-littered tables and book-strewn rooms. Thanks to my children Joey and Kellie, for their lack of patience and insistence that I play. Thanks to my sister Jean, who, like my friends, started every long-distance phone conversation with "Is IT done?" Thanks to Dr. Susan Hall for her proofreading, encouragement, and the many ideas she offered about learning activities for the Instructor's Manual. Thanks to all my friends who sat around the pool in Harmony Hills and told me to "Hurry up . . . so we can have fun." Thanks to my racquetball pals at the Incarnate Word gym for the hours of exercise and diversion . . . can't say enough about exercise and sanity. Last, but not least, many thanks to my little furry friend, Pretzyl, for the hundreds of hours she sat next to my computer as I typed away.

Barbara Herlihy

Nancy Maebius thanks her friends, students, and colleagues at The Health Institute of San Antonio. The vocational nursing students, from whom I learn so much, provided much inspiration and many ideas for inclusion of content; friends and colleagues who supplied encouragement include Bev Halter, Kiska Varela, Lea Ann Loftis, Donna Albee, Beryl Pixley, Collette Moreno, Michael Pleuger, Mary Ellen Proscia, and Peggy Richardson.

Nancy K. Maebius

Brief Contents

Detailed Contents

The
Human
Body
in
Health
and
Illness

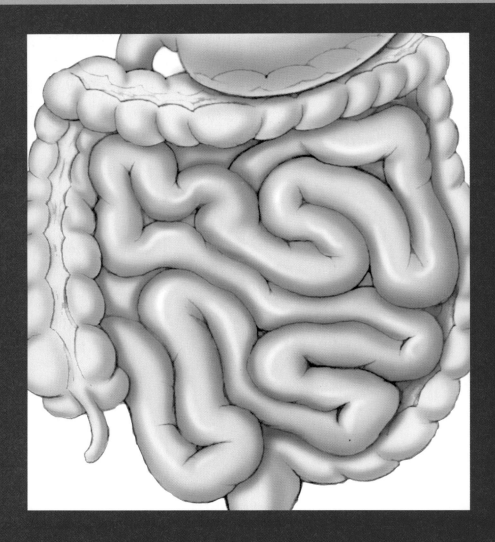

••• Key Terms

Abdominopelvic cavity
  (ăb-dŏm″-ĭ-nō-pĕl′vĭk kăv′ĭ-tē)
Anatomical position
  (ăn″-ə-tŏm′ĭ-kəl pə-zĭsh′ən)
Anatomy (ə-năt′ə-mē)
Cell (sĕl)
Cranial cavity (krā′nē-əl kăv′ĭ-tē)
Dorsal cavity (dôr′səl kăv′ĭ-tē)
Frontal plane (frŭn′tl plān)
Homeostasis (hō″mē-ō-stā′sĭs)
Organ (ôr′gən)

Organ system (ôr′gən sĭs′təm)
Physiology (fĭz″ē-ŏl′ə-jē)
Sagittal plane (săj′ĭ-tl plān)
Spinal (vertebral) cavity
  (spī′nəl or vûr′tə-brəl kăv′ĭ-tē)
Thoracic cavity (thə-răs′ĭk kăv′ĭ-tē)
Tissue (tĭsh′oo)
Transverse plane (trănz-vûrs′ plān)
Ventral cavity (vĕn′trəl kăv′ĭ-tē)

••• Selected terms in bold type in this chapter are defined in the Glossary.

1 INTRODUCTION TO THE HUMAN BODY

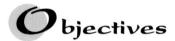

Objectives

1. Define the terms *anatomy* and *physiology.*
2. List the levels of organization of the human body.
3. Describe the 11 major organ systems.
4. Explain the word *homeostasis.*
5. Define the term *anatomical position.*
6. List common terms used for relative positions of the body.
7. Describe the three major planes of the body.
8. List anatomical terms for regions of the body.
9. Describe the major cavities of the body.

The human body is a wonderful creation. Millions of microscopic parts work together in a coordinated fashion to keep you going day in and day out for about 75 years. Most of us are curious about our bodies—how they work, why they do not work, what makes us tick, and what makes us sick. As you study about the body, you will sometimes feel like this cartoon character: "What is this? Why do I need it? How does it work? Why don't I have one?" As you study anatomy and physiology, you will learn the answers to these questions.

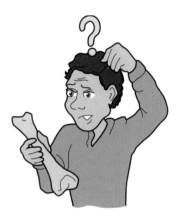

ANATOMY AND PHYSIOLOGY: WHAT THEY ARE

Anatomy (ə-năt′ə-mē) is the branch of science that studies the structure, or morphology, of the body. For instance, anatomy describes what the heart looks like, how big it is, what it is made of, how it is organized, and where it is located. The word *anatomy* comes from the Greek word meaning to dissect. The science of anatomy arose from observations made by scientists as they dissected the body.

Physiology (fĭz″ē-ŏl′ə-jē) is the branch of science that describes how the body works, or functions. For instance, physiology describes how the heart pumps blood and why the pumping of blood is essential for life. **Pathophysiology** is the branch of science that describes the consequences of the improper functioning of the body parts—how a body part functions when a person has a disease. For instance, pathophysiology describes what happens during a heart attack, when the heart functions poorly or not at all.

Why study anatomy and physiology as part of your professional curriculum? You need to know these subjects. Unless you gain a good understanding of normal anatomy and physiology, you cannot understand the diseases and disorders experienced by your patients. Nor can you understand the basis for the various forms of treatment such as drug therapy and surgical procedures.

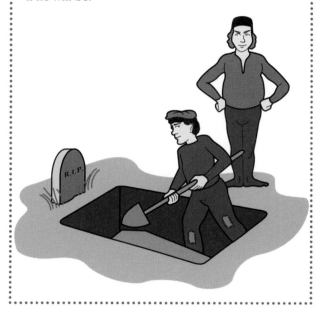

Do You Know...

Why is this grave being robbed, and why is the grave-robber in big, big trouble?

Dissection of the human body during medieval times was not allowed by either the church or the state. Thus, the only way that the early anatomists had of obtaining human bodies for dissection was to rob graves. Medieval scientists hired people to rob graves. Punishment for robbing graves was swift and severe. This lad will be in big, big trouble if he is caught, and it looks as if he will be.

You want to give your patients the best possible care, so you must have a sound understanding of the human body.

Anatomy and physiology are closely related. Structure and function go together. When you examine the anatomy of a body part, ask yourself how its structure relates to its function. For instance, the structure of the hand is related to its function, its ability to grasp an object (Fig. 1–1). The heart pumps blood, and the long, strong, flexible tail of the monkey allows it to hang from the tree. In all animals, structure and function go together.

THE BODY'S LEVELS OF ORGANIZATION

The body is organized from the very simple to the complex, from the microscopic atom to the complex human organism. Note the progression

Do You Know...

Why was this famous anatomy lab built over a small river in Italy?

Because dissection of the human body was illegal during the middle ages, the anatomy labs were routinely raided by the police. In the event of a police raid, the partially dissected body was lowered through a hole in the floor of the lab onto a barge on the river. The body (and incriminating evidence) then floated away.

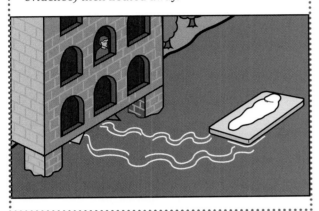

from simple to complex in Figure 1–2. Tiny atoms form molecules. These, in turn, form larger molecules. The larger molecules are eventually organized into **cells** (sĕlz), the basic unit of life. Specialized groups of cells form **tissues** (tĭsh'o͞oz). Tissues are then arranged into **organs** (ôr'gənz) such as the heart, stomach, and kidney. Each organ has a function, such as digestion, excretion, or reproduction. Groups of organs, in turn, create **organ systems** (ôr'gən sĭs'təmz). All of the organ systems together form the **human organism.** From simple to complex, the body is built from the tiny atom to the human being.

ORGANS AND ORGAN SYSTEMS

Definitions: Organs Becoming Organ Systems

An **organ** is a group of tissues arranged to accomplish a particular function. For instance, the tissues of the heart are arranged so that the heart can act as a pump. The heart, of course, pumps blood. An **organ system** is a group of organs that help each other to perform a particular function.

FIGURE 1–1 ● Structure and function: structure and function are closely related.

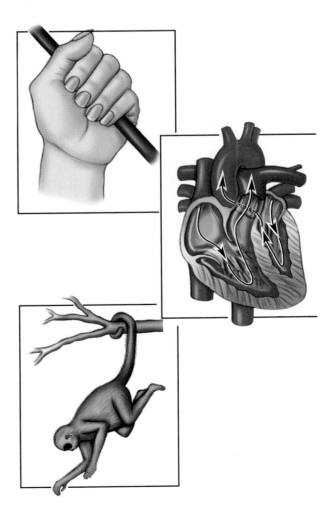

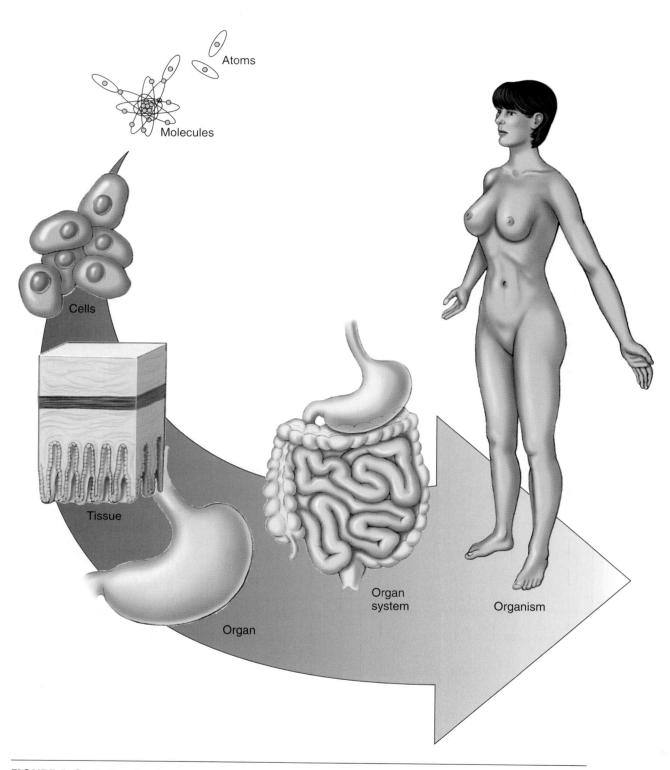

FIGURE 1–2 ● Levels of organization: from simple to complex, from atom to human organism.

Just as the heart is an organ that pumps blood, the blood vessels are organs that receive the blood from the heart, distribute it throughout the body, and return it to the heart. The heart and the blood vessels are both necessary to perform the function of the organ system. This organ system, the circulatory system, delivers oxygen and other nutrients to all the cells of the body. (You will learn about the circulatory system in Chapter 15.)

More Definitions: Major Organ Systems

Eleven major organ systems make up the human body. Each has a specific function. Refer to Figure 1–3 and identify the location and distribution of the organs of each system.

- The **integumentary system** consists of the skin and related structures, such as hair and nails. The integumentary system performs several important functions: it forms a covering for the body, helps to regulate body temperature, and contains some of the structures necessary for sensation.
- The **skeletal system** forms the basic framework of the body. It consists primarily of bones, joints, and cartilage. The skeleton protects and supports body organs.
- The **muscular system** consists of three types of muscles. Skeletal muscles attach to the bones and are responsible for movement of the skeleton and the maintenance of body posture. Two other types of muscles are found within the organs and are responsible for movement.
- The **nervous system** consists of the brain, spinal cord, nerves, and sense organs. Sensory nerves receive information from the environment and bring it to the spinal cord and brain, where it is interpreted. Decisions made by the brain and spinal cord are transmitted along other nerves to various body structures.
- The **endocrine system** consists of numerous glands that secrete hormones and chemical substances that regulate body activities such as growth, reproduction, and water balance.
- The **circulatory system** consists of the heart and blood vessels. This system pumps and transports blood throughout the body. Blood carries nutrients and oxygen to all the body's cells and also carries the waste away from the cells to the organs of excretion.
- The **lymphatic system** consists of the lymph nodes, lymphatic vessels, lymph, and other lymphoid organs (eg, tonsils, spleen). Lymph and lymphoid structures play an important role in the defense of the body against pathogens and other foreign material.
- The **respiratory system** consists of the lungs and other structures that conduct air to and from the lungs. Within the lungs, the respiratory gases, oxygen and carbon dioxide, move across a thin membrane. Oxygen moves into the blood from the lungs and then moves throughout the body. Carbon dioxide moves from the blood into the lungs and is exhaled as waste.
- The **digestive system** consists of organs designed to ingest (eat) food, break it down into substances that can be absorbed by the body, and eliminate the residue, or waste. Digestive organs include the stomach, intestines, and accessory organs such as the liver and gallbladder.
- The **urinary system** consists of the kidneys and other structures that help to excrete waste products from the body through the urine. The urinary system helps control the amount and composition of water and other substances in the body.
- The **reproductive system** consists of organs and structures that enable the human organism to reproduce. The female reproductive system produces the ovum and the hormones essential for pregnancy. The male reproductive system produces sperm and hormones and consists of structures necessary for the deposition of sperm into the female.

HOMEOSTASIS: STAYING THE SAME

Homeostasis (hō″mē-ō-stā′sĭs) literally means staying *(stasis)* the same *(homeo)*. The term refers to the body's ability to maintain a stable internal environment in response to a changing external environment. When your body achieves homeostasis, the conditions in your body remain the same, despite the many changes outside. For instance, your body temperature stays around 37°C (98.6°F) even when room temperature increases to 100°F or decreases to 60°F. The amount of water in your cells stays the same whether you drink 2, 3, or 4 liters of water per day. Your blood sugar remains within normal limits whether you have just eaten a turkey dinner or have fasted for 6 hours.

Homeostasis means that the body has a way of staying the same even when external conditions change. Mechanisms that help maintain homeostasis are called **homeostatic mechanisms**. The body has hundreds of homeostatic mechanisms, including mechanisms for temperature control, blood sugar control, water balance, blood pressure regulation, and regulation of plasma sodium levels. When homeostatic mechanisms do not work normally, the result can be disease or dysfunction. **Homeostatic imbalance** is therefore associated with various disorders.

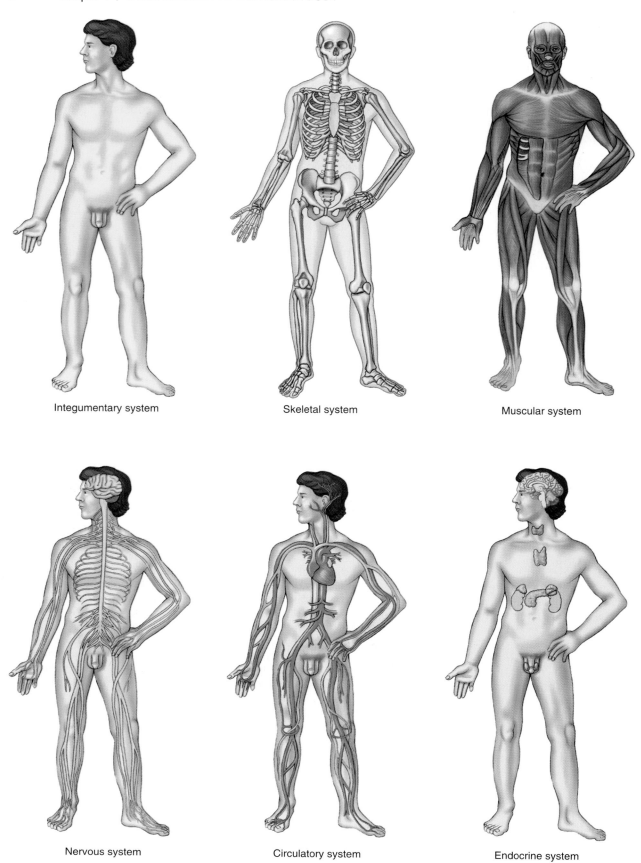

Integumentary system

Skeletal system

Muscular system

Nervous system

Circulatory system

Endocrine system

FIGURE 1–3 ● Major organ systems of the body.

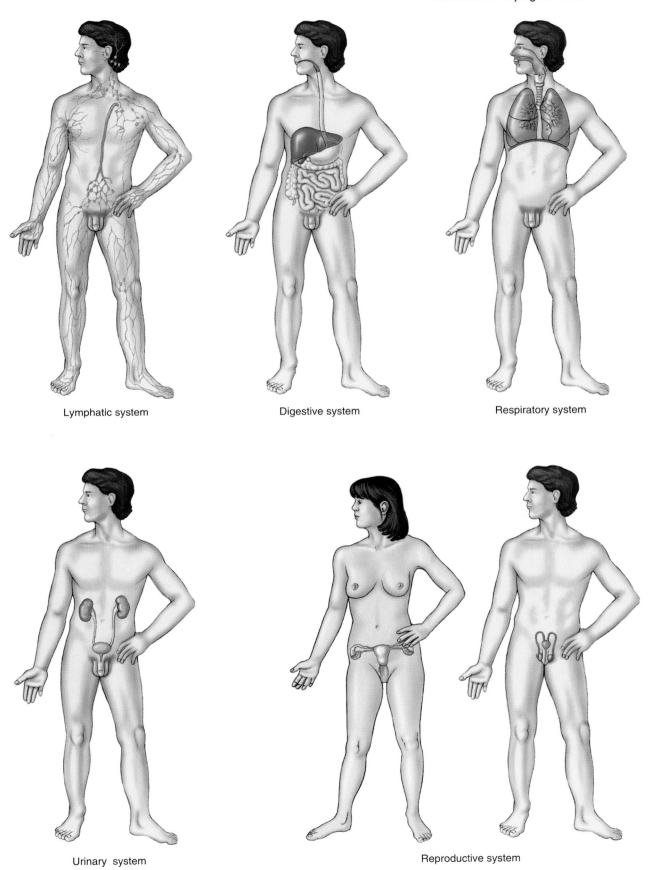

Lymphatic system

Digestive system

Respiratory system

Urinary system

Reproductive system

FIGURE 1–3 • *Continued*

ANATOMICAL TERMS: TALKING ABOUT THE BODY

Special terms describe the location, position, and regions of body parts. Because these terms are used frequently throughout this text (and in all of your medical courses), you should become familiar with them now. Persons in the medical field are often accused of speaking their own language. Indeed, we do! We always use these terms as if the body were standing in its anatomical position.

Anatomical Position

In its **anatomical position** (ăn″ə-tŏm′ĭ-kəl pə-zĭsh′ən), the body is standing erect, with the face forward, the arms at the sides, and the toes and palms of the hands directed forward (Fig. 1–4).

Relative Positions

Specific terms describe the position of one body part in relation to another body part. These are directional terms. They are like the more familiar directions: north, south, east, and west. While you can correctly describe Canada as located north of the United States, you would sound strange if you described the head as north of the chest. In locating body parts, therefore, we use other terminology. The terms come in pairs. Note that the two terms in each pair are generally opposites.

● Superior and inferior. **Superior** means that a part is above another part or is closer to the head. For example, the head is superior to the chest. **Inferior** means that a part is located below another part or is closer to the feet. The chest, for example, is inferior to the head.

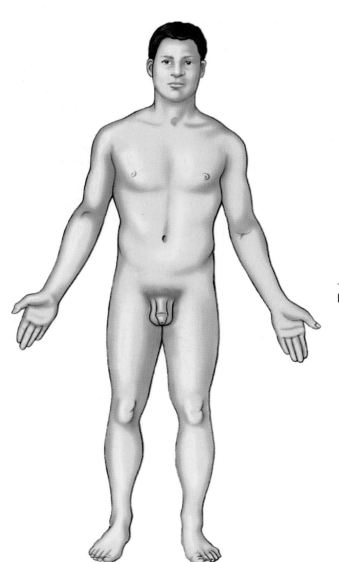

FIGURE 1–4 ● Anatomical position.

- Anterior and posterior. **Anterior** means toward the front surface (the belly surface). **Posterior** means toward the back surface. For example, the heart is anterior to the spinal cord. The heart is posterior to the breast bone. Another word for anterior is **ventral.** Another word for posterior is **dorsal.** If you are a fish lover, think of the dorsal fin of a fish. And if you swim in the ocean, think of the dorsal part of the shark that can be seen moving effortlessly and very quickly toward your surf board!
- Medial and lateral. Imagine a line drawn through the middle of your body, dividing it into right and left halves. This is the midline point. **Medial** means toward the midline of the body. The nose, for example, is medial to the ears. **Lateral** means away from the midline of the body. For example, the ears are lateral to the nose.
- Proximal and distal. **Proximal** means that the structure is nearer the trunk (main part) of the body or is closer to a point of attachment. Because the elbow is closer to the trunk of the body than is the wrist, it is described as proximal to the wrist. The wrist is proximal to the fingers, meaning that the wrist is closer to the trunk of the body than are the fingers. **Distal** means that a part is farther away from the trunk of the body (or point of attachment) than is another part. For example, the wrist is distal to the elbow, and the fingers are distal to the wrist.

 Do You Know...

Why can the wrist be described as both proximal and distal?

The terms *proximal* and *distal* are relational terms. In other words, these terms describe the location of the wrist in relation to another part of the body. For instance, the wrist is proximal to the fingers. This description means that the wrist is closer to the trunk of the body than are the fingers. The wrist is distal to the elbow. This description means that the wrist is farther away from the trunk of the body than is the elbow.

- Superficial and deep. **Superficial** means that a part is located on or near the surface of the body. The skin is superficial to the muscles. **Deep** means that the body part is away from the surface of the body. The bones, for example, are deep to the skin.
- Central and peripheral. **Central** means that the part is located in the center. **Peripheral** means away from the center. The heart, for example, is located centrally, while the blood vessels are located peripherally (away from the center and extending toward the limbs).

✳ **SUM IT UP!** Specific terms describe the relative positions of one body part to the other. The terms are paired as opposites and include superior and inferior, anterior (ventral) and posterior (dorsal), medial and lateral, proximal and distal, superficial and deep, central and peripheral.

Planes and Sections of the Body

When we refer to the left side of the body, the top half of the body, or the front of the body, we are referring to the planes, or sections, of the body. Each plane divides the body with an imaginary line in one direction. Figure 1–5 shows three important planes.

- Sagittal plane (Fig. 1–5A). The **sagittal plane** (săj′ĭ-tl plān) divides the body lengthwise into right and left portions. If the cut is made exactly down the midline of the body, the right and left halves of the body are equal. This division is a **midsagittal section.**
- Frontal plane (Fig. 1–5B). The **frontal plane** (frŭn′tl plān) divides the body into anterior (ventral) and posterior (dorsal) portions. This plane creates the front part of the body and the back part of the body. The frontal plane is also called the **coronal plane.** Why? *Coronal* means crown. The imaginary line for the coronal plane is made across the part of the head where a crown sits and then downward through the body.
- Transverse plane (Fig. 1–5C). The **transverse plane** (trănz-vûrs′ plān) divides the body horizontally, creating an upper (superior) and a lower (inferior) body. When the body or an organ is cut horizontally or transversely, it is called a **cross section.**

Regional Terms

Specific terms describe the different regions or areas of the body. Figure 1–6 illustrates the terms used to identify the regions on the anterior and posterior surfaces of the body.

On the anterior surface, identify the following regions:

Abdominal: anterior trunk just below the ribs
Antecubital: area in front of the elbow
Axillary: armpit
Brachial: arm
Buccal: cheek area
Cephalic: head
Cervical: neck region
Cranial: nearer to the head
Digital: fingers, toes
Femoral: thigh area
Inguinal: area where the thigh meets the trunk of the body

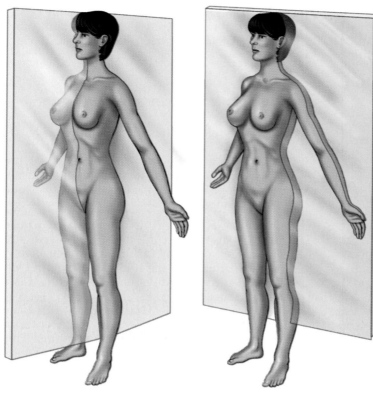

A Sagittal plane   B Frontal (coronal) plane

FIGURE 1–5 ● Planes of the body. A, Sagittal. B, Frontal (coronal). C, Transverse.

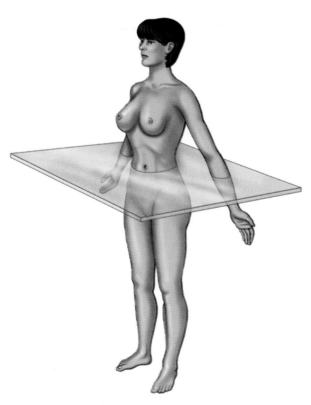

C Transverse plane

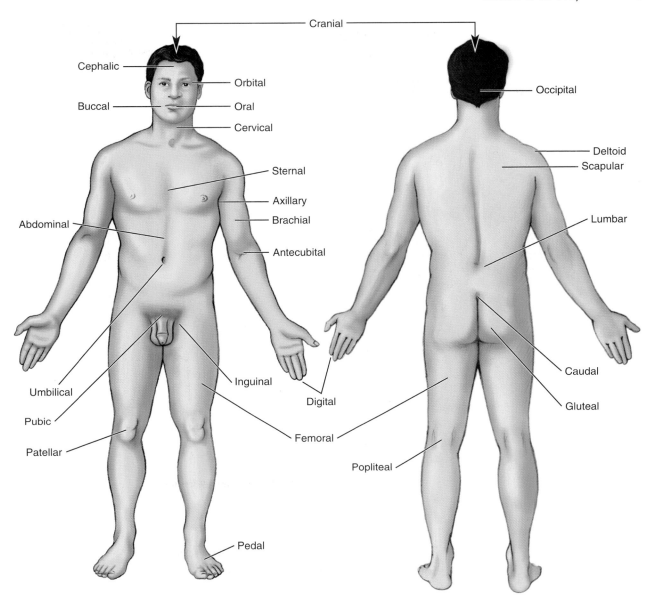

FIGURE 1-6 ● Regional terms. A, Anterior view. B, Posterior view.

Oral: mouth
Orbital: area around the eye
Patellar: front of the knee
Pedal: foot
Pubic: genital area
Sternal: middle of the chest (anterior)
Umbilical: navel

On the posterior surface, identify the following regions:

Caudal: nearer to the lower region of the spinal column (near your tail bone)
Deltoid: rounded area of the shoulder closest to the upper arm
Gluteal: buttocks
Lumbar: area of the back between the ribs and the hips

Occipital: back of the head
Popliteal: behind, or back of, the knee area
Scapular: shoulder blade area

CAVITIES OF THE BODY

Dorsal Cavity

The organs, called **viscera,** are located within the cavities of the body. Cavities are large internal spaces. The body contains two major cavities: the dorsal cavity and the ventral cavity (Fig. 1–7). The **dorsal cavity** (dōr′səl kăv′ĭ-tē) is located toward the back of the body and has two divisions: the **cranial cavity** (krā′nē-əl kăv′ĭtē) and the **spinal**

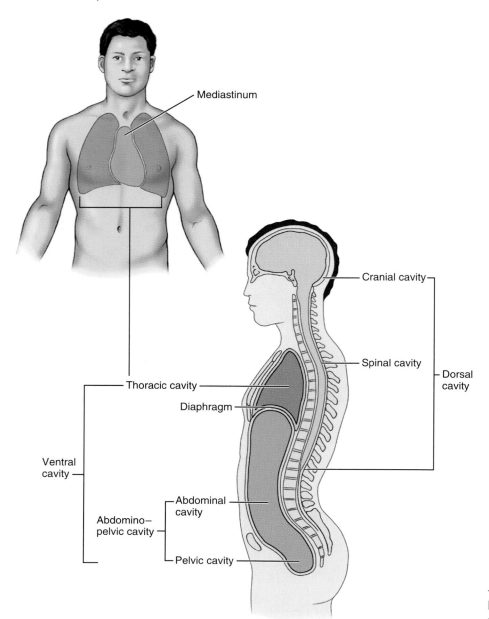

FIGURE 1-7 ● Major body cavities.

(vertebral) cavity (spī′nəl *or* vūr′tə-brəl kăv′ĭ-tē). The cranial cavity is located within the skull and contains the brain. The spinal, or vertebral, cavity extends downward from the cranial cavity and is surrounded by bony vertebrae; it contains the spinal cord. These two areas form one continuous space.

Ventral Cavity

The larger **ventral cavity** (věn′trəl kăv′ĭtē) is located toward the front of the body and has two divisions: the **thoracic cavity** (thə-răs′ĭk kăv′ĭ-tē) and the **abdominopelvic cavity** (ăb-dŏm″ĭ-nō-pĕl′vĭk kăv′ĭ-tē). The thoracic cavity is sur-

rounded by the rib cage and is separated from the abdominopelvic cavity by the diaphragm, a large muscle used in breathing. The thoracic cavity is located above the diaphragm. The lungs occupy most of the space within the thoracic cavity.

Four smaller cavities are located in the head. They include the oral cavity, nasal cavities, orbital cavities, and middle ear cavities. (These cavities are described in later chapters.)

Thoracic Cavity

The thoracic cavity is divided into two compartments by the **mediastinum,** a space that contains the heart, esophagus, trachea, thymus gland, and large blood vessels attached to the heart. The right and left lungs are located on either side of the mediastinum.

Abdominopelvic Cavity

The abdominopelvic cavity is located below, or inferior to, the diaphragm. The upper portion of this cavity is the **abdominal cavity.** It contains the stomach, most of the intestine, the liver, the gallbladder, the pancreas, the spleen, and the kidneys. The lower portion of the abdominopelvic cavity is called the **pelvic cavity.** It extends downward from the level of the hips and includes the rectum, the urinary bladder, and the internal parts of the reproductive system.

Because the abdominopelvic cavity is so large, it is subdivided into smaller areas for study. Quadrants and regions divide the abdominopelvic cavity. Note the organs located in each quadrant or region, as shown in Figure 1–8.

DIVISION INTO QUADRANTS. The abdominopelvic cavity can be divided into four **quadrants** (Fig. 1–8A). The quadrants are named for their positions: the right upper quadrant (RUQ), the left upper quadrant (LUQ), the right lower quadrant (RLQ), and the

left lower quadrant (LLQ). Note, for example, that the liver is located in the right upper quadrant.

A patient who presents in the emergency room with acute pain in the RLQ might be diagnosed with appendicitis. Note that the RLQ appears to be on your left. This is similar to looking in a mirror. Keep this in mind when you are studying the diagrams in the text.

DIVISION INTO REGIONS. A second system divides the abdominopelvic cavity into nine separate regions that resemble the squares for tic-tac-toe (Fig. 1–8B). The three central regions (from top to bottom) include the epigastric, umbilical, and hypogastric regions. The epigastric region is located below the breast bone. Epigastric literally means upon *(epi)* the stomach *(gastric).* The umbilical region is the centermost region and surrounds the umbilicus, or navel. The hypogastric region is located just below the umbilical region. Hypogastric literally means below *(hypo)* the stomach *(gastric).*

Six regions are located on either side of the central regions. They include the hypochondriac, lumbar, and iliac regions. The right and left hypochondriac regions are located on either side

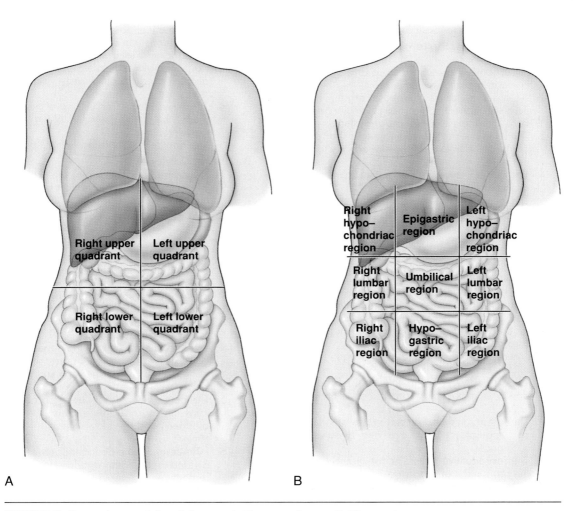

A

B

FIGURE 1–8 • Areas of the abdomen. A, Four quadrants. B, Nine regions.

of the epigastric region and overlie the lower ribs. The word hypochondriac literally means below *(hypo)* the cartilage *(chondro)* and refers to the composition of the ribs (cartilage). The right and left lumbar regions are located on either side of the umbilical region and are inferior to the hypochondriac regions. The right and left iliac regions are also called the right and left inguinal regions. They are located on either side of the hypogastric region and inferior to the lumbar regions. A knowledge of the these regions helps you to understand terms such as epigastric pain and inguinal hernia.

✳ **SUM IT UP!** The organs, or viscera, are located within body cavities. The two major cavities are the dorsal cavity, located toward the back of the body, and the larger ventral cavity, located in the front of the body. The dorsal cavity is subdivided into the cranial cavity and the spinal cavity and contains the brain and the spinal cord. The ventral cavity is subdivided into the thoracic cavity and the abdominopelvic cavity. The thoracic cavity contains the lungs. The mediastinum in the thoracic cavity contains the heart, trachea, esophagus, thymus gland, and the large blood vessels attached to the heart.

Summary Outline

Anatomy is the study of structure; physiology is the study of function.

I. Levels of Organization
A. From Simple to Complex
1. The body is arranged from simple to complex, from atom to molecules to larger molecules to cells to tissues to organs to organ systems to human organism (you).
2. Structure and function are related.

B. Organs, Organ Systems, and Homeostasis
1. An organ is a group of tissues arranged to perform a particular function.
2. An organ system is a group of organs that help each other to perform a particular function. There are 11 major organ systems.
3. The integumentary system provides the covering for the body and maintains body temperature.
4. The skeletal system provides support and protection.
5. The muscular system enables the body to move.
6. The nervous system is concerned with sensation, interpretation, and integration.
7. The endocrine system secretes hormones that help control body activities such as growth and reproduction.
8. The heart and circulatory systems transport nutrients and oxygen around the body.
9. The lymphatic system is concerned with defense against pathogens and foreign substances.
10. The respiratory system takes in oxygen and excretes carbon dioxide.
11. The digestive system takes in, breaks down, and absorbs food; it then excretes waste.
12. The urinary system excretes waste as urine and regulates body water and dissolved substances.
13. The reproductive system is concerned with the production of offspring.
14. Homeostasis means staying the same. The term refers to the body's ability to maintain a stable internal environment in response to a changing external environment.

II. Anatomical Terms and Body Cavities
A. Anatomical Position
1. The anatomical position is the body standing erect, arms by the side, with palms facing forward.
2. The anatomical terms describe the body in its anatomical position.
3. Paired terms that describe direction include superior and inferior, anterior and posterior, medial and lateral, proximal and distal, superficial and deep, central and peripheral.
4. The three planes, or cuts, are the sagittal plane, the frontal (coronal) plane, and the transverse plane.
5. Regional terms are listed in Figure 1–6.

B. Dorsal Cavity
1. The cranial cavity contains the brain.
2. The spinal cavity, or vertebral cavity, contains the spinal cord.

C. Ventral Cavity
1. The ventral cavity contains the thoracic and abdominopelvic cavity.
2. The thoracic cavity is above the diaphragm and contains the right and left lungs; it also contains the mediastinum (heart, trachea, esophagus, thymus gland, and the large blood vessels attached to the heart).
3. The abdominopelvic cavity is located below the diaphragm.
4. The abdominal cavity is the upper part that contains the stomach, most of the intestines, the liver, the spleen, and the kidneys.
5. The pelvic cavity is the lower part that contains the reproductive organs, the urinary bladder, and the lower part of the intestines.
6. For reference, the abdominopelvic cavity is divided into four quadrants and nine regions.

Review Your Knowledge

1. State whether the following descriptions refer to anatomy or physiology:
   a. What the heart looks like
   b. What the heart is made of
   c. Where the heart is located
   d. How the heart pumps blood
   e. Why the pumping of blood is necessary for life

2. How does the anatomical structure of a body part relate to its function?

3. State the levels of organization of the human body, going from simple to complex.

4. Explain the difference between an organ and an organ system.

5. Name 11 major organ systems and the primary function of each.

6. What term refers to the ability of the body to maintain a stable internal environment in response to a changing external environment?

7. Define anatomical position.

8. List the opposite term for the following directional terms:
   a. Inferior
   b. Anterior
   c. Caudal
   d. Lateral
   e. Distal
   f. Superficial
   g. Peripheral

9. Name the plane of the body that corresponds to the following descriptions:
   a. Divides the body into right and left
   b. Divides the body into front and back
   c. Divides the body into top and bottom

10. Define the terms *dorsal cavity* and *ventral cavity*.

11. Name the nine regions of the abdominopelvic cavity.

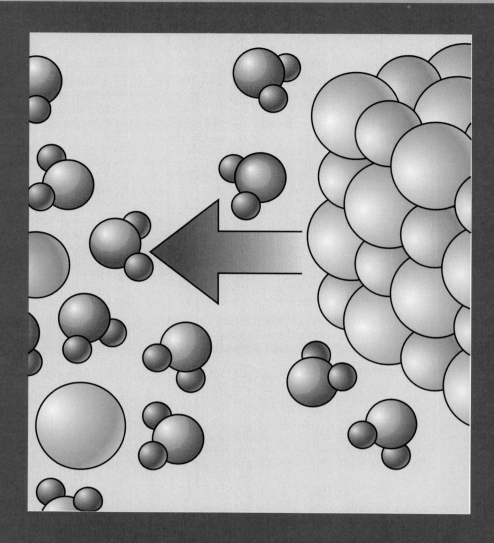

••• Key Terms

Acid (ăs′ĭd)

Adenosine triphosphate (ATP)
   (ə-dĕn′ə-sēn trī-fŏs′fāt)

Atom (ăt′əm)

Base (bās)

Buffer (bŭf′ər)

Catalyst (kăt′ə-lĭst)

Compound (kŏm′pound)

Covalent bond (kō-vā′lənt bŏnd)

Electrolyte (ĕ-lĕk′trō-līt″)

Element (ĕl′ə-mĕnt)

Energy (ĕn′ər-jē)

Enzyme (ĕn′zīm)

Hydrogen bond (hī′drə-jən bŏnd)

Ionic bond (ī-ŏn′ĭc bŏnd)

Isotope (ī′sə-tōp″)

Matter (măt′ər)

Molecule (mŏl′ĭ-kyōōl)

pH (pē″āch′)

Solution (sə-lōō′shən)

Suspension (səs-pĕn′shən)

••• Selected terms in bold type in this chapter are defined in the Glossary.

2 BASIC CHEMISTRY

Objectives

1. Define the words *matter* and *element*.

2. List the four elements that compose 96% of body weight.

3. Describe the three components of an atom.

4. Describe the role of electrons in the formation of chemical bonds.

5. Differentiate among ionic, covalent, and hydrogen bonds.

6. Explain the differences among ions, cations, and anions.

7. Describe the relationship of an electrolyte to an ion.

8. Explain the difference between a molecule and a compound.

9. List five reasons why water is essential to life.

10. Describe chemical reaction.

11. Differentiate between mechanical and chemical energy.

12. Explain the role of catalysts and enzymes.

13. Differentiate between an acid and a base.

14. List three mechanisms that regulate acid-base balance.

15. Describe pH in terms of hydrogen ion concentration.

16. State an example of a mixture, a solution, a suspension, and a colloidal suspension.

Why a chapter on chemistry? Because our bodies are made of different chemicals. The food we eat, the water we drink, and the air we breathe are all chemical substances. We digest our food, move our bodies, experience emotions, and think great thoughts because of chemical reactions. To understand the body, we must understand some general chemical principles.

MATTER, ELEMENTS, AND ATOMS

Matter

Chemistry is the study of matter. **Matter** (măt′ər) is anything that occupies space and has weight. Anything that you see as you look around is matter.

Matter exists in three states: solid, liquid, and gas. Solid matter has a definite shape and volume. Skin, bones, and teeth are examples of solid matter. Liquid matter takes the shape of, or conforms to, whatever container it is in. Liquid matter includes blood, saliva, and digestive juices. A gas, or gaseous matter, has neither shape nor volume. The air we breathe is matter that exists as gas.

Matter can undergo both physical and chemical changes. The logs in a fireplace illustrate the difference between a physical and a chemical change (Fig. 2–1). The logs can undergo a **physical change** by being chopped into smaller chips of wood with a hatchet. The wood chips are smaller than the log, but they are still wood. The matter (wood) has not essentially changed. Only the physical appearance has changed. A **chemical change** occurs when the wood is burned. When

burned, the wood ceases to be wood. The chemical composition of the ashes is essentially different from that of the wood when the wood is chemically changed.

The body contains many examples of physical and chemical changes. For example, digestion involves both physical and chemical changes. Chewing breaks the food into smaller pieces; this is a physical change. Chemicals called digestive **enzymes** (ĕn′zīmz) change the food into simpler substances; this is a chemical change.

Elements

All matter, living or dead, is composed of elements. An **element** (ĕl′ə-mĕnt) is a fundamental substance that cannot be broken down into a simpler form by ordinary chemical reactions. Even a very small amount of an element contains millions and millions of *identical* atoms. For example, all atoms of the element sodium are identical. (Note that the same name, sodium, is used for both the element and the atom.) Although there are more than 100 elements, only about 25 elements are required by living organisms.

The most abundant elements found in the body are listed in Table 2–1. Four elements—carbon, hydrogen, oxygen, and nitrogen—make up 96% of the body weight. The **trace elements** are present in tiny amounts. Despite the small amounts required, the trace elements are essential for life.

Each of the elements included in Table 2–1 is represented by a symbol. For example, the symbol O is for oxygen, N is for nitrogen, Na is for sodium, K is for potassium, and C is for carbon. The first letter of the symbol is always capitalized. These symbols are used frequently. You should memorize the symbols of the major elements. You will need to use them.

Atoms

Atomic Structure

Elements are composed of atoms. An **atom** (ăt′əm) is the smallest unit of an element with that element's chemical characteristics. It is the basic unit of matter. An atom is composed of three subatomic particles: protons, neutrons, and electrons.

The arrangement of the subatomic particles resembles the sun and planets (Fig. 2–2A). The sun is the center. The planets constantly move around the sun in orbits, or circular paths. The atom is composed of a nucleus (ie, the sun) and shells, or orbits, that surround the nucleus (Fig. 2–2B).

Where are the subatomic particles located? The protons and the neutrons are located in the

CHANGES IN MATTER

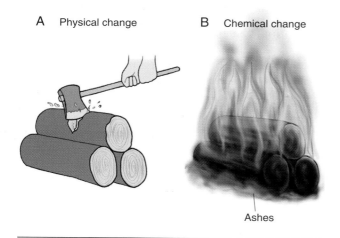

A Physical change

B Chemical change

Ashes

FIGURE 2–1 ● Changes in matter. A, Physical change (the wood is still wood). B, Chemical change (the wood is no longer wood).

Table 2 • 1	COMMON ELEMENTS IN THE HUMAN BODY

ELEMENT	SYMBOL	PERCENTAGE OF BODY WEIGHT
Oxygen	O	65.0%
Carbon	C	18.5%
Hydrogen	H	9.5%
Nitrogen	N	3.2%
Calcium	Ca	
Phosphorus	P	
Potassium	K	
Sulfur	S	
Sodium	Na	
Chlorine	Cl	
Magnesium	Mg	
Iodine	I	
Iron	Fe	
Chromium	Cr	
Cobalt	Co	
Copper	Cu	
Fluorine	F	
Selenium	Se	
Zinc	Zn	

nucleus (Fig. 2–2C). **Protons** carry a positive (+) electrical charge; **neutrons** carry no electrical charge. The electrons are located in the shells, or orbits, surrounding the nucleus like planets. **Electrons** carry a negative (−) electrical charge. In each atom, the number of protons (+) is equal to the number of electrons (−). The atom is therefore electrically neutral; it carries no net electrical charge.

All protons are alike; all neutrons are alike; and all electrons are alike. So what makes one atom different from another atom? The difference is primarily due to the *numbers* of protons and electrons in each atom. For instance, hydrogen is the simplest and smallest atom. It has one proton and one electron. Helium has two protons and two electrons. Lithium has three protons and three electrons. Hydrogen, helium, and lithium are different atoms because of the different numbers of protons and electrons.

Two terms describe individual atoms. The **atomic number** is the number of *protons* in the nucleus. Thus, hydrogen has an atomic number of 1; helium has an atomic number of 2, and lithium has an atomic number of 3. The **atomic weight** of an atom is determined by adding the numbers of protons and neutrons in the nucleus. Thus, the atomic weight of hydrogen is also 1 because the hydrogen nucleus contains one proton and no neutrons. The atomic weight of helium is 4 because the nucleus contains two protons and two neutrons.

What is an isotope? An **isotope** (ī′sə-tōp″) is a different form of the same atom. For example, hydrogen has different forms. Hydrogen has an atomic number of 1 and an atomic weight of 1; it has one proton and no neutrons in the nucleus. A second and less common form of hydrogen is called "heavy" hydrogen. It has one proton *and* one neutron in its nucleus; thus, its atomic number is 1, but its atomic weight is approximately 2. Because its atomic number is 1, it is still a hydrogen atom. The additional neutron in the nucleus, however, makes it "heavy" and changes its atomic weight. "Heavy hydrogen" is an isotope of hydrogen. Remember: an isotope has the same atomic number as an atom but a different atomic weight. An isotope of an atom varies only in the number of neutrons.

Heavier isotopes of atoms are often unstable; their nuclei break down, or decay, giving off particles or energy waves. By emitting particles or energy waves, the unstable nuclei become more stable. Unstable isotopes are called **radioisotopes.** The process of spontaneous breakdown (decay) is called **radioactivity.** Radioisotopes are damaging to tissue and are used clinically to destroy cells. For instance, radioactive iodine is used to destroy excess thyroid tissue. Other radioisotopes are used to destroy cancer cells.

A

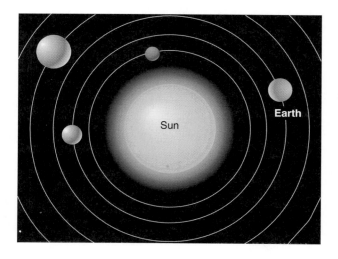

B

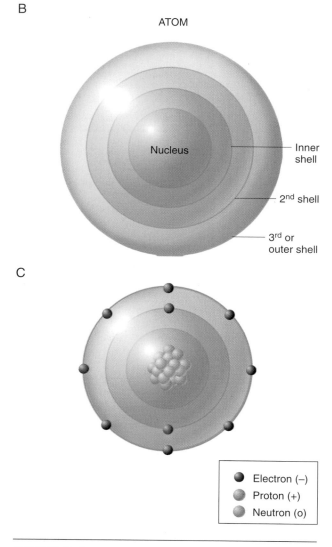

Electron Shells

Electrons surround the nucleus in orbits called energy levels or electron shells (see Fig. 2–2C). The number of shells varies from one atom to the next; some atoms, like hydrogen, have only one shell; other atoms, like sodium, have three shells. Each shell can hold a specific number of electrons. The inner shell closest to the nucleus can hold only two electrons. The second and third shells each hold eight electrons.

The only electrons that are important for chemical bonding are the electrons in the outermost shell. If it is not filled with its proper number of electrons, the outer shell becomes unstable. It then seeks either to give up electrons so as to empty the shell or to acquire electrons so as to fill the shell. The tendency of the outer shell to want to become stable forms the basis of chemical bonding.

CHEMICAL BONDS

Atoms are attracted to each other because they want to achieve a stable outer electron shell. In other words, they want either to fill or to empty the outer electron shell. The force of attraction between the atoms is similar to the force of two magnets. When you try to separate the magnets, you can feel the pull. The electrical attraction between atoms is a **chemical bond.** The three types of chemical bonds are ionic bonds, covalent bonds, and hydrogen bonds.

Ionic Bonds

The **ionic bond** (ī-ŏn′ĭc bŏnd) is caused by a transfer of electrons between atoms. The interaction of the sodium and the chlorine atoms illustrates an ionic bond (Fig. 2–3A). The sodium atom has 11 protons in the nucleus and 11 electrons in the shells. There are two electrons in the inner shell, eight electrons in the second shell, and only one electron in the outer shell. The single electron makes the outer shell unstable. To become more stable, the sodium atom would like to donate the single electron. Donating an electron forms a bond between the two atoms. Sodium often bonds with chlorine.

The chlorine (Cl) atom has 17 protons in the nucleus and 17 electrons orbiting in its shells. The electrons are positioned as follows: two electrons in the inner shell, eight electrons in the second shell, and seven electrons in the outer shell. The seven electrons make the outer shell unstable. The chlorine atom would like to add a single electron. The electrical attraction occurs between the outer shells of the sodium and chlorine atoms.

The single electron in the outer shell of the sodium atom is attracted, or pulled, toward the

FIGURE 2–2 ● Structure of the atom. A, Subatomic particles arranged like the sun and the planets. B, Nucleus (sun) and electron shells (orbits of planets). C, Protons and neutrons located in the nucleus (sun) and electrons (planets) encircling the nucleus (sun) in orbits.

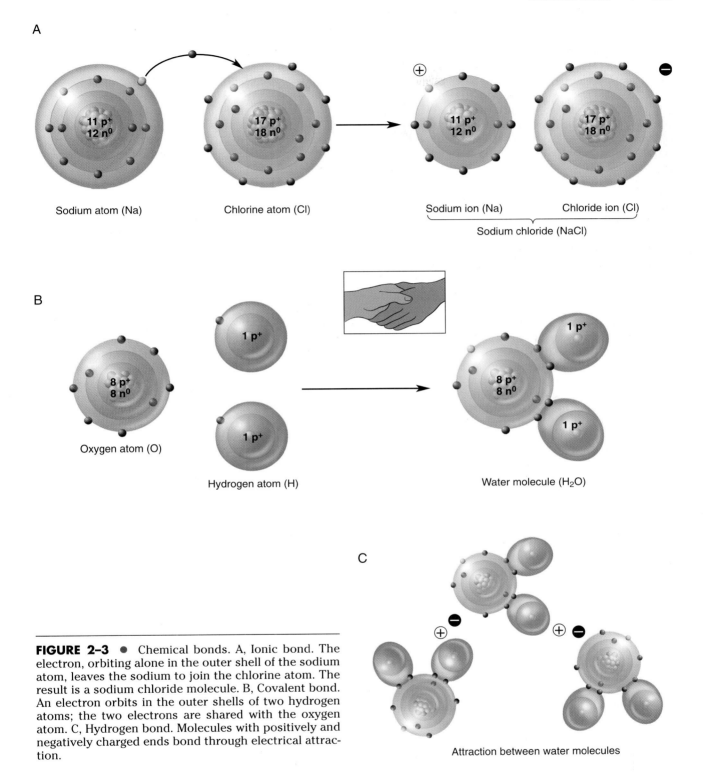

A

Sodium atom (Na)   Chlorine atom (Cl)   Sodium ion (Na)   Chloride ion (Cl)

Sodium chloride (NaCl)

B

Oxygen atom (O)

Hydrogen atom (H)

Water molecule (H_2O)

C

Attraction between water molecules

FIGURE 2–3 ● Chemical bonds. A, Ionic bond. The electron, orbiting alone in the outer shell of the sodium atom, leaves the sodium to join the chlorine atom. The result is a sodium chloride molecule. B, Covalent bond. An electron orbits in the outer shells of two hydrogen atoms; the two electrons are shared with the oxygen atom. C, Hydrogen bond. Molecules with positively and negatively charged ends bond through electrical attraction.

seven electrons in the outer shell of the chlorine atom. Sodium and chlorine form an ionic bond because the electron in the outer shell of the sodium atom leaves the sodium, while the incomplete outer shell of the chlorine atom accepts the single electron from the sodium. Thus, the sodium atom and the chlorine atom bond ionically to form NaCl, table salt.

Covalent Bonds

A second type of chemical bond is the **covalent bond** (kō-vā′lənt bŏnd). Covalent bonding involves a *sharing* of electrons by the outer shells of the atoms. Covalent bonding is like joining hands (Fig. 2–3B). The formation of water from hydrogen and oxygen atoms illustrates covalent bonding. Oxygen has eight electrons, two in the inner shell and only six in the outer shell. An oxygen atom needs two electrons to complete the outer shell. Hydrogen has only one electron and requires one electron to complete its inner shell.

Water is formed when two hydrogen atoms, each with one electron, share those electrons with one oxygen atom. By sharing the electrons of the oxygen, each of the two hydrogen atoms has completed the inner shells (capacity is two electrons). By sharing the electrons of two hydrogen atoms, the outer shell of the oxygen is completed with eight electrons. Water is represented as H_2O (two hydrogen and one oxygen).

Carbon atoms always form covalent bonds. A carbon atom has four electrons in the outer shell. Carbon can bond with hydrogen (H), oxygen (O), nitrogen (N), and other carbon (C) atoms. Carbon is one of the major elements in the body. Covalent bonding of carbon with hydrogen, oxygen, and nitrogen forms complex molecules such as proteins and carbohydrates. Covalent bonds are strong and do not break apart in aqueous (water) solution. The strength of these bonds is important because the protein produced by the body must not "fall apart" when exposed to water.

For instance, many proteins, such as hormones, are transported around the body in blood, which is mostly water. If the covalent bonds of the protein broke apart in water, the hormones would be unable to accomplish their tasks. So many chemical reactions in the body involve carbon that a separate branch of chemistry studies only carbon-containing substances. The study of carbon-containing substances is called **organic chemistry.** In contrast, **inorganic chemistry** studies non–carbon-containing substances.

Hydrogen Bonds

A third type of bond is a **hydrogen bond** (hī′drə-jən bŏnd) (Fig. 2–3C). It differs from the ionic and covalent bonds in that the hydrogen bond is not caused by either the transfer or the sharing of electrons of the outer shells of atoms. Hydrogen bonding is best illustrated by the attraction of one water molecule for another water molecule. Because of the sharing of electrons within a water molecule, a slight positive (+) charge occurs around the hydrogen end of the water and a slight negative (−) charge occurs around the oxygen end. Consequently, the positive (+) end of one water molecule is attracted to the negative (−) end of a second molecule. This attraction between water molecules is a hydrogen bond.

Although hydrogen bonds are weak, they play an important role in the body. For example, they help to form the shape of large molecules such as DNA. By determining the shape of DNA, the hydro-

gen bonds also affect its function. Hydrogen bonds also determine some of the characteristics of water. For instance, water is considered the universal solvent, meaning that most substances can dissolve in water. This ability to dissolve substances is due to the electrical charges on the water molecules. For instance, the plasma protein albumin carries a negative (−) charge. It is attracted to the positive (+) end of the water molecule. The attraction of the electrical charges allows albumin to dissolve in water.

IONS

Cations, Anions, and Electrolytes

Several other terms are related to the activity of the electrons in the outer shells of the atoms. If the negatively charged electrons are lost from or gained by the outer shell of an atom, the electrical charge of the atom changes. In other words, the electrical charge of the atom or element changes from a neutral charge (ie, no charge) to either a positive (+) charge or a negative (−) charge. Elements that carry an electrical charge are called **ions.** If the ion is positively charged, it is a **cation.** If the ion is negatively (−) charged, it is an **anion.**

An **electrolyte** (ĕ-lĕk′trō-līt″) is a substance that forms ions when it is dissolved in water. Electrolytes, as the name implies, are capable of conducting an electrical current. For instance, the electrocardiogram (ECG) and the electroencephalogram (EEG) record electrical events in the heart and brain. Movement of ions through the tissues causes the electrical events recorded on the ECG and EEG.

Ion Formation

Ions are formed when electrons in the outer shell are either lost or gained. For instance, the sodium atom has 11 protons (positive charge) and 11 electrons (negative charge). If a single electron is lost, the sodium is left with 11 positive (+) charges and only 10 negative (−) charges. Sodium is said to carry a net charge of +1. The sodium ion is therefore a **cation.** It is represented as Na^+.

The chlorine atom has 17 protons (positive charge) and 17 electrons (negative charge). If an electron is gained, the chlorine then contains 17 (+) charges and 18 (−) charges. Chlorine is said to carry a net charge of −1 and is called an **anion.** The chlorine anion is called chloride and is represented as Cl^-. Some atoms may give up more than one electron and have a stronger positive charge. Calcium, for instance, gives up two electrons. It is represented as Ca^{2+}. Table 2–2 presents other important ions.

Table 2•2   COMMON IONS

NAME	SYMBOL	FUNCTION
Cations		
Sodium	Na^+	Fluid balance (principal extracellular cation); nerve and muscle function
Calcium	Ca^{2+}	Component of bones and teeth; blood clotting; muscle contraction
Iron	Fe^{2+}	Component of hemoglobin (oxygen transport)
Hydrogen	H^+	Important in acid-base balance
Potassium	K^+	Nerve and muscle function; principal intracellular cation
Anions		
Chloride	Cl^-	Primary extracellular anion
Bicarbonate	HCO_3^-	Important in acid-base regulation
Phosphate	HPO_4^{2-}	Component of bones and teeth; component of ATP (energy)

Ionization

When an electrolyte splits, or breaks apart in solution, the electrolyte is said to **dissociate** (Fig. 2–4). For example, sodium chloride (table salt) is an electrolyte. In the solid state it appears as tiny white granules. When dissolved in water, however, the table salt dissociates. What is happening?

$$NaCl \longrightarrow Na^+ \quad + \quad Cl^-$$

NaCl	Na⁺	Cl⁻
salt	sodium ion (cation)	chloride ion (anion)

When the salt is placed in water, the **ionic bonds** holding the sodium and chlorine together weaken. The solid NaCl then splits into Na^+ (sodium ion) and Cl^- (chloride ion). In other words, the NaCl dissociates. Because the products of this dissociation are ions, this dissociation process is referred to as **ionization.** Only electrolytes **ionize.**

MOLECULES AND COMPOUNDS

Molecules

When two or more atoms bond together, they form a **molecule** (mŏl′ĭ-kyōōl). Two identical atoms may bond. For instance, one atom of oxygen may bond with another atom of oxygen to form a molecule of oxygen, designated O_2. The same bonding is true for nitrogen (N_2) and hydrogen (H_2) (Fig. 2–5). A molecule can also be formed when atoms of different elements combine. For instance, when two atoms of hydrogen combine with one atom of oxygen, a molecule of water (H_2O) is formed.

Compounds

A substance that contains molecules formed by two or more *different* atoms is called a **com-**

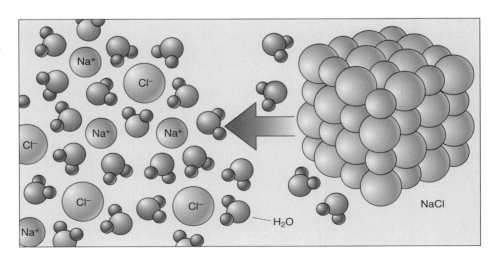

FIGURE 2–4 • Ionization. Electrolyte (NaCl) dissociates into ions (Na^+ and Cl^-) when placed in water.

A

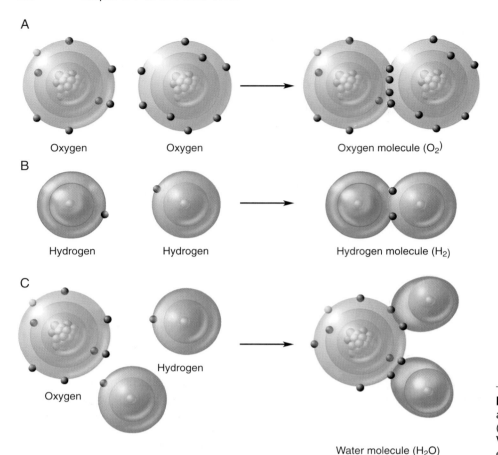

Oxygen   Oxygen   Oxygen molecule (O_2)

B

Hydrogen   Hydrogen   Hydrogen molecule (H_2)

C

Oxygen   Hydrogen

Water molecule (H_2O)

FIGURE 2–5 ● Molecules and compounds. A, Oxygen (O_2). B, Hydrogen (H_2). C, Water. Water is both a molecule and a compound.

pound (kŏm′pound). For instance, if two atoms of hydrogen combine with one atom of oxygen, water is formed. Water is considered both a molecule and a compound.

Some Important Compounds and Molecules

Water

Water is the most abundant compound in the body. It constitutes approximately two thirds of an adult's body weight and even more of a child's body weight. Water is essential for life. While we can last for many weeks without food, we can last only a few days without water. What makes water so special?

- *Water as the universal solvent.* Water is called the universal solvent because most substances dissolve in water. Its use as a solvent is one of the most important characteristics of water. By dissolving in water, most substances can move faster and more easily. They also can participate in many chemical reactions. Glucose, for instance, dissolves in blood (which is mostly water) and then moves quickly to every cell in the body.

- *Water as temperature regulator.* Water has the ability to absorb large amounts of heat without the temperature of the water itself increasing dramatically. This ability means that heat can be removed from heat-producing tissue, like exercising muscle, while the body maintains a normal temperature. Water, therefore, plays an important role in the body's temperature regulation.

- *Water as an ideal lubricant.* Water is a major component of mucus and other lubricating fluids. Lubricating fluids decrease friction as two structures slide past each other.

- *Water in chemical reactions.* Water often plays a crucial role in chemical reactions. For instance, water is necessary to break down carbohydrate during digestion. Water is also necessary in the buildup of substances such as protein.

- *Water as a protective device.* Water may also be used to protect an important structure. For instance, the cerebrospinal fluid (which is mostly water) surrounds and cushions the delicate brain and spinal cord. Likewise, the amniotic fluid surrounds and cushions the developing infant in the mother's womb.

Oxygen

Oxygen (O_2), a molecule composed of two oxygen atoms, exists in nature as a gas. The air we breathe contains 21% oxygen. Oxygen is essential for life; without a continuous supply we would quickly die. The oxygen we breathe in is used by the cells to extract, or liberate, the energy from the food we eat. This energy runs, or powers, the body. Like an engine, if the body has no energy, it stops running. The importance of oxygen accounts for the urgency associated with cardiopulmonary resuscitation (CPR). If the heart stops beating, the delivery of oxygen to the tissue ceases. CPR must, therefore, be started immediately. Otherwise, irreversible brain damage will occur.

Carbon Dioxide

Carbon dioxide (CO_2) is a compound that consists of one carbon atom and two oxygen atoms, hence the name carbon dioxide (*di* means two). Carbon dioxide is a waste product, so it must be eliminated from the body. Carbon dioxide is made when food is chemically broken down for energy.

✳ **SUM IT UP!** Chemistry is the study of matter. Matter is composed of elements such as hydrogen, oxygen, carbon, and nitrogen. Each element is composed of millions of identical atoms. Atoms are composed of subatomic particles called protons, neutrons, and electrons. Chemical bonds are formed through the interaction of one atom with another, particularly with electrons. The three chemical bonds are ionic, covalent, and hydrogen bonds. The transfer of electrons is also responsible for the formation of ions (cations and anions). Molecules and compounds are formed when atoms interact in a particular fashion.

CHEMICAL REACTIONS

A **chemical reaction** is a process whereby the atoms of molecules or compounds interact to form new chemical combinations. For instance, glucose interacts with oxygen to form carbon dioxide, water, and energy. This chemical interaction is characterized by the breaking of the chemical bonds of glucose and oxygen and the making of new bonds as carbon dioxide and water are formed. The reaction is represented as follows:

$$C_6H_{12}O_6 + O_2 \longrightarrow CO_2 + H_2O + Energy$$
glucose oxygen carbon water
dioxide

The rates of chemical reactions (ie, how fast they occur) are important. Most chemical reactions take place very slowly. Chemical substances called **catalysts** (kăt′ə-lĭsts) can speed up the rate of a chemical reaction. When proteins perform the role of catalysts, they are called enzymes. Most chemical reactions need a catalyst or an enzyme.

ACIDS AND BASES

A normally functioning body requires a balance between substances classified as acids and as bases. Acid-base balance is important because the chemical reactions in the body occur only when these substances are in balance. Imbalances of acids and bases cause life-threatening clinical problems. An understanding of the chemistry of acids, bases, and buffers is crucial to understanding acid-base balance.

Acids

We all recognize the sour taste of an acid. Grapefruit juice, lemon juice, and vinegar are acids. In addition to a sour taste, very strong acids, such as hydrochloric acid (HCl), can actually cause severe burns. Acid splashed in your eye, for instance, can damage the eye tissue to the point of blindness.

An **acid** (ăs′ĭd) is an electrolyte that dissociates into hydrogen ion (H^+) and an anion. Its dissociation is represented as follows:

$$HCl \longrightarrow H^+ + Cl^-$$
hydrochloric   hydrogen   chloride
acid   ion   ion

In this reaction, hydrochloric acid (HCl) dissociates into hydrogen ion (H^+) and the chloride ion (Cl^-). For our purposes, the most important component is the H^+. The amount of H^+ in solution determines the acidity of a solution.

A **strong acid** dissociates completely into hydrogen ion (H^+) and an anion. Hydrochloric acid (HCl), found within the stomach, is a strong acid; it yields many H^+. Strong acids are capable of causing severe tissue injury. A **weak acid** does not dissociate completely. Vinegar, or acetic acid, is a weak acid. Vinegar dissociates *slightly* into H^+. Most of the vinegar remains in its undissociated form. Its dissociation is represented as follows:

$$Vinegar \rightleftharpoons H^+ + acetate$$

The heavy arrow pointing to the left indicates that the vinegar remains as vinegar, forming very little H^+. Because the number of hydrogen ions (H^+) determines the acidity of a solution, vinegar is classified as a weak acid. This weakness is the

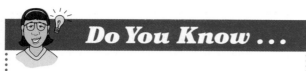

Do You Know . . .

Why are antacids used?

Patients with ulcers often have excess stomach acid. The stomach acid (hydrochloric acid) can be neutralized with a drug that contains a base. Because these drugs oppose acids, they are called **antacids.** One of the most commonly used antacids contains aluminum hydroxide. The hydroxyl ion of the drug combines with the H^+ of the stomach acid, thereby converting the acid (H^+) to salt and water. The acid has been neutralized by the antacid. Both the salt and the water are then excreted from the body. Thus the acid, which has been burning a hole in the stomach lining as an ulcer, has been eliminated.

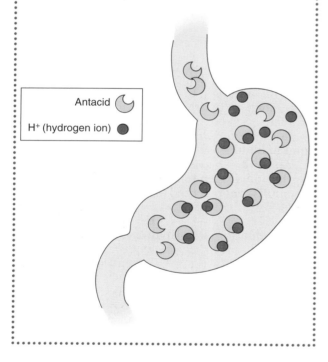

Antacid

H^+ (hydrogen ion)

reason that vinegar does not burn your hand. HCl is so strong that it can actually burn a hole through your hand.

Bases

A **base** (bās) has a bitter taste and is slippery like soap. Bases are substances that combine with H^+. Bases usually contain the hydroxyl ion, represented as OH^-. Sodium hydroxide (NaOH) is an example of a base. NaOH dissociates into sodium ion (Na^+) and the hydroxyl ion (OH^-) as follows:

$$NaOH \longrightarrow Na^+ + OH^-$$

The hydroxyl ion (OH^-) is a hydrogen ion eliminator. In other words, the OH^- looks for and soaks up a hydrogen ion. The addition of a base makes a solution less acidic.

Neutralization of Acids and Bases

When an acid is mixed with a base, the H^+ of the acid combines with the OH^- of the base to form water. In addition, the Na^+ and the Cl^- combine to form a salt, NaCl. The reaction is important because the H^+ is converted to water. In other words, the acid has been **neutralized.** This chemical reaction is represented as follows:

$$\underset{\text{acid}}{HCl} + \underset{\text{base}}{NaOH} \longrightarrow \underset{\text{water}}{H_2O} + \underset{\text{salt}}{NaCl}$$

In a neutralization reaction, an acid combines with a base to form a salt and water.

Measurement: The pH Scale

pH (pē″āch′) is a unit of measurement that indicates how many H^+ are in a solution. The **pH scale** ranges from 0 to 14 (Fig. 2–6). At the midpoint of the scale, pH 7, the number of H^+ in pure water is equal to the number of OH^-. Therefore, the solution is neutral. A pH that measures less than 7 on the scale indicates that the solution has more H^+ than OH^-. The solution is then said to be acidic.

Note the pH of lemon juice and vinegar on the scale. They are both less than 7. A pH measuring more than 7 indicates fewer H^+ than OH^-. These substances are bases, and the solution is said to be **basic,** or **alkaline.** The pH scale measures the degree of acidity or alkalinity.

Reading the pH Scale

Each pH unit represents a 10-fold change in H^+ concentration. For instance, a change in 1 pH unit (from 7 to 6) represents a 10-fold increase in H^+, whereas a change in 2 pH units (from 7 to 5) represents a 100-fold increase in H^+ concentration. The important point is this: very small changes in the pH reading indicate very large changes in the H^+ concentration.

pH of Body Fluids

Note the pH of some of the body fluids. The stomach contents are very acidic, with a pH of 1 to 4. The pH of urine is normally acidic, with a pH range of 5 to 8, although a number of conditions,

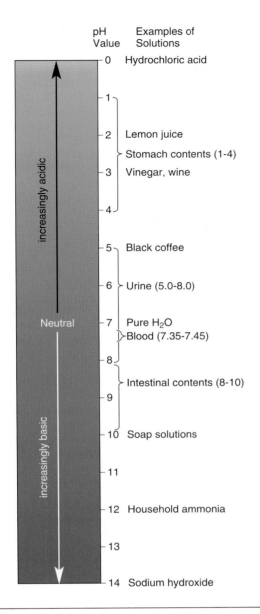

pH Value / Examples of Solutions

- 0 — Hydrochloric acid
- 1
- 2 — Lemon juice
  - Stomach contents (1-4)
- 3 — Vinegar, wine
- 4
- 5 — Black coffee
- 6 — Urine (5.0-8.0)
- 7 — Pure H$_2$O / Blood (7.35-7.45)
- 8
  - Intestinal contents (8-10)
- 9
- 10 — Soap solutions
- 11
- 12 — Household ammonia
- 13
- 14 — Sodium hydroxide

increasingly acidic / Neutral / increasingly basic

FIGURE 2–6 • pH scale. The scale indicates the H$^+$ concentration. A pH of 0 is most acidic (has the greatest concentration of H$^+$), while a pH of 14 is least acidic (has no H$^+$). The pink coloring indicates the acidic range. The blue coloring indicates the basic, or alkaline, range. Note the pH of various substances.

including diet, can change urinary pH. Urine can even become alkaline in response to diet. The intestinal secretions are alkaline, with a pH range of 8 to 10.

Blood pH is maintained within a narrow range of 7.35 to 7.45, a slightly alkaline pH. Because the blood pH is normally slightly alkaline (7.35 to 7.45), a blood pH of less than 7.35 is more acidic than normal, and the patient is said to be acidotic. If the patient's blood pH is greater than 7.45, the patient is said to be alkalotic. Because all of the body enzymes work best at a normal blood pH, both **acidosis** and **alkalosis** cause serious clinical problems and must be corrected. The need to maintain the body's normal alkaline state is the reason for monitoring blood pH closely during the course of a patient's illness.

Regulation of Blood pH

The blood pH is regulated on a minute-by-minute basis by three means: a buffer system, the lungs, and the kidneys. The buffer system is the first line of defense against changes in blood pH. A **buffer** (bŭf′ər) is a chemical substance that prevents large changes in pH. A buffer acts in two ways. If the H$^+$ concentration in the blood increases, the buffer removes excess H$^+$, thereby restoring pH to normal. If instead, the H$^+$ concentration decreases, the buffer donates H$^+$ to the blood, thereby restoring blood pH. (A more detailed description of buffer function is presented in Chapter 21.) The second and third lines of defense in the regulation of blood pH are the lungs and the kidneys. (These processes of regulation are described in Chapters 18, 20, and 21.)

✳ **SUM IT UP!** Millions of chemical reactions occur in the body every minute. Chemical reactions are processes whereby one chemical substance is converted into a different chemical substance. Chemical reactions either use energy or release energy. The speed, or rate, of a chemical reaction can be increased by a catalyst, or enzyme. A normally functioning body requires a balance between acids and bases. Hydrogen ion concentration is measured by pH. Normal blood pH is 7.35 to 7.45 and is therefore slightly alkaline. When pH falls below 7.35, the person is said to be acidotic; when pH rises above 7.45, the person is said to be alkalotic. Blood pH is regulated within normal limits by three mechanisms: buffers, the lungs, and the kidneys.

ENERGY

Unlike matter, energy cannot be seen or weighed. Energy can be measured only by observing its effect on matter. **Energy** (ĕn′ər-jē) is the ability to do or perform work. The body depends on a continuous supply of energy. Even at rest, the body is continuously working and using up energy. Heart muscle, for instance, is contracting and forcing blood throughout a large network of blood vessels. Nerve and muscle cells are continuously pumping sodium out of the cells. This effort sets the stage for the formation of nerve impulses. The cells of the pancreas are continuously making enzymes so that we can digest our food. Without energy, the body ceases to function.

Forms of Energy

There are six forms of energy, summarized in Table 2–3. **Mechanical energy** is expressed as movement. For instance, when the leg muscles contract, you are able to walk. Walking is an expression of mechanical energy. **Chemical energy** is stored within the chemical bonds. The energy holds the atoms together. When the chemical bonds are broken, chemical energy is released. The released energy can then be used to perform other kinds of work, such as digesting food. This process is similar to the running of a car's engine. The energy released from the burning, or breakdown, of the gas is used to turn the engine; the running engine then moves your car.

Conversion of Energy

Energy is easily converted from one form to another. For instance, when a log burns, the chemical energy stored in it is converted to heat **(thermal energy)** and light **(radiant energy)**. In a similar way, the chemical energy stored in the muscle is converted into mechanical energy when the muscle contracts and moves your leg.

The conversion of energy in the body is generally accompanied by the release of heat. For instance, when muscles contract during strenuous exercise, chemical energy is converted into both mechanical energy (running) and heat. Recall how hot you get while exercising. Your body heat (body temperature) is caused by conversion of energy. (Body temperature is further described in Chapter 6.)

Energy Transfer: The Role of Adenosine Triphosphate

The energy used to power the body comes from the food we eat (Fig. 2–7A). As the food is broken down, the energy is released. This energy, however, cannot be used *directly* by the cells of the body. The energy must first be transferred to another substance called **adenosine triphosphate** (ə-děn′ə-sēn trī-fŏs′fāt), abbreviated **ATP**. ATP is an energy transfer molecule.

ATP is composed of three parts: a base, a sugar, and three phosphate groups (Fig. 2–7B). For our purposes, the phosphate groups are the most important part of the ATP molecule. The phosphate groups have unique chemical bonds. The "squiggly" lines connecting the second and third phosphate groups indicate that these bonds are **high-energy bonds.** When these bonds are broken, a large amount of energy is released. More importantly, the energy released from ATP can be used directly by the cell. The cell uses this energy to perform its tasks.

The energy stored within the high-energy bonds is similar to the energy stored in a loaded mouse trap (Fig. 2–7C). Energy is stored in the trap when you set the metal bar in its loaded position. When the trap is set off by the mouse, the metal bar snaps back into its original position, thereby releasing the stored energy. Similarly, when energy is needed by the body, ATP is split. The energy that was stored in ATP is released. In other words, the bond that holds the end phosphate group is broken, and energy is released. With the release of energy, the splitting of ATP also yields ADP

Table 2 • 3	**FORMS OF ENERGY**	
FORM OF ENERGY	**DESCRIPTION**	**EXAMPLE**
Mechanical	Energy that causes movement	Movement of legs in running, walking Contraction of heart muscle, causing movement of blood
Chemical	Energy that is stored in chemical bonds	Fuel to do work, like running
Electrical	Energy that is released from the movement of charged particles	Electrical signal involved in the transmission of information along nerves
Radiant	Energy that travels in waves	Light: stimulates the eyes for vision; ultraviolet radiation from the sun for tanning
Thermal	Energy that is transferred because of a temperature difference	Responsible for body temperature
Nuclear	Energy that is released during the decay of radioactive substances such as isotopes	Not useful physiologically

A

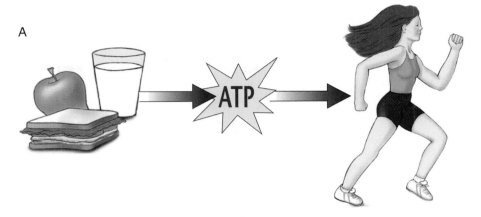

B

Structure of ATP:

High-energy
chemical bonds

P   P   P

Phosphate

Base

Sugar

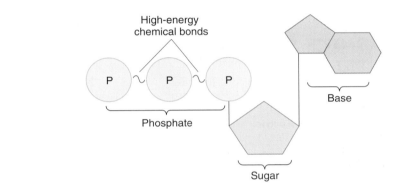

FIGURE 2-7 ● Energy. A, We get energy from food. B, Energy is stored within the high-energy bonds of ATP (adenosine triphosphate). C, Energy is stored in the loaded trap and released when the trap is sprung.

C

Stored energy

Energy
released

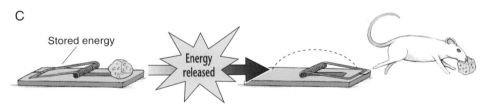

(adenosine diphosphate) and P (phosphate). This process is indicated as follows:

$$ATP \longrightarrow Energy + ADP + P$$

ADP is identical to ATP, but the molecule now has one less phosphate group. ATP is replenished, or restored, when energy, obtained from burning food, reattaches the end phosphate to ADP as follows:

$$ADP + P + Energy \longrightarrow ATP$$

MIXTURES, SOLUTIONS, AND SUSPENSIONS

You will encounter several other chemical terms in clinical situations.

Mixtures are combinations of two or more substances that can be separated by ordinary physical means. When separated, the substances keep, or retain, their original properties. For instance, imagine that you have a mixture of sugar and little bits of iron. A magnet is then moved close to this sugar-iron mixture. The magnet pulls all of the iron away from the sugar, thereby separating the two substances. Note that the two substances have retained their original properties. The sugar is still sugar, and the iron is still iron.

Solutions (sə-lōō'shənz) are mixtures. In a solution, the particles that are mixed together remain evenly distributed. Salt water is an example of a solution. A solution has two parts: a solvent and a solute. The **solute** is the substance present in the smaller amount; it is the substance being dissolved. The salt in the salt water is the solute. The solute can be solid, liquid, or gas.

The **solvent** is the part of the solution present in the greater amount. It does the dissolving. Water is the solvent in salt water. The solvent is usually liquid or gas. If water is the solvent, the solution is referred to as an **aqueous solution.** If alcohol is the solvent, the solution is referred to as a **tincture.** A solution is always clear, and the solute does not settle to the bottom.

Suspensions (səs-pĕn′shənz) are mixtures. In a suspension, the particles are relatively large and tend to settle to the bottom unless the mixture is shaken continuously. For instance, if sand and water are shaken together and then allowed to sit undisturbed, the sand gradually settles to the bottom.

In a **colloidal suspension,** the particles do not dissolve, but they are so small that they remain suspended within the liquid, even when not being shaken. A colloid is a glue-like substance that re-sembles gelatin or mucus. The body contains many colloidal substances. Blood plasma is a colloidal suspension because the proteins remain suspended within the plasma. Other examples of colloidal suspensions include mayonnaise, egg white, and jellies.

✳ **SUM IT UP!** Energy is the ability to do work. Without an adequate supply of energy, the body cannot work, and it dies. Energy is derived from food and transferred to high-energy bonds in ATP. When needed, the energy is released from the ATP and used to power the body. Chemical combinations include mixtures, solutions, and suspensions.

Summary Outline

Our bodies are made of different chemicals. To understand the body, you need to understand some general chemical principles.

I. Matter, Elements, and Atoms

A. Matter
1. Matter is anything that occupies space and has weight. Matter exists in three states: solid, liquid, and gas.
2. Matter can undergo physical and chemical changes.

B. Elements
1. An element is a fundamental substance that cannot be broken down into a simpler form by ordinary chemical means.
2. Four elements (carbon, hydrogen, oxygen, and nitrogen) make up 96% of the body cells.

C. Atoms
1. An atom is the basic unit of matter; it is the smallest unit of an element that has that element's chemical characteristics.
2. An atom is composed of three subatomic particles: neutrons and protons that are located in the nucleus of the atom and electrons that encircle the nucleus in orbitals.
3. The atomic number is the number of protons in the nucleus. The atomic weight is the weight of the neutrons and protons in the nucleus.
4. An isotope is an atom with the same atomic number but a different atomic weight. A radioisotope is an unstable isotope that decays into a more simple substance by giving off waves, or particles.

II. Chemical Interactions

A. Electron Shells and Bonding
1. Each electron shell, or orbital, holds a specific number of electrons. The inner shell holds two electrons, and the outer shells hold eight electrons each.
2. Ionic bonds are formed as electrons are transferred to stabilize the shells of the atoms.
3. Covalent bonds are formed as the electrons of the outer shells are shared by the interacting atoms.
4. Hydrogen bonds are intermolecular bonds and do not involve transfer, or sharing, of the electrons.

B. Ion Formation
1. An ion is an atom that gains or loses an electron or electrons and therefore carries an electrical charge. A cation is a positively charged ion. An anion is a negatively charged ion.
2. An electrolyte is a substance that forms ions when dissolved in water. This process is called ionization.

C. Molecules and Compounds
1. A molecule is a substance formed from two or more atoms (eg, O_2, H_2O).
2. A compound is a substance that forms when two or more different atoms bond (eg, H_2O).
3. Important molecules and compounds include water, oxygen, and carbon dioxide.

D. Acids and Bases
1. An acid is an electrolyte that dissociates into hydrogen ion (H^+). The amount of H^+ in solution determines the acidity.
2. A base is a substance that combines with H^+ and eliminates H^+; a base neutralizes an acid by producing a salt and water.
3. The pH scale measures acidity and alkalinity. A pH of 7 is neutral. A pH less than 7 is acidic, and a pH greater than 7 is basic, or alkaline.
4. The normal pH of the blood is 7.35 to 7.45. A person with a pH less than 7.35 is acidotic, and a person with a pH greater than 7.45 is alkalotic.
5. Blood pH is regulated by buffers, the respiratory system, and the kidneys.

Summary Outline, *continued*

III. Energy
Energy is defined as the ability to do work.

A. Forms of Energy
1. The six forms of energy are mechanical, chemical, electrical, radiant, thermal, and nuclear.
2. Most energy is dissipated as heat.

B. Role of adenosine triphosphate (ATP)
1. ATP transfers energy from one chemical substance to another.

2. The energy is stored in the phosphate bonds of the ATP.

IV. Mixtures, Solutions, and Suspensions
A mixture is a blend of two or more substances that can be separated by ordinary physical means. Solutions, suspensions, and colloidal suspensions are types of mixtures.

Review Your Knowledge

1. Explain the difference between a physical and a chemical change.

2. What are the four major elements that make up 96% of the body?

3. Explain why radioisotopes are radioactive.

4. Describe three types of chemical bonds.

5. State the types of bonds formed in the following compounds: NaCl (table salt) and $C_6H_{12}O_6$ (glucose).

6. How are electrolytes capable of conducting an electric current?

7. What is the difference between a molecule and a compound?

8. List five reasons water is an essential compound for the body.

9. What is the role of enzymes and catalysts in chemical reactions?

10. What is the difference between a strong acid and a weak acid?

11. What happens when an acid is mixed with a base?

12. What is the meaning of the following pH measurements: 6.0, 7.0, and 8.5?

13. List three ways in which blood pH is regulated.

14. What do the terms *acidosis* and *alkalosis* mean?

15. What is the difference between mechanical energy and chemical energy?

16. How is energy in food converted to a form of energy that can be used by the body?

17. What is the difference between the following terms: mixtures, solutions, suspensions, and colloidal suspensions?

18. What is the solute in salt water? What is the solvent in salt water?

19. State whether each of the following is a mixture, solution, suspension, or colloidal suspension: iron filings sprinkled throughout sugar, salt water, sand in water, and blood plasma.

20. Explain why antacids are used to treat patients with ulcers.

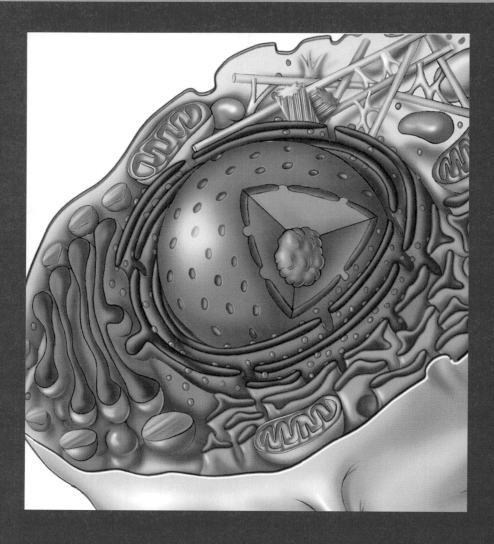

••• Key Terms

Active transport (ăk′tĭv trănz′pôrt)

Cell membrane (sĕl mĕm′brān)

Cytoplasm (sī′tə-plăz″əm)

Differentiation (dĭf′ər-ĕn″shē-ā′shən)

Diffusion (dĭ-fyōō′zhən)

Endocytosis (ĕn″dō-sī-tō′sĭs)

Endoplasmic reticulum
(ĕn″dō-plăs′mĭk rĕ-tĭk′yōō-lŭm)

Exocytosis (ĕk″sō-sī-tō′sĭs)

Facilitated diffusion
(fə-sĭl′ə-tā″təd dĭ-fyōō′zhən)

Filtration (fĭl-trā′shən)

Golgi apparatus (gôl′jē ăp″ə-rā′təs)

Hypertonic solution (hī″pər-tŏn′ĭk sə-lōō′shən)

Hypotonic solution (hī″pō-tŏn′ĭk sə-lōō′shən)

Isotonic solution (ī″sō-tŏn′ĭk sə-lōō′shən)

Lysosomes (lī′sə-sōmz)

Mitochondria (mī″tō-kŏn′drē-ə)

Mitosis (mī-tō′sĭs)

Nucleus (nōō′klē-əs)

Organelle (ôr″gə-nĕl′)

Osmosis (ŏz-mō′sĭs)

••• Selected terms in bold type in this chapter are defined in the Glossary.

3 CELLS

*O*bjectives

1. Label a diagram of the main parts of a typical cell, with the cell membrane, cytoplasm, nucleus, and organelles.

2. Describe the functions of the main organelles of the cell.

3. Explain the role of the nucleus.

4. Identify the structure of the cell membrane, including the lipid layers, the proteins, and the pores.

5. Differentiate between active and passive transport.

6. Describe the movement of substances across a cell membrane: diffusion, facilitated diffusion, osmosis, filtration, and active transport.

7. Compare isotonic, hypotonic, and hypertonic solutions.

8. Describe the five stages of mitosis (cell division).

9. Explain what is meant by cell differentiation.

hat do this monk and a cell have in common? While looking at a piece of cork under a microscope one day, Robert Hooke, in the 1600s, observed cube-like structures that resembled the rooms, or cells, occupied by monks in a monastery. Hooke therefore called his structures **cells.**

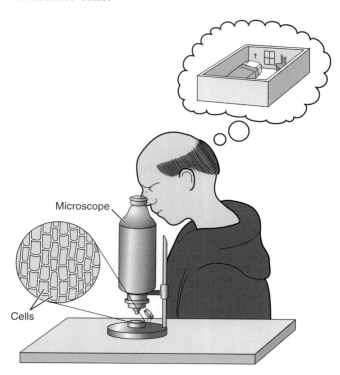

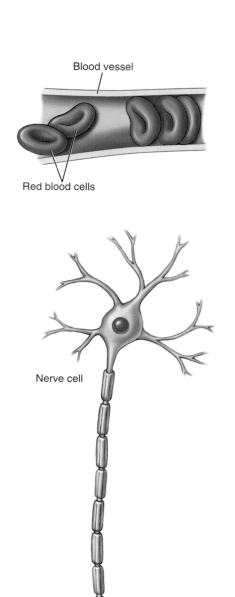

Blood vessel

Red blood cells

Nerve cell

The cell is the structural and functional unit of all living matter. Cells vary considerably in size, shape, and function. The red blood cell, for instance, is tiny, whereas a single nerve cell may measure 4 feet in length (Fig. 3–1). The shapes and structures of the cells are also very different. The red blood cell is shaped like a Frisbee and is able to bend. The shape allows it to squeeze through tiny blood vessels and deliver oxygen to every cell in the body. Some nerve cells are very long and many resemble bushes or trees. Their shapes enable them to conduct electrical signals quickly over long distances. Cell structure and cell function are closely related.

A TYPICAL CELL

Despite the differences, cells have many similarities. Figure 3–2 is a typical cell with all known cellular components. Each specialized cell, such as a nerve cell or a red blood cell, for example, possesses some or all of the properties of the typical cell.

The cell is encased by a membrane. Many smaller structures are inside the cell. Table 3–1 summarizes the functions of these cellular components.

FIGURE 3–1 • Cells come in all different shapes and sizes.

Table 3 • 1	CELL STRUCTURE AND FUNCTION

CELL STRUCTURE	FUNCTION
Cell membrane	Contains cellular contents; regulates what enters and leaves the cell
Cytoplasm	Surrounds and supports organelles; medium through which nutrients and waste move
Nucleus	Contains genetic information; control center of the cell
Nucleolus	Forms ribosomes
Endoplasmic reticulum (ER)	Transports material through the cytoplasm
Rough	Contains the ribosomes where protein is synthesized
Smooth	Site of steroid synthesis
Mitochondria	Convert energy in nutrients to ATP (power plants of the cell)
Golgi apparatus	Packages protein with membrane; puts the finishing touches on protein
Ribosomes	Site of protein synthesis
Lysosomes	"Housekeeping" within the cell; phagocytosis through powerful enzymes
Cytoskeleton	Provides for intracellular shape and support
Centrioles	Help separate the chromosomes during mitosis
Cilia	Create movement over the cell surface
Flagella	Create movement of cell (allow the sperm to swim)

Cell Membrane

The cell is encased by a cell membrane. The **cell membrane** (sĕl mĕm′brān) separates intracellular (inside the cell) material from extracellular (outside the cell) material. In addition to physically holding the cell together, the cell membrane performs other important functions. One of its chief functions is the selection of substances allowed to enter or leave the cell. Because the membrane selects, or chooses, the substances allowed to cross it, the membrane is said to be **selectively permeable,** or **semipermeable.** Only selected substances can penetrate, or pass through, the membrane.

What makes a cell membrane? The cell membrane is composed primarily of phospholipids and protein (Fig. 3–3). The phospholipids are arranged in two layers. The protein molecules in the membrane perform several important functions: they provide structural support for the membrane, act as a binding site for hormones, and poke holes, or pores, through the lipid membrane. These pores form channels through which water and dissolved substances flow.

Substances move across the selectively permeable membrane either by dissolving in the lipid portion of the membrane as oxygen and carbon dioxide do or by flowing through the pores. Electrically charged substances, such as sodium and chloride, cannot penetrate the lipid membrane and must use the pores. The size of the pores also helps select which substances cross the membrane. Substances larger than the pores cannot cross the membrane, while smaller substances, such as sodium and chloride, flow through easily.

Inside the Cell

The inside of the cell is divided into two compartments: the nucleus and the cytoplasm. The inside of the cell resembles the inside of a raw egg. The yellow yolk is like the nucleus, and the white is like the cytoplasm.

Nucleus

The **nucleus** (noo′klē-əs) is the control center of the cell; it controls the workings of the entire cell (see Fig. 3–2). Most adult cells have one nucleus. Mature red blood cells have no nucleus, while other cells, such as some white blood cells, may have several nuclei.

Surrounding the nucleus is a double-layered **nuclear membrane.** The nuclear membrane contains large pores, or holes. These allow for the free movement of certain substances between the nucleus and the cytoplasm. For example, a large molecule called messenger ribonucleic acid (mRNA) is made in the nucleus but functions within the cytoplasm. The large pores in the nuclear membrane enable the mRNA to move from the nucleus to the cytoplasm.

The nucleus is filled with a gel-like substance called **nucleoplasm.** It also contains two other structures: (1) the nucleolus or little nucleus,

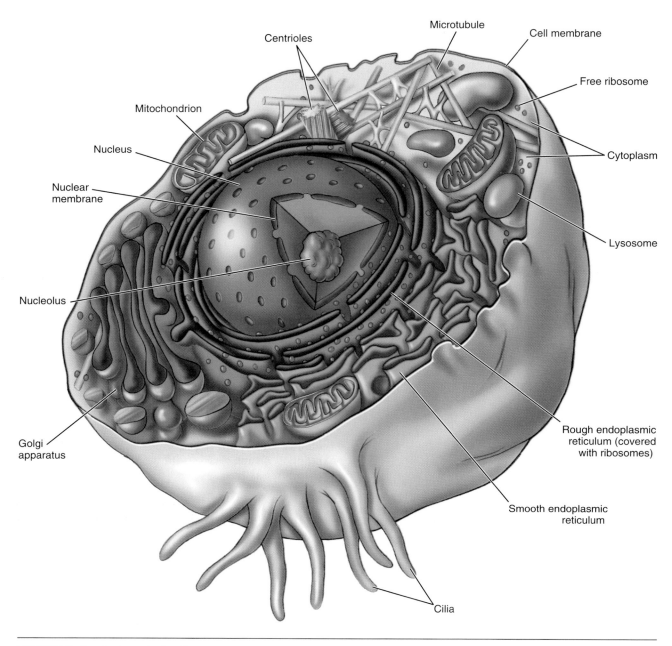

FIGURE 3-2 ● A typical cell.

which is concerned with the synthesis, or production, of ribosomes and (2) chromatin, thread-like structures that contain genes.

Cytoplasm

CYTOPLASMIC GEL. The **cytoplasm** (sī'tō-plăz"əm) is a gel-like substance inside the cell but outside the nucleus (it is like the white of a raw egg). The gel is composed primarily of water, electrolytes, nutrients, and metabolic waste products. The cytoplasm contains numerous cytoplasmic organelles and inclusion bodies. The **organelles** (ōr"gə-nĕlz'), or little organs, each have a specific role. The **inclusion bodies** are temporary structures that appear and disappear. These include

water vacuoles, secretory vesicles, and various granules. Locate the organelles in Figure 3–2.

CYTOPLASMIC ORGANELLES

Mitochondria. The **mitochondria** (mī"tō-kŏn'drē-ə) are tiny, slipper-shaped organelles located in the cytoplasm. The number of mitochondria per cell varies, depending on the metabolic activity of the cell (ie, how hard the cell works). The more metabolically active the cell, the greater the number of mitochondria. The liver, for instance, is very active and therefore has many mitochondria per cell. Bone cells are less active metabolically and have fewer mitochondria.

The mitochondrial membrane has two layers (Fig. 3–4). The outer layer is smooth, while the

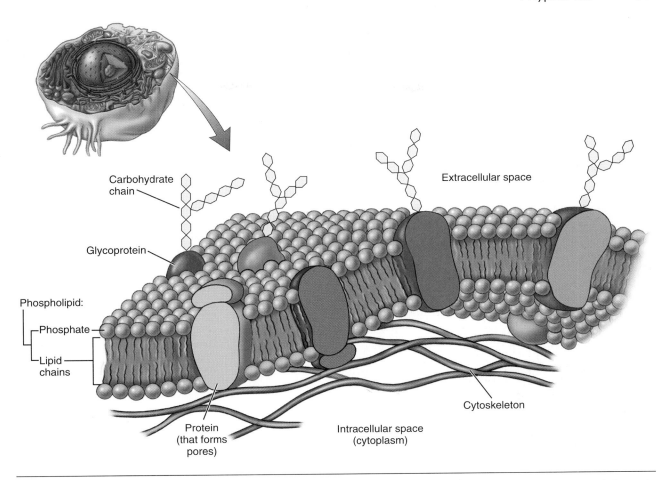

Carbohydrate chain

Extracellular space

Glycoprotein

Phospholipid:

Phosphate

Lipid chains

Cytoskeleton

Protein (that forms pores)

Intracellular space (cytoplasm)

FIGURE 3–3 • Structure of the cell membrane. Note the phospholipid bilayer and the proteins scattered throughout the phospholipids. The proteins create the pores.

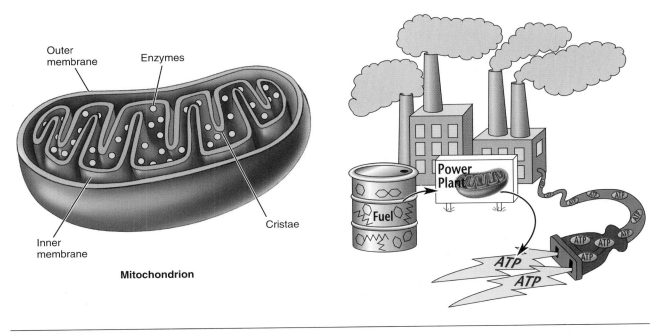

Outer membrane

Enzymes

Cristae

Inner membrane

Mitochondrion

Power Plant

Fuel

ATP

FIGURE 3–4 • Mitochondrion. Because most of the ATP is produced in the mitochondria, they are referred to as the power plants of the cell.

inner layer has many folds, referred to as **cristae.** The enzymes associated with adenosine triphosphate (ATP) production are located along the cristae. Because the mitochondria produce most of the energy (ATP) in the body, they are referred to as the "power plants" of the cell. (See Chapter 2 for an explanation of ATP.)

Ribosomes. **Ribosomes** are cytoplasmic organelles concerned with protein synthesis, which is explained in Chapter 4. Some ribosomes are attached to the endoplasmic reticulum. Others float freely within the cytoplasm.

Endoplasmic Reticulum. The **endoplasmic reticulum** (ĕn″dō-plăz′mĭk rĕ-tĭk′yōō-lŭm) (ER) is

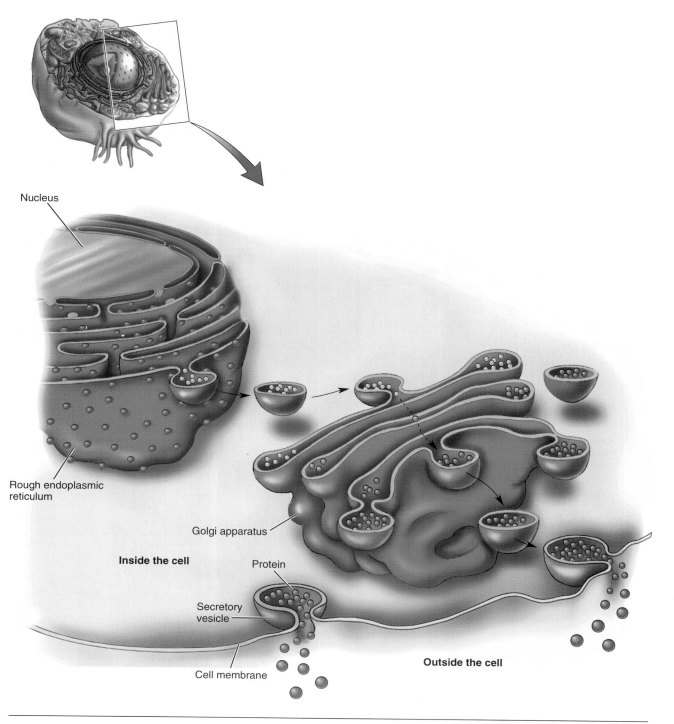

Nucleus

Rough endoplasmic reticulum

Golgi apparatus

Inside the cell

Protein

Secretory vesicle

Cell membrane

Outside the cell

FIGURE 3–5 ● Golgi apparatus. It adds the finishing touches to the proteins, preparing them for export to another part of the body.

a network of membranes within the cytoplasm (see Fig. 3–2). These long, folded membranes form channels through which substances move. There are two types of ER. The ER that contains ribosomes along its surface is called rough endoplasmic reticulum, or RER, because of its rough, sandpaper-like appearance. The RER is primarily concerned with protein synthesis. The ER that does not contain ribosomes on its surface appears smooth; it is therefore called smooth endoplasmic reticulum (SER). SER is primarily concerned with the synthesis of lipids and steroids. Protein synthesized along the RER is transported through the channels to the Golgi apparatus for further processing.

Golgi Apparatus. The **Golgi apparatus** (gōl′jē ăp″ə-rā′təs) is a series of flattened membranous sacs (Fig. 3–5). Proteins synthesized along the RER are transported to the Golgi through channels formed by the ER. The Golgi put the finishing touches on the protein. For example, a glucose molecule may be attached to a protein within the Golgi apparatus. A segment of the Golgi membrane then wraps itself around the protein and pinches itself off to form a secretory vesicle. In this way the Golgi apparatus packages the protein for secretion.

Lysosomes. **Lysosomes** (lī′sə-sōmz) are membranous sacs containing powerful hydrolytic enzymes. Lysosomes are digestive organelles. Lysosomal enzymes break down intracellular waste and debris and thus help to "clean house." Lysosomal enzymes perform several other functions. They participate in the destruction of bacteria, a process called phagocytosis. They also assist in reducing organ size. In the weeks after delivery of a baby, for instance, uterine size diminishes partly in response to lysosomal activity.

Cytoskeleton. The **cytoskeleton** is composed of thread-like structures called microfilaments and microtubules (tiny tube-like structures). The cytoskeleton helps to maintain the shape of the cell and assists the cell in various forms of cellular movement. Cellular movement is particularly evident in muscle cells, which contain large numbers of microfilaments.

Centrioles. **Centrioles** are paired, rod-shaped microtubular structures that play a key role in cellular reproduction.

On the Cell Membrane

Cilia

Cilia are short, hair-like projections that are visible on the outer surface of the cell. Cilia engage in a wave-like motion, which moves substances across the surface of the cell. Cilia are abundant on the cells that line the respiratory passages. The cilia help move mucus and trapped dust and dirt toward the throat, away from the lungs. Once in the throat, the mucus can then be cleared by coughing. The cilia therefore help to keep the respiratory passages clean and clear. Cigarette smoking damages the cilia and thus deprives the smoker of this benefit.

Flagella

Flagella are similar to cilia in that both are hair-like projections. Flagella, however, are thicker, longer, and fewer in number; they help move the cell. The tail of the sperm is an example of a flagellum; the tail enables the sperm to swim.

✳ **SUM IT UP!** The cell is the structural and functional unit of all living matter. While cells differ considerably, they also share many similarities. The cell is surrounded by a cell membrane. The inside of the cell is divided into the nucleus and the cytoplasm. The nucleus is the control center of the cell; it directs the cell's inner workings. The cytoplasm contains many little organs, or organelles, each of which has a special task to perform.

MOVEMENT ACROSS THE CELL MEMBRANE

As shown below, cells are bathed in an extracellular fluid that is rich in nutrients such as oxygen, glucose, and amino acids. These nutrients are needed within the cell and must therefore cross the cell membrane. The cell's waste, such as carbon dioxide that accumulates within the cell, must also cross the cell membrane. Wastes are eventually eliminated from the body.

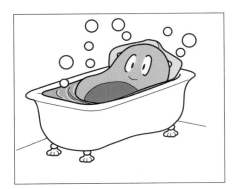
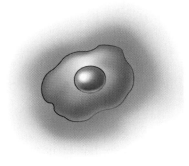

Table 3 • 2

TRANSPORT MECHANISMS

MECHANISM	DESCRIPTION
Passive	
Diffusion	Movement of a substance from an area of high concentration to an area of low concentration.
Facilitated diffusion	A helper molecule within the membrane assists the movement of substances from an area of high concentration to an area of low concentration.
Osmosis	Movement of water (solvent) from an area where there is more water to an area where there is less water.
Filtration	Movement of water and dissolved substances from an area of high pressure to an area of low pressure; the water and dissolved substances are pushed.
Active	
Active transport pumps	Movement of a substance uphill (from an area of low concentration to an area of high concentration). Requires an input of energy (ATP).
Endocytosis	Taking in or ingestion of substances by the cell membrane.
Phagocytosis	Engulfing of solid particles by the cell membrane (cellular eating).
Pinocytosis	Engulfing of liquid droplets (cellular drinking).
Exocytosis	Secretion of cellular products (eg, protein, debris) out of the cell.

A number of mechanisms assist in the movement of water and dissolved substances across the cell membrane. The transport mechanisms can be divided into two groups: the **passive transport** mechanisms and the **active transport** (ăk′tĭv trănz′pôrt) mechanisms. Table 3–2 summarizes both kinds of transport.

The passive transport mechanisms require no additional energy in the form of ATP. Passive transport is something like the downward movement of a ball (Fig. 3–6). The ball is at the top of the hill.

Once released, the ball rolls downhill. The ball does not need to be pushed; it moves passively, without any input of energy. Passive transport mechanisms cause water and dissolved substances to move without additional energy, like a ball rolling downhill.

Active transport mechanisms require an input of energy in the form of ATP. Active transport is like the upward movement of a ball (see Fig. 3–6). For the ball to move uphill, it must be pushed, therefore requiring an input of energy.

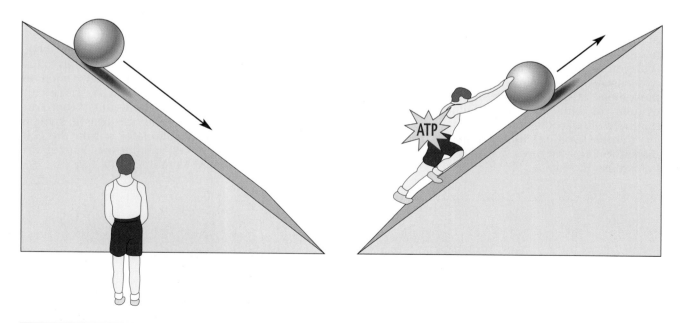

A Passive (downhill)

B Active (uphill)

ATP

FIGURE 3–6 ● Transport mechanisms: passive and active. A, Passive transport mechanisms do not require an input of energy. The ball rolls downhill on its own. B, Active transport requires an input of energy. The ball must be pushed uphill with energy invested.

Passive Transport Mechanisms

The passive mechanisms that move substances across the membrane include diffusion, facilitated diffusion, osmosis, and filtration.

Diffusion

Diffusion (dĭ-fyoo′zhən) is the most common transport mechanism. Diffusion is the movement of a substance from an area of higher concentration to an area of lower concentration. For instance, a tablet of red dye is placed in a glass of water (Fig. 3–7A). The tablet dissolves, and the dye moves from an area where it is most concentrated (glass #1) to an area where it is less concentrated (glasses #2 and #3). Diffusion continues until the dye is evenly distributed throughout the glass.

The scent of our pet skunk also illustrates diffusion (Fig. 3–7B). The skunk scent does not take long to permeate the area! Diffusion is involved in

A

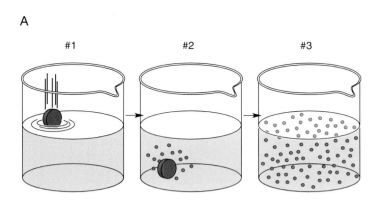

B

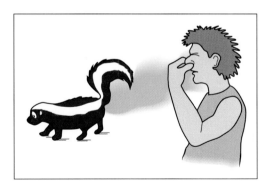

C

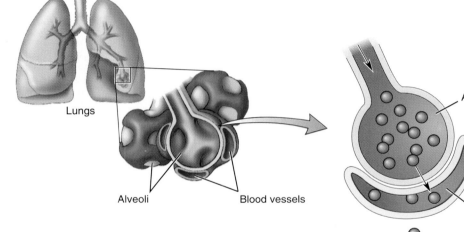
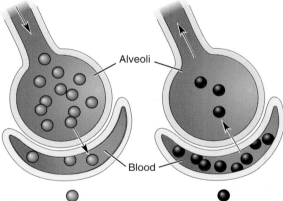

FIGURE 3–7 ● Diffusion. A, A tablet is placed in glass #1. Given enough time, the tablet dissolves and is evenly scattered throughout glass #3. B, The odor from the skunk has rapidly diffused. C, Another example of diffusion: oxygen diffuses from the lung (alveoli) into the blood, and carbon dioxide diffuses from the blood into the alveoli of the lung.

many physiologic events. For instance, diffusion causes oxygen to move across the membrane of the alveolus of the lung into the blood (Fig. 3–7C). Oxygen diffuses from the alveolus into the blood because the concentration of oxygen is greater within the alveolus than within the blood. Conversely, carbon dioxide, a waste product that accumulates within the blood, diffuses in the opposite direction (ie, carbon dioxide moves from the blood into the alveolus). The lungs then exhale the carbon dioxide, thereby eliminating waste from the body. Thus the process of diffusion moves oxygen into the blood and carbon dioxide out of the blood.

Facilitated Diffusion

Facilitated diffusion (fə-sĭl′ə-tā″təd dĭ-fyōo′zhən) is a special case of diffusion. As in diffusion, substances move from a higher concentra-tion toward a lower concentration (Fig. 3–8). In facilitated diffusion, however, the substance (eg, glucose) is helped across the membrane by a molecule within the membrane. (*Facilitate* means to help.) The substance (glucose) hops on the "helper" molecule on the external surface of the cell, is carried across the membrane, and then hops off inside the cell. Facilitated diffusion is a commonly used transport mechanism within the body. Remember: even though glucose is helped across the membrane, facilitated diffusion is considered passive.

Osmosis

Osmosis (ŏz-mō′sĭs) is a special case of diffusion. Osmosis is the diffusion of *water* through a selectively permeable membrane. A selectively permeable membrane allows the passage of some substances while restricting the passage of others.

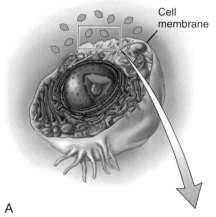

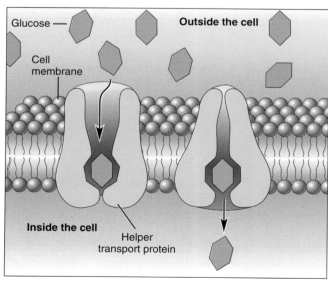

A

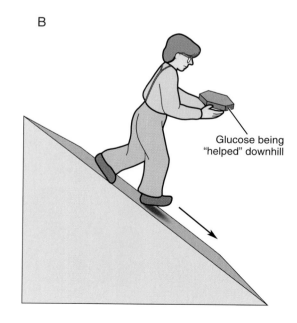

B

FIGURE 3–8 ● Facilitated diffusion ("diffusion with help"). A, Like diffusion, the substances diffuse from an area of high concentration to an area of low concentration. A helper protein molecule in the membrane assists in the movement. B, The helper carries the glucose downhill.

During osmosis, the water diffuses from an area with more water to an area where there is less water. The dissolved substances, however, do not move.

Two different solutions in the glass illustrate osmosis. The glass is divided into two compartments (A and B) by a semipermeable membrane (Fig. 3–9). Compartment A contains a dilute glucose solution, while compartment B contains a more concentrated glucose solution. Remember: The membrane is permeable *only* to water. The glucose cannot cross the membrane and is therefore confined to its compartment.

During osmosis, the water moves from compartment A to compartment B (ie, from the area where there is more water to the area where there is less water). Two effects occur: (1) the amount, or volume, of water in compartment B becomes greater than the volume in compartment A, and (2) the concentrations of the solutions in both compartments change. The solution in compartment A becomes more concentrated, while the solution in compartment B becomes more dilute.

Whenever dissolved substances such as glucose or protein are confined in a space by a selectively permeable membrane, they can pull water into the compartment by osmosis. This capacity to pull water is referred to as the **osmotic pressure.** The strength of the osmotic pressure is related directly to the concentration of the solution. The greater the concentration, the greater is the osmotic, or pulling, pressure. Because osmotic pressure pulls water into a compartment, it can cause swelling.

For instance, tissue injury causes leakage and accumulation of proteins within the tissue spaces.

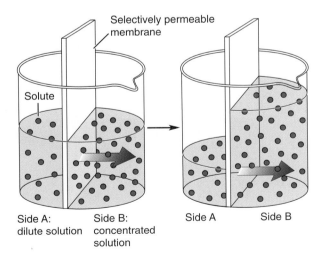

FIGURE 3–9 ● Osmosis. The glass is sectioned into side A and side B by a selectively permeable membrane; the membrane is permeable only to water. The water moves from side A to side B, thereby creating unequal volumes.

Do You Know...

Why may a blood clot continue to expand even when the bleeding stops?

The components of the blood clot are osmotically active substances. The blood clot pulls water into itself, thereby expanding. If the expanding blood clot is located within the brain, it presses on the brain tissue, causing a variety of neurologic deficits.

The confined proteins act osmotically, pulling water toward them. This process causes an accumulation of water in the tissue spaces. The accumulation of water is referred to as **edema.** The osmotically induced flow of water causes injured or inflamed tissue to swell.

Tonicity

Note what happens when two compartments containing different concentrations of solute (dissolved substances) interact (Fig. 3–10). To describe the water movement, three terms are used: isotonic, hypotonic, and hypertonic.

ISOTONIC SOLUTIONS. An **isotonic solution** (ī″sō-tŏn′ĭk sə-lōō′shən) has the same concentration as the solution to which it is compared (*iso* means same). For instance, the inside of a red blood cell (RBC) has a concentration similar to that of a 0.9% salt solution (normal saline). If an RBC is submerged in a 0.9% salt solution, the concentrations on both sides of the membrane are the same. The solution in the glass is said to be isotonic with respect to the inside of the RBC. Because it is isotonic, there is no *net* movement of water; the cell neither gains nor loses water.

Why is water movement an important consideration? If the cell gains water, the RBC membrane bursts, or lyses. If the RBC loses water, the cell shrinks. In both cases, RBC function is severely impaired. Isotonic solutions do not cause cells to swell or shrink. Isotonic solutions are commonly administered intravenously. Commonly used isotonic solutions include normal saline (0.9% NaCl), 5% D/W (dextrose or glucose in water), and Ringer's solution.

HYPOTONIC SOLUTIONS. If an RBC is placed in pure water (ie, a solution containing no salt), water moves into the cell by osmosis (from where there is more water to where there is less water). The pure water, being more dilute than the inside of the cell, is said to be hypotonic. **Hypotonic solutions** (hī″pō-tŏn′ĭk sə-lōō-shənz) cause the RBCs to burst, or lyse. This process is referred to as hemolysis. Because of hemolysis, pure water is not administered intravenously.

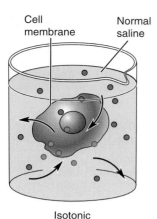
Cell membrane   Normal saline

Isotonic

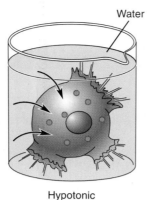
Water

Hypotonic

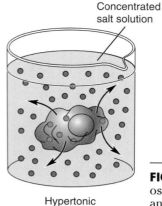
Concentrated salt solution

Hypertonic

FIGURE 3–10 ● Effects of osmosis: Isotonic, hypotonic, and hypertonic solutions.

A boiled hot dog may also illustrate this bursting effect. The hot dog, which contains much salt, is boiled in plain water. Because the plain water is hypotonic relative to the hot dog, water diffuses into the hot dog and bursts it.

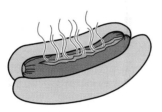

HYPERTONIC SOLUTIONS. If an RBC is placed within a very concentrated salt solution, water diffuses out of the RBC into the bathing solution, causing the RBC to shrink, or **crenate.** The salt solution is referred to as a **hypertonic solution** (hī″pər-tŏn′ĭk sə-loo′shən) . (Under special conditions, hypotonic or hypertonic solutions may be administered intravenously. Most IV solutions, however, are isotonic.)

Filtration

With diffusion and osmosis, water and dissolved substances move across the membrane in response to a difference in concentrations. With **filtration** (fĭl-trā′shən), however, water and dissolved substances cross the membrane in response to differences in pressures. In other words, a pressure, or force, pushes the substances across the membrane.

A syringe can illustrate filtration (Fig. 3–11). Syringe #1 is filled with water. If a force is applied to the plunger, the water is pushed out through the needle. The water moves in response to a pressure difference, with greater pressure at the plunger than at the tip of the needle. In the second syringe, tiny holes are made in the sides of the barrel. When force is applied to the plunger, water squirts out the sides of the syringe and out the tip of the needle.

Where does filtration occur in the body? The movement of fluid across the capillary wall can be compared to the movement of water in the syringe with holes on the side (syringe #2). The capillary is a tiny vessel that contains blood. The capillary wall is composed of a thin layer of cells with many little holes, or pores. The pressure in the capillary pushes water and dissolved substances out of the blood and through the pores in the capillary wall into the tissue spaces. This process is filtration; it is movement caused by pushing. (Capillary filtration is further explained in Chapter 15.)

Do You Know...

What would happen if pure water were administered intravenously?

Pure water is a hypotonic solution (it has fewer solute particles than the inside of a red blood cell does). If pure water were infused intravenously, the water would enter the red blood cells, causing swelling of the cells and hemolysis. Among other effects, the hemoglobin that is liberated from the burst red blood cells would severely damage the kidneys.

Do You Know...

Why may a hypertonic solution be administered intravenously to decrease cerebral edema or swelling (fluid in the brain tissue)?

Because a hypertonic solution contains more solute than is present in the interstitial or tissue fluid of the brain, water would leave the brain tissue (in response to osmosis) and move into the blood. As the blood is carried away from the brain, the swelling, or edema, decreases.

Active Transport Mechanisms

The active transport mechanisms include active transport pumps, endocytosis, and exocytosis.

Active Transport Pumps

Active transport refers to a transport mechanism that requires an input of energy (ATP) to achieve its goal. Why is it necessary to pump certain substances? Because the amount of some substances in the cell is already so great that the only way to move additional substances into the cell is to pump them in. For instance, the cell normally contains a large amount of potassium (K^+). The only way to move additional potassium (K^+) into the cell is to pump it in. To move the K^+ from an area of low concentration to an area of high concentration (pumping uphill), energy is invested (Fig. 3–12A). The energy ultimately comes from the food we eat.

A

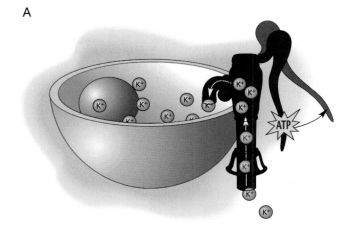

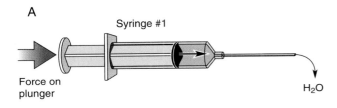

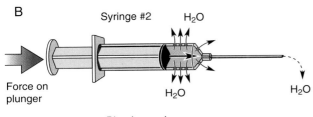

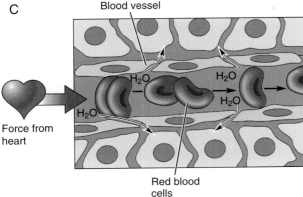

FIGURE 3–11 • Filtration. Water moves because it is pushed. A, The plunger of syringe #1 is pushed, causing water to flow out of the tip of the needle. B, Holes are punched into the side of syringe #2. When the plunger is pushed, water squirts through the holes in the sides of the syringe. C, Like syringe #2, the capillaries have holes. When the blood is pushed through the capillaries, some of the water from the blood squirts through the holes into the tissue spaces.

B
Endocytosis

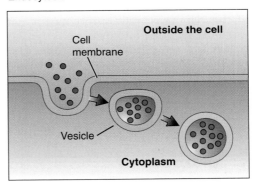

C
Exocytosis

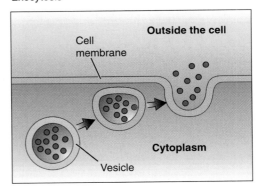

FIGURE 3–12 • Active transport. A, active transport pumps uphill. Potassium (K^+) must be pumped because it is moving uphill, from an area of low concentration to an area of high concentration. An investment of energy (ATP) is required. B, Endocytosis. A cell engulfs a particle by surrounding it with the cell's own membrane. C, Exocytosis. A vesicle within the cell moves toward and fuses with the cell membrane. The contents of the vesicle are released from the cell.

Endocytosis

Endocytosis (ĕn″dō-sī-tō′sĭs) is a transport mechanism that involves the intake of food or liquid by the cell membrane (Fig. 3–12B). In endocytosis, the particle is too large to move across the membrane by diffusion. Instead, the particle is surrounded by the cell membrane, which engulfs its and takes it into the cell. There are two forms of endocytosis. If the endocytosis involves a solid particle, it is called **phagocytosis** (*phago* means eating). For instance, white blood cells eat, or phagocytose, bacteria, thereby helping the body to defend itself against infection. If the cell ingests a water droplet, the endocytosis is called **pinocytosis,** or "cellular drinking."

Exocytosis

Whereas endocytosis brings substances into the cell, **exocytosis** (ĕk″sō-sī-tō′sĭs) moves substances out of the cell (Fig. 3–12C). For instance, the cells of the pancreas make proteins for use outside the pancreas. The pancreatic cells synthesize the protein and wrap it in a membrane. This membrane-bound vesicle moves toward and merges with the cell membrane. The protein is then expelled from the vesicle into the surrounding space. This process is exocytosis.

✳ **SUM IT UP!** Water and dissolved substances must be able to move from one body compartment to another. This movement usually involves passage across cell membranes. Movement of water and dissolved substances is achieved through both passive and active transport mechanisms. Passive transport mechanisms require no investment of energy (ATP) and include diffusion, facilitated diffusion, osmosis, and filtration. The active transport mechanisms include the active transport pumps, endocytosis, and exocytosis. The transport mechanisms are summarized in Table 3–2.

CELL DIVISION

Cell division, or cell reproduction, is necessary for bodily growth and repair. The frequency of cell division varies considerably from one tissue to the next. Some cells reproduce very frequently, while other cells reproduce very slowly or not at all. For instance, the cells that line the digestive tract are replaced every few days, and

A

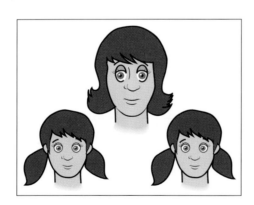

B

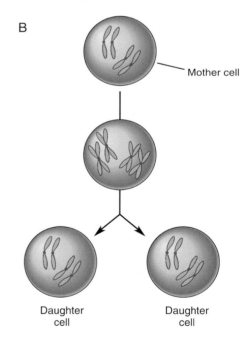

Mother cell

Daughter cell

Daughter cell

C

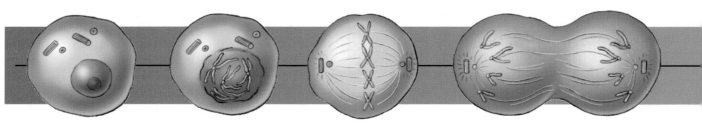

INTERPHASE   PROPHASE   METAPHASE   ANAPHASE

over 2 million red blood cells are replaced every second. Certain nerve cells in the brain and spinal cord, however, do not reproduce at all.

Two types of cell division are mitosis and meiosis. Meiosis occurs only in sex cells and will be discussed in Chapter 22. **Mitosis** (mī-tō′sĭs) is involved in bodily growth and repair. Mitosis is the splitting of one mother cell into two identical "daughter cells." The key word is *identical.* In other words, an exact copy of genetic information, stored within the chromosomes, must be passed from the mother cell to the two daughter cells.

What is happening during mitosis? Mitosis is divided into five phases: interphase, prophase, metaphase, anaphase, and telophase (Fig. 3–13). The most important point about mitosis is this: one cell splits into two genetically identical cells.

Interphase

The cell spends most of its time in interphase, during which it grows and carries on its daily activ-

ities. This phase is sometimes called the resting phase, an inaccurate term because the cell is very active during this phase. It is called resting only because the cell is not dividing. During interphase, the chromosomes in the nucleus double. The chromosomes contain the genes and therefore store and pass on our hereditary characteristics, or traits.

Prophase, Metaphase, Anaphase, and Telophase

During three phases of mitosis (prophase, metaphase, and anaphase), the pairs of identical chromosomes line up in the middle of the cell. Spindles attach to the chromosomes. As the spindles pull on the chromosomes, each pair of chromosomes splits and is pulled to the left or the right. The result is the separation of chromosomes into two identical sets, one set at one end of the dividing cell and a second identical set at the other end. Each end of the

FIGURE 3–13 ● Mitosis. A, Like mother, like daughters! During mitosis, the mother cell splits into two identical daughter cells. B, The arrangement of chromosomes that cause the formation of identical daughter cells. C, Cell division: stages of mitosis. The mother cell goes through the following stages as it divides into two identical daughter cells: interphase → prophase → metaphase → anaphase → telophase.

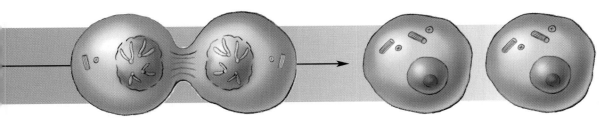

TELOPHASE   DAUGHTER CELLS

cell therefore contains the same genetic information.

During telophase, the outer cell membrane constricts and pinches the cell in half, forming two individual and genetically identical cells. The interior of the cell then reorganizes until it resembles the cell in interphase. Telophase completes mitosis.

CELL DIFFERENTIATION

Mitosis assures us that the division of one cell produces two *identical* cells. How do we account for the differences in cells, such as muscle cells, red blood cells, and bone cells? In other words, how do cells differentiate, or develop different characteristics?

An embryo begins life as a single cell, the fertilized ovum. Through mitosis, the single cell divides many times into identical cells. Then, sometime during their development, the cells start to specialize, or differentiate (Fig. 3–14). The exact way that specialization, or **differentiation** (dĭf″ər-ĕn″shē-ā′shən), occurs is not known. One cell, for instance, may switch on enzymes that produce red blood cells. Other enzymes are switched on and produce bone cells. Whatever the mechanism, you started life as a single adorable cell and ended up as billions of specialized cells.

ORDER, DISORDER, AND DEATH

Most cell growth is orderly. Cells normally reproduce at the proper rate and align themselves in the correct positions. At times, however, cell growth becomes uncontrolled and disorganized. Too many cells are produced. This process is experienced by the patient as a lump or tumor (*tumor* means swelling).

Tumors may be classified as benign (noncancerous) or malignant (**cancerous**). Cancer cells grow rapidly and invade surrounding tissue. Cancer cells are appropriately named. Cancer means "crab"; cancer cells, like a crab, send out claw-like extensions. Cancer cells also detach from the original tumor and spread throughout the body. The widespread invasion of the body by cancer cells often causes death. The spreading of cancer cells is referred to as **metastasis.**

A Papanicolaou test (Pap smear) is a type of diagnostic procedure. A sample of cells is obtained, usually from around the cervix in the female. The sample of cells (the smear) is then examined under the microscope for signs of cancerous changes. A positive Pap smear may detect early cancer, which is associated with a very high cure rate. This is the reason for the annual Pap smear for many women.

Sometimes the cells are injured so severely that they die, or necrose (from the Greek word *necros,* meaning death). For instance, the cells may be deprived of oxygen for too long a period,

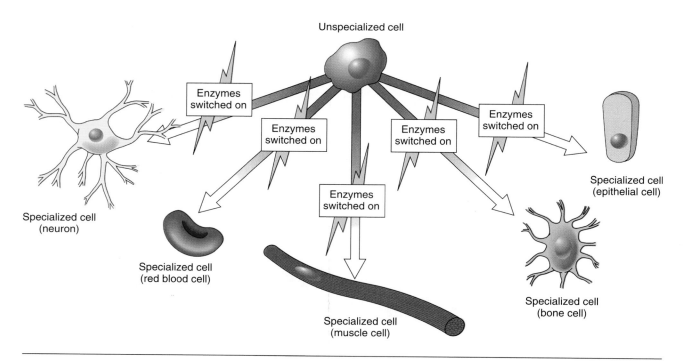

FIGURE 3–14 ● Cell differentiation: the ability of cells to specialize into different shapes and sizes to perform different functions. Note that the different cells all originated from a single cell.

may be poisoned (eg, by mercury), damaged by bacterial toxins, or suffer the damaging effects of radiation.

✳ **SUM IT UP!** The union of the sperm and egg forms a single cell that divides by mitosis into billions of identical cells. The cells then specialize, or differentiate, into many different types of cells, all of which are needed to perform a wide variety of functions. Most cells grow in an orderly way. Cells can, however, grow abnormally. The result is sometimes a tumor, which may be benign or malignant.

As You Age

1. All cells show changes as they age. The cells are larger, and their capacity to divide and reproduce tends to decrease.
2. Normal cells have built-in mechanisms to repair minor damage; this ability to repair declines in aging cells.
3. When DNA is damaged, changes in membranes and enzymes occur in the cell. Changes in the transport of ions and nutrients occur at the cell membrane. The chromosomes in the nucleus undergo such changes as clumping, shrinkage, and fragmentation.
4. Certain genetic disorders such as Down syndrome are more common in children born to older women.
5. Organelles such as mitochondria and lysosomes are present in reduced numbers as a person ages. In addition, cells function less efficiently.

Disorders of Cellular Growth

Atrophy — Without nourishment. Atrophy is a decrease in the size of the cells, leading to a wasting away of tissues and organs.

Dysplasia — Abnormal growth. Dysplasia is an alteration in cell size, shape, and organization. The concern is that these alterations can result in cancer.

Hyperplasia — Overgrowth. Hyperplasia is an increase in the numbers of cells, resulting in an increase in the size of tissues and organs.

Metaplasia — Transformation of one cell type into another (eg, the change of columnar cells in the breathing passages of a smoker into a different cell type).

Necrosis — Death of cells or groups of cells.

Neoplasm — Abnormal new growth, also called a tumor. A malignant neoplasm is a cancerous tumor. A benign neoplasm is a noncancerous tumor. Malignant neoplasms tend to metastasize, or spread, from an original (primary) site to another (secondary) site.

Summary Outline

I. The Typical Cell: Structures and Functions
The cell is the structural and functional unit of all living matter that contains protein.

A. Cell Membrane (Plasma Membrane)
1. The cell membrane is composed of a phospholipid bilayer that contains protein.
2. The cell membrane is selectively permeable; it regulates what enters or leaves the cell.

B. Structures Inside the Cell
1. The nucleus is the control center of the cell; it stores the genetic information.
2. The cytoplasm is a gel-like substance inside the cell membrane but outside of the nucleus.
3. Many different organelles are in the cytoplasm: mitochondria, ribosomes, endoplasmic reticulum, Golgi apparatus, lysosomes, cytoskeleton, and centrioles.
4. The mitochondria are the power plants of the cell because they are the sites of most ATP production.
5. Ribosomes are concerned with protein synthesis.
6. The endoplasmic reticulum has two types. The rough endoplasmic reticulum (RER) is concerned with protein synthesis, and the smooth endoplasmic reticulum (SER) is concerned with the synthesis of lipids and steroids.
7. The Golgi apparatus puts the finishing touches on the newly synthesized protein and then wraps the protein in a membrane.
8. Lysosomes are digestive organelles that act as intracellular scavengers, or housekeepers.
9. The cytoskeleton is composed of microfilaments and microtubules that give shape and support to the cell.
10. Centrioles are rod-shaped microtubular structures that play a role in cell reproduction.

C. Structures on the Cell Membrane
1. Cilia are short, hair-like projections on the outer surface of some cells.
2. Flagella are long hair-like projections that help move some cells.

II. Movement of Substances Across the Membrane

A. Passive Transport Mechanisms
1. Passive transport mechanisms require no input of energy (ATP).
2. Diffusion causes a substance to move from an area of greater concentration to an area of lesser concentration.
3. Facilitated diffusion is the same as diffusion but uses a helper molecule to increase the rate of diffusion.
4. Osmosis is a special case of diffusion using a semipermeable membrane. Osmosis involves the diffusion of water from an area with more water to an area of less water. The concentrations of a solution are expressed as tonicity. Solutions are isotonic, hypotonic, or hypertonic.
5. Filtration is the movement of water and dissolved substances from an area of high pressure to an area of low pressure.

B. Active Transport Mechanisms
1. Active transport requires an input of energy (ATP).
2. Active transport pumps move substances from an area of low concentration to an area of high concentration.
3. Endocytosis moves substances into a cell; pinocytosis is cellular "drinking" and phagocytosis is cellular "eating."
4. Exocytosis moves substances out of a cell.

III. Cell Division (Cell Reproduction)

A. Mitosis
1. Mitosis is the splitting of one mother cell into two *identical* daughter cells.
2. The five phases of mitosis are interphase, prophase, metaphase, anaphase, and telophase.

B. Meiosis and Differentiation
1. Meiosis occurs only in sex cells.
2. Cell differentiation refers to cellular specialization.

Review Your Knowledge

1. Cells vary considerably in size, shape, and function. How do red blood cells and nerve cells differ in structure and function?

2. Explain the meaning of *semipermeable* as it applies to the cell wall.

3. List three functions of protein in the cell membrane.

4. Which substances cannot penetrate the lipid membrane of the cell wall and must use the pores?

5. List two structures found in the nucleus.

6. What is found in the colloidal suspension of cytoplasm?

7. Explain why the liver has more mitochondria per cell than bone cells.

8. Which part of the cell produces ATP? What is the function of RER and SER? Which organelle packages the protein for secretion from the cell?

9. List three functions of lysosomes in the cell.

10. Which part of the cell helps to maintain the shape of the cell and assists the cell in cellular movement? What are the functions of cilia and flagella?

11. Explain how substances move across the cell membrane by active transport, diffusion, osmosis, and filtration. Define *pinocytosis* and *phagocytosis*.

12. Explain how glucose moves across the cell membrane.

13. Describe how osmotic pressure is related to swelling.

14. What happens to red blood cells that are placed in hypertonic and hypotonic solutions?

15. Explain why pure water is not administered intravenously.

16. Explain how filtration works like a syringe in the movement of blood through capillaries.

17. How is the movement of potassium into the cell similar to the action of a pump?

18. Define *mitosis*. What are five phases in the cell life cycle?

19. What word describes the process by which cells (such as muscle cells, red blood cells, and bone cells) develop different characteristics?

20. How do "poorly differentiated cells" relate to cancer cells?

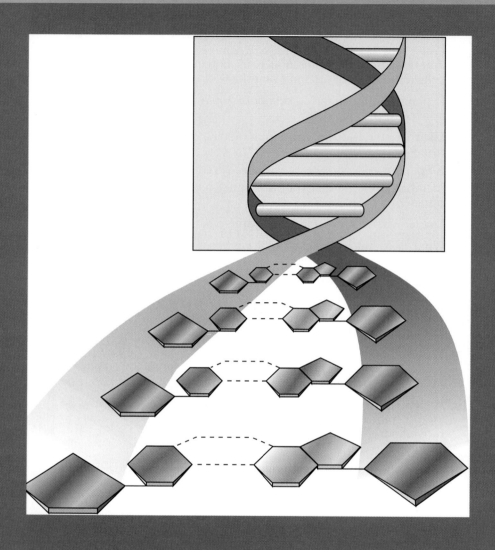

••• Key Terms

Aerobic catabolism (âr-ō'bĭk kə-tăb'ə-lĭz-əm)

Amino acids (ə-mē'nō ăs'ĭdz)

Anabolism (ə-năb'ə-lĭz-əm)

Anaerobic catabolism
  (ăn'âr-ō'bĭk kə-tăb'ə-lĭz-əm)

Base-pairing (bās pâr'ĭng)

Base-sequencing (bās sē'kwĕn-sĭng)

Carbohydrates (kär"bō-hī'drāts)

Catabolism (kə-tăb'ə-lĭz-əm)

Chromosomes (krō'mə-sōmz)

Deoxyribonucleic acid (DNA)
  (dē-ŏk"sē-rī"bō-nōō-klē'ĭk ăs'ĭd)

Glucose (glōō'kōs)

Glycogen (glī'kə-jĕn)

Glycolysis (glī-kŏl'ĭ-sĭs)

Lipid (lĭp'ĭd)

Metabolism (mĕ-tăb'ə-lĭz'əm)

Monosaccharides (mŏn"ō-săk'ə-rīdz)

Organic compound (ôr-găn'ĭk kŏm'pound)

Peptide bond (pĕp'tĭd bŏnd)

Protein (prō'tēn)

Ribonucleic acid (RNA) (rī"bō-nōō-klē'ĭk ăs'ĭd)

••• Selected terms in bold type in this chapter are defined in the Glossary.

4 CELL METABOLISM

*O*bjectives

1. Define *metabolism, anabolism,* and *catabolism.*

2. Explain the use of carbohydrates in the body.

3. Differentiate between the anaerobic and aerobic metabolism of carbohydrates.

4. Explain the use of lipids in the body.

5. Explain the use of proteins in the body.

6. Describe the structure of a nucleotide.

7. Describe the roles of DNA and RNA in protein synthesis.

8. Explain what is meant by the blueprint of life.

9. Differentiate between base-pairing and base-sequencing.

10. Describe protein synthesis.

To carry on its function, the cell, like a factory, must bring in and use raw material. The raw material comes from the food we eat. It includes carbohydrates, protein, and fat (Fig. 4–1).

METABOLISM: ANABOLISM AND CATABOLISM

Once inside the cell, the raw materials undergo thousands of chemical reactions. The

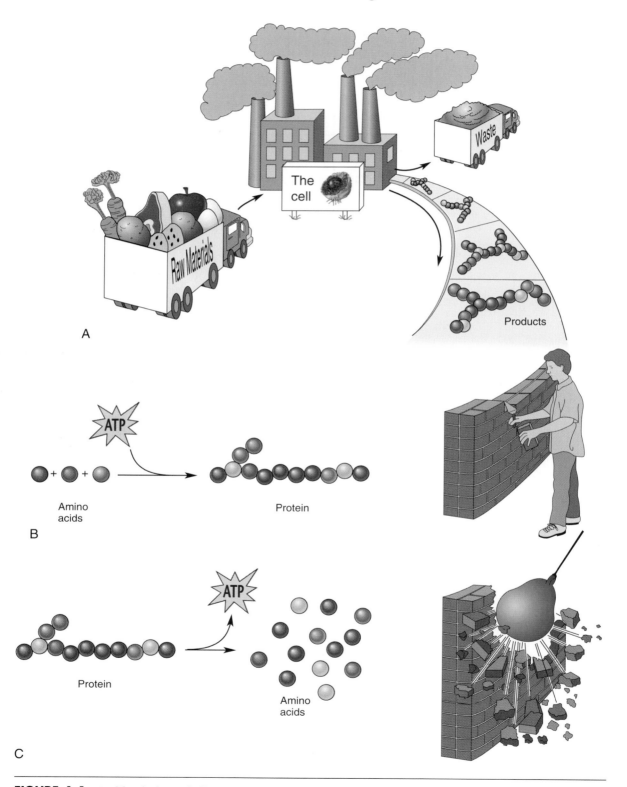

FIGURE 4–1 ● Metabolism. A, Raw materials (food) to run the factory (body). B, Anabolism, or building up. C, Catabolism, or breaking down.

series of chemical reactions necessary for the use of the raw material is called **metabolism** (mĕ-tăb′ə-lĭz-əm). Metabolism can be divided into two parts: anabolism and catabolism (see Fig. 4–1).

Anabolism (ə-năb′ə-lĭz-əm) includes reactions that build larger, more complex substances from simpler substances. The building of a large protein from individual amino acids is an example of anabolism. The process is similar to the building of a brick wall from individual bricks. Anabolic reactions generally require an input of energy in the form of adenosine triphosphate (ATP). (Energy transfer and ATP are explained in Chapter 2.)

Catabolism (kə-tăb′ə-lĭz-əm) includes reactions that degrade, or break down, larger, more complex substances into simpler substances. The breakdown of a large protein into individual amino acids is an example of catabolism. This process is similar to the dismantling, or knocking down, of a brick wall. Catabolism is generally associated with the release of energy, which is eventually converted into ATP.

CARBOHYDRATES

We have all eaten sugars and starchy food. Bread, potatoes, rice, pasta, and jelly beans are among our favorite foods. These are all carbohydrates. **Carbohydrates** (kär″bō-hī′drāts) are **organic compounds** (ôr-găn′ĭk kŏm′poundz) composed of carbon (C), hydrogen (H), and oxygen (O). Carbohydrates are classified according to size (Fig. 4–2). **Monosaccharides** (mŏn″ō-săk′ərīdz) are single *(mono)* sugar *(saccharide)* compounds. **Disaccharides** are double *(di)* sugars, and **polysaccharides** are many *(poly)* sugar com-

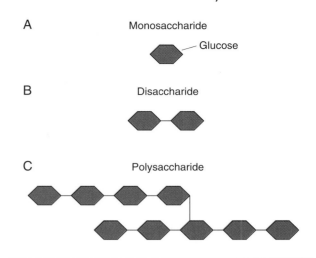

FIGURE 4–2 • Carbohydrates. A, Monosaccharide. B, Disaccharide. C, Polysaccharide.

pounds. The shorter monosaccharides and disaccharides are called **sugars,** and the longer chain polysaccharides are called **starches.** The carbohydrates are listed in Table 4–1.

Monosaccharides

Monosaccharides are sugars containing three to six carbons. The six-carbon simple sugars include glucose, fructose, and galactose (see Fig. 4–2A). **Glucose** (gloo′kōs) is the most important of the three and is used by the cells as an immediate source of energy.

There are also five-carbon monosaccharides. They include **ribose** and **deoxyribose.** These

Table 4 • 1	CARBOHYDRATES
NAME	**FUNCTION**
Monosaccharides (simple sugars)	
Glucose	Most important energy source
Fructose	Converted to glucose
Galactose	Converted to glucose
Deoxyribose	Sugar in DNA
Ribose	Sugar in RNA
Disaccharides (double sugars)	
Sucrose	Split into monosaccharides
Maltose	Split into monosaccharides
Lactose	Split into monosaccharides
Polysaccharides (many sugars)	
Starches	Found in plant foods; digested to monosaccharides
Glycogen	Animal starch; excess glucose stored in liver and skeletal muscle
Cellulose	Nondigestable by humans; forms dietary fiber or roughage

sugars are used in the synthesis of the nucleic acids, RNA and DNA.

Disaccharides

Disaccharides are double sugars. They are made when two monosaccharides are linked together (see Fig. 4–2B). The disaccharides include sucrose (table sugar), maltose, and lactose. Disaccharides are present in the food we eat. They must be digested, or broken down, into monosaccharides before they can be absorbed across the walls of the digestive tract and used by the cells. For instance, sucrose is broken down into the monosaccharides glucose and fructose. Both monosaccharides are absorbed. The glucose is used immediately by the cells, but the fructose is first changed to glucose and then is used by the cells.

Polysaccharides

Polysaccharides are made of many (poly) glucose molecules linked together. Some are linked together in straight chains, others in branched chains (see Fig. 4–2C). The three polysaccharides of interest to us are the starch found in plants, animal starch, and cellulose. **Starch** is the storage polysaccharide in plants. It is a series of glucose molecules linked together in a branched

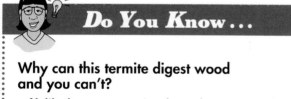

Why can this termite digest wood and you can't?

Unlike humans, termites have the enzymes that digest cellulose. The ability to make this enzyme enables the mighty termite to eat your house plank by plank.

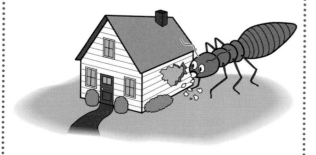

pattern. The starchy foods, such as potatoes, peas, grains, and pasta, contain this type of starch.

Glycogen (glī′kə-jĕn) is also called animal starch and is a highly branched polysaccharide similar to plant starch. Glycogen is the form in which humans store glucose. Glycogen is stored primarily in the liver and skeletal muscle. When blood sugar levels become low, the glycogen is converted in the liver to glucose. The glucose is then released into the blood, where it restores normal blood sugar levels.

Cellulose is a straight-chained polysaccharide found in plants. Although we do not have the enzymes to digest cellulose as a source of nutrients, this polysaccharide plays an important role in our digestive process. The cellulose provides the fiber in our diet and improves digestive function in many ways.

Uses of Glucose

What about that mound of jelly beans, those colored, oval globs of glucose, that you just ate? Glucose is used by the body primarily as a fuel. In this way, glucose provides the energy, in the form of ATP, that the cell needs to do its work. Glucose is used by the body in three ways: (1) it can be burned immediately as fuel for energy; (2) it can be stored as glycogen and burned as fuel at a later time; and (3) it can be stored as fat and burned as fuel at a later time. The "stored as fat" phrase is the most distressing!

Glucose is broken down under two different conditions: in the absence of oxygen (the process is called **anaerobic catabolism** [ăn′âr-ō′bĭk kə-tăb′ə-lĭz-əm]) and in the presence of oxygen (the process is called **aerobic catabolism** [âr-ō′bĭk kə-tăb′ə-lĭz-əm]). In the absence of oxygen, glucose is broken down through a series of chemical reactions, first into pyruvic acid and then into lactic acid. This anaerobic process occurs in the cytoplasm and is called **glycolysis** (glī-kŏl′ĭ-sĭs). Because most of the energy is still locked up in the lactic acid molecule, glycolysis produces only a small amount of ATP (Fig. 4–3A).

If oxygen is available, glucose is completely broken down to form carbon dioxide, water, and energy (ATP) (Fig. 4–3B). The glucose is first broken down to pyruvic acid in the cytoplasm. The pyruvic acid molecules then move into the mitochondria, the power plants of the cell. In the presence of oxygen and special enzymes in the mitochondria, the pyruvic acid fragments are completely broken down to carbon dioxide and water. This process is accompanied by the release of a large amount of energy (ATP). The enzymes in the mitochondria include the enzymes of the citric acid cycle, also called the Krebs cycle.

Three important points about aerobic catabolism (with oxygen) should be remembered. First, the chemical reactions occurring in the mitochondria require oxygen. If the cells are deprived of oxygen, they soon become low in energy and cannot carry out their functions. This need for oxygen is the reason we need to breathe continuously—to ensure a continuous supply of oxygen to the cells. Second, when glucose is broken down completely to CO_2 and H_2O, all of the stored energy is released. Thus, the aerobic breakdown of glucose produces much more ATP than does the anaerobic (without oxygen) breakdown of glucose. Third, if oxygen is not available to the cell, the pyruvic acid cannot enter the mitochondria. Instead, the pyruvic acid is converted to lactic acid in the cytoplasm. The buildup of lactic acid is the reason that a lack of oxygen in a critically ill patient causes lactic acidosis.

The Making of Glucose

As we have seen, carbohydrates can be broken down in the cells as a source of energy. Cells can also make, or synthesize, glucose from noncarbohydrate substances. Protein, for instance, can be broken down and the breakdown products used to make glucose. Glucose synthesis is an important mechanism in the regulation of blood sugar. For example, if blood sugar declines, protein is converted to glucose in the liver and released into the blood, thereby restoring blood sugar to normal.

Clinicians see abnormal conditions involving glucose utilization and glucose synthesis. In the diabetic person, the lack of the insulin hormone affects glucose metabolism in two ways. First,

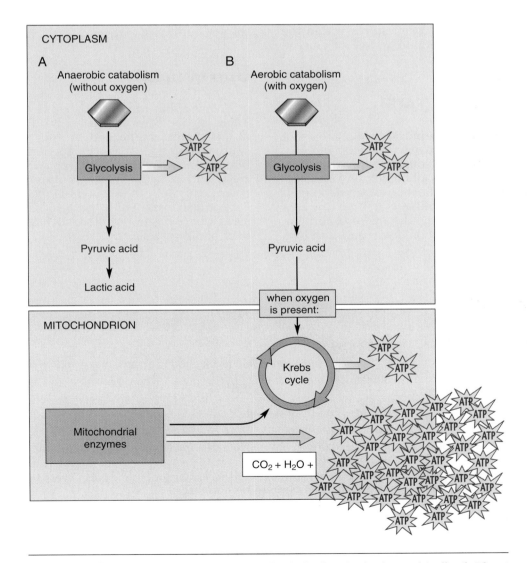

FIGURE 4–3 ● Breakdown of glucose (carbohydrate). A, Anaerobically (without oxygen) to lactic acid (glycolysis). B, Aerobically (with oxygen) to carbon dioxide and water. Note the greater amount of energy (ATP) associated with aerobic breakdown.

because insulin is needed for the transport of glucose into the cell, a lack of insulin deprives the cells of glucose and, thus, the energy that glucose provides. Second, the lack of insulin causes body protein to be broken down and then converted into glucose. Because the diabetic cells cannot utilize it, the glucose accumulates in the blood, making the person hyperglycemic (having excess glucose in the blood). Thus, the diabetic person ends up with most of the glucose in the blood and not in the cells, where it is needed for energy.

Glucose is stored in the form of glycogen. If excess glucose is present, the glucose molecules are linked together into a long, branch-like glycogen molecule (a polysaccharide as in Fig. 4–2). Glycogen, or animal starch, is the storage form of glucose and is found primarily in the liver and skeletal muscle. When needed, the glycogen can be broken down into individual glucose molecules. For instance, in an exercising muscle, ATP is used up quickly. The glycogen stores within the muscle provide an immediate source of glucose that can be burned as fuel.

LIPIDS (FATS)

Most of the **lipids** (lĭ′pĭdz), or fats, are eaten as fatty meats, egg yolk, dairy products, and oils. The lipids found most commonly in the body include triglycerides, phospholipids, and steroids. Other derivatives, or relatives, of lipids (lipoid substances) are listed in Table 4–2.

Like carbohydrates, lipids are organic compounds composed of carbon, hydrogen, and oxygen. Lipids, however, are longer and have a more complex arrangement than carbohydrates. The building blocks of lipids are the long-chain fatty acids and glycerol.

The lipid illustrated in Figure 4–4A is a **triglyceride.** It has three (tri) long fatty acid chains attached to one small glycerol molecule. A phospholipid is formed when a phosphorus-containing group attaches to one of the glycerol sites (Fig. 4–4B). Phospholipids are important components of the cell membrane.

The steroid is a third type of lipid. The most important steroid in the body is cholesterol (Fig. 4–4C). While most cholesterol is consumed as meat, eggs, and cheese, the body can also synthesize cholesterol in the liver. Despite all the bad press about it, cholesterol performs several important functions. For instance, cholesterol is found in all cell membranes and is necessary for the synthesis of vitamin D in the skin. It is also used in the ovaries and testes in the synthesis of the sex hormones.

Uses of Lipids

What about the bacon you ate for breakfast? There is good news and bad news. The good news is this: lipids are needed by the body (1) as a source of energy, (2) as a component of cell membranes and myelin sheath (coverings of nerve cells), and (3) in the synthesis of steroids. The bad news is this: fat can be put into long-term storage. Fat can make you fat! It can also be deposited in areas where it is not wanted, such as the inside of your blood vessels.

Table 4 • 2	LIPIDS
LIPID TYPE	**FUNCTION**
Triglycerides	In adipose tissue: protect and insulate body organs; major source of stored energy
Phospholipids	Found in cell membranes
Steroids	
Cholesterol	Used in synthesis of steroids
Bile salts	Assist in digestion of fats
Vitamin D	Synthesized in skin on exposure to ultraviolet radiation; contributes to calcium and phosphate homeostasis
Hormones from adrenal cortex, ovaries, and testes	Adrenal cortical hormones are necessary for life and affect every body system; ovaries and testes secrete sex hormones
Lipoid substances	
Fat-soluble vitamins (A, D, E, K)	Variety of functions (identified in later chapters)
Prostaglandins	Found in cell membranes; affect smooth muscle contraction
Lipoproteins	Help transport fatty acids. High density lipoprotein (HDL) is "good cholesterol"; Low density lipoprotein (LDL) is "bad cholesterol"

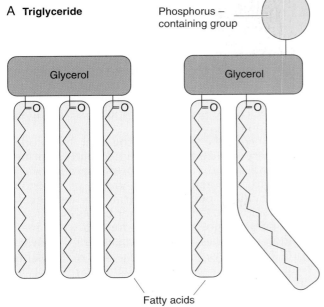

A **Triglyceride**

B **Phospholipid**

Phosphorus – containing group

Glycerol

Glycerol

Fatty acids

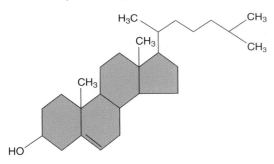

C **Steroid (cholesterol)**

H₃C · CH₃ · CH₃ · CH₃ · CH₃ · HO

FIGURE 4–4 ● Lipids. A, Triglyceride (formed from three fatty acid molecules and one glycerol molecule). B, Phospholipid (formed from two fatty acid molecules and a phosphorus-containing molecule). C, A steroid (cholesterol).

Metabolism of Lipids

How are fatty acids broken down? Like glucose, fatty acids and glycerol can be broken down so as to release the stored energy. Because the fatty acids are long structures, however, they must be chopped into tiny units before entering the mitochondria and becoming part of the citric acid cycle (Krebs cycle). The aerobic burning of the fatty acid units in the mitochondria releases a huge amount of energy (ATP). Because the fatty acids are much longer than the glucose molecules, the amount of energy released in the burning of fatty acids is much greater than the amount released in the burning of glucose.

Do You Know...

Why does a comatose person have a fruity odor to his breath?

Occasionally, fatty acid catabolism becomes disturbed. In the diabetic person, for instance, glucose is not available for cellular metabolism. Instead, fats are broken down rapidly and incompletely. The fatty acid units are produced faster than they can be transported into the mitochondria. They form **ketone bodies** and eventually find their way into the blood.

There are three types of ketone bodies: acetone and two very strong acids (ketoacids). The acids are responsible for the development of diabetic ketoacidosis. The acetone is not an acid; it forms a gas that is exhaled from the lungs. The breath of a diabetic person in ketoacidosis has a sweet fruity odor because of the acetone. The smell of acetone on the person's breath is a strong indication that fatty acid metabolism is out of control.

Knowing her lipid metabolism, Mother Nature encourages the grizzly bear to overeat and gain weight. By doing so, the grizzly is able to hibernate during the winter months because he is able to live off the fat stored during the summer and autumn feeding frenzies. While hibernating, the bear's fat is gradually broken down, and the ATP that is released is sufficient to keep him alive.

How are fatty acids made? As we all know, fat can also be made, or synthesized. The extra donut eaten today is worn on your hip tomorrow! When excess calories (energy) are consumed, the enzymes that synthesize fat are stimulated. The fat is deposited in adipose tissue throughout the body. In males, a large amount of the fat is deposited in the abdominal region, while in females, most of the fat appears on the hips and thighs.

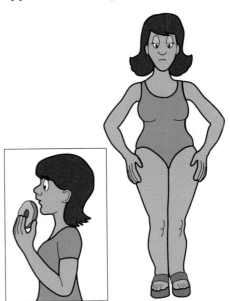

PROTEINS

Protein is the most abundant organic matter in the body. Because proteins are present in so many physiologically important compounds, it is safe to say that they participate in every body function. For instance, almost every chemical reaction in the body is regulated by an enzyme, which is a protein substance. Most hormones are proteins; they exert important widespread effects throughout the body. Hemoglobin, which delivers oxygen to every cell in the body, is a protein. Finally, muscles contract because of their contractile proteins, actin and myosin. As you can see, proteins are essential to life.

Amino Acids

The building blocks of protein are **amino acids** (ə-mē′nō ăs′ĭdz). About 20 amino acids are used to build body protein. Most amino acids come from protein foods. Foods such as lean meat, milk, and eggs are excellent sources of protein. More than half of the amino acids can be synthesized by the body. If the diet lacks the amino acid alanine, for instance, alanine can be synthesized within the liver.

Some amino acids, however, cannot be synthesized by the body and must be obtained from dietary sources. Because dietary intake of these amino acids is essential, these amino acids are called **essential amino acids.** The amino acids that can be synthesized by the liver are called **nonessential amino acids,** meaning that these amino acids are not absolutely necessary in the diet. See Table 4–3 for a list of common amino acids. (Note: the word *nonessential* does not mean that these amino acids are not essential to the body. The term refers to the ability of the body to

synthesize these amino acids when they are not included in the diet.)

Like carbohydrates and lipids, amino acids are composed of carbon, hydrogen, and oxygen. In addition to these three elements, amino acids also contain nitrogen. The nitrogen appears as an amine group (NH_2). At the other end of the amino acid is the acid group (COOH): hence the name amino acid. Note the amine group and the acid group in Figure 4–5A, which includes the amino acid alanine.

Amino acids are joined together by peptide bonds. A **peptide bond** (pĕp′tīd bŏnd) is formed when the amine group (NH_2) of one amino acid joins with the acid (COOH) group of a second amino acid. A **peptide** is formed when several amino acids are joined together by peptide bonds (Fig. 4–5B). A **polypeptide** is formed when many amino acids are joined together. **Proteins** (prō′tēnz) are very large polypeptides. Most proteins are composed of more than one polypeptide chain.

Uses of Proteins

Proteins are used in three ways. The most important use is in the synthesis of hormones, enzymes, antibodies, plasma proteins, muscle proteins, hemoglobin, and most cell membranes. In one way or another, proteins play a key role in every physiologic function. The various types of proteins and their functions are listed in Table 4–4. With such a large demand for protein, most of the amino acids are carefully conserved by the body and used in the synthesis of protein.

There are two other less common uses of protein. First, protein can be broken down and used as fuel, as a source of energy for ATP production. This process, however, is not desirable. The preferred energy sources are carbohydrate and fat. Second, protein can be broken down and converted to glucose. This mechanism is used by the body to ensure that the blood glucose level does

Table 4•3	COMMON AMINO ACIDS	
Alanine	Leucine
Arginine	Lysine
Asparagine	Methionine
Aspartic acid	Phenylalanine
Cysteine	Proline
Glutamic acid	Serine
Glutamine	Threonine
Glycine	Tryptophan
Histidine	Tyrosine
Isoleucine	Valine

Do You Know...

What does a BUN measure?

Urea is made in the liver and circulates in the blood. The nitrogen in the blood urea is called blood urea nitrogen (BUN). Urea is excreted in the urine. If the kidneys are unable to make urine, the urea cannot be eliminated from the body. Instead, the urea remains in the blood. An elevated BUN therefore indicates kidney disease.

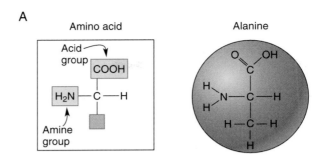

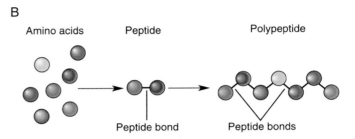

FIGURE 4–5 ● Amino acids and proteins. A, The general structure of an amino acid with the amino group on one end and an acid group on the other end. Alanine is an example of an amino acid. B, The assembly of several amino acids to form a peptide. A longer peptide is called a polypeptide. Longer polypeptides are called proteins.

not become too low to sustain life. Use of protein for glucose synthesis occurs when the blood glucose level cannot be maintained by dietary carbohydrate and glycogen stores.

Breakdown of Protein

Because amino acids contain nitrogen as well as carbon, hydrogen, and oxygen, the breakdown of protein poses a special problem. Although the breakdown of an amino acid is similar to that of glucose, the presence of nitrogen creates a major difference. Carbon, hydrogen, and oxygen can be broken down into carbon dioxide and water and eliminated from the body. The nitrogen part of the amino acid, however, must be handled in a special

way, primarily by the liver. Nitrogen is either recycled and used to synthesize different amino acids or converted to urea and excreted.

Conversion of Protein to Urea

Some of the nitrogen released by the breakdown of amino acids is ultimately removed from the body. The process occurs when the nitrogen-containing amine group NH_2 is removed from the amino acid and the liver converts the compound to urea (Fig. 4–6). Blood then carries the urea from the liver to the kidneys, and urea is eliminated in the urine. Most nitrogen, however, is recycled rather than excreted in urine.

Table 4 • 4   PROTEINS

TYPE	FUNCTION
Structural proteins	
Components of cell membranes	Perform many functions: determine pore size; allow hormones to "recognize" cell
Collagen	Structural component of muscle and tendons
Keratin	Part of skin and hair
Peptide hormones (eg, insulin, growth hormone)	Many hormones are proteins and have widespread effects on many organ systems
Hemoglobin	Transport of oxygen
Antibodies	Protect body from disease-causing microorganisms
Plasma proteins	Blood clotting; fluid balance
Muscle proteins	Enable muscle to contract
Enzymes	Regulate the rates of chemical reactions

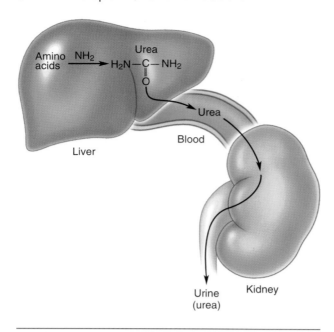

FIGURE 4–6 • Urea. Conversion of nitrogen, which is toxic, to urea in the liver. The urea flows by way of the blood to the kidney, where it is eliminated in the urine.

✳ **SUM IT UP!** The body, like a factory, requires raw material for growth, repair, and operation. The raw materials for the body come in the form of food—the carbohydrates, proteins, and fats. Carbohydrates and fats are the body's primary fuel. The proteins are used primarily in the synthesis of many vital substances, such as hormones, enzymes, antibodies, plasma proteins, and structural components of cells. Metabolism refers to the millions of chemical reactions that make the body run. The anabolic reactions are involved in the buildup, or synthesis, of complex substances from simpler substances. Anabolic reactions generally require input of energy. Catabolic reactions break down complex substances into simpler substances, generally in an effort to

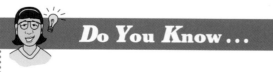

Why can liver failure alter level of consciousness?

Under normal conditions, the liver extracts ammonia (NH_3) from the blood and converts it to urea. In liver failure, the extraction of ammonia from the blood is diminished, so blood levels of ammonia rise. Because ammonia is toxic to the brain cells, the person becomes disoriented and may lose consciousness.

liberate energy stored within the food substances. Often the energy liberated from catabolic reactions is used to power anabolic reactions.

GENETIC INFORMATION AND PROTEIN SYNTHESIS

Heredity

Specific types of protein synthesized by cells largely determine body structure and function. These proteins are present in cell membranes, control thousands of metabolic reactions as enzymes, and regulate organ function as hormones. Although much structure and function are common to all people, some characteristics, or traits, are inherited.

Heredity causes parents and children to resemble each other. You look like your parents because your proteins are similar to your parents' proteins (Fig. 4–7). Each genetically related person might, for example, have blue eyes, brown hair, and light skin. A growing child's stature and appearance will also come to resemble the parents'. The similarity is caused by the action of specific proteins.

DNA: Blueprint for Life

The information concerning protein synthesis is stored in the nucleus of the cell, and more specifically within the **chromosomes** (krō′mə-sōmz) (see Fig. 4–7). Each chromosome is composed of a series of genes. A **gene** is a segment of **deoxyribonucleic acid (DNA)** (dē-ŏk″sē-rī″bō-nōō-klē′ĭk ăs′ĭd). DNA contains the information for making a particular protein. In other words, DNA is the blueprint for protein synthesis. And, because proteins control the life activities of the cell, DNA is considered the blueprint for life. (Remember that protein synthesis refers to the proper assembly of amino acids. Each protein's amino acids must be strung together in an exact order.)

Each gene carries information in its strand of DNA. For example, one gene might carry information for blue eyes. A second gene might contain DNA for straight hair. Because this information is stored within the genes, it is called **genetic information.**

DNA Structure

DNA (*deoxyribonucleic acid*) is a nucleic acid. **Nucleic acids** are composed of smaller units called **nucleotides** (Fig. 4–8A). A nucleotide has three parts: a sugar, a phosphate group, and a base. Nucleotides are joined together to form long strands. Two strands of nucleotides are arranged in a twisted ladder formation to form DNA (Fig. 4–8B). Note the ladder structure of DNA. The two sides of the DNA ladder are composed of sugar-phosphate molecules. The rungs, or steps, of the

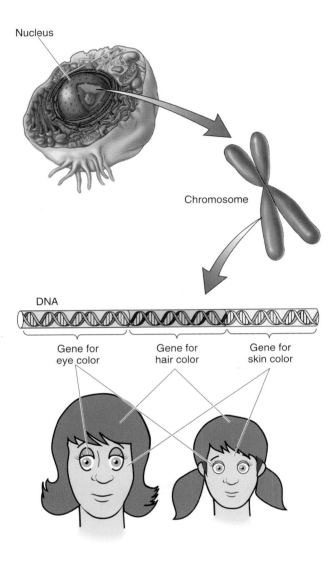

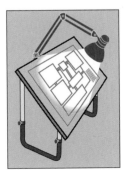

FIGURE 4–7 ● Chromosomes, genes, and the blueprint of life.

ladder are composed of bases, one base from each side.

The names of the bases in DNA are adenine (A), cytosine (C), guanine (G), and thymine (T). Note the different shapes (colors) of the bases in the rungs of the ladder. Note also that the bases of the rungs of the ladder have a particular arrangement. Adenine can pair, or join, only with thymine, while cytosine can pair only with guanine. Adenine and thymine are called **base-pairs;** cytosine and guanine are base-pairs. This system is called **base-pairing** (bās pâr´ĭng).

The Genetic Code

The **genetic code** refers to the information about protein synthesis within DNA. More specifically, the information is stored, or encoded, within the *sequence* of bases along one strand (one side of the ladder) of DNA (Fig. 4–9).

READING THE GENETIC CODE. A single strand of DNA reads vertically (according to the bases in the rungs) GTCGCCCTT. GTC (a sequence of three bases) codes for a particular amino acid. GCC codes for another amino acid, and CTT codes for a third amino acid. The list of bases in triplicate *(in threes)* is called **base-sequencing** (bās sē´kwĕn-sĭng). In this way, DNA codes for the proper assembly of amino acids and therefore the synthesis of protein.

Note: Do not confuse base-pairing with base-sequencing. Base-pairing describes the way in which two strands of DNA are linked together by the bases. Base-sequencing describes the sequence, or order, of the bases along a single strand of DNA. The genetic code is stored within the *sequence* of bases.

COPYING THE GENETIC CODE: MRNA. The genetic code for protein synthesis is stored in the nucleus in the DNA. DNA does not leave the nucleus. Protein synthesis, however, occurs on the ribosomes in the cytoplasm. How does the code get out of the nucleus and into the cytoplasm? The copying and delivery of the genetic code is done by a second nucleic acid called RNA (ribonucleic acid) (Fig. 4–10).

Ribonucleic acid (RNA) (rī´bō-noo-klē´ĭk ăs´ĭd) is a nucleic acid composed of nucleotides and resembling the structure of DNA. RNA differs from DNA in three ways:

- The sugars are different. The sugar in DNA is deoxyribose, whereas the sugar in RNA is ribose.
- DNA has two strands, whereas RNA has only one strand.
- There is a difference in one of the bases. Both DNA and RNA contain cytosine (C), guanine (G), and adenine (A). The fourth base differs. DNA contains thymine (T), whereas RNA contains uracil (U). The uracil in RNA base-pairs with adenine.

Text continued on page 69

A

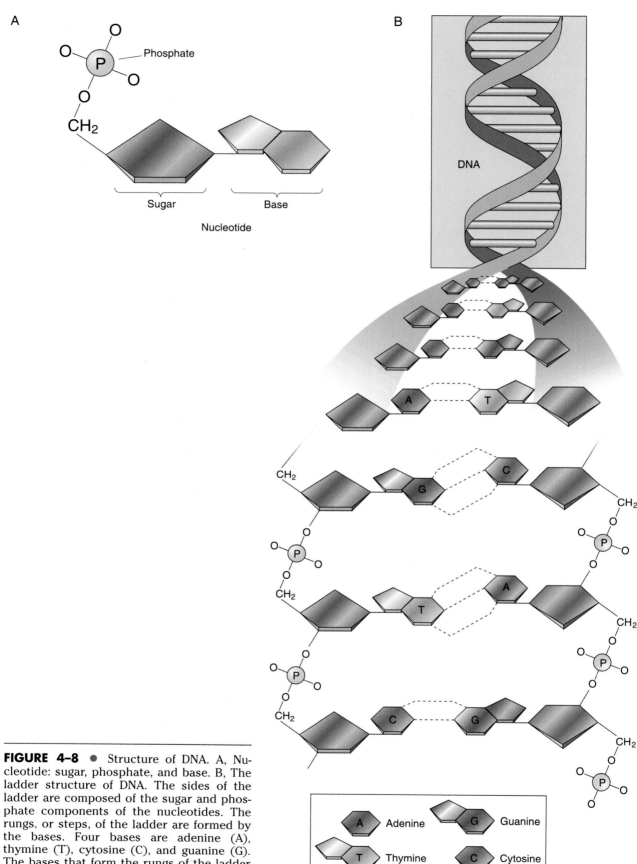

Phosphate

Sugar   Base

Nucleotide

B

DNA

A --- T

CH2   G --- C   CH2

T --- A

C --- G

A   Adenine   G   Guanine

T   Thymine   C   Cytosine

FIGURE 4–8 ● Structure of DNA. A, Nucleotide: sugar, phosphate, and base. B, The ladder structure of DNA. The sides of the ladder are composed of the sugar and phosphate components of the nucleotides. The rungs, or steps, of the ladder are formed by the bases. Four bases are adenine (A), thymine (T), cytosine (C), and guanine (G). The bases that form the rungs of the ladder do so by base-pairing.

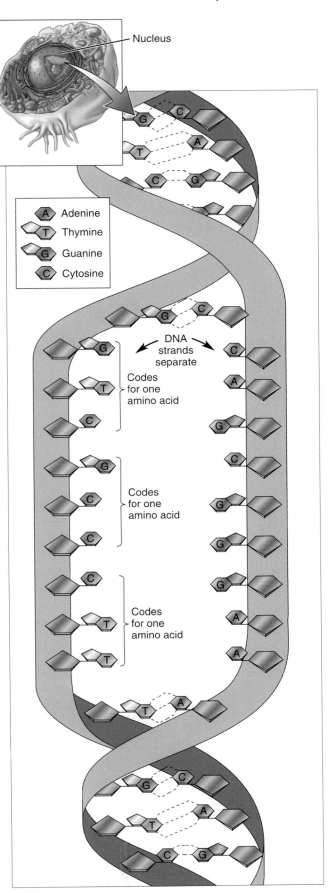

FIGURE 4-9 ● DNA. A piece of DNA separates into two strands. A single strand of DNA shows a sequence of bases: GTCGCCCTT. Three bases (triplicate) code for one amino acid. Note the code for three amino acids. This is called base-sequencing; it stores the genetic code.

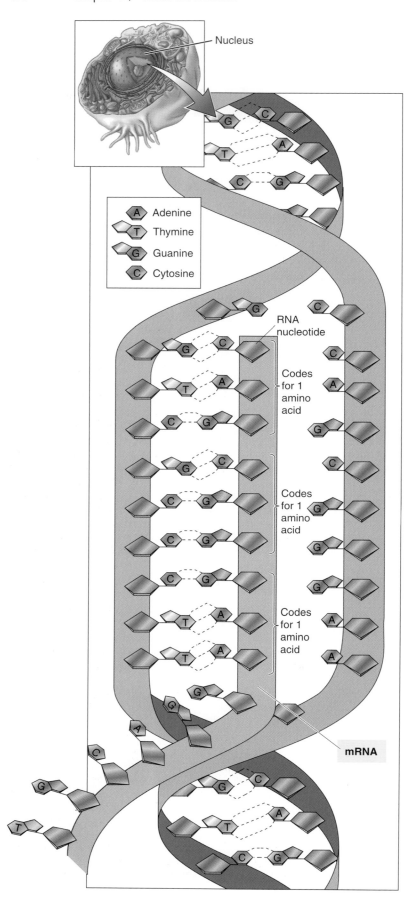

Nucleus

A Adenine
T Thymine
G Guanine
C Cytosine

RNA nucleotide

Codes for 1 amino acid

Codes for 1 amino acid

Codes for 1 amino acid

mRNA

FIGURE 4–10 • Transcription: the copying of the genetic code from DNA by mRNA. The code on the DNA strand reads GTCGCCCTT. Because of base-pairing, the RNA strand must read CAGCGGGAA.

Table 4•5	COMPARISON OF DNA AND RNA STRUCTURES	
	DNA	**RNA**
Sugar	Deoxyribose	Ribose
Base	Adenine	Adenine
	Guanine	Guanine
	Cytosine	Cytosine
	Thymine	Uracil
Strands	Double (2)	Single (1)

The differences between DNA and RNA are summarized in Table 4–5.

There are three types of RNA, but we are concerned with only two types: messenger RNA (mRNA) and transfer RNA (tRNA). Messenger RNA copies the genetic code from DNA in the nucleus and then carries the code, or message, to the ribosomes in the cytoplasm. Because this type of RNA acts as a messenger by carrying the code from the nucleus to the cytoplasm, it is called messenger RNA.

tRNA is found attached to individual amino acids within the cytoplasm. tRNA carries the amino acids to the ribosomes and helps to assemble the amino acids in the proper sequence as the polypeptide (protein) is formed. (Remember that protein synthesis refers to the proper assembly of amino acids. Each protein's amino acids must be strung together in an exact order.)

Steps in Protein Synthesis

How do DNA and RNA control protein synthesis? Five steps are involved (Fig. 4–11).

STEP #1 IN PROTEIN SYNTHESIS. When a particular protein is to be synthesized, one strand of DNA in the nucleus separates from its complementary strand (the second side of the ladder). The exposed sequence of bases (the genetic code) on the separated DNA strand is copied onto a strand of mRNA. The copying of the strand occurs by base-pairing. For instance, if the first sequence of bases is GTC on the DNA, then the only bases that can pair with the GTC are CAG. The second sequence reads GCC. The only bases that can pair with this sequence are CGG. This is the way that the mRNA copies the code on the strand of DNA. The copying of the genetic code by mRNA is called **transcription** (see Fig. 4–10).

STEP #2 IN PROTEIN SYNTHESIS. The mRNA leaves the nucleus and travels to the ribosomes in the cytoplasm. Thus the genetic code is transferred from the nucleus to the cytoplasm.

Do You Know...

How do anticancer drugs affect protein synthesis?

Many anticancer drugs interfere with protein synthesis. If a drug can block the protein synthesis in a cancer cell, the functioning of the cell will be impaired, causing cellular death. Anticancer drugs interfere at many points along the synthetic pathway of proteins: they may (1) interfere with the synthesis of healthy DNA, (2) block the synthesis of mRNA, or (3) interfere with the assembly of amino acids along the ribosome.

While anticancer drugs are effective in blocking protein synthesis and therefore growth in cancer cells, they also block synthesis in many healthy fast-growing cells. Destruction of normal cells accounts for the many serious toxic reactions associated with these agents.

STEP #3 IN PROTEIN SYNTHESIS. The code on the mRNA (now sitting on a ribosome) determines what amino acids can attach to it. For instance, the code may specify that only the amino acid alanine can bind to site number 1 and only the amino acid cysteine can bind to site number 2.

How does alanine (located in the cytoplasm) know that it should move to the ribosome for protein assembly? Alanine is attached to tRNA. The tRNA contains bases that can recognize and pair with the bases on mRNA (ribosomes). For example, if mRNA contains the base sequence GCA, then only a tRNA with the base sequence of CGU can attach to that site. tRNA transfers amino acids in the cytoplasm to the ribosome, where they are placed in the exact order dictated by the genetic code. The reading of the mRNA genetic code by tRNA is called **translation.** Note: *Transcription* refers to the copying of the genetic code of DNA in the nucleus by mRNA. *Translation* refers to the recognition of the genetic code of mRNA by tRNA. This process occurs along the ribosomes in the cytoplasm.

STEP #4 IN PROTEIN SYNTHESIS. The amino acids are lined up in proper sequence along the ribosome. A peptide bond forms between each amino acid, creating a growing peptide chain.

STEP #5 IN PROTEIN SYNTHESIS. When all of the amino acids have been assembled in the exact sequence dictated by the genetic code, the protein chain is terminated. A complete protein has been created. The protein is now ready for use in the cell or for export to another site outside the cell.

✻ **SUM IT UP!** Body structure and function are largely determined by the specific proteins synthesized by the cells. It is safe to say that you are what your proteins are. Because of the crucial roles played by proteins, an elaborate cellular mechanism guides the assembly of the various amino acids into proteins. Your protein blueprint, or genetic code, is stored in the DNA (nucleus). When there is need for protein synthesis, the code must be transported to the ribosome, where amino acid assembly takes place. Protein synthesis occurs in five steps: (1) separation of the two strands of DNA and the copying of the code by mRNA, called transcription; (2) the movement of mRNA out of the nucleus to the ribosomes in the cytoplasm; (3) the translation of the code on mRNA by tRNA, so that amino acids are delivered to the ribosomes by tRNA; (4) the formation of peptide bonds between the amino acids arranged in proper sequence along the ribosome; and (5) termination of the new protein chain.

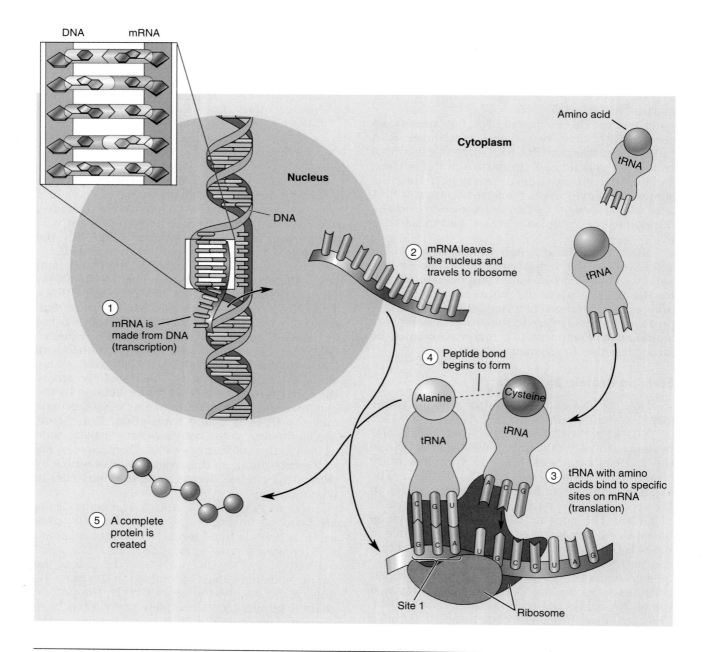

FIGURE 4–11 • Steps in protein synthesis: (1) Transcription, the copying of the genetic code by mRNA; (2) mRNA transfers the code from the nucleus to the ribosome (cytoplasm); (3) translation, (tRNA recognizes the code on mRNA); (4) formation of peptide bonds between the amino acids assembled along the ribosome; and (5) termination of the completed protein.

As You Age

1. Age brings a decrease in the number and function of organelles such as mitochondria. Because mitochondria play a key role in metabolism, a decrease in mitochondrial function affects metabolism.

2. In general, metabolism slows with aging. This effect is secondary to a decrease in hormonal secretion, particularly the thyroid hormones. A decreased metabolism has several effects: less tolerance to cold, a tendency to gain weight, and metabolic effects such as a decreased efficiency in using glucose.

3. The rate of protein synthesis decreases. Tissue growth and repair slow, as does the synthesis of other proteins such as digestive enzymes.

Disorders of Metabolism

Cyanide poisoning

Cyanide is a poison that acts by inactivating some of the enzymes in the mitochondria. As a result, oxygen cannot be used, production of ATP stops, and the person dies. A commonly used cardiac drug produces cyanide as a side effect. Unless monitored closely, the patient taking this drug could die of cyanide poisoning.

Enzyme deficiency diseases

Many diseases are caused by the lack of an enzyme or a defective enzyme. Phenylketonuria is caused by a deficiency of an enzyme that metabolizes the amino acid phenylalanine. Phenylalanine is excreted in the urine, producing phenylketonuria (PKU), a condition that causes severe mental retardation. Cystic fibrosis is caused by defective transporter membrane proteins. This deficiency causes the production of a thick and salty mucus, sweat, and pancreatic enzymes. The thick mucus in the lungs causes difficulty in breathing. The thick mucus in the pancreas plugs the pancreatic ducts, thereby decreasing the flow of digestive enzymes. Glycogen storage disease is due to an enzyme deficiency that causes excess glycogen to be deposited in the liver and skeletal muscle.

Hormonal changes

Because metabolism is greatly affected by hormones, hormonal changes cause metabolic changes. For example, the fasting and starved states are associated with many hormonal adjustments. One is an increase in growth hormone. Growth hormone stimulates protein synthesis, causes the mobilization of fats, and slows carbohydrate use. Infection causes the release of glucagon. Glucagon, in turn, stimulates the metabolic pathways in the liver to use protein to make sugar. Stress causes the release of many stress hormones, including cortisol and epinephrine. Both hormones cause profound changes in metabolism.

Hormonal disorders

All hormonal disorders are characterized by metabolic changes. In diabetes mellitus, the lack of insulin affects carbohydrate, protein, and fat metabolism; the body burns fat and wastes protein and carbohydrates. Hyperthyroidism increases the metabolic rate; the body speeds up its metabolism, sometimes to the point of causing the heart to fail.

Hypermetabolic state

The hypermetabolic states also develop in patients who have sustained severe burns, in patients with life-threatening infections, and in cachexic patients (patients with advanced cancer who appear wasted).

Lactic acidosis

The amount of oxygen severely decreases in the tissues of a patient in shock. This decrease in oxygen causes the metabolism to shift from an aerobic (with oxygen) to an anaerobic (without oxygen) metabolism. The anaerobic burning of glucose produces lactic acid. An accumulation of lactic acid causes a severe disturbance in blood pH called lactic acidosis.

Summary Outline

To carry on its functions, the cell must metabolize its fuel: the carbohydrates, proteins, and fats.

I. Metabolism

A. Anabolism

1. Anabolism includes the chemical reactions that build larger, more complex substances from simpler substances.
2. The synthetic or anabolic processes require an input of energy (ATP).

B. Catabolism

1. Catabolism includes those chemical reactions that degrade, or break down, larger, more complex substances into simpler substances.
2. Catabolic reactions are usually accompanied by the release of energy.

II. Raw Materials

A. Carbohydrates: Structure and Function

1. Carbohydrates are composed of monosaccharides, disaccharides, and polysaccharides.
2. The most important monosaccharide is glucose. The body uses glucose as the primary source of energy. Glucose can also be stored as glycogen and converted to and stored as fat.
3. Ribose and deoxyribose are five-carbon monosaccharides used in the synthesis of DNA and RNA.
4. Disaccharides are double sugars and must be broken down into monosaccharides.
5. Glycogen is a polysaccharide; it is the storage form of glucose. Glycogen is stored primarily in the liver and skeletal muscle.
6. Glucose can be catabolized anaerobically and aerobically. Anaerobically, glucose is incompletely broken down (glycolysis) into lactic acid and small amounts of ATP. Aerobically, glucose is broken down completely (glycolysis and the citric acid cycle) into CO_2 and H_2O and large amounts of energy (ATP).
7. Glucose can be synthesized from nonglucose substances.

B. Lipids

1. The most common lipids are triglycerides, phospholipids, and steroids.
2. Lipids are used primarily as a source of energy and in the synthesis of membranes.
3. The long fatty-acid chains are broken down into two-carbon units in the cytoplasm. The small units are fed into the mitochondria where the enzymes of the citric acid (Krebs) cycle help to catabolize them completely to CO_2 and H_2O, releasing large amounts of energy.
4. Lipids can be stored in adipose tissue as fat.

C. Protein

1. Protein is composed of a series of amino acids linked together by peptide bonds in a specific sequence.
2. Proteins are used primarily in the synthesis of hormones, enzymes, antibodies, plasma proteins, muscle proteins, hemoglobin, and cell membranes. Proteins are also used as fuel and as raw material for the making of glucose.
3. Protein is metabolized in a manner similar to glucose. There is special handling of nitrogen by the urea cycle.

III. Genetic Information and Protein Synthesis

A. DNA

1. Deoxyribonucleic acid, DNA, is the "blueprint for life."
2. Information concerning protein synthesis is stored in the DNA of genes (a series of genes forms a chromosome).
3. DNA is a double-stranded series of nucleotides, arranged in a twisted-ladder formation.
4. A nucleotide is composed of a sugar, a phosphate group, and a base. For DNA, the sugar is deoxyribose, and the bases are adenine, thymine, cytosine, and guanine.
5. Each strand of DNA is linked according to base-pairing (adenine links with thymine; cytosine links with guanine).
6. The genetic code is stored in the sequence of three bases along a strand of DNA.

B. RNA

1. The structure of ribonucleic acid (RNA) is similar to the structure of DNA, with the following differences: in RNA the sugar is ribose; RNA is single stranded; and the RNA bases are adenine, uracil, cytosine, and guanine.
2. Two types of RNA include messenger RNA (mRNA) and transfer RNA (tRNA).

C. Protein Synthesis: Five Steps

1. The genetic code on DNA is copied by mRNA. This process is called transcription.
2. mRNA transfers the genetic code from the nucleus to the ribosomes into the cytoplasm.
3. The genetic code of mRNA is read by tRNA (attached to individual amino acids in the cytoplasm). This process is called translation.
4. A peptide bond between each amino acid in the peptide chain grows along the ribosome.
5. The protein chain is terminated.

Review Your Knowledge

1. What are the two phases of metabolism?

2. Name the three elements which make up carbohydrates.

3. Describe the structure of sugars and starches.

4. What are three simple sugars, or monosaccharides? Which monosaccharide is used by the cells as the immediate source of energy?

5. Name three disaccharides.

6. Which polysaccharide found in plants is not digested, but forms the fiber of our diet?

7. What are three ways in which the body uses glucose?

8. What are three ways in which anaerobic and aerobic catabolism are different? What is the cause of lactic acid buildup?

9. Name two ways in which the lack of the insulin hormone affects glucose metabolism.

10. What are the three most common forms of lipids found in the body? State three ways in which lipids are used in the body.

11. What is the most abundant organic matter found in the body?

12. How are essential amino acids different from nonessential amino acids? How are amino acids joined together to form protein?

13. Name seven components of the body that are made of protein. What is the relationship of protein to urea?

14. How are chromosomes, genes, and DNA involved with protein synthesis? What is the structure of DNA?

15. Contrast base-pairing with base-sequencing.

16. Describe how the genetic code is copied so that it can get out of the nucleus into the cytoplasm?

17. Explain how alanine (located in the cytoplasm) knows that it should move to the ribosome for protein assembly. List the five steps of protein synthesis.

18. How does a sweet, fruity odor on a person's breath relate to fatty acid metabolism?

19. What is the significance of an elevated BUN?

20. What are three ways in which anticancer drugs may affect protein synthesis?

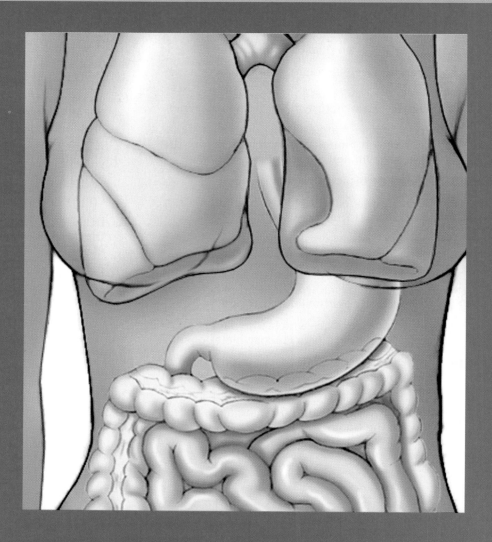

••• Key Terms

Adipose tissue (ăd″ĭ-pōs tĭsh′o͞o)

Areolar tissue (ə-rē′ō-lər tĭsh′o͞o)

Chondrocyte (kŏn′drō-sīt)

Columnar cells (columnar epithelium)
(kə-lŭm′nər sĕlz *or* ĕp″ĭ-thē′lē-əm)

Connective tissue (kə-nĕk′tĭv tĭsh′o͞o)

Cuboidal cells (cuboidal epithelium)
(kyo͞o-boi′d′l sĕlz *or* ĕp″ĭ-thē′lē-əm)

Endocrine gland (ĕn′də-krĭn glănd)

Epithelial tissue (ĕp″ĭ-thē′lē-əl tĭsh′o͞o)

Exocrine gland (ĕk′sə-krĭn glănd)

Ligament (lĭg′ə-mĕnt)

Mucous membrane (myo͞o′kəs mĕm′brān)

Muscle tissue (mŭs′əl tĭsh′o͞o)

Nervous tissue (nûr′vəs tĭsh′o͞o)

Osseous tissue (ŏs′ē-əs tĭsh′o͞o)

Parietal layer (pə-rī′ĭ-təl lā′ər)

Serous membrane (sîr′əs mĕm′brān)

Simple epithelium (sĭm′pəl ĕp″ĭ-thē′lē-əm)

Squamous cells (squamous epithelium)
(skwā′məs sĕlz *or* ĕp″ĭ-thē′lē-əm)

Tendon (tĕn′dən)

Visceral layer (vĭs′ər-əl lā′ər)

••• Selected terms in bold type in this chapter are defined in the Glossary.

5 TISSUES AND MEMBRANES

*O*bjectives

1. List the four basic types of tissues.

2. Describe the functions of epithelial, connective, muscle, and nervous tissue.

3. Explain how epithelial tissue is classified.

4. Differentiate between endocrine and exocrine glands.

5. List the types of epithelial and connective tissue membranes.

6. Differentiate between mucous and serous membranes.

In Chapter 3 we studied a typical cell. We explained how it divides into millions of identical cells and how they differentiate into cells with unique shapes, sizes, and functions. In this chapter, we see how these cells are arranged to perform specific functions.

Tissues are groups of cells that are similar to each other in structure and function. Like the individual tiles arranged as a beautiful floor, cells are placed in various patterns to make different tissues. Four major types of tissues are epithelial, connective, nervous, and muscular (Table 5–1).

EPITHELIAL TISSUE

Epithelial tissue (ĕp″ĭ-thē′lē-əl tĭsh′ōō), also called the epithelium (plural, epithelia), forms large, continuous sheets. Epithelial tissue helps to form the skin and covers the entire outer surface of the body. Sheets of epithelium also line most of the inner cavities, such as the mouth, the respiratory tract, and the reproductive tracts (Fig. 5–1). Types of epithelial tissue are listed in Table 5–2.

What does epithelial tissue do? Epithelial tissue is primarily concerned with protection, absorption, filtration, and secretion. The skin, for instance, protects the body from sunlight and from invasion by disease-producing bacteria. The epithelial tissue lining the respiratory passages helps to clean the inhaled air. The epithelium of the respiratory tract secretes mucus and is lined with cilia. The mucus traps the dust inhaled in the air, and the constantly waving cilia move the dust and mucus toward the throat. The dust and mucus

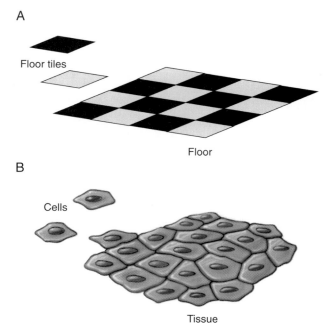

A

Floor tiles

Floor

B

Cells

Tissue

FIGURE 5–1 • Assembly of identical tiles to form a beautiful floor. This arrangement is analogous to the assembly of identical cells to form a sheet of tissue.

are then either coughed up or swallowed and eliminated in the stools.

Epithelial tissue also functions in the transport of substances across membranes. Epithelium is abundant in organs like those in the digestive tract, which must absorb large amounts of water and digested food. Lastly, epithelial tissue forms glands that secrete a variety of hormones and enzymes.

Epithelial tissue has a number of characteristics:

• Epithelial tissue forms continuous sheets. The cells fit together snugly like tiles.
• Epithelial tissue has two surfaces. One surface is always unattached, or free, like the surface of the outer skin or the inner lining of the mouth. The undersurface, or bottom, of the epithelium is attached to a **basement membrane.** The basement membrane is a very thin material that anchors the epithelium to the underlying structure.
• Epithelial tissue has no blood supply of its own; it is avascular. It depends for its nourishment on the blood supply of underlying connective tissue.
• Because epithelial tissue is so well nourished from the underlying connective tissue, it is able to regenerate, or repair, quickly if injured.

Epithelial tissue is classified according to its shape and the numbers of layers. Epithelial tissue has three shapes: squamous, cuboidal, and columnar (Fig. 5–2). The **squamous cells** (skwā′məs sĕlz) are thin and flat and look like fish scales.

Table 5 • 1	TYPES OF TISSUES	
MAJOR TYPE	**SPECIFIC TYPE**	
Epithelial tissue	Simple squamous	
	Simple cuboidal	
	Simple columnar	
	Pseudostratified columnar	
	Stratified squamous	
	Transitional	
Connective tissue	Loose (areolar)	
	Adipose	
	Dense fibrous	
	Reticular	
	Cartilage	
	Bone	
	Blood	
Nervous tissue	Neurons	
	Neuroglia	
Muscle tissue	Skeletal	
	Smooth	
	Cardiac	

Table 5•2 TYPES OF EPITHELIAL TISSUE

TYPE	LOCATION	FUNCTION
Simple		
Simple squamous	Walls of blood vessels (capillaries) Alveoli (air sacs in lungs) Kidneys	Permits the exchange of nutrients and wastes Allows diffusion of O_2 and CO_2 Filtration of water and electrolytes
Simple cuboidal	Lining of kidney tubules Various glands (thyroid, pancreas, salivary glands)	Absorption of water and electrolytes Secretion of enzymes and hormones
Simple columnar	Digestive tract	Protection, absorption, and secretion of digestive juice; often contains goblet cells (mucus)
Pseudostratified columnar	Lining of respiratory tract Lining of reproductive tubes (fallopian tubes)	Protection and secretion; cleans respiratory passages; sweeps egg toward uterus
Stratified		
Stratified squamous	Outer layer of skin Lining of mouth, esophagus, anus, and vagina	Protects body from invading microorganisms; withstands friction
Transitional	Urinary bladder	Permits expansion of an organ without tearing

Looks like: **Cell Shapes:**   **Types of cell layers:**

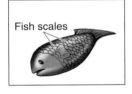

Fish scales

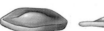

Squamous

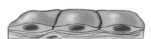

Simple

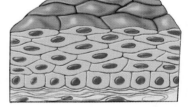

Stratified

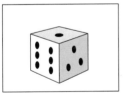

Cuboidal

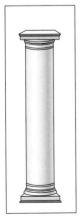

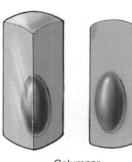

Columnar

FIGURE 5–2 ● Classification of epithelial tissue according to the shape of the cells (squamous, cuboidal, and columnar) and the numbers of layers of cells (simple or stratified).

Do You Know...

What causes a bed sore?

A bed sore is another name for a pressure ulcer, or a decubitus ulcer. The ulcer is caused by an interruption of the blood supply to a tissue. Pressure ulcers frequently develop in patients who have been bedridden for long periods. They are caused by the weight of the body on the skin overlying a bony area (eg, elbow, heel, hip). The weight of the body compresses, or squeezes, the blood vessels, cutting off the supply of blood to the tissues. Deprived of its blood supply, the tissue dies, forming an ulcer.

Do You Know...

What is the difference between a carcinoma and a sarcoma?

Both are malignant (cancerous) tumors. The difference between the two lies in the types of tissue involved. A **carcinoma** is a malignant tumor involving epithelial tissue. A **sarcoma** involves connective tissue.

(The word squamous comes from *squam,* meaning scale.) The **cuboidal cells** (kyōō-boi′d′l sĕlz) are cube-like and look like dice. The **columnar cells** (kə-lŭm′nər sĕlz) are tall and narrow and look like columns.

Epithelial cells are arranged in either a single layer or multiple layers (see Fig. 5–2). One layer of cells is a **simple epithelium** (sĭm′pəl ĕp″ĭ-thē′lē-əm). Two or more layers of cells are a **stratified epithelium.**

Both the shape and the number of layers are used to describe the various types of epithelium. For instance, simple squamous epithelium refers to a single layer of squamous cells. Stratified squamous epithelium contains multiple layers of squamous cells. Note that Figure 5–2 shows stratified squamous epithelium but not stratified cuboidal or columnar tissue. Stratified cuboidal and stratified columnar epithelium are found in very few organs.

Simple Epithelia

Because **simple epithelia** are so thin, they are concerned primarily with the movement, or transport, of various substances across the membranes from one body compartment to another (Fig. 5–3).

Simple squamous epithelium is a single layer of squamous cells with an underlying basement membrane. Because this tissue is so thin, simple squamous epithelium is found where substances move by rapid diffusion or filtration. For instance, the walls of the capillaries (the smallest blood vessels) are composed of simple squamous epithelium. The walls of the alveoli (air sacs of the lungs) are also composed of simple squamous epithelium. This tissue allows the rapid diffusion of oxygen from the alveoli into the blood.

Simple cuboidal epithelium is a single layer of cuboidal cells resting on a basement mem-

brane. This epithelial layer is most often found in glands and in the kidney tubules, where it functions in the transport and secretion of various substances.

Simple columnar epithelium refers to a single layer of columnar cells resting on its basement membrane. These tall, tightly packed cells line the entire length of the digestive tract and play a major role in the absorption of the products of digestion. A lubricating mucus is produced by **goblet cells,** which are common in this type of tissue.

Pseudostratified columnar epithelium is a single layer of columnar cells. Because the cells are so irregularly shaped, the cells appear multilayered; hence the name *pseudostratified,* meaning falsely stratified. Their function is similar to the function of simple columnar cells: they facilitate absorption and secretion. A ciliated pseudostratified epithelium lines the respiratory passages. The mucus secreted by mucus-secreting cells of this tissue helps to trap the dust and debris of the inhaled air. The cilia then propel the mucus toward the throat.

Stratified Epithelia

Stratified epithelia are multilayered (having two layers or more) and are therefore stronger than simple epithelia. They perform a protective function and are found in tissue exposed to everyday wear and tear, such as the mouth, the esophagus, and the skin. **Stratified squamous epithelium** is the most common of the stratified epithelia. It withstands friction well and is found in the lining of the mouth and on the outer surface of the skin.

Transitional epithelium is found primarily in organs that need to stretch. The urinary bladder is one such organ. This epithelium is called transitional because the cells slide past one another when the tissue is stretched. The cells appear stratified when the urinary bladder is empty (ie, unstretched) and simple when the bladder is full (ie, stretched).

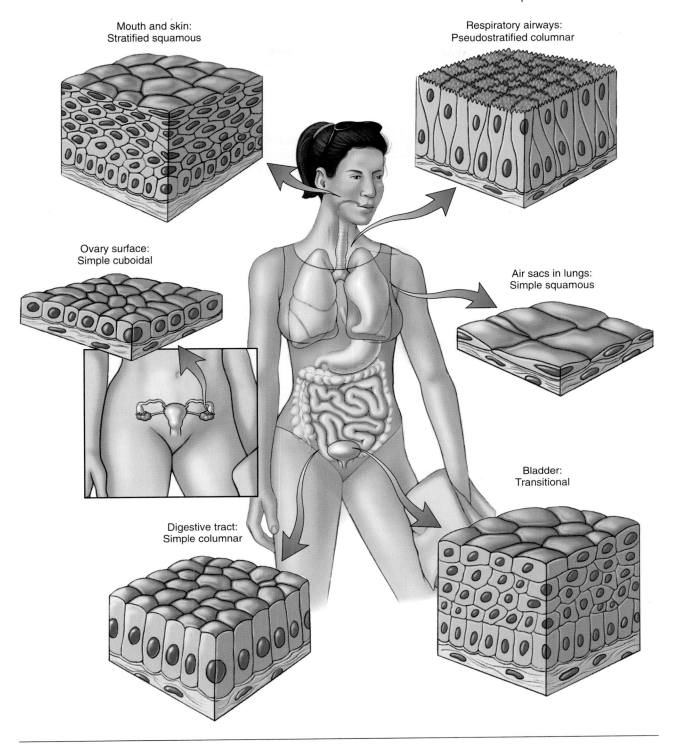

Mouth and skin:
Stratified squamous

Respiratory airways:
Pseudostratified columnar

Ovary surface:
Simple cuboidal

Air sacs in lungs:
Simple squamous

Bladder:
Transitional

Digestive tract:
Simple columnar

FIGURE 5–3 ● Location of epithelial tissue. Epithelial tissue forms the skin and the linings of the inner cavities, such as the digestive tract, the respiratory tract, and the urinary tract.

Glandular Epithelia

A **gland** is made up of one or more cells that secrete a particular substance. Much of the glandular tissue is composed of simple cuboidal epithelium.

Two types of glands are the exocrine glands and the endocrine glands. The **exocrine glands** (ĕk′sə-krĭn glăndz) have ducts, or tiny tubes, into which the exocrine secretions are released before reaching body surfaces or body cavities. The exocrine secretions include mucus, sweat, saliva,

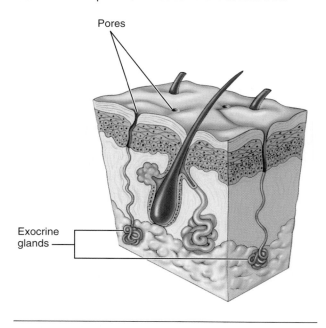

FIGURE 5–4 ● Exocrine gland. The gland secretes its substance (eg, sweat) into a duct that directs the secretion outside the body.

and digestive enzymes. The ducts carry the exocrine secretions outside the body. For instance, sweat flows from the sudoriferous glands through ducts onto the surface of the skin for evaporation (Fig. 5–4).

The **endocrine glands** (ĕn′də-krĭn glăndz) secrete hormones, such the thyroid hormones. Endocrine glands do not have ducts and so are called ductless glands. Because endocrine glands are ductless, the hormones are secreted directly into the blood. The blood then carries the hormones to their sites of action. The pituitary, thyroid, and adrenal glands are examples of endocrine glands.

CONNECTIVE TISSUE

Connective tissue (kə-nĕk′tĭv tĭsh′o͞o) is the most abundant of the four tissue types and is widely distributed throughout the body. Connective tissue is found in blood, under the skin, in bone, and around many organs. As the name suggests, connective tissue connects, or binds together, the parts of the body. Other functions include support, protection, storage of fat, and transport of substances.

Although connective tissue types may not resemble each other very closely, they share two characteristics. First, most connective tissue—with the exception of ligaments, tendons, and car-

tilage—has a good blood supply. Ligaments and tendons have a poor blood supply, and cartilage has no blood supply. As any athlete knows, an injury to these structures usually heals very slowly. The second characteristic shared by most connective tissue is an abundance of intercellular matrix.

The **intercellular matrix** is what makes the various types of connective tissue so different. Intercellular matrix is material located outside the cell. It fills the spaces *between* the cells (intercellular space). The cell makes the matrix and secretes it into the intercellular spaces. The hardness of the intercellular matrix varies from one cell type to the next. The intercellular matrix may be liquid (as in blood), gel-like (as in fat tissue), or hard (as in bone). The amount of matrix also varies from one cell type to the next. In fat tissue, the cells are close together, with little intercellular matrix. Bone and cartilage, however, have few cells and large amounts of intercellular matrix.

Also found in the matrix of most connective tissue are protein **fibers.** The fiber types include collagen (white), elastin (yellow), and reticular fibers (fine collagen). Collagen fibers are strong and flexible but only slightly elastic. Elastic fibers are not very strong, but they are stretchy, like a rubber band. They can be stretched and will return to their original length when tension on the fibers is relaxed.

Recently, injections of collagen have been used cosmetically to remove unwanted lines and wrinkles. Collagen is obtained from cattle or, more often, from the patient's own hips, thighs, and abdomen. The collagen is then injected under the patient's skin. Acting as a filler, the collagen smoothes out unwanted wrinkles, creating a surgical fountain of youth. Tex, here, could use some collagen filler.

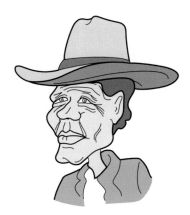

The many types of connective tissue are loose (areolar), adipose, dense fibrous, reticular connective, cartilage, bone, and blood (Fig. 5–5). Table 5–3 describes these types.

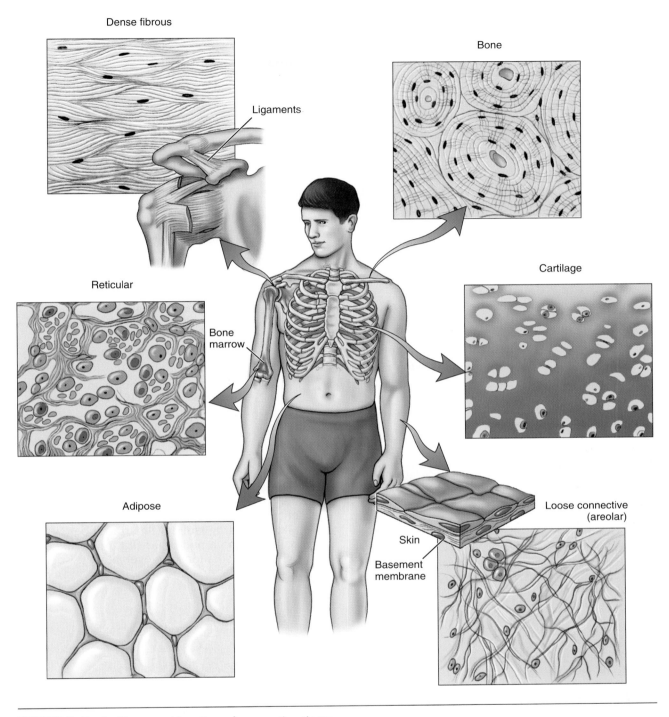

Dense fibrous

Ligaments

Bone

Cartilage

Reticular

Bone
marrow

Skin

Basement
membrane

Loose connective
(areolar)

Adipose

FIGURE 5–5 ● Types and location of connective tissue.

Loose Connective Tissue

Loose connective tissue, or **areolar tissue** (ə-rē′ō-lər tĭsh′oo) (see Fig. 5–5), is made up of fibroblasts and a gel-like intercellular matrix. Fibroblasts are large, star-shaped cells that secrete collagen and elastic fibers into the intercellular space. Loose connective tissue is soft and surrounds, protects, and cushions many of the organs. It acts like "tissue glue" because it holds the organs in position. Loose connective tissue is the most widely distributed type of connective tissue. A layer of this tissue underlies all mucous membranes.

Table 5•3	TYPES OF CONNECTIVE TISSUE	
TYPE	**LOCATION**	**FUNCTION**
Loose (areolar)	Beneath skin and most epithelial layers; between muscles	Binds together, protects, cushions; "tissue glue"
Adipose	Beneath skin (subcutaneous) Around kidney and heart Behind eyeballs	Cushions, insulates, stores fat
Dense fibrous	Tendons, ligaments, capsules, and fascia Skin (dermis)	Binds structures together
Reticular	Lymphoid tissue such as lymph nodes, spleen, and bone marrow	Forms internal framework of lymphoid organs
Cartilage		
Hyaline	Ends of long bone at joints Connects ribs to sternum Rings in trachea of respiratory tract Nose Fetal skeleton	Supports, protects, provides framework
Fibrocartilage	Intervertebral discs (in backbone) Pads in knee joint Pad between pubic bones (symphysis pubis)	Cushions, protects
Elastic cartilage	External ear and part of larynx	Supports, provides framework
Bone	Bones of the skeleton	Supports, protects, provides framework
Blood	Blood vessels throughout the body	Transports nutrients, hormones, respiratory gases (O_2 and CO_2), waste

Do You Know...

Why can an improperly applied tourniquet cause gangrene?

Gangrene is local death, or necrosis, of soft tissue. If the blood supply to an area is stopped for too long, the tissue distal to the tourniquet is deprived of oxygen and nutrients, and it dies.

Adipose tissue (ăd′ĭ-pōs tĭsh′ o͞o), or fat, is a type of loose connective tissue in which the fibroblasts enlarge and store fat (see Fig. 5–5). Adipose tissue forms the tissue layer underlying the skin, the subcutaneous layer. Because of its location, adipose tissue can insulate the body from extremes of outside temperature. For instance, in a cold environment, the adipose tissue prevents the loss of heat from the body. This protection is best appreciated in observing the fat content of animals living in arctic conditions. The walrus, for instance, has huge layers of fat tissue called blubber. Because of the insulating qualities of the blubber, the walrus can swim in deep cold waters without freezing to death. Think of how long you could sit on an iceberg, even if you had a few extra pounds!

Adipose tissue is also deposited around certain organs. The kidney, for instance, has a layer of fat tissue that helps hold it in place. In extremely thin individuals, this fat tissue may be absent, allowing the kidney to move around. This is called a floating kidney (illustrated below). The eyeball also has a pad of fat that performs a protective role: it cushions the eyeball in its socket.

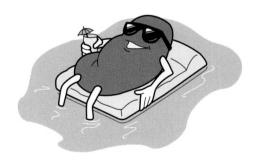

Dense Fibrous Tissue

Dense fibrous tissue is composed of fibroblasts and intercellular matrix that contains many collagen and elastic fibers. The main type of fiber in dense fibrous tissue is collagen. The fibroblasts secrete the fibers into the intercellular matrix. The

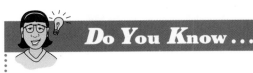

Do You Know...

Why do overweight men and women "round out" into different shapes?

Overeating results in the storage of fat in adipose tissue. Because fat metabolism is affected by the sex hormones estrogen and testosterone, storage sites differ for males and females. In the male, excess fat is stored primarily in the abdominal region, while in the female, excess fat is stored around the breasts and hips.

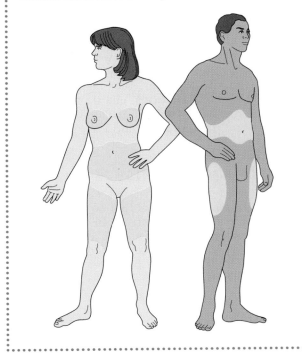

fibers form strong, supporting structures such as tendons, ligaments, capsules, and fascia.

Tendons (tĕn′dənz) are cord-like structures composed of dense fibrous connective tissue that attach muscles to bones. **Ligaments** (lĭg′ə-mĕnts) are dense fibrous connective tissue that cross joints and attach bone to bone. Because ligaments contain more elastic fibers than tendons do, they stretch more easily. The ability to stretch is important; it prevents tearing of the ligaments when the joints bend. Dense fiber also forms tough **capsules** around certain organs, such as the kidney and the liver. Lastly, dense fibrous connective tissue forms bands, or sheets, of tissue called **fascia.** Fascia covers muscles, blood vessels, and nerves; it covers, supports, and anchors the organs to nearby structures.

If stretching is excessive (eg, in athletic injuries), however, tendons and ligaments can tear, causing severe pain and impaired mobility. A ruptured Achilles tendon, for example, is a serious injury. The Achilles tendon attaches the leg muscles to the heel region of the foot. If excessive force is exerted on the tendon, it may snap or rupture, causing severe pain and loss of foot movement.

Reticular Connective Tissue

Reticular connective tissue is characterized by a network of delicately interwoven reticular (fine collagen) fibers. It forms the internal framework for lymphoid tissue such as the spleen, lymph nodes, and bone marrow.

Cartilage

Cartilage is formed by **chondrocytes** (kŏn′drō-sīts), or cartilage cells. The chondrocytes secrete a protein intercellular matrix that is firm, smooth, and flexible. Although the matrix of cartilage is solid, it is not as hard as that of bone. Three types of cartilage are hyaline cartilage, elastic cartilage, and fibrocartilage.

Hyaline cartilage is found in only a few places in the body: the larynx, or voicebox, in the throat region; the ends of long bones at joints; the nose; and the area between the breastbone and the ribs. Figure 5–5 illustrates the attachment of the breastbone to the ribs by the hyaline cartilage. Hyaline cartilage is also found in large quantities in the fetal skeleton. As the fetus matures, however, the cartilage ossifies, or is converted to bone.

The shark skeleton is composed entirely of cartilage. Unlike in the human skeleton, ossification does not occur in the shark. In recent years, shark cartilage has been sold as a tumor suppressant. Because sharks do not develop cancer, it is assumed that the shark cartilage contains a tumor-suppressing agent. As yet, however, no scientific information exists to suggest that shark cartilage conveys cancer immunity.

Do You Know...

Why does meat simmered in soup become more tender?

The large number of collagenous fibers in meat makes the meat tough. When the collagen is boiled, the fibers turn into a soft gelatin. Thus the meat becomes more tender.

Bone

Bone tissue is also called **osseous tissue** (ŏs'ē-əs tĭsh'o͞o). Bone cells are called **osteocytes.** Bone cells secrete an intercellular matrix that includes collagen, calcium salts, and other minerals. The mineral-containing matrix makes the bone tissue hard. The hardness of the bone enables it to protect organs, such as the brain, and to support the weight of the body for standing and moving. Bone also acts as a storage site for mineral salts, especially calcium. (Bone structure is further explained in Chapter 7.)

When mineralization of bone tissue is diminished, as in osteoporosis, the bone is weakened and tends to break easily. Adequate dietary intake of calcium is essential for strong bones. Calcium is needed throughout the life cycle but is especially important during childhood, when bones are growing, and after menopause, when estrogen levels in women decline. Estrogen normally encourages the deposition of calcium in bone tissue. Exercise and weight bearing also encourage the deposition of calcium within bones.

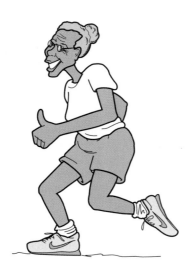

Blood

Blood is a unique type of connective tissue that consists of blood cells surrounded by a fluid matrix called **plasma.** Unlike other connective tissues, which contain collagen and elastin fibers in the intercellular matrix, plasma contains nonfibrous plasma proteins. Blood plays an important role in the transport of substances throughout the body. Blood also carries heat and so plays a key role in the regulation of body temperature. (Blood is described in more detail in Chapter 13.)

NERVOUS TISSUE

Nervous tissue (nûr'vəs tĭsh'o͞o) makes up the brain, the spinal cord, and the nerves. Nervous tissue consists of two types of cells: the neurons and the neuroglia (Fig. 5–6).

Neurons are nerve cells that transmit electrical signals to and from the brain and spinal cord. Neurons have many shapes and sizes. The neuron has three parts: (1) the **dendrites,** which receive information from other neurons and then transmit the information *toward* the cell body; (2) the **cell body,** which contains the nucleus and is essential to the life of the cell; and (3) the single **axon,** which transmits information *away from* the cell body.

Neuroglia, or glia, are cells that support and take care of the neurons. The word *glial* means glue-like and refers to the ability of these cells to support, or glue together, the vast network of neurons. Unlike the neurons, glia do not transmit electrical signals. (Nervous tissue is described more fully in Chapters 9, 10, and 11.)

MUSCLE TISSUE

Muscle tissue (mŭs'əl tĭsh'o͞o) is composed of cells that shorten, or contract. In doing so, they cause movement of a body part. Because the cells are long and slender, they are called fibers rather than cells. The three types of muscle are skeletal, smooth, and cardiac (Fig. 5–7).

Skeletal Muscle

Skeletal muscle is generally attached to bone (the skeletal system). Because skeletal muscle can be controlled voluntarily ("I *choose* to move my leg"), it is also called **voluntary muscle.** Because of the appearance of striations, or stripes, skeletal muscle is also called striated muscle. The stripes, or striations, are due to the arrangement of the muscle proteins in the muscle fibers. Skeletal muscles move the skeleton, maintain posture, and stabilize joints.

Smooth Muscle

Smooth muscle is generally found in the walls of the viscera, or organs, such as the stomach, intestines, and urinary bladder. It is also found in tubes, such as the bronchioles (breathing passages) and blood vessels. The function of smooth muscle is related to the organ in which it is found. For instance, smooth muscle in the stomach helps to mash and churn food, while the smooth muscle in the urinary bladder helps to expel urine.

A Neuron

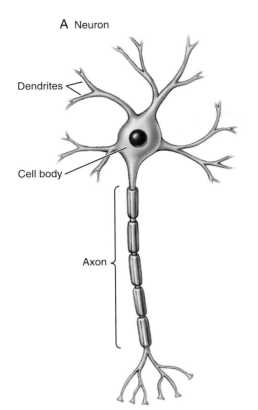

Dendrites

Cell body

Axon

B Neuroglia (glia)

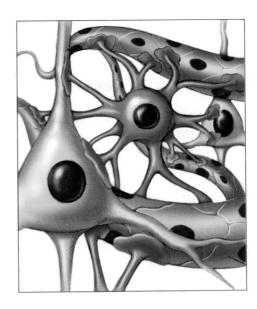

FIGURE 5–6 ● The two types of nervous tissue. A, Neuron. B, Neuroglia.

Skeletal

Cardiac

Smooth

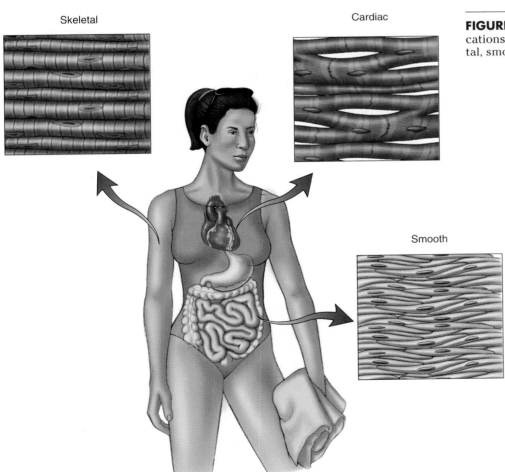

FIGURE 5–7 ● Types and locations of muscle tissue: skeletal, smooth, and cardiac.

Smooth muscle is not voluntarily controlled and is called **involuntary muscle.** For instance, you usually do not make a conscious effort to raise your blood pressure when you exercise. Unlike skeletal muscle, smooth muscle does not appear striped, or striated. Smooth muscle is therefore called **nonstriated muscle.**

Cardiac Muscle

Cardiac muscle is found only in the heart, where it functions to pump blood into a vast network of blood vessels. Cardiac muscle is striated and involuntary. Cardiac muscle fibers are long branching cells that fit together tightly at junctions. These tight-fitting junctions are called **intercalated discs** and promote rapid conduction of electrical signals throughout the heart. The three types of muscle are illustrated in Figure 5–7.

TISSUE REPAIR

How does tissue repair itself after an injury? Two types of tissue repair are regeneration and fibrosis. **Regeneration** refers to the replacement of tissue by cells that are identical to the original cells. Regeneration occurs only in tissues whose cells undergo mitosis, such as the skin.

Fibrosis is the replacement of injured tissue by the formation of fibrous connective tissue, or scar tissue. The fibers of scar tissue pull the edges of the wound together and strengthen the area. Damaged skeletal muscle, cardiac muscle, and nervous tissue do not undergo mitosis and must be replaced by scar tissue. The steps involved in tissue repair are illustrated and described in Figure 5–8.

✳ **SUM IT UP!** Tissues are groups of cells that are similar to each other in structure and function. The four types of tissues are epithelial, connective, nervous, and muscle. Epithelial tissue

FIGURE 5–8 ● Steps in tissue repair. A, A deep wound to the skin severs blood vessels, causing blood to fill the wound. B, A blood clot forms, and as it dries, it forms a scab. C and D, The process of tissue repair begins. Scar tissue forms in the deep layers. E, At the same time, surface epithelial cells multiply and fill the area between the scar tissue and the scab. F, When the epithelium is complete, the scab detaches. The result is a fully regenerated layer of epithelium over an underlying area of scar tissue.

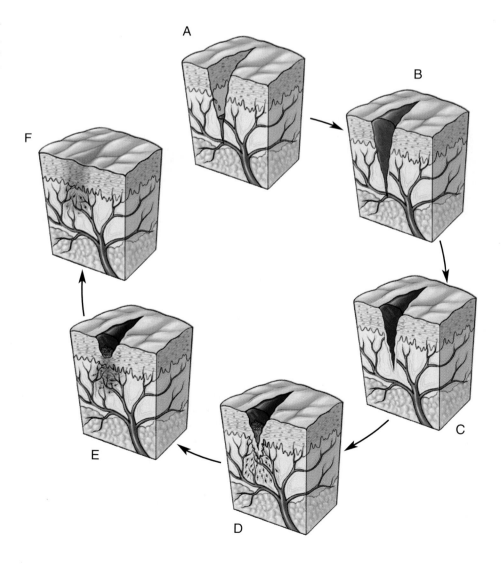

covers and lines; it is primarily concerned with the processes of secretion, filtration, and absorption. Connective tissue is the most widespread and diverse of the tissue types; it connects and binds together parts of the body. Nervous tissue is found in the brain, spinal cord, and nerves and is concerned with the transmission of information throughout the entire body. Two types of cells form the nervous tissue: neurons and neuroglia. Muscle tissue is composed of cells that can shorten, or contract, and thus produce movement of body parts. The three types of muscle are skeletal, smooth, and cardiac.

MEMBRANES

Classification of Membranes

Membranes are thin sheets of tissue that cover surfaces, line body cavities, and surround organs. Membranes are classified as epithelial or connective tissue. The epithelial membranes include the cutaneous membrane (skin), mucous membranes, and serous membranes. The connective tissue membranes include the synovial membrane and those listed in Table 5–4. (The connective tissue membranes are described later in the text. For example, the synovial membrane is described in Chapter 7.)

Epithelial Membranes

The **epithelial membranes** include the cutaneous membrane (skin), the mucous membranes, and the serous membranes (Fig. 5–9). Although called epithelial, these membranes contain both an epithelial sheet and an underlying layer of connective tissue.

Cutaneous Membrane

The **cutaneous membrane** is the skin. The outer layer of skin **(epidermis)** is stratified squamous epithelium. This layer protects the body from invading microorganisms. It also prevents the body from drying out, or dehydrating, because the squamous epithelial cells contain a water-

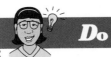

Do You Know...

Why should tumors be biopsied?

A **biopsy** refers to the removal of tumor tissue for microscopic examination. By viewing the tumor specimen under a microscope, the pathologist can determine whether the tumor is malignant (cancerous) or benign (noncancerous).

Table 5 • 4   TYPES OF MEMBRANES

TYPE	LOCATION
Epithelial Membranes	
Cutaneous membrane	Skin (outer layer)
Mucous membrane	Digestive tract lining
	Urinary tract lining
	Reproductive tract lining
	Respiratory tract lining
Serous membrane	
Pleura	Thoracic cavity
Pericardium	Thoracic cavity around the heart
Peritoneum	Abdominal cavity
Connective Tissue Membranes	
Synovial	Lines joint cavities; secretes synovial fluid
Periosteum	Covers bone; contains the blood vessels that supply the bone
Perichondrium	Covers cartilage; contains capillaries that nourish the cartilage
Meninges	Covers brain and spinal cord
Fascia (various kinds)	Throughout body

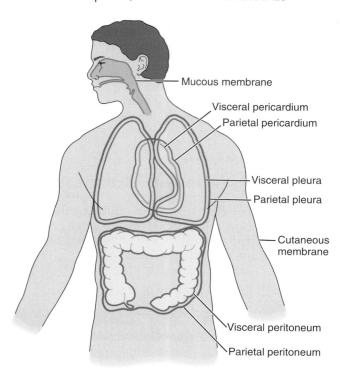

- Mucous membrane
- Visceral pericardium
- Parietal pericardium
- Visceral pleura
- Parietal pleura
- Cutaneous membrane
- Visceral peritoneum
- Parietal peritoneum

FIGURE 5–9 ● Epithelial membranes: cutaneous membrane (skin), mucous membranes, and serous membranes (pleura, pericardium, and peritoneum).

proofing substance. The underlying layer **(dermis)** is composed of dense fibrous connective tissue. It strengthens and helps anchor the epidermal layer. (The cutaneous membrane is described more fully in Chapter 6.)

Mucous Membranes

Mucous membranes (my o͞o′kəs měm′ brānz) line all body cavities that open to the exterior of the body (see Fig. 5–9). They include the digestive, the urinary, the reproductive, and the respiratory tracts. For instance, the digestive tract opens to the exterior of the body at the mouth and at the anus, while the respiratory tract opens to the exterior at the nose and at the mouth. Mucous membranes, often called **mucosae,** usually contain stratified squamous epithelium or simple columnar epithelium. Most mucous membranes are adapted for absorption and secretion. Most mucous membranes secrete mucus. The mucus keeps the membrane moist and also lubricates the membrane. For instance, in the digestive tract, the mucus allows the food to move through the tract with little friction.

Serous Membranes

Serous membranes (serosae) (sîr′əs měm′brānz) line the ventral body cavities, which are not open to the exterior of the body. For instance, if you were to enter the abdominal or thoracic cavity surgically, you would be looking at

serous membranes. Serous membranes secrete a thin, watery fluid **(serous fluid).** The fluid allows the membranes to slide past one another with little friction.

A serous membrane is composed of simple squamous epithelium resting on a thin layer of loose connective areolar tissue. Serous membranes line a cavity and then fold back onto the surface of the organs within that cavity. Thus, part of the membrane lines the wall of the cavity, while the other part covers the organ or organs within that cavity. The part of the membrane that lines the walls of the cavity is the **parietal layer** (pə-rī′ě-təl lā′ər) (*parie* means wall), while the part of the membrane that covers the outside of an organ is the **visceral layer** (vĭs′ər-əl lā′ər) (*viscera* means organ).

The three serous membranes are the pleura, the pericardium, and the peritoneum (see Fig. 5–9).

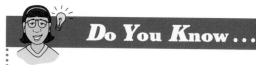

Do You Know...

Why is pleurisy so painful?

Pleurisy refers to an inflammation of the pleura and a decrease in serous fluid. As the inflamed and "dry" pleural membranes slide past one another during breathing movements, the person experiences pain.

- The **pleura** is found in the thoracic cavity. The **parietal pleura** lines the wall of the thoracic cavity. The **visceral pleura** covers each lung.
- The **pericardium** is found in the thoracic cavity and is associated with the heart. The **parietal pericardium** lines the sling (pericardium), that supports the heart. The **visceral pericardium** forms the outside lining of the heart.
- The **peritoneum** is found within the abdominal cavity. The **parietal peritoneum** lines the walls of the abdominal cavity. The **visceral peritoneum** covers the abdominal organs. (These will be described further in Chapter 19.)

Infection in the abdominal cavity often involves the peritoneum. For instance, a ruptured appendix allows the escape of intestinal contents, loaded with bacteria, into the peritoneal cavity. This leakage causes a life-threatening infectious condition called **peritonitis.** Aggressive treatment with antibiotics is required. Occasionally, the pus must be drained from the abdominal cavity.

✳ **SUM IT UP!** Membranes are sheets of tissue. Membranes cover surfaces, line body cavities, and surround organs. Membranes are classified as epithelial membranes or connective tissue membranes. The epithelial membranes include the cutaneous membrane (skin), mucous membranes, and serous membranes. The connective tissue membranes include the synovial membrane, which lines the cavities of freely movable joints.

As You Age

1. Because tissues consist of cells, cellular aging alters the tissues formed by the cells. Alterations in tissues, in turn, affect organ function. For instance, by the age of 85 years, lung capacity has decreased by 50%; muscle strength has decreased by about 45%; and kidney function has decreased by 30%.

2. Collagen and elastin decrease in connective tissue. Consequently, tissues become stiffer, less elastic, and less efficient in their functioning.

3. Lipid and fat content of tissues change. In men, there is a gradual increase in tissue lipids and fat until age 60, and then there is a gradual decrease. In women, lipids and fats accumulate in the tissues continuously; there is no decline as in men.

4. The total amount of water in the body gradually decreases. The change in body fat and the decrease in water are major reasons that the elderly population responds differently to drugs than the younger population does.

5. Tissue atrophy causes a decrease in the mass of most organs.

Disorders of Tissues and Membranes

Adhesion	An abnormal joining of tissues by fibrous scar tissue. Adhesions may bind or constrict organs, causing obstruction (especially in the abdomen) and decreased flexibility.
Cancer	Abnormal growth that can affect all types of tissues and membranes. Tumors are named according to the type of tissue involved. A carcinoma involves epithelial tissue (eg, adenocarcinoma—cancer arising from glandular tissue). A sarcoma involves connective tissue (eg, osteosarcoma—a cancer involving bone).
Collagen diseases	For unknown reasons, collagen can be destroyed, causing damage to the connective tissue of the body. Because collagen is a main component of connective tissue, the effects of collagen diseases are widespread. Examples of collagen disease include rheumatoid arthritis, systemic lupus erythematosus (SLE), and scleroderma. Many of the collagen diseases are autoimmune disorders, in which the patient's own immune system attacks and destroys collagen.

continued

Disorders of Tissues and Membranes *continued*

Gangrene	Death (necrosis) of the soft tissues of a body part, such as the toes, fingers, or intestines. Gangrene occurs when the blood supply to the tissue is cut off. Diabetic patients experience gangrene of the toes when their arteries become clogged with fat deposits. Infection can also impede blood flow to a body part and therefore cause gangrene.
Neoplasm	A neoplasm (tumor) may be malignant (cancerous) or benign (noncancerous). Examples of benign connective tissue neoplasms include adenoma (glandular tissue), osteoma (bone), chondroma (cartilage), fibroma (fibroblasts), lipoma (fat tissue), and polyps (adenomas commonly found in vascular areas such as the nose, rectum, and uterus).

Summary Outline

Tissues are groups of cells that are similar to each other in structure and function. Membranes are thin sheets of tissue that cover surfaces, line body cavities, and surround organs.

I. Types of Tissue
A. Epithelial Tissue
1. Epithelial tissue covers surfaces and lines cavities.
2. Simple squamous epithelium is a single layer of flat cells, generally found where the exchange of gases and nutrients is important (eg, alveoli in the lungs, in the capillaries).
3. Simple cuboidal epithelium is a single layer of cube-shaped cells found primarily in glands and the kidney tubules.
4. Simple columnar epithelium is a single layer of column-shaped cells found primarily in the lining of the digestive tract.
5. Pseudostratified columnar epithelium is a single layer of columnar cells that appears multilayered. It functions in absorption and secretion.
6. Stratified squamous epithelium is multilayered and performs a protective function in tissue exposed to everyday wear and tear (eg, lining of the mouth and outer surface of the skin).
7. Transitional epithelium is a modification of stratified squamous epithelium and is found primarily in organs that need to stretch (eg, urinary bladder).
8. Glandular epithelium is generally composed of simple cuboidal epithelium. Glandular epithelium forms exocrine glands (have ducts) and endocrine glands (do not have ducts).

B. Connective Tissue
1. Connective tissue is the most abundant of the four tissue types and is widely distributed throughout the body.
2. The primary function of connective tissue is to bind together the parts of the body. Other functions include support, protection, storage of fat, and transport of substances.
3. Connective tissue has intercellular matrix that fills spaces between cells. The intercellular matrix may be liquid, gel-like, or hard. The matrix often contains protein fibers that are secreted by the cells. The fiber types include collagen (white), elastin (yellow), and reticular (fine).
4. Loose connective (areolar) tissue is soft and surrounds, protects, and cushions many organs (acts like tissue glue).
5. Adipose (fat) is a type of loose connective tissue that stores fat. It forms the subcutaneous layer (under the skin) and cushions the kidneys and eyeballs.
6. Dense fibrous connective tissue is composed of fibroblasts and intercellular matrix that contains collagen and elastic fibers. It forms tendons, ligaments, capsules, and fascia.
7. Reticular connective tissue is characterized by a network of delicately interwoven reticular (fine) fibers. It forms the framework for lymphoid tissue.
8. Cartilage is connective tissue formed by chondrocytes. The three types of cartilage are hyaline, elastic, and fibrocartilage.
9. Bone (osseous tissue) is connective tissue formed by osteocytes. Bone cells secrete an intercellular matrix that includes collagen, calcium salts, and other minerals.
10. Blood is connective tissue that consists of blood cells surrounded by a fluid matrix called plasma.

Summary Outline, continued

C. Nervous Tissue
1. Nervous tissue is found in peripheral nerves, brain, and spinal cord.
2. The two types of nervous tissue are neurons (which transmit electrical signals), and neuroglia (which support and take care of the neurons).

D. Muscle Tissue
1. Muscle cells shorten, or contract, thereby causing movement.
2. The three kinds of muscle are skeletal, smooth, and cardiac.

II. Tissue Repair
A. Tissue Repair by Regeneration
1. Regeneration refers to the replacement of tissue by cells that are identical to the original cells.
2. Regeneration occurs only in cells that undergo mitosis.

B. Tissue Repair by Fibrosis
1. Fibrosis refers to replacement of injured tissue by the formation of fibrous connective tissue, or scar tissue.
2. Fibrosis occurs in cells that do not undergo mitosis.

III. Membranes
A. Epithelial Membranes
1. The cutaneous membrane is the skin; it is composed of an outer epidermis and an inner dermis.
2. Mucous membrane is an epithelial membrane that lines all body cavities that open to the exterior of the body (eg, respiratory and digestive tracts).
3. Serous membranes are epithelial membranes that line the ventral body cavities not open to the exterior of the body.
4. Serous membranes form two layers: a parietal layer that lines the wall of the cavity and a visceral layer that covers the outside of an organ.
5. The three serous membranes are the pleura (found in the thoracic cavity and associated with the lungs), the pericardium (found in the thoracic cavity and associated with the heart), and the peritoneum (found in the abdominal cavity).

B. Connective Tissue Membranes
1. Synovial membranes are connective tissue membranes.
2. Other connective tissue membranes are listed in Table 5–4.

Review Your Knowledge

1. Define *tissue*. What are four different kinds of tissue?

2. What are four functions of epithelial tissue? What is the thin material that anchors the epithelium to the underlying structure?

3. Of the four types of tissue, which type regenerates most quickly?

4. State two ways in which epithelium is classified. What is the type of epithelium that contains multiple layers of thin, flat cells?

5. Which type of epithelium is found where there is movement of substances by rapid diffusion or filtration? Where is cuboidal epithelium found in the body? Which type of epithelium plays a major role in the absorption of the products of digestion? Where is pseudostratified columnar epithelium found in the body?

6. State the function of transitional epithelium.

7. How are exocrine glands different from endocrine glands?

8. Of the four types of tissue, which one is the most abundant and most widely distributed throughout the body?

9. Which type of loose connective tissue is most common in the body, as it underlies all mucous membranes and holds organs in position? Which type of loose connective tissue serves as an insulator?

10. What is the difference between tendons and ligaments?

11. What are three types of cartilage?

12. What is the name of the condition in which mineralization of bone tissue is diminished?

13. What are the three parts of a neuron?

14. What are the three types of muscle tissue?

15. Which type of tissue repair occurs only in tissues whose cells undergo mitosis?

16. What is the difference between mucous and serous membranes?

17. Which membrane would be affected by a ruptured appendix?

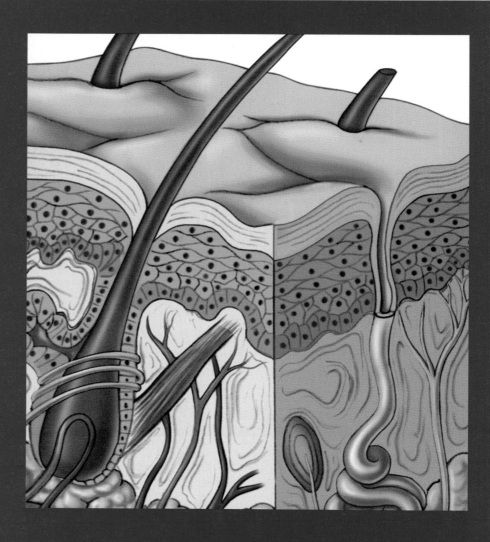

Selected terms in bold type in this chapter are defined in the Glossary.

6 INTEGUMENTARY SYSTEM AND BODY TEMPERATURE

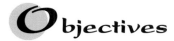

Objectives

1. Describe the two layers of skin: epidermis and dermis.

2. Define *stratum germinativum* and *stratum corneum.*

3. List the two major functions of the subcutaneous layer.

4. List the factors that influence the color of the skin.

5. Describe the accessory structures of the skin: hair, nails, and glands.

6. List six functions of the skin.

7. Describe how the skin helps to regulate temperature.

8. List three factors that affect the amount of heat produced in the body.

9. Explain four processes by which the body loses heat.

10. Describe factors that affect variations in body temperature.

11. List three structures in the skin that assist in temperature regulation.

12. Describe ways in which the skin is affected by partial-thickness and full-thickness burns.

Oh no, a pimple! How many times have you looked in the mirror only to see a pimple, rash, wrinkle, or unwanted hair? No other organ in the body is so scrutinized, scrubbed, lifted, and painted over as the skin. Yet year after year, the skin withstands the effects of harsh weather, the burning rays of the sun, constant bathing, friction, injury, and microorganisms that are constantly trying to penetrate its surface.

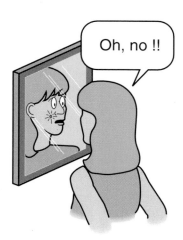

Oh, no !!

The skin, the accessory structures (sweat glands; sebaceous, or oil glands; hair; and nails) and the subcutaneous tissue below the skin form the integumentary system. The **integumentary system** (ĭn-tĕg″yōō-mĕn′tə-rē sĭs′təm) performs many roles, most of which protect the body from harm or act as a barrier against the external environment.

STRUCTURES OF THE SKIN

The skin, or **cutaneous membrane** (kyōō-tā′nē-əs mĕm′brān), is considered an organ. (An organ is two or more kinds of tissues grouped together to perform specialized tasks.) The skin has two distinct layers: the outer, or surface, layer is the **epidermis** (ĕp″ĭ-dûr′mĭs) and the inner layer is the **dermis** (dûr′mĭs). The dermis is anchored to a subcutaneous layer (Fig. 6–1).

Layers of the Skin

Epidermis

The epidermis is the thin outer layer of the skin. The epidermis is composed of stratified squamous epithelium. Like all epithelial tissue, the epithelium is avascular; it has no blood supply of its own. Oxygen and nutrients, however, diffuse into the lower epidermis from the rich supply of blood in the underlying dermis. The epidermis can be divided into five layers. Two layers are the

Do You Know...

What is a callus?

A callus is a response to excessive pressure or irritation. If the skin is subjected to pressure, the rate of mitosis will increase in the stratum germinativum, creating a thicker epidermis. The thickening is called a callus.

deeper stratum germinativum and the more superficial stratum corneum.

The **stratum germinativum** (strā′təm jûr″mĭ-nə-tĭv′əm) lies close to the dermis and thus has access to a rich supply of blood. The cells of this layer are continuously dividing, producing millions of cells per day. As the cells divide, they push the older cells up toward the surface of the epithelium. As the cells move away from the dermis, two changes take place. First, as they move away from their source of nourishment, the cells begin to die. Second, the cells undergo a process of keratinization, whereby a tough protein, **keratin** (kĕr′ə-tĭn), is deposited within the cell. The keratin hardens and flattens the cells as they move

Do You Know...

Did Toad do it?

Did Toad have anything to do with the wart on Helga's nose? No. A wart is an epidermal growth on the skin and is caused by a virus. Toad is innocent of this charge!

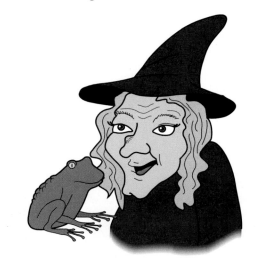

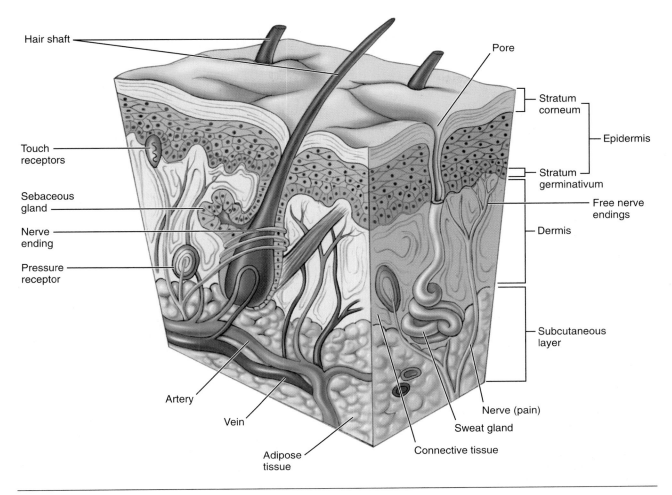

Hair shaft

Touch receptors

Sebaceous gland

Nerve ending

Pressure receptor

Artery

Vein

Adipose tissue

Pore

Stratum corneum

Epidermis

Stratum germinativum

Free nerve endings

Dermis

Subcutaneous layer

Nerve (pain)

Sweat gland

Connective tissue

FIGURE 6–1 ● The skin. Two layers of skin are the epidermis and the dermis. The dermis lies on the subcutaneous layer, or the hypodermis.

toward the outer surface of the skin. In addition to hardening the cells, the keratin performs a second important role: it waterproofs the skin. Have you ever noticed that your hand does not dissolve when you place it in water? A waterproofed skin neither absorbs nor loses much water.

The **stratum corneum** (strā′təm kôr′nē-əm) is the surface layer of the epidermis. It is composed of about 30 layers of dead, flattened, keratinized cells. This layer makes up three fourths of the epidermal thickness. The dead cells are continuously sloughed off through wear and tear. These cells are replaced by other cells that are constantly moving up from the deeper layers.

Because the skin is continuously exposed to the harsh effects of the environment, it is apt to dry out and become damaged. The skin may be cut, burned, and frozen. It may also be irritated by chemicals such as poison ivy and invaded by pathogens. Perhaps the most recent and dramatic example of pathogenic invasion of the skin is the flesh-eating bacterium, Group A *Streptococcus*.

The skin can also reflect disease processes in the body. For example, a person allergic to penicillin may develop hives, or urticaria. A person with herpes zoster (shingles), inflammation of nerves caused by the chickenpox virus, will develop painful skin lesions along the path of the nerve.

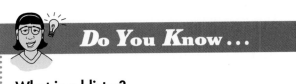

Do You Know...

What is a blister?

A blister is a fluid-filled pocket between the dermis and the epidermis. When the skin is injured by constant rubbing or irritation, some plasma leaks from the blood vessels into the dermis and accumulates between these layers.

Do You Know...

What are stretch marks?

If the skin is overstretched from pregnancy or obesity, the dermis may be damaged. The damaged dermis forms pink lines that gradually turn white. These are called stretch marks.

Dermis

The dermis, or **corium,** is also called the true skin. It is located under the epidermis and is thicker than the epidermis. The dermis is composed of dense fibrous connective tissue and contains numerous collagenous and elastic fibers, which are surrounded by a gel-like substance. The fibers make the dermis strong and stretchable. The thickness of the epidermis and dermis varies according to location in the body. Look at the skin in the palms of your hands and the soles of your feet; it is much thicker here than it is over your inner arm or your eyelids.

Although derived from the epidermis, the accessory structures such as the hair, nails, and certain glands are imbedded within the dermis. Also located in the dermis are blood vessels, nervous tissue, and some muscle tissue. Many of the nerves have specialized endings called sensory receptors, which detect pain, temperature, pressure, and touch.

Do You Know...

What is your leather jacket made of?

Your leather jacket is the dermis of an animal's skin. The collagen in the dermis becomes very tough when treated with tannic acid.

Subcutaneous Layer

The dermis lies on the subcutaneous layer. This layer is not considered part of the skin; it lies under the skin and so is called the **subcutaneous layer** (sŭb″kyōō-tā′nē-əs lā′ər), or the hypodermis. The subcutaneous layer is composed primarily of loose connective and adipose tissue. The subcutaneous tissue performs two main roles: it helps to insulate the body from extreme temperature changes in the external environment, and it anchors the skin to the underlying structures. A few areas of the body have no subcutaneous layer;

Do You Know...

How do you inject a medication into the subcutaneous layer?

When injecting medication subcutaneously, you need to use the correct-size needle and to insert the needle at the proper angle. The needle penetrates the epidermis and dermis so that the tip of the needle is located in the subcutaneous layer, where the medication is deposited.

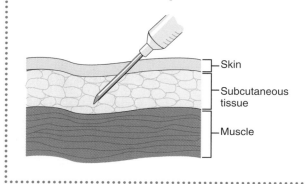

the skin anchors directly to the bone. Look at the skin over your knuckles. It is wrinkled and creased because it attaches directly to bone. Imagine what you would look like if all your skin were anchored directly to underlying bone.

Skin Color

Why are there different colors of skin? Skin color is determined by many factors: some genetic, some physiologic, and some due to disease. When we think of skin color, we generally think of black, brown, yellow, and white—and the many shades in between! These skin colors are genetically determined.

Deep within the epidermal layer of the skin are cells called **melanocytes.** Melanocytes secrete a skin-darkening pigment called **melanin** (mĕl′ə-nĭn); the melanin stains the surrounding cells, causing them to darken. The more melanin secreted, the darker the skin color. Interestingly, we all have the same numbers of melanocytes. What determines our skin color is not the numbers of melanocytes but the amount of melanin secreted.

Can melanocytes increase their secretion of melanin? Yes! When exposed to the ultraviolet radiation of sunlight, the melanocytes secrete more melanin. The skin darkens in an attempt to protect the deeper layers from the harmful effects of radiation. Lighter-skinned people often bake in the sun for hours trying to boost melanin production. This effort creates the famous summer tan.

A number of conditions involve malfunctioning melanocytes. What happens if the melanocytes completely fail to secrete melanin? In these persons, the skin, hair, and the colored part of the eye (iris) are white. This condition is referred to as **albinism.** Other persons develop a condition called **vitiligo.** This condition involves a loss of pigment (melanin) in certain areas of the skin, creating patches of white skin. Melanin can also stain unevenly. **Freckles** and **moles** are examples of melanin that becomes concentrated in local areas.

Moles are a normal occurrence; most people have 10 to 20 moles. Unfortunately, a mole may undergo malignant (cancerous) change, forming a **malignant melanoma.** A previously smooth mole that becomes darker and develops a rough or notched edge should be evaluated immediately. Malignant melanoma tends to metastasize (spread) very rapidly and is one of the cancers most difficult to treat. Exposure to sunlight increases the risk of malignant melanoma.

In addition to melanin, skin also contains a yellow pigment called **carotene.** The yellowish tint of carotene in most persons is hidden by the effects of melanin. Because persons of Asian descent have little melanin in their skin, the carotene gives their skin a yellow tint. What accounts for the pinkish color of fair-skinned persons? Because these persons produce so little melanin, the dermis is visible; it is the blood in the dermal capillaries that provides the pinkish tinge to the skin.

The ability of blood in the dermis to affect skin color also accounts for a number of other conditions. Poorly oxygenated blood causes the skin to look blue. This condition is called **cyanosis.** Embarrassment causes the blood vessels in the skin to dilate. This condition increases blood flow to the skin, causing the person to blush or flush. What about the saying "He was white as a sheet"? A person who is scared experiences a constriction of the blood vessels in the skin. This condition causes a decrease in the amount of blood and a loss of the pinkish tinge.

Skin color may also change in response to disease processes. Assessment of skin color provides valuable clues to underlying pathology. A person with liver disease is unable to excrete a pigment called bilirubin. This pigment is instead deposited in the skin, causing yellow jaundice. A person with a poorly functioning adrenal gland may deposit excess melanin in the skin and appear to be bronzed. A black-and-blue discoloration (bruise) indicates that blood has escaped from the blood vessels and clotted under the skin.

Skin color may also change in response to diet. For instance, it is possible to achieve a carotene-induced yellow tint to the skin by overeating carotene-rich vegetables such as carrots.

ACCESSORY STRUCTURES OF THE SKIN

The skin is the home of several accessory structures, including the hair, nails, and glands.

Hair

Thousands and thousands of years ago, we humans were a hairy lot. Like our furry pets, we depended on a thick crop of hair to keep us warm. Today, most of the hair covering our bodies is sparse and very fine, with the exception of the hair on our heads (and for some, that too is sparse). The main function of our sparse body hair is to sense insects on the skin before they can sting us. Some body parts are hairless. These include the palms of the hands, soles of the feet, lips, nipples, and parts of the external reproductive organs.

Some areas of hair perform important functions. For instance, the eyelashes and eyebrows protect the eyes from dust and perspiration. The nasal hairs trap dust and prevent it from being inhaled into the lungs. The hair of the scalp helps to keep us warm and, of course, plays an immensely important cosmetic role.

Hair growth is influenced by the sex hormones estrogen and testosterone. The onset of puberty is heralded by the growth of hair in the axillary and pubic areas in both males and females. In the male, the surge of testosterone also produces a beard and hairy chest. Estrogen, of course, does not have this effect.

The chief parts of a hair are the **shaft,** the part above the surface of the skin, and the **root,** the part that extends from the dermis to the surface (Fig. 6–2). Each hair arises from a group of epidermal cells that penetrate, or project down, into the dermis. This downward extension of epithelial cells forms the **hair follicle.** The epidermal cells at the base of the hair follicle receive a rich supply of blood from the dermal blood vessels. As these cells divide and grow, the older cells are pushed toward the surface of the skin. As they move away from their source of nourishment, the cells die. Like other cells that compose the skin, the hair cells also become keratinized. The hair that we brush, blow dry, and curl every day is a collection of dead keratinized cells.

Hair color is genetically controlled and is determined by the type and the amount of melanin. An abundance of melanin produces dark hair, whereas less melanin produces blond hair. With age, the melanocytes become less active; the absence of melanin produces white hair. Gray hair is due to a mixture of pigmented and nonpigmented hairs. Interestingly, red hair is due to a modified type of melanin that contains iron.

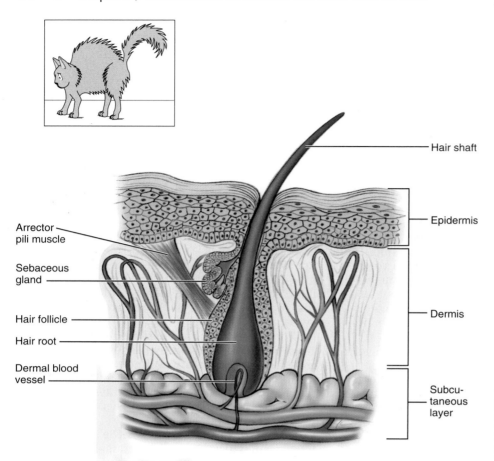

FIGURE 6–2 ● Hair follicle. A hair is composed of a hair shaft and a hair root. Note the relationship of the blood vessels, glands, and muscle to the hair follicle.

Curly, wavy, or straight—the shape of the hair shaft determines the appearance of the hair. A round shaft produces straight hair, whereas an oval shaft produces wavy hair. Curly and kinky hair are the result of flat hair shafts. Chemically, one can make the hair curly by flattening the hair shafts.

How does the frightened kitty get her hair to stand on end? Attached to the hair follicle is a bundle of smooth muscle cells called the arrector pili muscles (see Fig. 6–2). Contraction of these muscles causes the hair to stand on end. When frightened, the cat's brain sends its panic message along the nerves to the arrector pili muscles. The muscles then contract and pull the hair to an upright position. Kitty looks more ferocious with her hair standing on end, which helps in frightening off her attacker. Her hair also stands on end when she is cold. The raised hair traps heat and therefore helps to keep her warm.

Although humans may not benefit as much from hair as our furry friends do, we respond to fear and cold in the same way. Contraction of the arrector pili muscles also causes our hair to stand on end. As the hair stands, it pulls the skin up into little bumps. This reaction is the basis of goose flesh, or goose bumps. The erect hair does not do much to conserve our heat, but the contraction of the arrector pili muscles increases heat production. This response is called shivering. This is about as interesting as a hair can get.

Cosmetically, hair is important. Hair loss to the point of baldness is very distressing to some people. The loss of hair is called **alopecia.** The most common type of baldness is male-pattern baldness. It is a hereditary condition characterized by a gradual loss of hair with aging. A second common cause of hair loss is related to drug toxicity, as with chemotherapy or radiation therapy. Anticancer drugs are so toxic that they often destroy hair-producing cells. When drug therapy is terminated, the cells regenerate and start to grow hair again. Curiously, the new hair may be a different color or texture from the original (pre-drug) hair.

Nails

Nails are thin plates of stratified squamous epithelial cells that contain a very hard form of keratin (Fig. 6–3). The nails are found on the distal ends of the fingers and toes and protect these structures from injury.

A

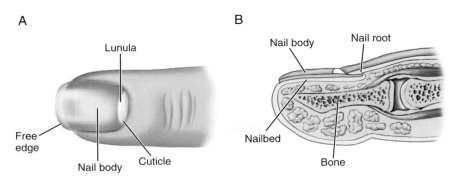

B

FIGURE 6–3 ● Nail. Three parts of the nail are the free edge, the nail body, and the nail root.

Each nail has the following structures: a free edge, a **nail body** (fingernail), and a **nail root.** The cells of the nail body develop and are keratinized in the nail root. The extent of nail growth is represented by the half-moon-shaped **lunula,** located at the base of the nail. As the nail body grows, it slides over a layer called the nailbed, a part of the epidermis. The pink color of nails is due to the blood vessels in the underlying dermal layer beneath the nail. The cuticle is a fold of stratum corneum that grows onto the proximal portion of the nail body.

Glands

Two major exocrine glands are associated with the skin. They are the sebaceous glands and the sweat glands (Fig. 6–4).

Most **sebaceous glands** (sĭ-bā′shəs glăndz), or **oil glands,** are associated with hair follicles and are found in all areas of the body that have hair. They secrete an oily substance called **sebum** that flows into the hair follicle and then out onto the surface of the skin. A small number of sebaceous glands open directly onto the surface of the skin.

FIGURE 6–4 ● Skin glands. Two types of skin glands are the sebaceous glands and the sweat glands. Two types of sweat glands are the apocrine glands and the eccrine glands. This tennis shoe is the home of one sweaty foot.

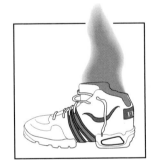

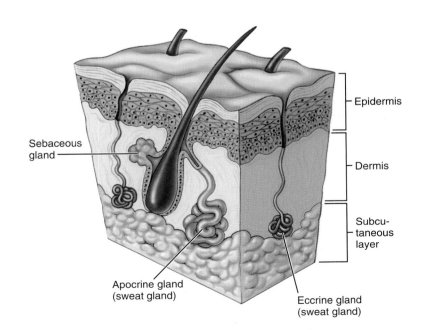

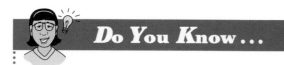

Do You Know...

What is cradle cap?

Cradle cap is also called seborrhea. It forms on the scalp of an infant, hence the name *cradle cap*. It is due to the oversecretion of sebaceous glands, which causes the formation of oily scales.

The sebum lubricates and helps waterproof the hair and skin. The sebum also inhibits the growth of bacteria on the surface of the skin. With aging, sebum production gradually decreases. This change accounts, in part, for the dry skin and brittle hair seen in older persons. The sebaceous glands play a unique role in the fetus. Babies are born with a covering that resembles cream cheese. The covering is called the **vernix caseosa** and is secreted by the sebaceous glands.

Sometimes the sebaceous glands become blocked by accumulated sebum and other debris. When the sebum is exposed to the air and dries out, it turns black, forming a **blackhead.** When the blocked sebum becomes infected it is a **pimple** (pustule). You have seen the contents of a pimple. Blackhead and pimple formation is common among adolescents because sebaceous gland activity responds to the hormonal changes associated with puberty.

The **sweat glands,** or **sudoriferous glands** (soo″də-rĭf′ər-əs glǎndz), are located in the dermis and the subcutaneous layer (see Fig. 6–4). They are found in all regions of the skin and are particularly abundant on the palms and soles. As the name implies, these glands secrete sweat. An individual has approximately three million sweat glands.

Two types of sweat glands are the apocrine and the eccrine sweat glands. The **apocrine glands** (ǎp′ə-krĭn glǎndz) are usually associated with hair follicles and are found in the axillary and genital areas. The apocrine glands respond to emotional stress and become active when the person is frightened, upset, in pain, or sexually excited. Because the development of these glands is stimulated by the sex hormones, they become more active during puberty. The sweat produced by these glands does not have a strong odor. If allowed to accumulate on the skin, however, the substances in sweat are degraded by bacteria into chemicals with a strong unpleasant odor. This is called body odor (B.O.) and is the reason we use deodorants.

In animals such as the dog, these secretions act as sex attractants. Watch how eagerly Rover sniffs when a potential mate is in the immediate area!

The **eccrine glands** (ĕk′rĭn glǎndz) are the more numerous and widely distributed of the sweat glands. They are located throughout the body and are especially numerous on the forehead, upper lip, palms, and soles. Unlike apocrine glands, the eccrine glands are not associated with hair follicles.

The sweat secreted by the eccrine glands plays an important role in temperature regulation. As sweat evaporates from the skin surface, heat is lost. These are the glands that make you sweat profusely on hot days or during periods of strenuous exercise. Unlike the apocrine glands, which become active during puberty, the eccrine glands function throughout your entire lifetime. Eccrine secretion is composed primarily of water and a few salts.

Modified sweat glands include the mammary glands and the ceruminous glands. The mammary glands are located in the breasts; they secrete milk. (The secretion of milk is discussed further in Chapter 23). The **ceruminous glands** (sĕ-roo′mən-əs glǎndz) are found in the external auditory canal of the ear. They secrete cerumen, or ear wax. This yellow, sticky, wax-like secretion repels insects and traps foreign material.

✳ **SUM IT UP!** The integumentary system is composed of the skin and accessory organs (hair, nails, and glands). The skin is composed of two layers: the epidermis and the dermis. The dermis sits on a subcutaneous layer called the hypodermis.

FUNCTIONS OF THE SKIN

The skin is a complex organ that performs many different functions. The skin

- Keeps harmful substances out of the body and helps to retain water and electrolytes. The skin prevents excessive loss of water. A patient who suffers extensive burns very quickly becomes dehydrated because there is no skin to prevent water loss.
- Protects the internal structures and organs from injuries due to blows, cuts, harsh chemicals, sunlight, burns, and pathogenic microorganisms. The skin acts as a physical barrier and its acidic secretion discourages the growth of pathogens on its surface.
- Performs an excretory function. Although excretion is a minor role, the skin is able to excrete water, salt, and small amounts of waste such as urea.
- Acts as a gland by synthesizing and secreting vitamin D. Skin cells contain a molecule that is converted to vitamin D when exposed to sunlight. Vitamin D plays an important role in the utilization of calcium by bone tissue.

- Performs a sensory role by housing the sensory receptors for touch, pressure, pain, and temperature. In this way, the skin helps to detect information about the environment.
- Plays an important role in the regulation of body temperature.

Regulation of Body Temperature

Body Temperature: Heat Production

Heat is a form of energy (thermal) and is produced by the millions of chemical reactions occurring in the cells of the body. The heat produced by metabolizing cells is the basis of the body temperature. The greatest amount of heat is produced in the muscles and liver. At rest, the muscles produce about 25% of the total body heat, while the liver may produce up to 25% of the heat. The resting brain produces only about 15% of the heat. Interestingly, the studying brain does not produce much more heat.

The amount of heat produced can be affected by many factors: food consumption, the amounts and types of hormones that are secreted, and physical activity. With exercise, the amount of heat produced by the muscles may increase enormously (hundreds of times). The heat produced in the cells is picked up and distributed throughout the body by the blood. To repeat: the heat produced by the metabolizing cells is the basis of the body temperature.

Body Temperature: Heat Loss

The body constantly produces heat and constantly loses heat. Most of the heat loss (80%) occurs through the skin. The remaining heat (20%) is lost through the respiratory system (lungs) and in the excretory products (urine and feces). Heat loss occurs by four means: radiation, conduction, convection, and evaporation.

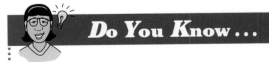

What is a cold sweat?

Sweating is regulated by the sympathetic nervous system. When a person is emotionally upset (eg, because of fright, embarrassment, or nervousness), the sympathetic nervous system is stimulated. This stimulation results in sweating. Because the sweating is not associated with exercise and an elevated body temperature, it is called a cold sweat.

Why do your ears get red in very cold temperatures?

Normally, as body temperature declines, the blood vessels constrict so as to conserve heat in the deeper layers of tissue. When the temperature drops too low, however, the blood vessels dilate in an attempt to prevent irreversible tissue damage. The dilated ear lobes appear red because of the increased flow of blood.

The amount of blood in the dermal blood vessels influences the amount of heat that can be lost or dissipated by radiation, conduction, and convection. **Radiation** (rā″dē-ā′shən) means that heat is lost from a warm object (eg, the body) to the cooler air surrounding the warm object. Thus, a person loses heat in a cold room. **Conduction** (kən-dŭk′shən) is the loss of heat from a warm body to a cooler object in contact with the warm body. For example, a person (warm object) becomes cold when sitting on a block of ice (cooler object). Clinically, a cooling blanket may be used to reduce a dangerously high fever. The warm body of a feverish patient loses heat to the cooler object, the cooling blanket. **Convection** (kən-věk′shən) is the loss of heat by air currents moving over the surface of the skin. For example, a fan moves air across the surface of the skin, thereby constantly removing the layer of heated air next to the body.

Finally, heat may be lost through evaporation. **Evaporation** (ē-văp″ə-rā′shən) occurs when a liquid becomes a gas. For example, when liquid alcohol is rubbed on the skin, it evaporates and cools the skin. Likewise, during strenuous exercise, sweat on the surface of the skin evaporates and cools the body. Note that the evaporation of water is associated with a loss of heat. On a hot, humid day, water cannot evaporate from the surface of the skin. Hence, heat loss is diminished. This is why we feel the heat so intensely on a hot, humid day.

Normal body temperature ranges between 97°F and 100°F, with an average of 98.6°F (36.2°C to 37.6°C, average 37°C). A higher-than-normal body temperature is referred to as **hyperthermia,** or **fever,** and usually accompanies an infection. A lower-than-normal body temperature is called **hypothermia** and is most apt to develop when a person is exposed to cold environmental temperatures.

Body temperature varies in different parts of the body. If you take a person's temperature orally (under the tongue), by axillary means (armpit), or rectally, you will get slightly different readings.

The axillary temperature is lower than the oral temperature, which, in turn, is lower than a rectal temperature.

Body temperature also varies with the time of day. The change in temperature is related to physical activity and eating. For example, body temperature is lowest in the early morning because we have been resting and have not eaten. As our physical activity and food consumption increase throughout the day, body temperature rises, so that it is highest in the late afternoon and early evening.

Body Temperature: Regulation

Body temperature is normally maintained at 98.6°F (37°C). The thermostat of the body is located in a part of the brain called the **hypothalamus.** When body temperature deviates from normal, information is sent from the hypothalamus to the skin. Three structures within the skin assist in temperature regulation: the blood vessels, the sweat glands, and the arrector pili muscles (Fig. 6–5).

With exercise and temperature elevation, the blood vessels dilate, thereby allowing more blood to flow to the skin. This activity transfers heat from the deeper tissues to the surface of the body. Note how flushed our jogger is because of the blood coming to the surface (see Fig. 6–5). Temperature elevation also stimulates the activity of the sweat glands. As the sweat evaporates from the surface of the body, heat is lost. Under extreme conditions of heat, 12 liters of sweat can be secreted in a 24-hour period. These two activities lower body temperature.

What about the gentleman awaiting the arrival of a bus during a snowfall? His body temperature is dropping. How does the body respond? First, the blood vessels constrict, reducing blood flow to the skin. This response traps the blood and heat in the deeper tissues, preventing heat loss. Second, the sweat glands become less active, also preventing heat loss. Third, the arrector pili muscles contract, causing shivering and an increase in the production of heat. These three activities raise body temperature to more normal levels.

When Skin Is Burned

Tragically, large areas of skin are often lost because of burns. Burns are classified according to both the depth of the burn and the extent of the surface area burned (Fig. 6–6A). On the basis of depth, burns are classified as either partial-thick-

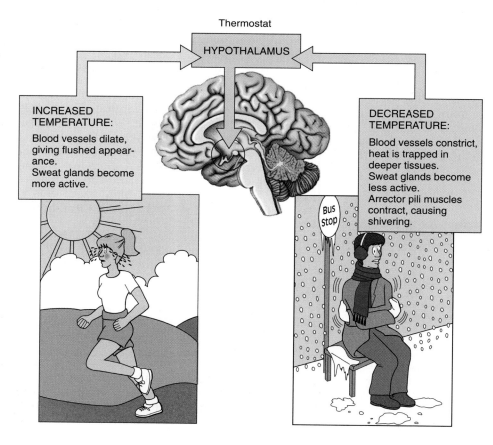

FIGURE 6–5 • Temperature regulation. The thermostat of the body is the hypothalamus. Two mechanisms, vasodilation and sweating, are involved in lowering temperature to normal. Three mechanisms that restore a lowered temperature toward normal are vasoconstriction, a lack of sweating, and shivering.

A

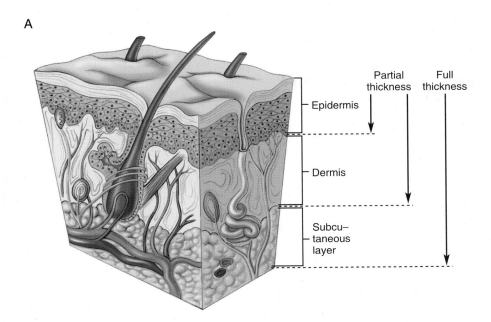

FIGURE 6-6 ● A, Burns: parts of the skin damaged by burns. Partial-thickness (first- and second-degree burns) and full-thickness burns (third-degree burns). B, The rule of nines for estimating the extent of burns.

B

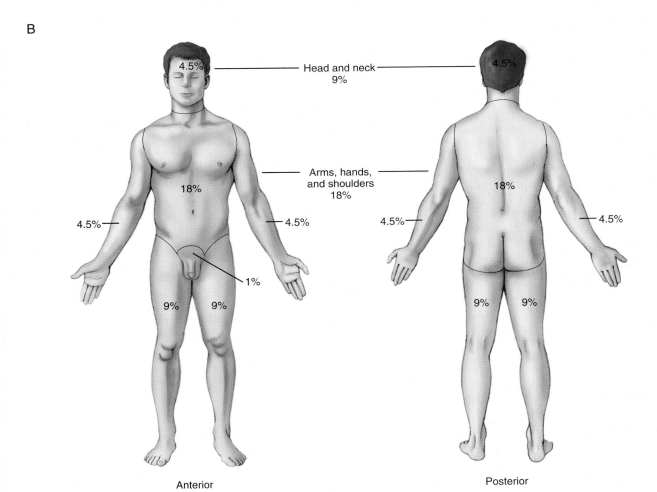

ness burns or full-thickness burns. Partial-thickness burns are further divided into first-degree and second-degree burns. A first-degree burn is red, painful, and slightly edematous (swollen). Only the epidermis is involved. A sunburn is an ex-

ample of a first-degree burn. A second-degree burn involves damage to both the epidermis and the dermis. With little damage to the dermis, the symptoms of a second-degree burn include redness, pain, edema, and blister formation. With greater damage to the dermis, the skin may appear red, tan, or white.

Full-thickness burns are also called third-degree burns. With a burn this severe, both the epidermis and the dermis are destroyed, often with destruction of the deeper underlying layers. Although first- and second-degree burns are painful, third-degree burns are painless because the sensory receptors have been destroyed. Third-degree burns may appear white, tan, brown, black, or a deep cherry red.

The extent of the burn injury is initially evaluated according to the rule of nines (Fig. 6–6B). In this system, the total body surface area is divided into regions. The assigned percentages are related to the number 9. For instance, the head and neck are considered 9% of the total body surface area. Each upper limb is 9%, while each lower limb is 18% (9 × 2). Note the percentages assigned to each specific body region. To determine proper treatment, the clinician needs to evaluate both the depth and the extent of the burn injury.

A Note About Skin Care

The skin is constantly exposed to all sorts of insults: the drying effects of soap and water, the damaging effects of the ultraviolet radiation of the sun, friction, numerous bumps, and exposure to sharp objects. While we cannot avoid normal wear and tear, we can protect the skin in several ways. For instance, we can lessen exposure of the skin to ultraviolet radiation. Sunbathing is deadly to the skin. Sun exposure both dries and irreversibly damages the skin. It also makes the skin leather-like, and, more importantly, it increases the risk of skin cancer and malignant melanoma.

Skin care is particularly important in the elderly. The skin of an elderly person is normally drier, more easily injured, and slower to heal. Because the skin is so dry, excessive use of soap should be discouraged. Limiting the use of soaps and excessive bathing prevents additional drying of the skin. Moreover, maintaining the acid surface of the skin serves to discourage the growth of bacteria (discussed further in Chapter 17). In addition to becoming drier with aging, the skin changes in another important way. Both the dermis and the underlying subcutaneous layer become thinner. As a result, the elderly bruise more easily because the blood vessels are not as well protected. In addition, heat is lost from the blood vessels so that older people often feel cold.

✳ **SUM IT UP!** The skin is a complex organ that performs many functions: it affords protection for the entire body, acts as a barrier, regulates temperature, detects sensations (touch, pressure, temperature, and pain), synthesizes vitamin D, and acts as an excretory organ. Because the skin protects us from and presents us to the external environment, we must take care of this marvelous organ.

As You Age

1. Aging causes a generalized thinning of the epidermis; the epidermal cells reproduce more slowly and are larger and more irregular. These changes result in thinner, more translucent skin.

2. Melanocyte activity decreases, resulting in decreased protection from ultraviolet light and greater susceptibility to sunburn and skin cancer. Selected melanocytes increase melanin production, resulting in brown spots, or age spots, especially in areas exposed to the sun.

3. The dermis becomes thinner, with a decreased amount of collagen and decreased number of elastic fibers. The result is increased fragility of the skin, as well as increased wrinkles. The skin also heals more slowly.

4. Vascularity of the dermis decreases (a decreased number of blood vessels) with a slower rate of repair. This change causes the skin to become more susceptible to small hemorrhages and to pressure ulcers.

5. Vascularity and circulation in the subcutaneous tissue decrease, so that drugs administered subcutaneously are absorbed more slowly.

6. The amount of adipose tissue in the subcutaneous layer decreases, resulting in folded and wrinkled skin that has a decreased ability to maintain body temperature. The person tends to feel cold.

7. Sebaceous gland activity decreases, resulting in dry, coarse, itchy skin.

8. Sweat gland activity decreases, resulting in decreased ability to regulate body temperature and intolerance to cold.

9. The rate of melanin production by the hair follicle decreases. As a result, hair becomes lighter in color, turning gray or white. Hair does not replace itself as often and becomes thinner.

10. Vascular supply to the nailbed decreases. Consequently, the nails become dull, brittle, hard, and thick; growth rate also slows.

Disorders of the Integumentary System

Acne	A disorder of the skin in which the sebaceous glands oversecrete sebum. The sebum and dead keratinized cells become clogged in a follicle and appear as blackheads or whiteheads. The clogged follicle may become infected with bacteria, thereby producing a pimple. The most common form of acne occurring during adolescence is acne vulgaris.
Athlete's foot	A fungal infection characterized by vesicles, fissures, ulcers, and pruritus (itching). It most commonly affects the toes but may also involve the fingers, palms, and groin area.
Boil	Also called a furuncle; a localized collection of pus caused by staphylococcal infection of hair follicles and sebaceous glands. A carbuncle is multiple, interconnecting furuncles.
Cold sore	Also called a fever blister; a collection of watery vesicles caused by infection with the herpes simplex virus.
Cyst	Sac-like structures containing fluid or semisolid material and surrounded by a strong capsule.
Dermatitis	Inflammation of the skin that may be caused by a variety of irritants such as chemicals, plants, and acids. Dermatitis is characterized by erythema (redness), papules (pimple-like lesions), vesicles (blisters), scabs, and crusts. Poison ivy is a form of contact dermatitis. Skin irritation occurs when contact is made with the irritating substance.
Eczema	From the Greek word meaning to erupt. Eczema is an inflammatory condition (atopic dermatitis) characterized by redness, papular and vesicular lesions, crusts, and scales.
Hives	Urticaria. Hives are due to an allergic reaction characterized by red patches (wheals) and generally accompanied by intense itching (pruritus).
Impetigo	A contagious infection of the skin generally caused by the *Staphylococcus* bacterium.
Psoriasis	From the Greek word meaning to itch. Psoriasis is a chronic condition characterized by lesions that are red, dry, elevated, and covered by silvery scales.
Skin cancer	There are several kinds of skin cancer, all related to excessive exposure to sun. The two most common types are basal cell carcinoma and squamous cell carcinoma. Basal cell carcinoma spreads locally and is successfully treated. The most serious and less successfully treated form of skin cancer is malignant melanoma, a cancer of the pigment-producing melanocytes.

Summary Outline

The integumentary system includes the skin; it covers the body, protects the internal organs, and plays an important role in the regulation of body temperature.

I. Structures: Organs of the Integumentary System

The integumentary system includes the skin, accessory structures, and subcutaneous tissue beneath the skin.

A. Skin

1. The skin is called the cutaneous membrane.
2. The skin has two layers, an outer layer called the epidermis and an inner layer called the dermis.

3. The epidermis has five layers. The stratum germinativum is the layer in which cell division takes place. The new cells produce keratin (waterproofing) and die as they are pushed toward the surface. The outer layer is the stratum corneum and consists of flattened, dead, keratinized cells.
4. The dermis is the corium, or true skin. It lies on the subcutaneous tissue.
5. Skin color is determined by many factors: some genetic, some physiologic, and some due to disease. Melanin causes skin to

continued

Summary Outline *continued*

A. Skin, *continued*

darken. Carotene causes skin to appear yellow. The amount of blood in the skin affects skin color (eg, flushing) as does the appearance of abnormal substances such as bilirubin (jaundice) and a low blood oxygen content (cyanosis).

B. Accessory Structures of the Skin

1. Hair is unevenly distributed over the skin. The location of the hair determines its function. Sparse body hair does little more than sense the presence of insects on the skin, while eyebrows and eyelashes protect the eyes from dust and perspiration.
2. The main parts of a hair are the shaft, the root, and the follicle.
3. Hair color is determined by the amount and type of melanin.
4. Nails are thin plates of stratified squamous epithelial cells that contain a hard form of keratin.
5. There are two major exocrine glands in the skin: the sebaceous glands and the sweat glands.
6. The sebaceous glands (oil glands) secrete sebum into the hair follicle or onto the surface of the skin. The sebum helps to waterproof the hair and skin. In the fetus, these glands secrete vernix caseosa, a cheese-like substance that coats the skin of a newborn.
7. There are two types of sweat glands (sudoriferous glands): the apocrine glands and the eccrine glands. The eccrine sweat glands play a crucial role in temperature regulation.
8. The mammary glands (secrete milk) and the ceruminous glands (secrete ear wax) are modified sweat glands.

C. Subcutaneous Tissue

1. Subcutaneous tissue anchors the dermis to underlying structures.
2. Subcutaneous tissue acts as an insulator; it prevents heat loss.

II. Regulation of Body Temperature

A. Heat Production

1. Heat produced by the metabolizing cells constitutes the body temperature.
2. Most of the heat is produced by the muscles and the liver.

B. Heat Loss

1. Most of the heat (80%) is lost through the skin.
2. Heat loss occurs through radiation, conduction, convection, and evaporation.
3. Normal body temperature is set by the body's thermostat in the hypothalamus. When body temperature rises above normal, heat is lost through sweating and vasodilation. When body temperature falls below normal, heat is conserved by vasoconstriction and produced by shivering.

III. When Skin Is Burned

A. Physiologic Effects

These include short-term effects (fluid and electrolyte losses, shock, inability to regulate body temperature, infection) and long-term effects (scarring, loss of function, and cosmetic and emotional problems).

B. Classification of Burns

1. Partial-thickness burns are first- or second-degree burns.
2. Full-thickness burns are third-degree burns.
3. The rule of nines is a way to evaluate burns.

Review Your Knowledge

1. What is the difference between the epidermis and the dermis?

2. Which protein waterproofs the skin?

3. In which layer of the skin are blood vessels and nerves found? What is the name of the layer found beneath the dermis?

4. How does the amount of melanin produced affect skin color? What is the relationship of albinism, vitiligo, freckles, and moles to melanin?

5. How are blood vessels in the dermis related to cyanosis, blushing, and looking "white as a sheet"?

6. What causes goose bumps?

7. What are two causes of alopecia?

8. Which layer of the epidermis forms the cuticle?

9. What is the difference between sebaceous and sudoriferous glands? Which gland secretes a substance that forms vernix caseosa in newborns?

10. What is the difference between apocrine and eccrine glands?

11. List six functions of the skin.

12. What are four types of heat loss from the body?

13. What factors affect variations in body temperature?

14. Explain the relationship between vasoconstriction and vasodilation in body temperature regulation.

15. What is the difference between a first-degree, second-degree, and third-degree burn? What is the rule of nines?

16. What is the effect of repeated sun exposure on the skin?

17. How does aging affect the skin?

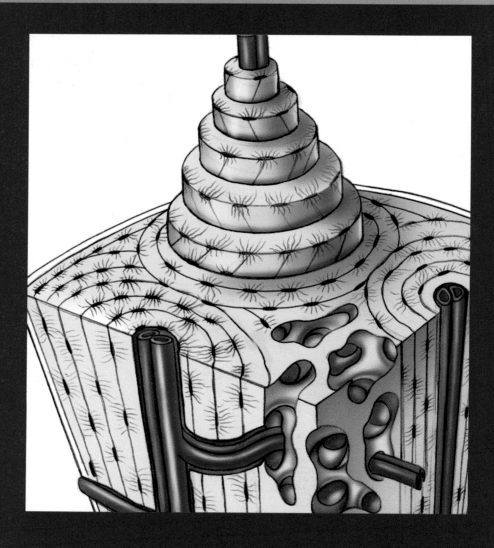

7 SKELETAL SYSTEM

Objectives

1. List the functions of the skeletal system.

2. Describe the structure of a long bone.

3. Differentiate between red and yellow bone marrow.

4. Describe the roles of osteoblasts and osteoclasts.

5. Contrast the axial skeleton and the appendicular skeleton.

6. List the bones of the axial skeleton.

7. List the bones of the appendicular skeleton.

8. Label important landmarks for selected bones on the skeleton.

9. List the main types of joints.

10. Describe the functions of joints.

11. Describe the types of movement that occur at diarthrotic, or synovial, joints.

The skeletal system consists of the bones and joints as well as the cartilage and the ligaments associated with the joints. Bone tissue is living and metabolically active, but because it contains much nonliving material such as calcium and phosphorus, it appears dead or dried up. In fact, the word *skeleton* comes from a Greek word meaning "dried up body."

The skeletal system, however, is anything but dead. It contains 206 bones that are very much alive and perform a number of important functions.

ARRANGEMENT AND FUNCTIONS OF BONES

As you can see from Figure 7–1, the bones of the skeletal system are arranged to provide a framework for our bodies. The skeletal system gives us our basic shape. Imagine what you would look like without bones!

The Skeletal System: What It Does

In addition to shaping us up, the skeletal system performs other functions:

- The bones of the lower extremities support the weight of the body.
- The bones support and protect the soft body organs. The skull, for instance, encases the brain, protecting it from injury.
- With the assistance of muscles, the skeletal system enables the body to move about.
- Bones store a number of minerals, the most important being calcium and phosphorus.
- Red bone marrow produces blood cells.

Many Sizes and Shapes of Bones

Bones come in many sizes and shapes, from the pea-sized bones in the wrist to the 24-inch-long femur in the thigh. The size and shape of a bone reflect its function (Fig. 7–2). The long, strong femur in the thigh, for instance, supports a great deal of weight and can withstand considerable force. Some of the skull bones, on the other hand, are thin, flat, and curved. Their function is to encase and protect the brain.

Bones are classified as follows:

- *Long bones.* Long bones are longer than they are wide. They are found in the arms and the legs.
- *Short bones.* Short bones are shaped like cubes and are found primarily in the wrists and ankles.
- *Flat bones.* Flat bones are thin, flat, and curved. They form the ribs, breastbone, and skull.
- *Irregular bones.* Irregular bones are differently shaped and are not classified as long, short, or flat. They include the hip bones, vertebrae, and various bones in the skull.

BONE TISSUE AND BONE FORMATION

Bone is also called **osseous tissue.** Bone cells, called **osteocytes,** secrete an intercellular substance, called **matrix**, containing calcium and other minerals. These minerals are deposited around protein fibers. The protein fibers provide elasticity. The minerals make bone tissue hard and strong. Bone tissue is the hardest of the connective tissues.

Compact and Spongy Bone

Two types of bone, or osseous tissue, are compact and spongy (Fig. 7–3). **Compact bone** refers to dense, hard bone tissue found primarily in the shafts of long bones and on the outer surfaces of other bones. **Spongy,** or **cancellous, bone** is less dense. Spongy bone is located primarily at the ends of long bones and in the center of other bones.

Compact and spongy bone look different under the microscope. Compact bone is tightly packed, so that its density can provide a great deal of strength. The microscopic unit of compact bone is the **osteon,** or **haversian system** (hə-vūr′zhən sĭs′təm). Each haversian system consists of mature osteocytes arranged in concentric circles around large blood vessels. The area surrounding the osteocytes is filled with protein fibers, calcium, and other minerals. Each haversian system looks like a long cylinder.

Compact bone consists of many haversian systems running parallel to each other. Communicating blood vessels run laterally and connect the haversian systems with each other and with the periosteal lining that surrounds the bone. The network of blood vessels ensures that the bone tissue receives an adequate supply of blood. Blood supplies tissues with oxygen and necessary nutrients.

Spongy, or cancellous, bone has a much different structure from compact bone (see Fig. 7–3B). Unlike compact bone, spongy bone does not contain haversian systems. In spongy bone, the bone tissue is arranged in plates called **trabeculae.** These bony plates are separated by irregular spaces, or holes, and give spongy bone a punched-out "Swiss cheese" appearance. The spaces in the bone are important for two reasons: they decrease the weight of the bone, making it lighter, and they contain red bone

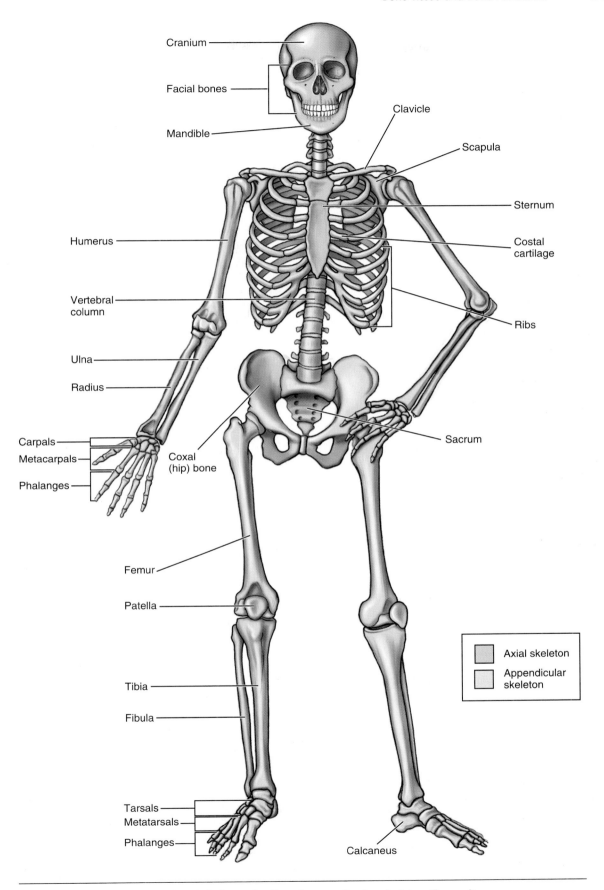

FIGURE 7-1 • Skeleton. Axial skeleton (red) and appendicular skeleton (brown).

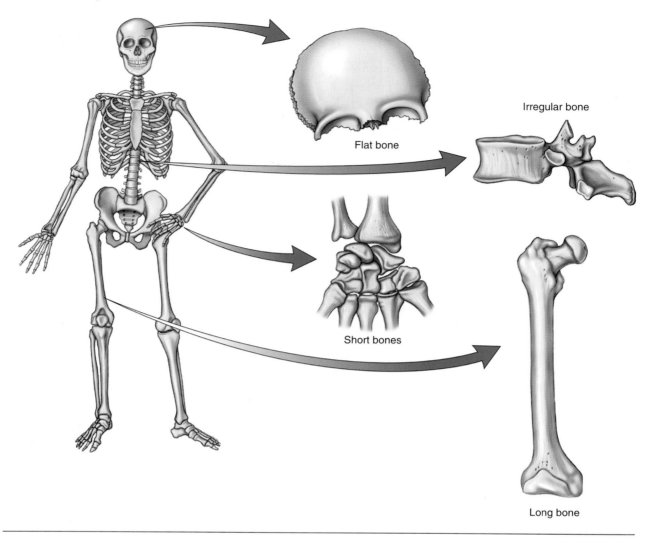

Irregular bone

Flat bone

Short bones

Long bone

FIGURE 7–2 ● Types of bones: long, short, flat, and irregular bones.

marrow. The red bone marrow richly supplies the spongy bone with blood and also produces blood cells for use throughout the body.

Long Bone

The arrangement of the compact and spongy tissue in a long bone accounts for its strength. Long bones contain sites of growth and reshaping and structures associated with joints (Fig. 7–3A). The parts of a long bone include the following:

- *Diaphysis.* The **diaphysis** (dī-ăf′ĭ-sĭs) is the long shaft of the bone. It is composed primarily of compact bone and therefore provides considerable strength.
- *Epiphysis.* The enlarged ends of the long bone are the epiphyses. The **epiphysis** (ĕ-pĭf′ĭ-sĭs) of a bone articulates, or meets, with a second bone

at a joint. Each epiphysis consists of a thin layer of compact bone overlying spongy bone. The epiphyses are covered by cartilage.
- *Epiphyseal disc.* A growing bone contains a band of hyaline cartilage located at the ends of long bones, between the epiphysis and the diaphysis. This band of cartilage is the **epiphyseal disc,** or **growth plate.** It is here that longitudinal bone growth occurs.
- *Medullary cavity.* The **medullary cavity** is the hollow center of the diaphysis. In infancy, the cavity is filled with red bone marrow for blood cell production. In the adult, the medullary cavity is filled with yellow bone marrow and functions as a storage site for fat; at this stage it is not associated with blood cell production. The inside of the medullary cavity is lined with connective tissue called the **endosteum.**
- *Periosteum.* The **periosteum** (pĕr″ē-ŏs′tē-əm) is a tough fibrous connective tissue membrane

that covers the outside of the diaphysis. It is anchored firmly to the outside of the bone on all surfaces except the articular cartilage. The periosteum protects the bone, serves as a point of attachment for muscle, and contains the blood vessels that nourish the underlying bone. Because the periosteum carries the blood supply to the underlying bone, any injury to this structure has serious consequences to the health of the bone. Like any other organ, the loss of blood supply can cause its death.

- *Articular cartilage.* The **articular cartilage** is found on the outer surface of the epiphysis. It

forms a smooth, shiny surface that decreases friction within a joint. Because a joint is also called an articulation, this cartilage is called articular cartilage.

Ossification

How does bone form? The 3-month-old fetus has an early skeleton-like frame composed of cartilage and connective tissue membrane (Fig. 7–4). As the fetus matures, the cartilage and connective

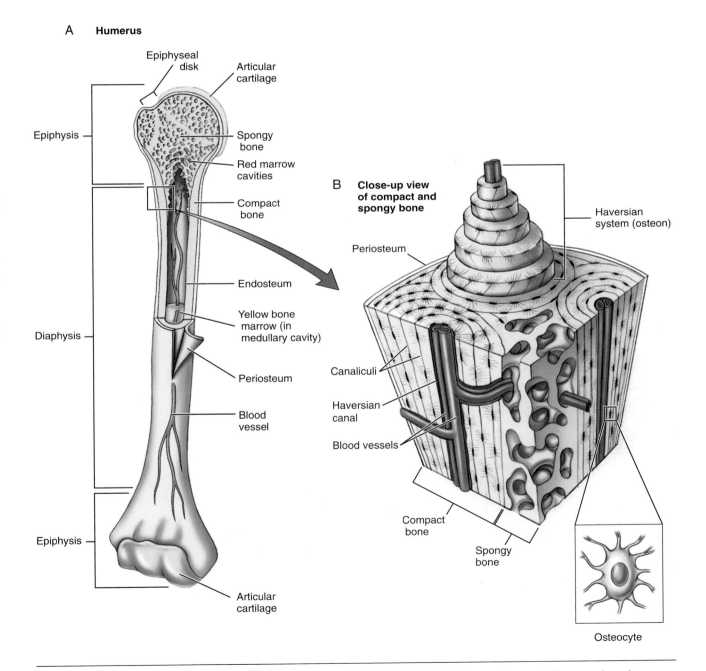

FIGURE 7–3 ● Bone. A, Anatomy of a long bone. B, Types of bone tissue (compact bone and spongy bone).

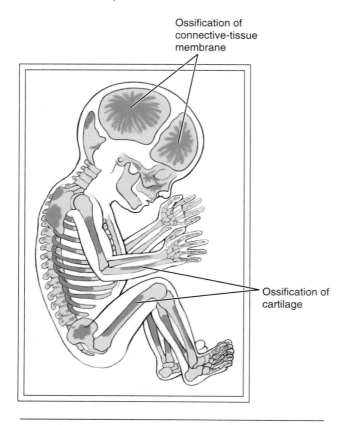

Ossification of connective-tissue membrane

Ossification of cartilage

FIGURE 7–4 ● Ossification of connective-tissue membrane (skull) and cartilage.

tissue change into bone. The formation of bone is called **ossification** (from the Latin *os,* meaning bone). Ossification occurs in different ways in flat and long bones.

Ossification of Flat Bones

In the fetus, the flat bones (eg, those in the skull) consist of a thin connective tissue membrane. Ossification begins when **osteoblasts** (ŏs′tē-ə-blăsts″), or bone-forming cells, migrate to the region of the flat bones. The osteoblasts secrete calcium and other minerals into the spaces between the thin connective tissue membranes, thereby forming bone. This type of ossification involves the replacement of thin membrane with bone.

Ossification of Long Bones

Ossification of long bones occurs as bone tissue replaces cartilage. The fetal skeletal is composed largely of cartilage, and the layout of the cartilage in the fetus provides a model for bone formation (see Fig. 7–4). As the baby matures, osteoblasts invade the cartilage and gradually replace the cartilage with bone. This process continues in each long bone until all but the articular

cartilage and the epiphyseal disc have been replaced by bone. By the time the fetus has fully matured, most cartilage of the body has been replaced by bone. Only isolated pieces of cartilage, such as the bridge of the nose and the parts of the ribs, remain.

Growing Bones

Maturation from infancy to adulthood is characterized by two types of bone growth. Bones grow longitudinally and determine the height of an individual. Bones also grow thicker and become wider so as to support the weight of the adult body.

Growing Taller

Longitudinal bone growth occurs at the epiphyseal disc (also called the growth plate) (see Fig. 7–3A). The cartilage adjacent to the epiphysis continues to multiply and grow toward the diaphysis. The cartilage next to the diaphysis, however, is invaded by osteoblasts and becomes ossified. As long as the cartilage continues to form within the epiphyseal disc, the bone continues to lengthen. Longitudinal bone growth ceases when the epiphyseal disc becomes ossified.

The epiphyseal disc is sensitive to the effects of certain hormones, especially growth hormone and the sex hormones. Growth hormone stimulates growth at the epiphyseal disc, making the child taller. The sex hormones estrogen and testosterone, however, cause the epiphyseal disc to seal, or fuse, thereby inhibiting further longitudinal growth. Because the epiphyseal disc is especially sensitive to the effects of the female hormone estrogen, girls tend to be shorter than boys. After puberty, which is associated with increasing plasma levels of sex hormones, longitudinal growth eventually ceases.

Because the epiphyseal disc plays such a crucial role in longitudinal bone growth, injury to the

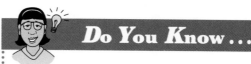

Do You Know . . .

Why are females generally shorter than males?

The epiphyseal disc is generally more sensitive to the effects of estrogen than to those of testosterone. During puberty in the female, the rising levels of estrogen seal the epiphyseal disc earlier than testosterone does in the male. The effects of the male hormone, testosterone, are felt at a later age. Thus, females stop growing at an earlier age than males do.

disc can severely retard bone growth. A child who injures the disc in a leg bone, for instance, may end up with that leg considerably shorter than the noninjured leg.

Growing Thicker and Wider

Long after longitudinal bone growth ceases, bones continue to increase in thickness and width. The bones are continuously being reshaped. Bone remodeling is accomplished by the combined actions of osteoblasts, which are bone-forming cells, and **osteoclasts** (ŏs'tē-ə-klăsts″), which are bone-destroying cells. Osteoblasts within the periosteum continuously deposit bone on the external bone surface.

Figure 7–5 shows the way in which osteoblastic activity works like a bricklayer. While osteoblasts build new bone, osteoclasts, found on the inner bone surface surrounding the medullary cavity, break down bone tissue, thereby hollowing out the interior of the bone. Osteoclastic activity is like sculpting. The bricklayer and the sculptor gradually create a large wide hollow bone that is strong but not too heavy.

One of the factors that stimulates bone growth is weight-bearing. Exercise keeps calcium in the bone and increases bone mass. The bones of bedridden or sedentary people tend to lose mass and are easily broken when stressed.

Bumps and Grooves

The surface of bone appears irregular and bumpy. This appearance is due to numerous

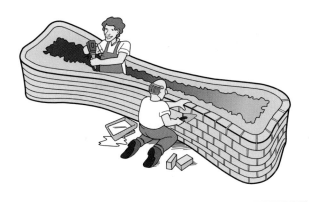

FIGURE 7–5 ● Bone remodeling. Osteoblasts (bricklayer) on the external bone lay down deposits of bone. Osteoclasts (sculptor) within the medullary cavity hollow out, or destroy, bone.

ridges, projections, depressions, and grooves called **bone markings.** The projecting bone markings (the markings that stick out) serve as points of attachment for muscles, tendons, and ligaments. The grooves and depressions form the routes traveled by blood vessels and nerves as they pass over and through the bones and joints. The projections and depressions also help to form joints. The head of the upper arm bone, for instance, fits into a depression in a shoulder bone, forming the shoulder joint. The specific bone markings are summarized in Table 7–1. Note the various markings on individual bones as they are described.

Table 7 • 1	BONE MARKINGS

BONE MARKINGS	DEFINITION
Projections/Processes	
Condyle	A large rounded knob that usually articulates with another bone
Epicondyle	An enlargement near or above a condyle
Head	An enlarged and rounded end of a bone
Facet	A small, flattened surface
Crest	A ridge on a bone
Process	A prominent projection on a bone
Spine	A sharp projection
Tubercle (tuberosity)	A knob-like projection
Trochanter	A large tubercle (tuberosity) found only on the femur
Depressions/Openings	
Foramen	An opening through a bone; usually serves as a passageway for nerves, blood vessels, and ligaments
Fossa	A depression or groove
Meatus	A tunnel or tube-like passageway
Sinus	A cavity or hollow space

Do You Know...

Why is osteoporosis so serious?

Osteoporosis (ŏs″tē-ō-pə-rō′sĭs) is a common bone disorder, especially in postmenopausal women. Osteoporosis is characterized by a decline in bone-making activity and the loss of bone tissue. As tissue is lost, the bones weaken and break. Common sites of fracture due to osteoporosis are the hip, wrist, and vertebrae. Osteoporosis may also affect the vertebral column. As the vertebrae collapse, nerves may be pinched, causing severe pain. The collapsed vertebrae also cause a shortening of the vertebral column and a change in its curvature. This change in shape, in turn, often impairs the functioning of organs such as the lungs.

Broken Bones

Occasionally, a bone breaks, or fractures (Fig. 7–6). A **simple fracture** is a break in which the overlying skin remains intact. Local tissue damage is minimal. A **compound fracture** is a broken bone that has also pierced the skin. The ends of the broken bone usually cause extensive tissue damage. The risk of infection is a concern with a compound fracture.

A **greenstick fracture** is an incomplete break in the bone. It usually occurs in children. Why is it called a greenstick fracture? If you were to bend a branch of a young tree, the branch would not snap and break apart completely. It would instead bend and perhaps break incompletely. The branch responds this way because it is young and pliable, much like a child's bone. Children's bones still have enough cartilaginous material to make them flexible.

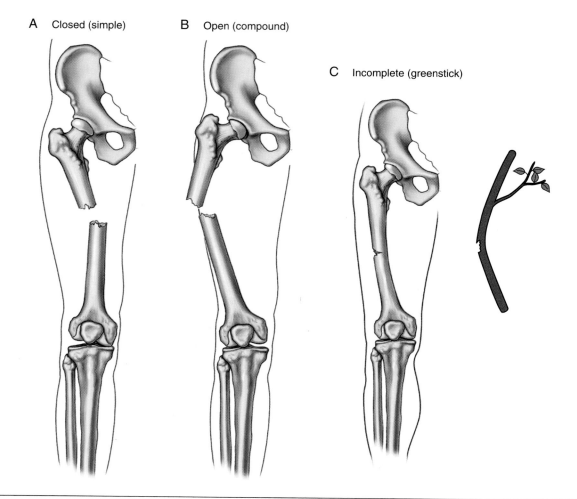

FIGURE 7–6 ● Common types of fractures: simple, compound, and greenstick fractures.

✳ **SUM IT UP!** The skeletal system consists of bones and joints as well as the cartilage and ligaments found in and around the joints. Bones are composed of two types of osseous tissue: compact (dense bone) and spongy (cancellous bone). Bones come in a variety of sizes and shapes. They are classified as long, short, flat, or irregular. We begin life in the womb as a skeleton-like frame made of cartilage and thin connective tissue membrane. With maturation, the process of ossification replaces most of the cartilage and certain connective tissue membrane. As a person matures, the skeleton enlarges, and bones grow longer, wider, and thicker.

 Do You Know...

What is a dislocation?

A dislocation, also called a **luxation,** is a displacement of a bone from its joint. As the bone slips out of its joint, ligaments and tendons are usually torn. Dislocations generally occur in response to an injury. Sometimes, however, the weight of a limb can cause a dislocation. For instance, a patient with paralysis involving the shoulder and arm may experience a **subluxation,** in which the weight of the paralyzed arm pulls the humerus out of the shoulder socket.

DIVISIONS OF THE SKELETAL SYSTEM

The skeleton is divided into the axial skeleton and the appendicular skeleton (see Fig. 7–1). The **axial skeleton** (ăk′sē-əl skĕl′ĭ-tn) includes the bones of the skull, the hyoid bone, the bones of the middle ear, the vertebral column, and the bony thorax. The **appendicular skeleton** (ăp″ən-dĭk′yə-lər skĕl′ĭ-tn) includes the bones of the extremities (arms and legs) and the bones of the hip and shoulder girdles. The names of the 206 bones of the skeleton are listed in Table 7–2.

Axial Skeleton

Skull

The skull is formed by two groups of bones: the cranium and the facial bones (Fig. 7–7). These bones also contain air spaces called **sinuses.**

CRANIUM. The **cranium** is a bony structure that encases and protects the brain. It is composed of eight bones.

Table 7•2	BONES OF THE ADULT SKELETON
BONES	**NUMBER**
Axial Skeleton (80)	
Skull (28)	
Cranium (8)	
Frontal	1
Parietal	2
Temporal	2
Occipital	1
Sphenoid	1
Ethmoid	1
Facial (14)	
Maxilla	2
Zygomatic	2
Palatine	2
Mandible	1
Lacrimal	2
Nasal	2
Inferior concha	2
Vomer	1
Middle Ear Bones (6)	
Malleus	2
Incus	2
Stapes	2
Hyoid Bone	1
Vertebral Column (26)	
Cervical vertebrae	7
Thoracic vertebrae	12
Lumbar vertebrae	5
Sacrum	1
Coccyx	1
Thoracic Cage (25)	
True ribs	14
False ribs	10
Sternum	1
Appendicular Skeleton (126)	
Pectoral girdle (4)	
Scapula	2
Clavicle	2
Upper limbs (60)	
Humerus	2
Radius	2
Ulna	2
Carpals	16
Metacarpals	10
Phalanges	28
Pelvic girdle (2)	
Os coxae	2
Lower limbs (60)	
Femur	2
Tibia	2
Fibula	2
Patella	2
Tarsals	14
Metatarsals	10
Phalanges	28
Total number of bones	**206**

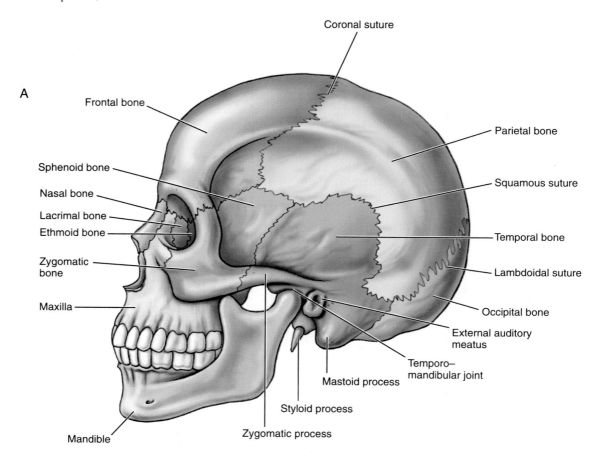

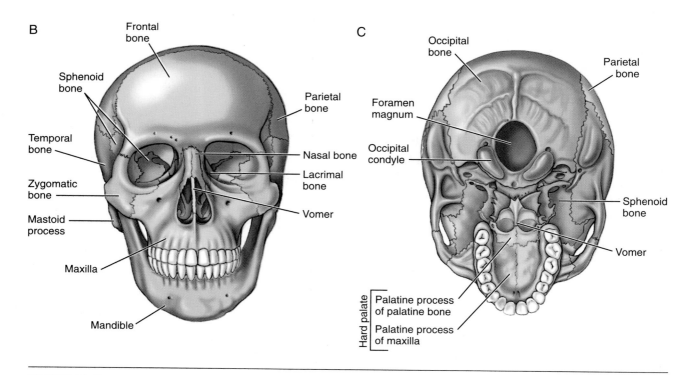

FIGURE 7–7 ● Bones of the skull. A, Side view. B, Front view. C, Base of the skull.

- *Frontal bone.* The **frontal bone** forms the forehead, part of the nose, and part of the bony structure surrounding the eyes.
- *Parietal bones.* The two **parietal bones** form most of the top of the head and part of the sides of the head.
- *Temporal bones.* The two **temporal bones** are on the sides of the head, close to the ears. Several important bone markings are found on the temporal bones. They include

External auditory meatus, the opening for the ear

Zygomatic process, which forms part of the cheekbone

Styloid process, a sharp projection used as a point of attachment for several muscles associated with the tongue and larynx

Mastoid process, which forms a point of attachment for some of the muscles of the neck

- *Occipital bone* (see Fig. 7–7C). The **occipital bone** is located at the base of the skull. The large hole in the occipital bone is called the **foramen magnum.** On either side of the foramen magnum are bony projections (occipital condyles) that sit on the first vertebra of the vertebral column.
- *Sphenoid bone.* The **sphenoid bone** is a butterfly-shaped bone that forms part of the floor and sides of the cranium (see Fig. 7–7C). The sphenoid bone also forms part of the orbits surrounding the eyes. In the midline of the sphenoid bone is a depression called the **sella turcica** (Turk's saddle); it forms the seat for the pituitary gland (not shown).
- *Ethmoid bone.* The **ethmoid bone** is an irregularly shaped bone that helps form the bony structure of the nasal cavity.

FACIAL BONES. There are 14 facial bones, most of which are paired (see Fig. 7–7). Only the mandible and the vomer are single bones.

- *Mandible.* The **mandible,** the lower jaw bone, forms the only freely movable joint in the skull. The anterior portion of the mandible forms the chin. Two posterior upright projections on the mandible have bony processes. These articulate with the temporal bones at the **temporomandibular joint.** These processes are points of attachment for chewing muscles. The lower teeth are located in this bone. Tension or stress often causes pain in the temporomandibular joint (TMJ). This condition is often associated with tooth grinding (bruxism) during sleep.
- *Maxilla.* Two maxillary bones fuse to form the upper jaw. The **maxilla** carries the upper teeth. An extension of the maxilla, the **palatine process,** forms the anterior portion of the hard palate (roof) of the mouth (see Fig. 7–7C). These bones also form parts of the nasal cavity and the eye orbits.

Do You Know...

What is TMJ discomfort?

The **temporomandibular joint (TMJ)** is the articulation of the mandible and the temporal bone. It can be felt as the depression immediately in front of the opening of the ear. TMJ discomfort is often attributed to stress, because "stressed out" persons tend to clench their jaws.

- *Palatine bones.* Two **palatine bones** form the posterior part of the hard palate and the floor of the nasal cavity. Failure of the palatine bones to fuse causes a cleft palate, making suckling very difficult for an infant. Fortunately, a cleft palate can be surgically repaired.
- *Zygomatic bones.* The **zygomatic bones** are the cheekbones. They also form a part of the orbits of the eyes.
- *Other Facial Bones.* Several other bones complete the facial structure. These bones include the lacrimal bones, the nasal bones, the vomer bone, and the inferior nasal conchae.

SINUSES. **Sinuses,** air-filled cavities located in several of the bones of the skull, perform two important functions. First, they lessen the weight of the skull because they are empty cavities rather than solid bone. Second, they amplify and increase the sound of the voice.

There are four sinuses (Fig. 7–8). They are called the **paranasal sinuses** because they surround and connect with the nasal structures. The names of the four sinuses reflect their location within the various skull bones: frontal sinus, ethmoidal sinus, sphenoidal sinus, and maxillary sinus.

Because the sinuses connect with the nasal passages and the throat, infections may spread from the nose and throat into the sinuses. Such infections are called sinusitis. They are experienced

Do You Know...

What is a cleft palate?

Occasionally, an infant is born with a hole in the roof of the mouth, a condition called cleft palate. Cleft palate is caused by the failure of the palatine processes of the maxilla and/or the palatine bones to fuse. With a hole in the roof of the mouth, the infant experiences considerable difficulty in suckling.

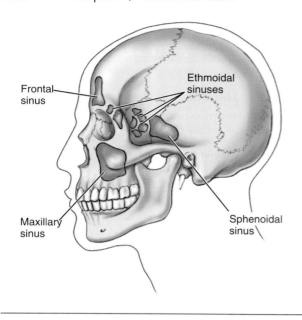

FIGURE 7–8 ● Sinuses: frontal, ethmoidal, maxillary, and sphenoidal.

as stuffiness and pain in the overlying facial regions.

HOW THE SKULL BONES HOLD TOGETHER. The bones of the adult skull form a unique kind of joint called a **suture** (see Fig. 7–7). The suture joins the bones of the skull much like a zipper. The major sutures include the coronal suture (meaning crown, from the Latin *corona*), the lambdoidal suture, and the squamosal suture. Unlike other bones in the body, no significant movement occurs between cranial bones.

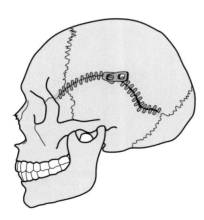

THE INFANT SKULL. The two major differences between the infant skull and the adult skull are fontanels and unfused sutures.

The infant skull has areas that have not yet been converted to bone. Instead, they are covered by fibrous membrane. Because these areas are soft to touch, they are called the baby's soft spots. Also, the rhythm of the baby's pulse can be felt in

Do You Know...

Why do allergies sometimes make your face hurt?

Allergies often cause the membranes that line the facial sinuses to oversecrete mucus. The mucus forms an excellent medium for bacterial growth. As the mucus accumulates and the membranes swell, pressure and discomfort are often experienced in the facial region, which overlies the sinuses (around the eyes and nose).

these soft spots, and so they are called **fontanels** (fŏn″tə-nĕlz′), meaning "little fountain(s)."

The two major fontanels are a larger diamond-shaped **anterior fontanel** and a smaller posterior triangular **occipital fontanel** (Fig. 7–9). By the time the child reaches 2 years of age, these fontanels have been gradually converted to bone and can no longer be felt.

The fontanels are one reason that the infant skull bones are more movable than those of the adult skull. Another reason is that the sutures of the infant skulls are not fused. Unfused sutures allow the skull to be compressed during birth. They also allow for the continued growth of the brain and skull after birth and throughout infancy.

Occasionally, the sutures of the infant skull fuse too early, preventing the growth of the brain. This condition is called **microcephalia** and is characterized by a small skull and impaired intellectual functioning. Sometimes, the skull expands too much. For instance, if excessive fluid accumulates within the brain of an infant, the bones are forced apart, and the skull enlarges. This condi-

Do You Know...

What does a bulging or sunken fontanel indicate?

If an infant suffers a severe head injury, the brain may swell. Because the fontanel is soft tissue, it will bulge outward in response to increasing pressure within the skull. Observation of the fontanels can therefore provide valuable information regarding the degree of brain swelling. Conversely, the fontanels may flatten out. If the infant is dehydrated, blood volume is low. In response to dehydration, the fontanels appear sunken. Thus the fontanels can indicate increases or decreases in pressure within the skull.

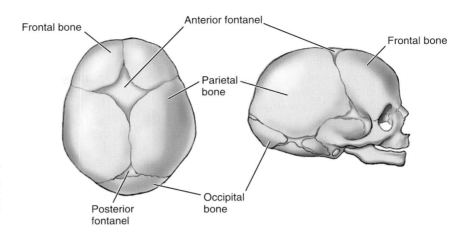

FIGURE 7-9 • Fontanels in the infant skull. The two largest fontanels are the anterior fontanel and the posterior fontanel.

tion is called **hydrocephalus** (or what laypersons call "water on the brain").

HYOID BONE. The **hyoid bone** is a U-shaped bone located in the neck. It anchors the tongue and is associated with swallowing. It is the only bone in the body that does not articulate with another bone.

BONES OF THE MIDDLE EAR. Each ear contains three small bones: the tiny ear bones are called **ossicles.** (They are described further in Chapter 11.)

Vertebral Column

The **vertebral column,** or backbone, extends from the skull to the pelvis (Fig. 7–10). The vertebral column consists of a series of bones called **vertebrae.** The vertebrae are stacked in a column, hence the term vertebral column. Sitting between each vertebra is a cartilaginous disc that acts as a shock absorber. The vertebral column performs four major functions: it forms a supporting structure for the head and thorax; it forms an attachment for the pelvic girdle; it encases and protects the spinal cord as it extends from the brain into the lumbar area; and it provides flexibility for the body.

The vertebrae are named according to their location in the body. For instance, the seven cervical vertebrae (C1 to C7) are located in the neck region; the 12 thoracic vertebrae (T1 to T12) are located in the chest region; and the five lumbar vertebrae (L1 to L5) are located in the lower back region. In addition, five sacral vertebrae fuse into one sacrum. The **sacrum** forms the posterior wall of the pelvis. Four to five small coccygeal verte-

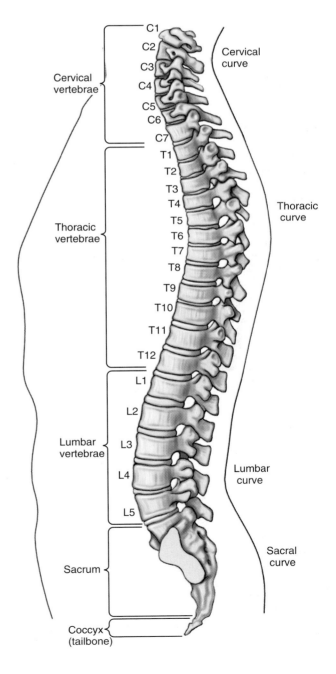

FIGURE 7-10 • Vertebral column, composed of seven cervical vertebrae, 12 thoracic vertebrae, five lumbar vertebrae, the sacrum, and the coccyx. The vertebral column has four curves: the cervical curve, the thoracic curve, the lumbar curve, and the sacral curve.

brae fuse into one **coccyx,** the tailbone. The adult has 26 vertebrae.

CURVATURES. When viewed from the side, the vertebral column has four normal curvatures (see Fig. 7–10): the cervical curve, the thoracic curve, the lumbar curve, and the sacral curve. The directions of the curvatures are important. The cervical and the lumbar curvatures are convex so that they bend forward, toward the front of the body. The thoracic and sacral curvatures are concave so that they bend backward, away from the front of the body. These curves center the head over the body, thereby providing the balance needed to walk in an upright position.

The curvature of the fetal spine is different. Its single curvature is concave, turned away from the front of the body. The cervical curvature develops about 3 to 4 months after birth as infants start to hold their heads up. The lumbar curvature develops at about 1 year of age, when the child begins walking

Figure 7–11 illustrates several abnormal curvatures of the spine. **Scoliosis** (skō″lē-ō′sĭs) refers to a lateral curvature, usually involving the thoracic vertebrae. If severe, a lateral curvature can compress abdominal organs. It can also diminish expansion of the rib cage and therefore impair breathing. **Kyphosis** is an exaggerated thoracic curvature. It is sometimes called hunchback. **Lordosis** is an exaggerated lumbar curvature and is sometimes called swayback. These abnormalities may be due to a genetic defect or may develop in response to disease or poor posture.

CHARACTERISTICS OF VERTEBRAE. The vertebra is an irregular bone that contains several distinct structures (Fig. 7–12). The body of the vertebra is padded by a cartilaginous disc and supports the weight of the vertebra sitting on top of it. Various processes provide sites of attachment for or articulation with ligaments, muscles, and other bones. The **vertebral foramen** is the opening for the spinal cord. The vertebrae are aligned so that, if you run your hand down your back, you will feel the spinous processes. For this reason, the vertebral column is also called the **spine.** Note that the vertebrae become larger as the vertebral column descends. The larger lower vertebrae carry a heavier load.

The vertebra has a bar-like lamina. A surgical procedure called a **laminectomy** may be performed to remove a damaged disc. Occasionally several vertebrae are fused together to stabilize a part of the vertebral column. This procedure is a **spinal fusion.**

TWO SPECIAL VERTEBRAE: ATLAS (C1) AND AXIS (C2). The first and second cervical vertebrae have several special features (see Fig. 7–12). The first cervical vertebra (C1) is called the **atlas.** The atlas has no body but does have depressions into which fit the bony projections of the occipital bone of the skull. The atlas supports the skull and allows you to nod "yes." The atlas is named after a figure in Greek mythology, Atlas, who carried the earth on his shoulders.

The second cervical vertebra (C2) is called the **axis.** The axis has a projection that fits into the atlas and acts as a pivot or swivel for the atlas. The axis allows your head to rotate from side to side as you say "no."

INTERVERTEBRAL DISCS. A layer of cartilage called a disc separates the vertebrae from each other. Because the discs are located between the vertebrae, they are called **intervertebral discs.** Discs create spaces for the spinal nerves. The disc

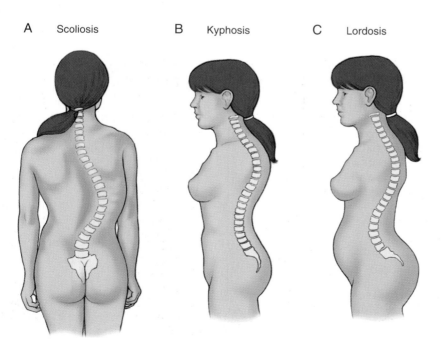

A Scoliosis   B Kyphosis   C Lordosis

FIGURE 7–11 ● Abnormal curvatures of the vertebral column. A, Scoliosis. B, Kyphosis ("hunchback"). C, Lordosis ("swayback").

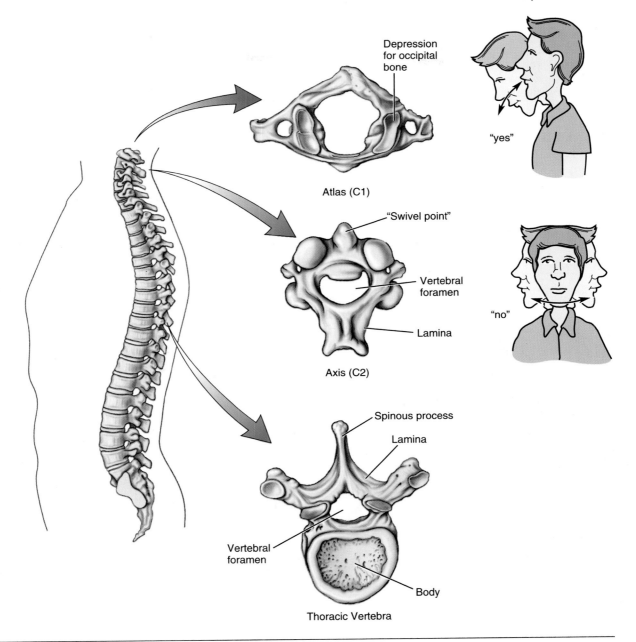

Depression for occipital bone

"yes"

Atlas (C1)

"Swivel point"

Vertebral foramen

Lamina

"no"

Axis (C2)

Spinous process

Lamina

Vertebral foramen

Body

Thoracic Vertebra

FIGURE 7-12 ● Anatomy of a vertebra: the atlas (C1), the axis (C2), and the thoracic vertebrae.

also acts like a cushion, preventing any grinding between vertebrae and absorbing the shock associated with running, jumping, and walking.

Occasionally, a disc slips out of place and puts pressure on a surrounding nerve. This pressure causes extreme pain and may require the surgical removal of the protruding disc.

Thoracic Cage

The thoracic cage is a bony cone-shaped cage that surrounds and protects the lungs, heart, and large blood vessels (Fig. 7–13). It plays a crucial role in breathing and helps to support the bones of the shoulder. The thoracic cage is composed of the sternum, the ribs, and thoracic vertebrae.

STERNUM. The **sternum,** or breastbone, is a dagger-shaped bone located on the anterior chest. The three parts are the **manubrium,** the **body,** and the **xiphoid process.** The xiphoid process is the tip of the sternum. It serves as a landmark for CPR (cardiopulmonary resuscitation).

RIBS. Twelve pairs of ribs attach posteriorly to the thoracic vertebrae. Anteriorly, the top seven pairs of ribs attach directly to the sternum by costal cartilage. They are called **true ribs.** The next five pairs attach indirectly to the sternum or do not attach at all. They are called **false ribs.** The bottom two pairs of false ribs lack sternal attachment and are therefore called **floating ribs.** Because of their location and lack of sternal support, the floating ribs are easily broken.

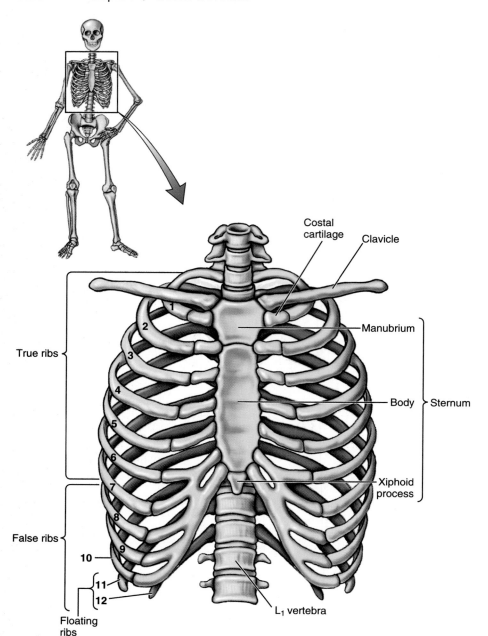

FIGURE 7–13 ● Thoracic cage. The sternum is composed of the manubrium, body, and xiphoid process. The ribs are both true and false.

Do You Know...

What is a sternal puncture?

Because the sternum is a site of red blood cell production and because it is so accessible by needle, the sternum is a common site of **bone marrow biopsy**. In this procedure, a needle is inserted into the sternum. A sample of bone marrow is aspirated, or withdrawn, from this site and analyzed under a microscope. The analysis of the bone marrow sample provides information on the numbers, types, and general health of the blood cells.

Located between the ribs are the intercostal muscles. Contraction of these muscles helps to move the thoracic cage during breathing. If you put your hand on your chest and take a deep breath, you will feel your thoracic cage move up and out.

Appendicular Skeleton

The appendicular skeleton is composed of the bones of the shoulder girdle, upper limbs (arms), pelvic girdle, and lower limbs (thighs and legs) (see Fig. 7–1).

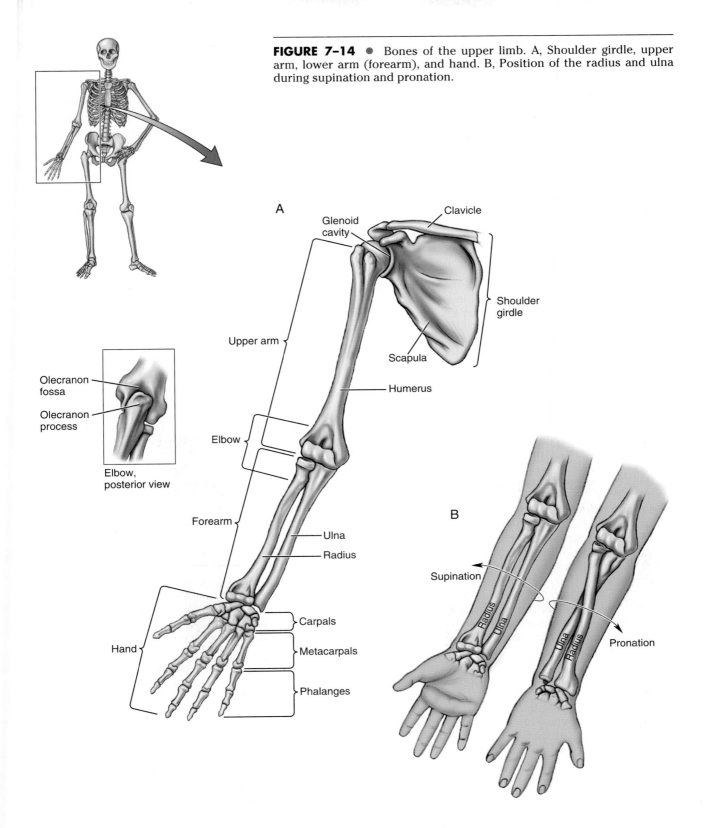

FIGURE 7–14 ● Bones of the upper limb. A, Shoulder girdle, upper arm, lower arm (forearm), and hand. B, Position of the radius and ulna during supination and pronation.

A

Glenoid cavity

Clavicle

Shoulder girdle

Scapula

Humerus

Upper arm

Olecranon fossa

Olecranon process

Elbow, posterior view

Elbow

Forearm

Ulna

Radius

B

Supination

Radius

Ulna

Ulna

Radius

Pronation

Hand

Carpals

Metacarpals

Phalanges

Shoulder Girdle

The **shoulder girdle** is also called the **pectoral girdle.** Each shoulder contains two bones: one clavicle and one scapula (Fig. 7–14). The shoulder supports the arms and serves as a place of attachment for the muscles. The shoulder girdle is designed for great flexibility. Move your shoulder and upper arm around and note how many different movements you can make. Compare this with the limited movement you have at the elbow and the knee.

CLAVICLE. The **clavicle** is also called the collarbone. It looks like a long rod and articulates with both the sternum and the scapula. The clavicle helps stabilize the shoulder. The attachment, how-

125

ever, is weak and is easily dislocated or broken. The clavicle is the most frequently broken bone in the body.

SCAPULA. The **scapula** is also called the shoulder blade or wing bone. Two large processes on the scapula allow it to articulate with the clavicle and serve as points of attachment for arm and chest muscles. The **glenoid cavity** on the scapula is the site where the head of the **humerus** (upper arm bone) fits, thereby allowing you to rotate your arm at the shoulder.

Upper Extremities (Arms)

The upper limb contains the bones of the upper arm (humerus), the forearm (ulna and radius), and the hand (carpals, metacarpals, and phalanges).

HUMERUS. The humerus is the long bone of the upper arm. The humerus contains a **head,** which fits into the glenoid cavity of the scapula, allowing the upper arm to rotate at the shoulder joint. At the other (distal) end of the humerus are several processes that allow it to articulate with the bones of the lower arm. The **olecranon fossa** is a depression of the humerus that holds the **olecranon process** of the ulna when the elbow is extended.

RADIUS. The **radius** is one of two bones of the forearm. It is located on the "thumb side" when the palm of the hand is facing forward. The head of the radius articulates with both the humerus and the ulna. The **radial tuberosity** at the proximal end of the radius is the site of attachment for the muscle, which is responsible for bending the forearm at the elbow.

ULNA. The **ulna** is the second bone of the forearm. The longer of the two bones, the ulna, is located on the little finger side of the forearm. It has processes and depressions that allow it to articulate with the humerus, radius, and bones of the wrist (the carpals). The olecranon process of the ulna is what you feel as the bony point of the elbow.

Note the relationship of the radius to the ulna when the hand moves from a palm up (supination) to a palm down (pronation) position. When the palm is up, the two bones are parallel. When the palm is down, the two bones cross to achieve this movement.

HAND. The hand is composed of a wrist, palm, and fingers. The wrist contains eight bones called **carpal bones,** which are tightly bound by ligaments. Five **metacarpal** bones form the palm of the hand; each metacarpal bone is in line with a finger. The 14 finger bones are called **phalanges,** or **digits.** Note that each digit has three bones except the thumb, which has only two bones. The heads of the phalanges are prominent as the knuckles when a fist is made.

Pelvic Girdle

The **pelvic girdle,** or **pelvis,** is composed of two coxal bones, the sacrum and the coccyx (Fig. 7–15A). The pelvic girdle performs three functions: it bears the weight of the body; it serves as a place of attachment for the legs; and it protects the organs located in the pelvic cavity, including the urinary bladder and the reproductive organs.

MALE AND FEMALE DIFFERENCES. The differences between the female and the male pelvis are related to the child-bearing role of the female. In general, the female pelvis is larger and shallower than the male pelvis. (See Fig. 7–15C and D.)

COXAL BONE. The **coxal bone** is called the **os coxae,** or hip bone (Fig. 7–15B). Each coxal bone is composed of three parts: the ilium, the ischium, and the pubis. The three bones join together to form a depression called the **acetabulum.** The acetabulum is important because it receives the head of the femur and therefore enables the thigh to rotate at the hip joint.

Ilium. The **ilium** is the largest part of the coxal bone. The ilium is the flared upper part of the bone and can be felt as the hip. The outer edge of the ilium is called the **iliac crest.** The ilium connects in the back with the sacrum, forming the **sacroiliac joint.** Like the sternum, the ilium produces blood cells and is a common site for bone marrow biopsy.

Ischium. The **ischium** is the most inferior part of the coxal bone. The ischium contains three important structures: the ischial tuberosity, the ischial spine, and the greater sciatic notch. The **ischial tuberosity** is the part of the coxal bone on which you sit. The **ischial spine** projects into the pelvic cavity and narrows the outlet of the pelvis. If the spines of a woman's two ischial bones are too close together, the pelvic outlet becomes too small to allow for the birth of a baby. The measurement of the distance between the two spines therefore provides valuable information as to the adequacy of the pelvis for child-bearing. The **greater sciatic notch** is the site where blood vessels and the sciatic nerve pass from the pelvic cavity into the posterior thigh region.

Pubis. The **pubis** is the most anterior part of the coxal bone. The two pubic bones join together in front as the **symphysis pubis.** A disc of cartilage separates the pubic bones at the symphysis pubis. In women, the disc expands in response to the hormones of pregnancy, thereby enlarging the pelvic cavity to provide a bigger space for the growing fetus.

A large hole called the **obturator foramen** is formed as the pubic bone fuses with a part of the ischium. The obturator is the largest foramen in the body. Blood vessels and nerves pass through the obturator foramen from the pelvic cavity into the anterior thigh.

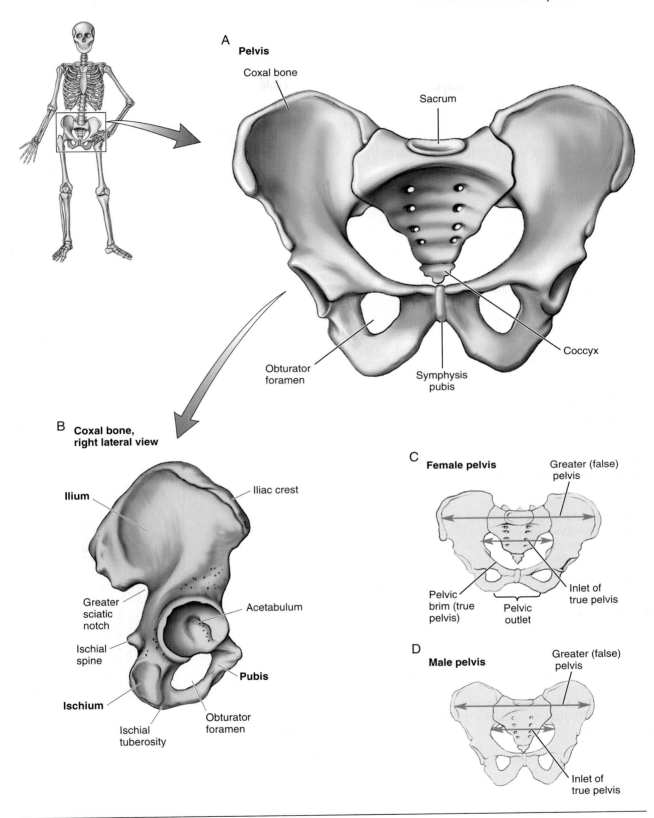

FIGURE 7-15 ● Pelvic cavity. A, Bones that make up the pelvic cavity. B, Coxal bone (ilium, ischium, and pubis). C, Female pelvis. D, Male pelvis.

What is meant by the true and false pelvis? The false pelvis is the area surrounded by the flaring parts of the two iliac bones (see Fig. 7–15C). The true pelvis lies below the false pelvis and is much smaller. The true pelvis is a ring formed by the fusion of the pelvic bones; it is also called the **pelvic brim.** The true pelvis has an inlet and an outlet area. In women, the dimensions of these areas are important because they must be large enough to allow for the passage of an infant during childbirth.

Lower Extremities

The lower limb includes the bones of the thigh (femur), the kneecap (patella), the lower leg (tibia and fibula), and the foot (tarsals, metatarsals, and phalanges) (Fig. 7–16).

FEMUR. The **femur** is the thighbone; it is the longest and strongest bone in the body. The femur articulates with the coxal bone to form the hip and with the bones of the lower leg to form the knee. The head of the femur sits in the acetabulum of the coxal bone and allows the thigh to rotate at the hip joint. The head of the femur continues as the neck. There are a number of bony processes on the femur. The most important are the **greater** and **lesser trochanters.** These trochanters provide sites of attachment for many muscles.

In older persons, the neck of the femur often breaks, causing a broken hip. Immobility may then cause serious complications. For example, because of the weight of the leg, an immobile, bedridden person may experience an outward rotation of the hip. If allowed to develop, this outward rotation makes walking very difficult and therefore delays rehabilitation. To prevent the outward rotation of the hip, a trochanter roll should be placed under the hip at the site of the greater trochanter.

PATELLA. The **patella** is the kneecap. It is located within a tendon that passes over the knee.

TIBIA AND FIBULA. The tibia and the fibula form the lower leg. The **tibia** is the shinbone and articulates with the femur at the knee. The tibia is the weight-bearing bone of the lower leg. A protuberance called the **tibial tuberosity** is the site of attachment for the ligaments from the thigh. At the distal end of the tibia, a protuberance called the **medial malleolus** articulates with the inner ankle bones.

FIGURE 7–16 • Bones of the lower limb, thigh, lower leg, and foot. The femur contains the head, neck, greater and lesser trochanters, and lateral condyle. The tibia, or shinbone, contains the tibial tuberosity and the medial malleolus. The fibula contains the lateral malleolus.

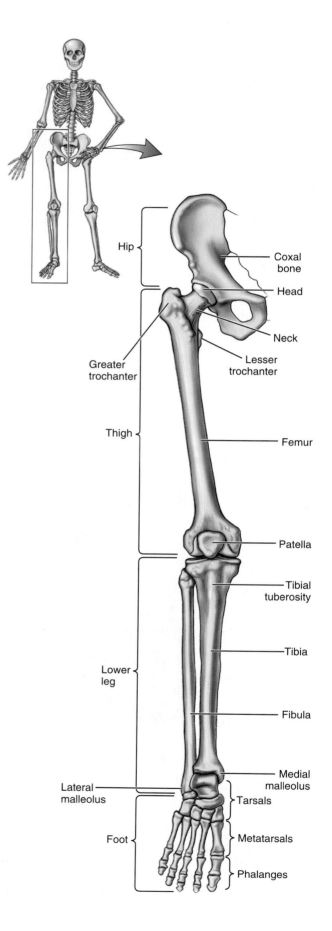

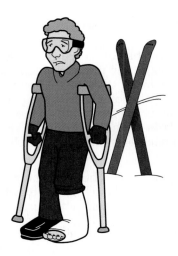

FOOT. Each foot (Fig. 7–17) has an ankle, an instep, and five toes. The seven **tarsal bones** form the ankle. These include the **calcaneus,** or heelbone, and the **talus,** the only freely movable tarsal bone. The talus articulates with the tibia and fibula. The weight of the body is supported primarily by the calcaneus and the talus. The instep of the foot is formed by five **metatarsal bones.** The ball of the foot is formed by the distal ends of the metatarsals. The tarsals, metatarsals, and associated tendons and ligaments form the arches of the foot. If the ligaments and tendons weaken, the arches can "fall," and the person is said to have flat feet. The toes contain 14 phalanges.

Footnotes: A person may develop a **heel spur.** A spur is excessive bone growth on the bottom of the calcaneus. The spur inflames the overlying tissue, making walking very painful. The footnote that many women know all too well: bunions develop in response to the continued abuse of poorly fitting high heels, whereby the big toe is compressed and forced toward the second toe. Over time, this position damages the joint, causing pain and deformity (see Fig. 7–17).

The **fibula** is the thinner bone positioned alongside the tibia in the lower leg. The proximal end of the fibula articulates with the tibia. The lower end forms the **lateral malleolus,** which articulates with the outer ankle bones.

Skiers frequently twist their ankles and break the fibula at the lateral malleolus.

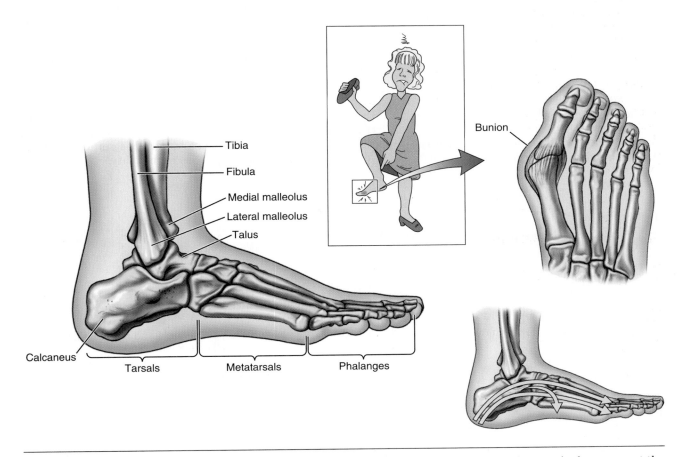

FIGURE 7–17 • Foot: tarsals (including the calcaneus and talus), metatarsals, and phalanges. Arches support the structure of the foot. Foot abuse: spiked heels lead to a bunion.

✳ **SUM IT UP!** The skeleton is divided into the axial and appendicular skeleton. The 206 bones of the skeleton appear in Table 7–2 and Figure 7–1.

JOINTS (ARTICULATIONS)

A joint, or **articulation** (är-tĭk″yə-lā′shən), is the site where two bones meet. Joints perform two functions: they hold the bones together, and they provide flexibility to a rigid skeleton. Without joints, we would move around stiffly like robots. Think of how awkward a basketball player would look if the entire skeleton were rigid! Joints can be classified into three groups according to the amount of movement: immovable, slightly movable, and freely movable (Table 7–3).

Immovable Joints

Immovable joints are called **synarthroses** (sĭn″är-thrō′sēz). The sutures in the skull are immovable joints. The sutures are formed as the irregular edges of the skull bones interlock and are bound by fibrous connective tissue.

Slightly Movable Joints

Slightly movable joints are called **amphiarthroses** (ăm″fē-är-thrō′sēz). Limited movement is usually achieved by bones connected by a cartilaginous disc. For instance, movement of the spinal column occurs at the intervertebral discs. Also, during pregnancy, the symphysis pubis allows the pelvis to widen.

Freely Movable Joints

Freely movable joints are called **diarthroses** (dī′är-thrō′sēz); they provide much more flexibility and movement than the other two types of joints. Most of the joints of the skeletal system are freely movable. All freely movable joints are **synovial joints** (sĭ-nō′vē-əl joints) (Fig. 7–18). A typical synovial joint includes the following structures:

- *Articular cartilage.* The articulating surface of each of the two bones is lined with **articular cartilage,** forming a smooth surface within the joint.
- *Joint capsule.* The **joint capsule** is made of fibrous connective tissue. It encloses the joint in a strong sleeve-like covering.
- *Synovial membrane.* Lining the joint capsule is the **synovial membrane.** This membrane secretes synovial fluid into the joint cavity.
- *Synovial fluid.* **Synovial fluid** lubricates the bones in the joint, thereby decreasing the friction within the joint.
- *Bursae.* Many synovial joints contain **bursae** (singular, bursa). Bursae are small sacs of synovial fluid between the joint and the tendons that cross over the joint. Bursae permit the tendons to slide as the bones move. Excessive use of a joint may cause a painful inflammation of the bursae, called **bursitis.** Tennis elbow is a bursitis caused by excessive and improper use of the elbow joint.
- *Supporting ligaments.* Surrounding the joint are **supporting ligaments.** These ligaments join the articulating bones together and stabilize the joint. Sometimes a ligament is stretched or torn, causing pain and loss of mobility.

Table 7 • 3	TYPES OF JOINTS		
TYPE	**DEGREE OF MOTION**	**DESCRIPTION**	**EXAMPLE**
Synarthrosis	Immovable	Suture/"zipper"	Cranial bones
Amphiarthrosis	Slightly movable	Disc of cartilage between two bones	Intervertebral discs; symphysis pubis
Diarthrosis	Freely movable	Ball and socket	Shoulder (scapula and humerus); hip (pelvic bone and femur)
		Hinge	Elbow (humerus and ulna); knee (femur and tibia); fingers
		Pivot	Atlas and axis; allows for rotation (side-to-side movement) of the head, indicating "no"
		Saddle	Thumb (carpometacarpal joint)
		Gliding	Carpals
		Condyloid	Temporal bone and mandible (jaw); knuckles

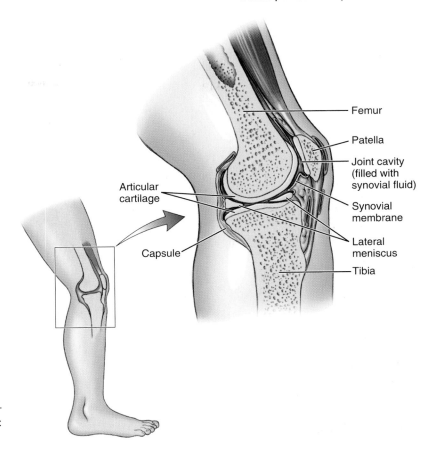

Femur
Patella
Joint cavity (filled with synovial fluid)
Synovial membrane
Lateral meniscus
Tibia
Articular cartilage
Capsule

FIGURE 7–18 ● Synovial joint (knee): structure and contents.

Knee: A Synovial Joint

The knee joint is an example of a synovial joint (see Fig. 7–18). In addition to all the structures contained in a synovial joint, the knee joint contains extra cushioning in the form of pads of cartilage. These pads absorb the shock of walking and jumping. Two crescent-shaped pads of cartilage, the **medial meniscus** and the **lateral meniscus,** rest on the tibia. Like other synovial joints, the knee joint is reinforced by supporting ligaments, the cruciate ligament in particular.

The medial meniscus and lateral meniscus are frequently injured or torn by athletes. A torn cartilage (usually the medial meniscus) is removed by arthroscopic surgery. An arthroscope is a viewing tube that allows the surgeon to see into the knee joint. The cruciate ligament is another structure that often requires surgical repair.

Moving Synovial Joints

There are many types of freely movable synovial joints. The type of motion and the degree of flexibility vary with each type of joint. For instance, if you move your elbow, your lower arm will move either up or down like two boards joined by a hinge. This motion is very different from the arm-swinging motion at the shoulder joint. Both the elbow and the shoulder joints are freely movable, but the types of movement differ.

Six types of freely movable joints are classified according to the type of movement allowed by the joint (Fig. 7–19 and see Table 7–3). Three of these joints are the hinge, the ball-and-socket, and the pivot joints.

Hinge Joint

The **hinge joint** allows movement similar to the movement of two boards joined together by a hinge. The hinge allows movement in one direction, where the angle at the hinge increases or decreases. Hinge joints include elbows, knees, and fingers. Move each of these joints to clarify the movement described here.

Ball-and-Socket Joint

A **ball-and-socket joint** is formed when the ball-shaped end of one bone fits into the cup-shaped socket of another bone, so that the bones can move in many directions around a central point. The shoulder and hip joints are ball-and-

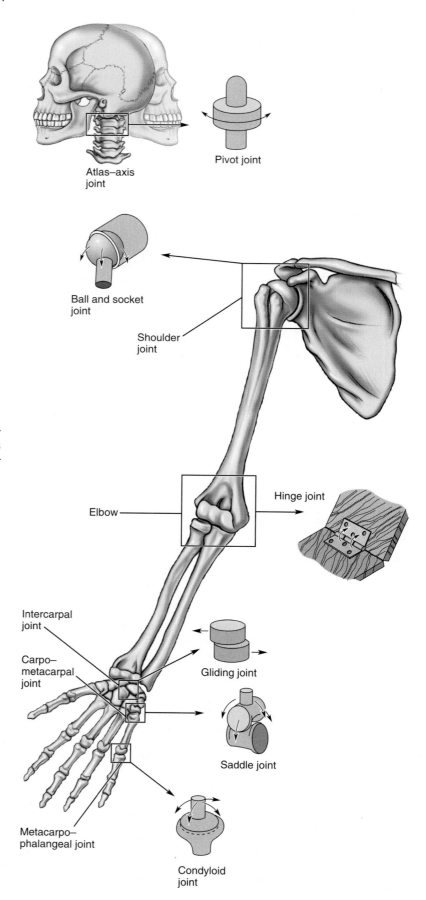

FIGURE 7–19 • Freely movable joints (diarthroses): ball-and-socket, hinge, gliding, saddle, condyloid, and pivot joints.

socket joints. The head of the humerus fits into the glenoid cavity of the scapula in the shoulder joint. The head of the femur fits into the acetabulum of the coxal bone in the hip joint.

Move your shoulder all around (as in pitching a softball) and note the freedom of movement. Compare this movement with the limited movement at the elbow or knee joints. While the arrangement of the ball-and-socket joints allow for a wide range of movement, it also allows for easy displacement of the joint structures. When a strong force is applied to the shoulder, for instance, a dislocation may occur. Dislocations occur frequently when football players are thrown to the ground.

Pivot Joint

A **pivot joint** allows for rotation around the length of a bone. The pivot joint allows only for rotation. An example is the side-to-side movement of the head indicating "no." This rotation occurs as the atlas (first cervical vertebra) swivels around, or pivots, on the axis (second cervical vertebra).

Aching Joints

A number of health problems affect joints, generally causing discomfort and impaired mobility. **Arthritis** refers to an inflammation of a joint. In time the joint may deteriorate to the point where it needs to be replaced. Synthetic joints have been designed for replacement of most joints, including the hip, knee, shoulder, and elbow joints. **Gout** can also affect joints. With this disease, the body overproduces a substance called uric acid. The excess uric acid accumulates in the joints and forms small, razor-sharp crystals. These crystals damage the joint and may also injure the kidney as the body attempts to excrete the uric acid in the urine.

Types of Joint Movements

Movements at synovial joints occur when the muscles that lie across the joints contract and exert pressure on the attached bone. These movements are illustrated in Figure 7–20.

- *Flexion* (flĕk'shən): the bending of a joint that decreases the angle between the bones (eg, bending the leg at the knee or bending the fingers)
- *Extension* (ĕk-stĕn'shən): the straightening of a joint so that the angle between the bones in-

creases (eg, straightening the leg at the knee, straightening the fingers to open the hand)
- *Plantar flexion:* bending the foot down, as in toe dancing
- *Dorsiflexion:* bending the foot up toward the leg
- *Hyperextension:* overextending the joint beyond its normally straightened position, as in moving the hand toward the upper surface of the wrist
- *Abduction* (ăb-dŭk'shən): movement away from the midline of the body (eg, move your leg sideways, away from your body)
- *Adduction* (ə-dŭk'shən): movement toward the midline of the body (eg, return your leg toward your body)
- *Inversion:* turning the sole of the foot inward so that it faces the opposite foot
- *Eversion:* turning the sole of the foot outward
- *Supination:* turning the hand so that the palm faces upward
- *Pronation:* turning the hand so that the hand faces downward
- *Circumduction:* a combination of movements, as in the circular arm movement that a softball pitcher makes while pitching the ball

✳ **SUM IT UP!** A joint, or articulation, is the place where two or more bones meet. Three types of joints are immovable joints (synarthroses), slightly movable joints (amphiarthroses), and freely movable joints (diarthroses). Freely movable joints are also called synovial joints. Types of freely movable joints include hinge, ball-and-socket, and pivot joints. Because of the diverse types of joints, the skeleton is capable of various movements.

As You Age

1. Because of loss of calcium and organic material, bones are less strong and more brittle. Many older women develop osteoporosis. As a result, bones fracture more easily. Moreover, fractured bones heal incompletely and more slowly.

2. Tendons and ligaments are less flexible. As a result, joints have a decreased range of motion. A thinning of the articular cartilage and bony overgrowths in the joints contributes to joint stiffness.

3. The intervertebral discs shrink. Because of the compressed discs and the loss of bone mass, body height decreases and the thoracic spine curves (causing kyphosis).

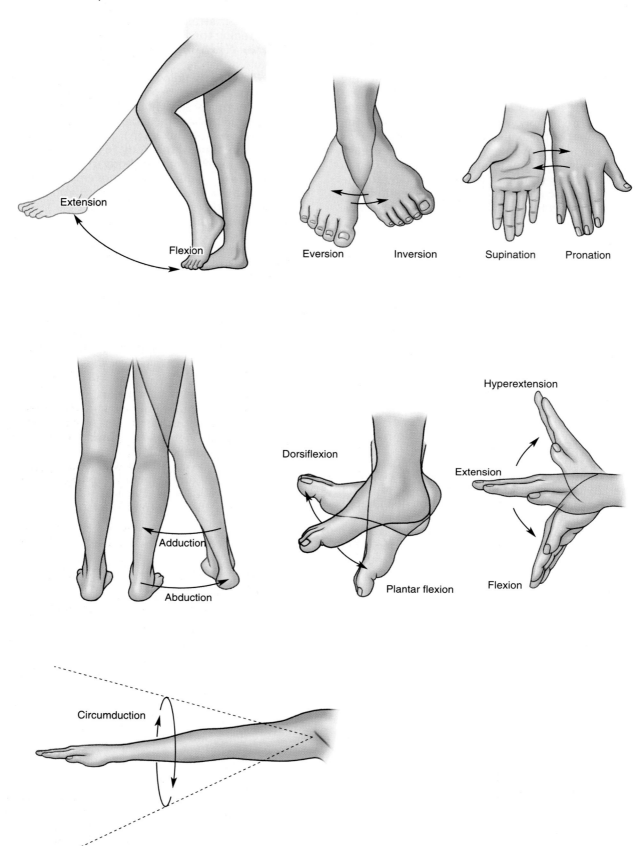

FIGURE 7–20 ● Types of movements at joints.

Disorders of the Skeletal System

Arthritis
Inflammation of a joint, usually accompanied by pain, swelling, and changes in structure. There are about 25 forms of arthritis. Osteoarthritis, also called degenerative arthritis or "wear-and-tear" arthritis, is the most common form. It is the result of degeneration of the articular cartilage. Rheumatoid arthritis, also called rheumatism, is an inflammation of the synovial membrane and is the most debilitating of the chronic forms of arthritis. Gouty arthritis, or gout, is a metabolic disorder and occurs when sharp uric acid crystals deposit in a joint.

Bursitis
Inflammation of one or more bursae, causing pain, swelling, and restriction of movement. Common forms include subacromial bursitis (painful shoulder), olecranon bursitis (miner's or tennis elbow), and prepatellar bursitis (housemaid's knee).

Cancer
Several types of cancer can occur in the skeletal system. Examples include osteosarcoma, a tumor of the bone, and chondrosarcoma, a tumor involving cartilage. The most common form of bone cancer is a myeloma, in which the malignant tumors in the bone marrow interfere with red blood cell production and cause destruction of bone.

Dislocation
Displacement, or luxation, of a bone from its joint with tearing of ligaments, tendons, and articular capsule. The shoulder joint is displaced more easily than other joints. The return of the bone into its joint is called a reduction. A partial dislocation is called a subluxation. When applied to the temporomandibular joint, a subluxation refers to the stretching of the capsule and ligaments that results in popping noises when the jaw moves.

Osteomalacia
Disease characterized by softening of the bones due to demineralization (loss of calcium and phosphorus). The demineralization is caused by vitamin D deficiency. The bone softening results in skeletal deformities. Osteomalacia in growing bones is called rickets.

Osteomyelitis
An inflammation of the bone and/or infection of the bone marrow most often caused by the *Staphylococcus* bacterium. Osteomyelitis often occurs as a complication of bone fractures and orthopedic surgery.

Osteoporosis
A loss of bone mass that makes the bones so porous that they crumble under the ordinary stress of moving about. Osteoporosis is related to loss of estrogen in older women, a dietary deficiency of calcium and vitamin D, and low levels of exercise.

Sprain
An injury to a joint caused by the twisting of the joint. A sprain causes pain, loss of mobility, swelling, and black-and-blue discoloration of the injured site. Ligaments may be torn, but there is no bone or joint damage.

Strain
An injury to a muscle or tendon at a joint. A strain is due to overuse or overstretching and is less serious than a sprain.

Tennis elbow
Also called lateral epicondylitis. Tennis elbow is an inflammation of the tissues around the lateral epicondyle of the humerus (elbow).

Summary Outline

The skeletal system supports the weight of the body, supports and protects body organs, enables the body to move, acts as storage site for minerals (especially calcium and phosphorus), and produces blood cells.

I. Bones: An Overview

A. Sizes and Shapes

1. Bones are classified into four groups: long, short, flat, and irregular.

2. Bone markings indicate sites of muscle attachments and passages for nerves and blood vessels.

3. A long bone has a long shaft (diaphysis) and two ends (epiphyses). Articular cartilage is found on the outer surface of the

continued

Summary Outline *continued*

I. Bones: An Overview, *continued*

A. Sizes and Shapes, *continued*

epiphyses. The diaphysis is surrounded by the periosteum.

4. The diaphysis is composed of compact or hard bone; its cavity contains yellow marrow. The epiphysis consists of spongy or soft bone; red marrow is found in the holes of spongy bone.

B. Bone Formation and Growth

1. Bones form, or ossify, in two ways. In the skull, osteoblasts replace thin connective tissue membrane, forming flat bones. Other bones form on hyaline cartilage models as osteoblasts replace cartilage with bone.
2. Bones grow longitudinally to determine height; bones also grow thicker and wider to support the weight of the body. Longitudinal bone growth occurs at the epiphyseal discs, bands of cartilage located at the ends of the diaphysis. The increase in the width and thickness is due to the coordinated actions of the osteoclasts and osteoblasts.
3. Bone growth and reshaping occur throughout life and depend on many factors, including diet, exercise, and hormones.

II. Divisions of the Skeletal System

The names of the 206 bones of the skeleton are listed in Table 7–2.

A. Axial Skeleton

1. The axial skeleton includes the bones of the skull (cranium and face), hyoid bone, bones of the middle ear, bones of the vertebral column, and the thoracic cage.
2. The skull of a newborn contains fontanels, which are membranous areas that allow brain growth.
3. The skull contains air-filled cavities called sinuses.
4. The vertebral column is formed from 24 vertebrae, the sacrum, and the coccyx. The vertebrae are separated by cartilaginous discs.

The vertebral column of the adult has four curves, or curvatures: the cervical, thoracic, lumbar, and sacral curves.

5. The thoracic cage is a bony cone-shaped cage formed by the sternum, 12 pairs of ribs, and thoracic vertebrae.

B. Appendicular Skeleton

1. The appendicular skeleton includes the bones of the extremities (arms and legs), and the bones of the hip and shoulder girdles.
2. The shoulder girdle consists of the scapula and the clavicle.
3. The pelvic girdle is formed by the two coxal bones and is secured to the axial skeleton at the sacrum.

III. Joints

A joint or articulation is the site where two bones meet.

A. Types of Joints (based on the degree of movement)

1. Immovable joints are called synarthroses (eg, sutures in the skull).
2. Slightly movable joints are called amphiarthroses (eg, symphysis pubis).
3. Freely movable joints are called diarthroses, or synovial joints. Structures within a synovial joint, such as the knee, include the articular cartilage of each bone, the joint capsule, the synovial membrane, synovial fluid, bursae, and supporting ligaments.
4. The types of freely movable joints include hinge, ball-and-socket, pivot, gliding, saddle, and condyloid.

B. Joint Movement

1. Freely movable joints are capable of different types of movement.
2. Types of movements at freely movable joints include flexion and extension, abduction and adduction, inversion and eversion, supination and pronation, and circumduction.

Review Your Knowledge

1. What are four types of bone classifications according to shape?

2. What are the differences among osteocytes, osteoblasts, and osteoclasts?

3. State the location of compact bone and spongy (cancellous) bone. Describe the diaphysis, epiphysis, and epiphyseal disc.

4. Define the following terms: *medullary cavity, endosteum, periosteum,* and *articular cartilage.*

5. What happens when the epiphyseal disk is injured?

6. What are the differences among simple, compound, and greenstick fractures?

7. What is the difference between the axial and the appendicular skeleton?

8. Name the eight bones of the cranium. List four bone markings found on the temporal bone. Which four bones communicate with the

Review Your Knowledge *continued*

paranasal sinuses? What is the only movable bone in the cranium?

9. Name the bones related to the following:
   a. Forehead
   b. Cheekbone
   c. Upper jaw
   d. Lower jaw

10. What are four functions of the vertebral column?

11. State the function of the atlas and the axis.

12. What are the differences among true, false, and floating ribs?

13. What are the two bones of the shoulder girdle? What is the name of the bony part of the elbow?

14. What is the longest bone of the body?

15. Give one example each of a synarthrotic, an amphiarthrotic, and a diarthrotic joint. What are four structures found at a diarthrotic joint?

16. Give one example each of a hinge, a ball-and-socket, and a pivot joint.

17. State the terms for the following movements:
    a. Bending the leg at the knee
    b. Straightening the fingers to open the hand
    c. Toe dancing
    d. Moving your leg sideways, away from your body
    e. Turning the sole of your foot outward
    f. Turning your hand so that the palm faces upward

18. What is a common site for bone marrow biopsy?

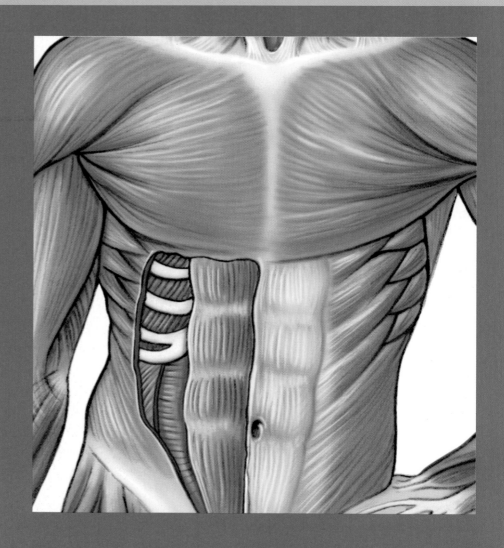

8 MUSCULAR SYSTEM

*O*bjectives

1. Identify three types of muscle tissue.

2. Describe the structure of a skeletal muscle.

3. Describe the sliding filament hypothesis of muscle contraction.

4. Describe the events that occur at the neuromuscular junction.

5. Explain the role of calcium and adenosine triphosphate in muscle contraction.

6. Identify the sources of energy for muscle contraction.

7. Trace the sequence of events from nerve stimulation to muscle contraction.

8. Define *twitch, summation, tetanus,* and *recruitment* as characteristics of muscle contraction.

9. Describe common types of movement.

10. State the basis for naming muscles.

11. Identify the major muscles.

12. List the actions of the major muscles.

The word *muscle* comes from the Latin word *mus* meaning little mouse. As muscles contract, the muscle movements under the skin resemble the movement of mice scurrying around. Thus the name *mus,* or muscle.

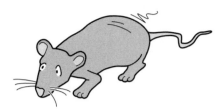

TYPES AND FUNCTIONS OF MUSCLES

The three types of muscles are skeletal, smooth, and cardiac (Fig. 8–1). Smooth muscle is discussed throughout the book and cardiac muscle in Chapter 14. In this chapter, the focus is on skeletal muscle.

Skeletal Muscle

Skeletal muscle (skĕl′ĭ-tl mŭs′əl) is generally attached to bone. Because skeletal muscle can be controlled by choice (ie, I *choose* to move my arm), it is also called **voluntary muscle.** The skeletal muscle cells are long, shaped like cylinders or tubes, and composed of proteins arranged to make the muscle appear striped, or **striated.** Skeletal muscles produce movement, maintain body posture, and stabilize joints. They also produce considerable heat and therefore help to maintain body temperature.

Cellular appearance:

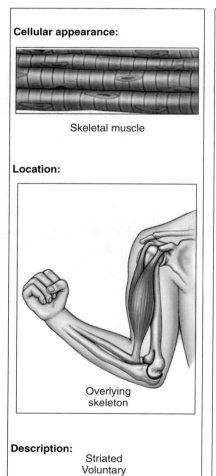

Skeletal muscle

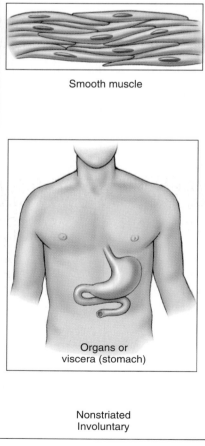

Smooth muscle

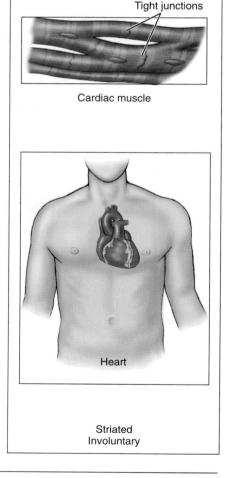

Tight junctions

Cardiac muscle

Location:

Overlying skeleton

Organs or viscera (stomach)

Heart

Description:

Striated
Voluntary

Nonstriated
Involuntary

Striated
Involuntary

◀ **FIGURE 8–1** ● Three types of muscle: skeletal, smooth, and cardiac. Skeletal muscle is striated (striped) and voluntary. Smooth muscle is nonstriated and involuntary. Cardiac muscle is striated and involuntary. Cardiac muscle has tight junctions called intercalated discs.

Smooth Muscle

Smooth muscle (smōŏth mŭs'əl) is generally found in the walls of the viscera (organs such as the stomach and bladder) and is called **visceral muscle.** It is also found in tubes and passageways such as the bronchioles (breathing passages) and blood vessels. Because smooth muscle functions automatically, it is called **involuntary muscle.** Unlike skeletal muscles, smooth muscle does not appear striped, or striated, and is therefore called **nonstriated muscle.**

The contraction of smooth muscle enables the viscera to perform their functions. Contraction of the stomach muscles, for instance, enables the stomach to mix solid food into a paste and then to push it forward into the intestine, where digestion continues.

Cardiac Muscle

Cardiac muscle (kär'dē-ăk mŭs'əl) is found only in the heart, where it functions to pump blood throughout the body. Like skeletal muscle, cardiac muscle is striated. Cardiac muscle cells are long branching cells that fit together tightly at junctions called **intercalated discs.** These tight-fitting junctions promote rapid conduction of electrical signals throughout the heart. Cardiac muscle is not under voluntary control and is classified as involuntary muscle.

STRUCTURE OF THE WHOLE MUSCLE

If you touch your thigh, you will feel a large muscle. This muscle is composed of thousands of single muscle fibers (muscle cells). The structure and function of the whole muscle differs in several ways from the structure and function of a single muscle fiber.

A large skeletal muscle is surrounded by layers of tough connective tissue called **fascia** (făsh'ē-ə) (Fig. 8–2A). This outer layer of fascia is called the **epimysium.** The fascia extends toward and attaches to the bone as a **tendon,** a strong cord-like structure. Another layer of connective tissue, called the **perimysium,** surrounds smaller bundles of muscle fibers. The bundles are called **fascicles.** Individual muscle fibers are found within the fascicles and are surrounded by a third layer of connective tissue called the **endomysium.**

Muscles form attachments to other structures in three ways. First, the tendon attaches the muscle to the bone. Second, muscles attach directly (without a tendon) to a bone or to soft tissue. Third, a flat, sheet-like fascia, called **aponeurosis** (ăp"ə-noo-rō'sĭs), may connect muscle to muscle or muscle to bone.

STRUCTURE AND FUNCTION OF A SINGLE MUSCLE FIBER

The muscle cell is an elongated muscle fiber (Fig. 8–2B). Some muscle fibers are 12 inches long. The muscle fiber has more than one nucleus and is surrounded by a cell membrane. At several points the cell membrane penetrates deep into the interior of the muscle fiber, forming **transverse tubules,** or **T tubules.** Within the muscle fiber is a specialized endoplasmic reticulum called the **sarcoplasmic reticulum** (sär'kə-plăz"mĭk rĭ-tĭk'yə-ləm).

Do You Know...

Why is beef red and chicken meat white?

Certain muscle fibers contain a reddish-brown pigment called **myoglobin.** The myoglobin stores oxygen in the muscle and gradually releases it when the muscle starts to work. Fibers that contain myoglobin are red because of the myoglobin pigment. This is the red meat of a steak. Fibers that do not contain myoglobin are white. This is the white meat in a chicken breast.

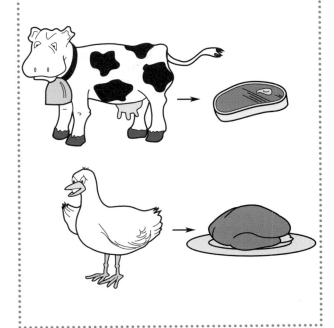

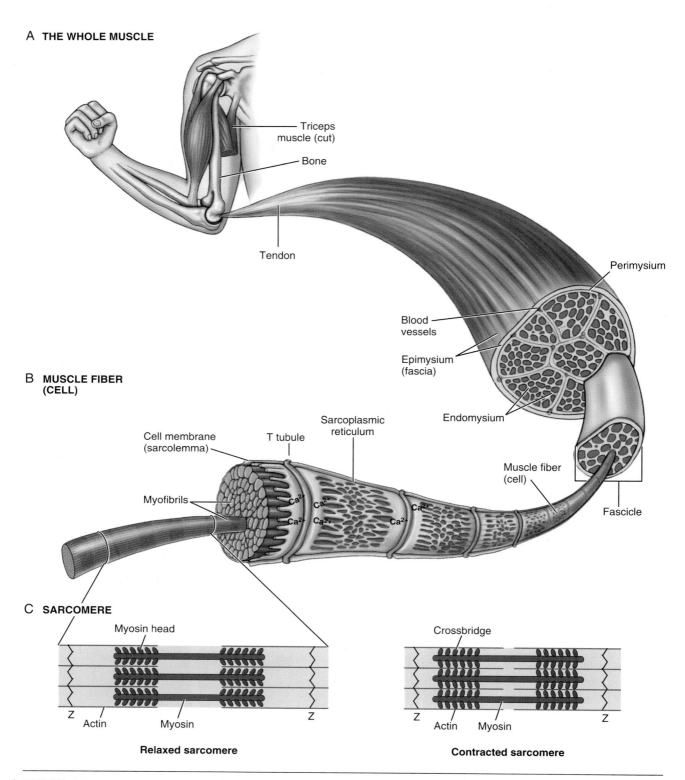

A **THE WHOLE MUSCLE**

Triceps muscle (cut)

Bone

Tendon

Perimysium

Blood vessels

Epimysium (fascia)

Endomysium

Muscle fiber (cell)

Fascicle

B **MUSCLE FIBER (CELL)**

Cell membrane (sarcolemma)

T tubule

Sarcoplasmic reticulum

Myofibrils

Ca²⁺ Ca²⁺ Ca²⁺
Ca²⁺ Ca²⁺ Ca²⁺

C **SARCOMERE**

Myosin head

Crossbridge

Z

Actin

Myosin

Z

Relaxed sarcomere

Z

Actin

Myosin

Z

Contracted sarcomere

◀ **FIGURE 8–2** • Structure of a whole muscle and a single muscle fiber. A, Structure of a whole muscle attached to the bone by a tendon. B, Structure of a muscle fiber showing cylinders of myofibrils and the arrangement of the sarcoplasmic reticulum. C, Sarcomeres (from Z line to Z line) showing the arrangement of the contractile proteins actin and myosin. The relaxed sarcomere is longer than the contracted sarcomere.

Each muscle fiber is composed of long cylindrical structures called **myofibrils.** Each myofibril is made up of a series of contractile units called **sarcomeres** (sär′kə-mîrz) (Fig. 8–2C). Each sarcomere extends from Z line to Z line and is formed by a unique arrangement of two contractile proteins, **actin** (ăk′tĭn) and **myosin** (mī′ə-sĭn). The Z lines occur at the ends of each sarcomere (see Fig. 8–2C). The thin actin filaments extend toward the center of the sarcomere from the Z lines. The thicker myosin filaments sit between the actin filaments. Extending from the myosin filaments are structures called **myosin heads.** The arrangement of the actin and myosin in each sarcomere gives skeletal and cardiac muscle its striped appearance.

HOW MUSCLES CONTRACT

When muscles contract, they shorten. Muscles shorten because the sarcomeres shorten, and the sarcomeres shorten because the actin and myosin filaments slide past each other. Note how much shorter the contracted sarcomere appears (see Fig. 8–2C).

How does the sarcomere shorten? When stimulated, the myosin heads make contact with the actin, forming temporary connections called **crossbridges.** Once the crossbridges are formed, the myosin heads rotate, pulling the actin toward the center of the sarcomere. The rotation of the myosin heads causes the actin to slide past the myosin. Muscle relaxation occurs when the crossbridges are broken and the actin and myosin return to their original positions. Because of this sliding activity of actin and myosin, muscle contraction is called the sliding filament hypothesis of muscle contraction.

Remember: The sarcomeres shorten not because the actin and myosin proteins shrink or shrivel up but because the proteins slide past one another. The sliding is like a trombone. The trombone shortens because the parts slide past one another, not because the metal shrinks or shrivels. Actin and myosin do the same thing—they slide.

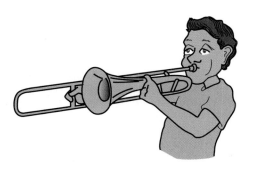

Contraction and Relaxation: The Role of Calcium and ATP

Adenosine triphosphate (ATP) and calcium play important roles in the contraction and relaxation of muscle. (See Chapter 2 for an explanation of ATP.) The ATP helps the myosin heads form and break crossbridges with the actin. The ATP, however, can perform its role only if calcium is present. When the muscle is relaxed, the calcium is stored in the sarcoplasmic reticulum, away from the actin and myosin. When the muscle is stimulated, calcium is released from the sarcoplasmic reticulum and causes the actin, myosin, and ATP to interact. Muscle contraction then occurs. When calcium is pumped back into the sarcoplasmic reticulum, away from the actin, myosin, and ATP, the crossbridges are broken, and the muscle relaxes. Note that the availability of calcium to the contractile proteins actin and myosin is necessary for muscle contraction.

 Do You Know…

What is rigor mortis?

Both the formation of crossbridges (muscle contraction) and the detachment of crossbridges (muscle relaxation) depend on ATP. When a person dies, the production of ATP ceases. The deficiency of ATP prevents the detachment of the crossbridges, so muscles remain contracted and become stiff. This change is called rigor mortis, or "stiffness of death." An assessment of rigor mortis often helps determine the exact time of death.

Skeletal Muscles and Nerves

Skeletal muscle contraction can take place only if the muscle is first stimulated by a nerve. The type of nerve that supplies the skeletal muscle is a **motor,** or **somatic nerve** (Fig. 8–3A). A motor nerve arises in the spinal cord and innervates, or supplies, several muscle fibers with nerve stimulation. The area where the motor nerve meets the muscle is called the **neuromuscular junction (NMJ)** (noŏr″ō-mŭs′kyə-lər jŭngk′shən) (Fig. 8–3B). Structures within the NMJ include the membrane at the end of the nerve, the space, or cleft, that exists between the nerve ending and muscle membrane, and the receptor sites on the muscle membrane.

The Neuromuscular Junction

What happens at the neuromuscular junction? The stimulated nerve causes the release of a

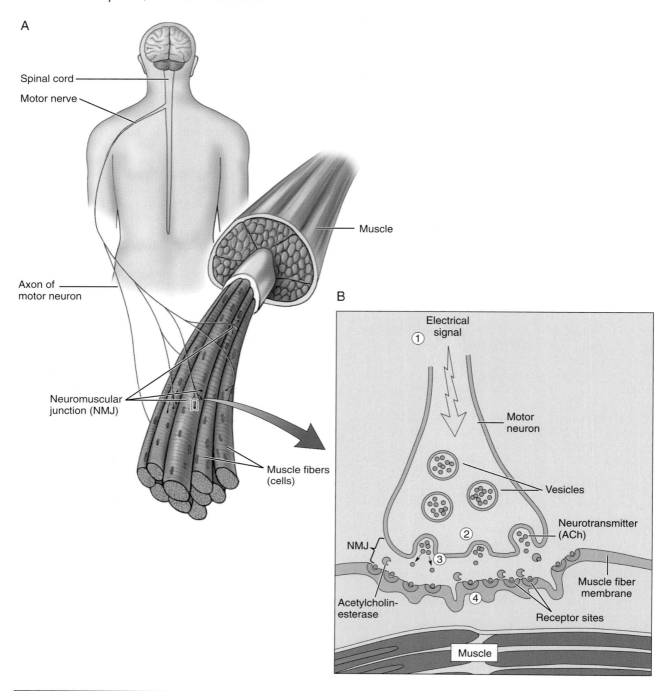

FIGURE 8–3 • Innervation of skeletal muscle and the neuromuscular junction (NMJ). A, Muscle fibers are innervated, or supplied, by a motor neuron. B, NMJ showing (1) the electrical signal; (2) the release of the neurotransmitter (ACh); (3) the diffusion of ACh across the junction (space); and (4) the binding of ACh to the receptors and the destruction of ACh by acetylcholinesterase.

chemical substance that diffuses across the NMJ and stimulates the muscle membrane. Four steps are involved in the transfer of the information from nerve to muscle at the NMJ (see Fig. 8–3).

- *Step 1:* Stimulation of the nerve causes an electrical signal, or nerve impulse, to move along the nerve toward the nerve ending. Stored

within the nerve ending are vesicles, or membranous pouches, filled with a chemical substance called a **neurotransmitter.** The neurotransmitter at the neuromuscular junction is **acetylcholine (ACh)** (ăs″ə-tĭl-kō′lēn).

- *Step 2:* The nerve impulse causes the vesicles to move toward and fuse with the nerve ending. ACh is released from the vesicles into the space between the nerve ending and the muscle membrane.

- *Step 3:* ACh diffuses across the space and binds to the receptor sites on the muscle membrane.
- *Step 4:* The ACh stimulates the receptors and causes an electrical signal to develop along the muscle membrane. The ACh then dissociates, or leaves, the binding site and is immediately destroyed by an enzyme that is found within the NMJ near the muscle membrane. The name of the enzyme is **acetylcholinesterase.** The free binding sites are then ready for additional ACh when the nerve is stimulated again.

The Stimulated Muscle Membrane

What happens to the electrical signal in the muscle membrane? It travels along the muscle membrane and triggers a series of events that result in muscle contraction (see Fig. 8–2B). Specifically, the electrical signal travels along the muscle

cell membrane and penetrates into its interior through the T tubules. The electrical signal stimulates the sarcoplasmic reticulum to release calcium. The calcium floods the sarcomeres and allows for the interaction of actin, myosin, and ATP, producing muscle contraction. Eventually, the calcium is pumped back into the sarcoplasmic reticulum, away from the actin and myosin, causing muscle relaxation.

Disorders of the Neuromuscular Junction

Certain conditions can cause problems at the NMJ (Fig. 8–4).

MYASTHENIA GRAVIS. Myasthenia gravis is a disease that affects the NMJ. The symptoms of the disease are thought to be due to damaged receptor sites on the muscle membrane. The receptor sites are altered so that they cannot bind ACh. Consequently, muscle contraction is impaired,

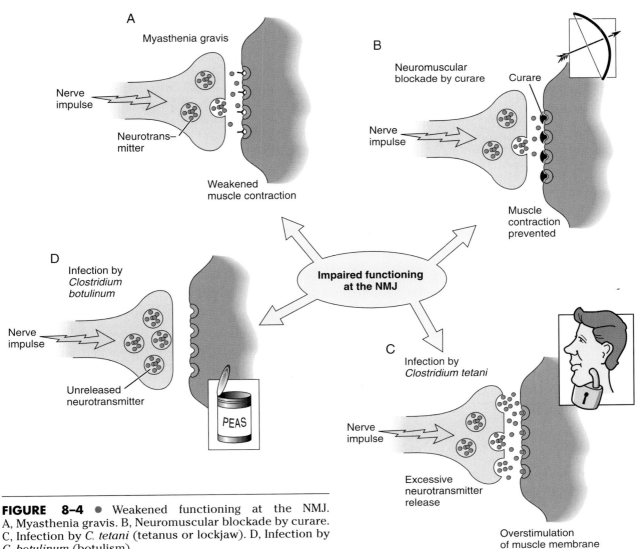

FIGURE 8–4 • Weakened functioning at the NMJ. A, Myasthenia gravis. B, Neuromuscular blockade by curare. C, Infection by *C. tetani* (tetanus or lockjaw). D, Infection by *C. botulinum* (botulism).

and the patient experiences extreme muscle weakness. (The word *myasthenia* literally means muscle weakness.) The muscle weakness becomes noticeable as low tolerance to exercise, difficulty raising the eyelids, and difficulty breathing.

NEUROMUSCULAR BLOCKADE CAUSED BY CURARE. Curare is a drug classified as a skeletal muscle blocker. Skeletal muscle blockers are frequently used during surgery to promote muscle relaxation. Curare works by blocking the receptor sites on the muscle membrane. Because the receptors are occupied by the drug, the ACh cannot bind with the receptor sites, and muscle contraction is prevented.

Because the respiratory muscles are also affected by curare, the patient must be mechanically ventilated until the effects of the drug disappear. Otherwise, the patient stops breathing and dies. Historically, curare was used as a poison in hunting animals. The tip of the arrowhead was dipped in curare. When the arrow pierced the skin of the animal, the curare was absorbed and eventually caused a fatal skeletal muscle blockade, in which respiratory muscle paralysis led to suffocation.

EFFECTS OF NEUROTOXINS ON MUSCLE FUNCTION. **Neurotoxins** are chemical substances that in some way disrupt normal function of the nervous system. Neurotoxins are produced by certain bacteria. For example, *Clostridium tetani* (a bacterium) secretes a neurotoxin that causes excessive firing of the motor nerves. This, in turn, causes excessive release of the neurotransmitter, overstimulation of the muscle membrane, and severe muscle spasm and tetanic contractions. Hence the name **tetanus** (tĕt′ə-nəs). Because the muscles of the jaw are frequently the first muscles affected, the disease is often called **lockjaw.**

A second neurotoxin is secreted by the bacterium *Clostridium botulinum.* This bacterium appears most often when food has been improperly processed and canned. Infection with this organism causes a disease known as **botulism,** a very serious form of food poisoning. The neurotoxin works by preventing the release of acetylcholine from the ends of the nerves within the NMJ. Without acetylcholine, the muscle fibers cannot contract, and the muscles, including the breathing muscles, become paralyzed.

✳ **SUM IT UP!** The three types of muscle are skeletal, smooth, and cardiac. A whole muscle is composed of muscle fibers (muscle cells). Each muscle fiber contains the contractile proteins actin and myosin, arranged into a series of sarcomeres. In accord with the sliding filament hypothesis, the interaction of the actin and myosin causes muscle contraction. Figure 8–5 summarizes the steps involved in the contraction and relaxation of skeletal muscle. Note the crucial role played by the motor nerve.

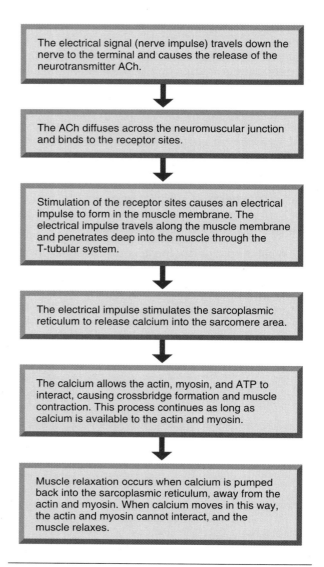

> The electrical signal (nerve impulse) travels down the nerve to the terminal and causes the release of the neurotransmitter ACh.

> The ACh diffuses across the neuromuscular junction and binds to the receptor sites.

> Stimulation of the receptor sites causes an electrical impulse to form in the muscle membrane. The electrical impulse travels along the muscle membrane and penetrates deep into the muscle through the T-tubular system.

> The electrical impulse stimulates the sarcoplasmic reticulum to release calcium into the sarcomere area.

> The calcium allows the actin, myosin, and ATP to interact, causing crossbridge formation and muscle contraction. This process continues as long as calcium is available to the actin and myosin.

> Muscle relaxation occurs when calcium is pumped back into the sarcoplasmic reticulum, away from the actin and myosin. When calcium moves in this way, the actin and myosin cannot interact, and the muscle relaxes.

FIGURE 8–5 ● Steps in contraction and relaxation of skeletal muscle.

RESPONSES OF A WHOLE MUSCLE

The sliding filament hypothesis explains the contraction and relaxation of a single muscle fiber. A whole skeletal muscle, however, is composed of thousands of muscle fibers. The contractile response of a whole muscle differs from that of a single muscle fiber in a number of ways.

Partial Versus All-or-Nothing Response

A single muscle fiber contracts in an all-or-nothing response. In other words, the single fiber contracts maximally (as strongly as possible), or it does not contract at all. It never partially contracts. A whole muscle, however, is capable of contracting partially; it can contract weakly or very strongly. For instance, only a small force of contraction is required to lift a pencil. A much greater force is required to lift a 100-pound weight.

How can a whole muscle vary its strength of contraction? Lifting the pencil may require the contraction of several hundred muscle fibers. These fibers contract in an all-or-nothing manner, but only a few fibers are contracting. Lifting a 100-pound weight, however, requires contraction of thousands of fibers, all contracting in an all-or-nothing manner. The greater muscle force is achieved by using, or recruiting, additional fibers. This process is called **recruitment** (rē-kroōt′měnt). Thus the strength of skeletal muscle contraction can be varied by recruitment of additional muscle fibers.

Twitch, Summation, and Tetanus

Several important terms describe whole-muscle contraction. They include twitch, summation, and tetanus. Of the three, tetanus is the most important.

TWITCH. If a single stimulus is delivered to a muscle, the muscle contracts and then fully relaxes. This single muscle response is termed a **twitch** (Fig. 8–6A). A certain amount of force is produced by a twitch. Twitches are not useful physiologically.

SUMMATION. If the frequency of stimulation increases (eg, three stimuli in rapid succession), the muscle cannot relax fully before it begins to contract for a second and third time. This ability of the muscle to contract without first experiencing

Do You Know...

What is hypocalcemic tetany?

Tetany is caused by low blood levels of calcium (hypocalcemia). The hypocalcemia triggers a continuous firing of the nerves that supply the skeletal muscles, resulting in sustained muscle contractions. Because this condition causes sustained muscle contraction, it is called tetanus or tetany. Tetany is life-threatening and demands immediate treatment, because it involves all skeletal muscles, including the breathing muscles. Immediate treatment includes ventilatory support and the intravenous administration of calcium.

full relaxation from the previous stimulus, is called **summation** (Fig. 8–6B).

TETANUS. If the frequency of stimulation is further increased (eg, 20 stimuli in rapid succession), the muscle has no time to relax. The muscle then remains in a contracted state. This sustained muscle contraction is called **tetanus** (Fig. 8–6C). Tetanic muscle contractions are smooth and sustained. They play an important role in maintaining posture. If, for instance, the muscles that maintain our upright posture merely twitched, we would be unable to stand and would instead twitch and flop around on the ground (not a pretty sight). Because the muscle is able to tetanize we are able to maintain an upright posture. Fatigue occurs if the muscle is not allowed to rest. (Do not confuse the tetanus described in this section with the disease called tetanus, or lockjaw.)

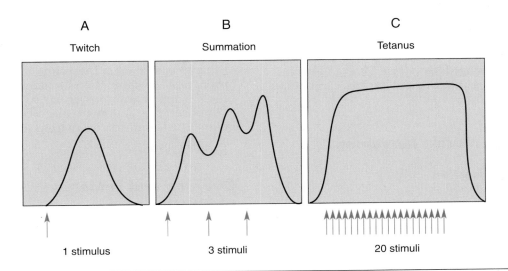

FIGURE 8–6 ● Contractile responses of skeletal muscle. A, Twitch. B, Summation. C, Tetanus.

Muscle Tone

Muscle tone, or **tonus** (tō′nəs), refers to a normal, continuous state of partial muscle contraction. Tone is due to the contraction of different groups of muscle fibers within a whole muscle. To maintain muscle tone, one group of muscle fibers contracts first. As these fibers begin to relax, a second group contracts. This pattern of contraction and relaxation continues so as to maintain muscle tone. Muscle tone plays a number of important roles. For instance, the muscle tone of the smooth muscle in blood vessels helps to maintain blood pressure. If the muscle tone were to decrease, the person might experience a life-threatening decline in blood pressure.

Energy Source for Muscle Contraction

Muscle contraction requires a rich supply of energy (ATP). The amount of ATP stored within a resting muscle is very small and is sufficient to maintain a contracting skeletal muscle for about 6 seconds. As ATP is consumed by the contracting muscle, it is replaced in three ways:

- *Aerobic metabolism.* In the presence of oxygen, fuel such as glycogen, glucose, and fats can be completely broken down to carbon dioxide, water, and energy (ATP). The yield of ATP is high. (See Chapter 4 for a review of aerobic and anaerobic metabolism.)
- *Anaerobic metabolism.* The body can also metabolize fuel in the absence of oxygen. When oxygen is not present, however, complete breakdown of the fuel is not possible, and lactic acid is produced. The accumulation of lactic acid may be responsible for some of the muscle soreness that accompanies heavy exercise.
- *Metabolism of creatine phosphate.* Creatine phosphate contains energy that the body can use to replenish ATP quickly during muscle contraction. As a storage form of energy, creatine phosphate ensures that skeletal muscle can operate for long periods.

Describing Muscle Movement

Origin and Insertion

The terms *origin* and *insertion* refer to the sites of muscle attachment. When muscle contracts across a joint, one bone remains relatively stationary or immovable. The **origin** (ôr′ə-jĭn) of the muscle attaches to the stationary bone, while the **insertion** (ĭn-sûr′shən) attaches to the more movable bone (Fig. 8–7). For instance, the origin of the biceps brachii is the scapula, while the inser-

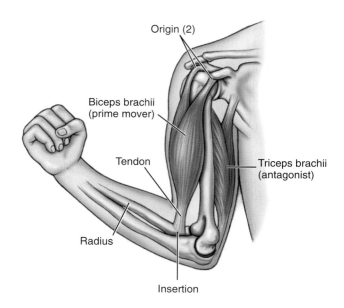

FIGURE 8–7 • Origin and insertion/antagonists. The location of the biceps brachii in the upper arm showing the insertion on the radius and the origin (two sites on the scapula). The triceps brachii exerts an antagonistic effect on the biceps brachii.

tion is on the radius. Upon contraction of the biceps brachii, the radius (insertion) is pulled toward the scapula (origin).

Prime Mover, Synergist, and Antagonist

Although most movement is accomplished through the cooperation of groups of muscles, a single muscle is generally responsible for most of the movement. The "chief muscle" is called the **prime mover** (prīm mōō′vər). Assisting the primer mover are "helper muscles" called **synergists** (sĭn′ər-jĭsts). Synergists are said to cooperate with other muscles. In contrast, **antagonists** (ăn-tăg′ə-nĭsts) are muscles that oppose the action of another muscle. For instance, contraction of the biceps brachii, the prime mover, pulls the lower arm toward the shoulder. The triceps brachii (upper arm, posterior) is the antagonist. It opposes the action of the biceps brachii by pulling the lower arm away from the scapula (see Fig. 8–7).

Overuse and Underuse of Muscles

Hypertrophy

Overused muscles will increase in size. This response to overuse or overwork is called **hypertrophy.** Athletes intentionally cause their muscles to hypertrophy. Weight lifters, for instance, de-

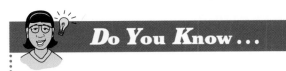

Do You Know...

What is wrong with bulking up?

Nothing is wrong with bulking up if it is done through weight lifting and exercise. Bulking up with the use of steroids, however, is dangerous. Steroids are thought to cause liver cancer, atrophy of the testicles in males, hypertension, and severe psychotic mood swings, among other health-related effects.

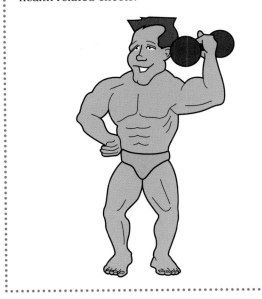

velop larger muscles than couch potatoes develop by watching television.

Like skeletal muscle, cardiac muscle can also hypertrophy. Cardiac hypertrophy is generally undesirable and usually indicates an underlying disease causing the heart to overwork. Hypertension, for instance, causes the heart to push blood into blood vessels that are very resistant to the flow of blood. This extra work causes the heart to enlarge.

Atrophy

If muscles are not used, they will waste away, or decrease in size. A person with a broken leg in a cast, for instance, is unable to bear weight or exercise that leg for several months. This lack of exercise will cause the muscles of the leg to **atrophy.** When weight bearing and exercise are resumed, muscle size and strength will be restored.

Contracture

If a muscle is immobilized for a prolonged period, it may develop a contracture. A **contracture** (kən-trăk′chər) is an abnormal formation of fibrous tissue within the muscle. It generally

"freezes" the muscle in a flexed position and severely restricts joint mobility.

NAMING SKELETAL MUSCLES

The names of the various skeletal muscles are generally based on one or more of the following characteristics: size, shape, orientation of the fibers, location, number of origins, identification of origin and insertion, and muscle action.

Size

These terms indicate size: vastus (huge), maximus (large), longus (long), minimus (small), and brevis (short). Examples of skeletal muscles include vastus lateralis and gluteus maximus.

Shape

Various shapes are included in muscle names: deltoid (triangular), latissimus (wide), trapezius (trapezoid), rhomboideus (rhomboid), and teres (round). Examples include the trapezius muscle, the latissimus dorsi, and the teres major.

Direction of Fibers

Fibers are oriented, or lined up, in several directions: rectus (straight), oblique (diagonal), transverse (across), and circularis (circular). Examples include rectus abdominis and the superior oblique.

Location

The names of muscles often reflect their location in the body: pectoralis (chest), gluteus (buttock), brachii (arm), supra (above), infra (below), sub (underneath), and lateralis (lateral). Examples include biceps brachii, pectoralis major, and gluteus maximus.

Number of Origins

The muscle may be named according to the number of sites to which it is anchored: biceps indicates two sites, triceps three, and quadriceps four. Examples include the biceps brachii, triceps brachii, and quadriceps femoris.

Origin and Insertion

Some muscles are named for sites of attachment both at the origin and the insertion. The sternocleidomastoid, for example, has its origin on the sternum and clavicle and its insertion on the mastoid. This information allows you to determine the function of the muscle. The sternocleidomastoid flexes the neck and rotates the head.

Muscle Action

The action of the muscle may be included in the name. For instance, an abductor muscle moves the limb away from the midline of the body,

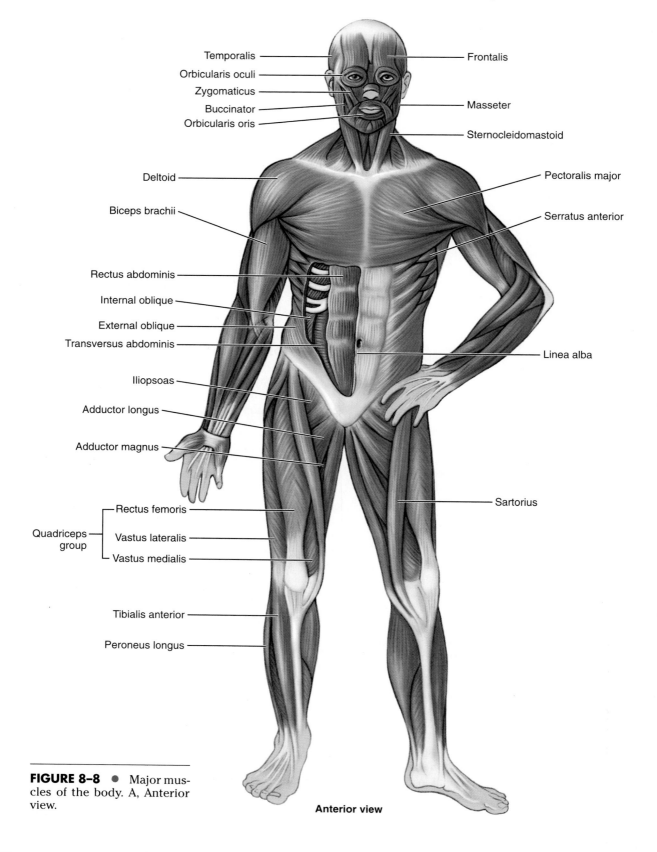

Temporalis

Orbicularis oculi

Zygomaticus

Buccinator

Orbicularis oris

Deltoid

Biceps brachii

Rectus abdominis

Internal oblique

External oblique

Transversus abdominis

Iliopsoas

Adductor longus

Adductor magnus

Rectus femoris

Quadriceps group

Vastus lateralis

Vastus medialis

Tibialis anterior

Peroneus longus

Frontalis

Masseter

Sternocleidomastoid

Pectoralis major

Serratus anterior

Linea alba

Sartorius

Anterior view

FIGURE 8–8 ● Major muscles of the body. A, Anterior view.

while an adductor moves the limb toward the midline. In the same way, a flexor muscle causes flexion, while an extensor muscle straightens the limb. A levator muscle elevates a structure, and a masseter muscle enables you to chew. Examples include the adductor magnus, flexor digitorum, and levator palpebrae superioris.

MUSCLES FROM HEAD TO TOE

Figure 8–8 shows the major skeletal muscles of the body. Details of muscle location and function are summarized in Table 8–1.

Text continued on page 154

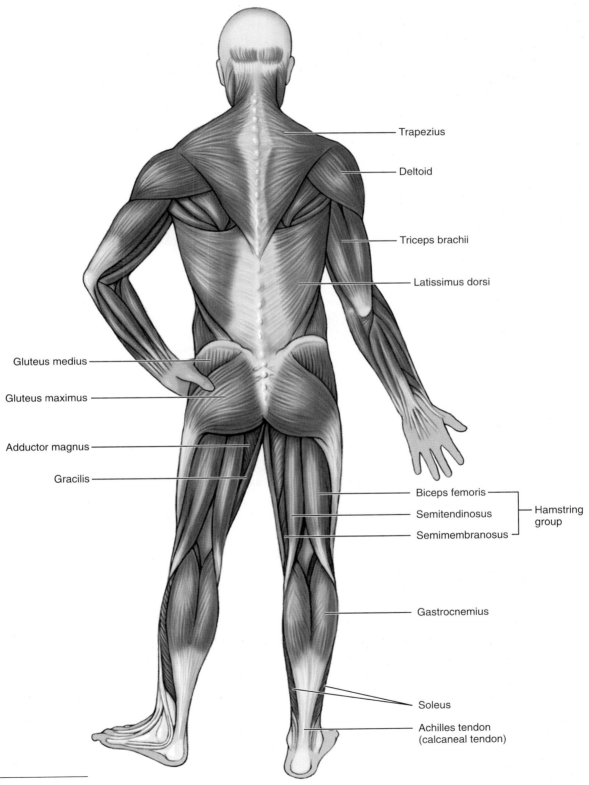

Trapezius

Deltoid

Triceps brachii

Latissimus dorsi

Gluteus medius

Gluteus maximus

Adductor magnus

Gracilis

Biceps femoris
Semitendinosus — Hamstring group
Semimembranosus

Gastrocnemius

Soleus

Achilles tendon (calcaneal tendon)

FIGURE 8–8 ● *Continued.* B, Posterior view.

Posterior view

Table 8•1 MUSCLES OF THE BODY

MUSCLE	DESCRIPTION	FUNCTION
Head		
Facial muscles		
Frontalis	Flat muscle covering the forehead	Raises eyebrows; surprised look; wrinkles forehead
Orbicularis oculi	Circular muscle around eye	Closes eyes; winking, blinking, and squinting
Levator palpebrae superioris	Back of eye to upper eyelid	Opens eyes
Orbicularis oris	Circular muscle around mouth	Closes/purses lips; kissing muscle
Buccinator	Horizontal cheek muscle	Flattens the cheek; trumpeter's muscle; Whistling muscle; helps with chewing
Zygomaticus	Extends from the corner of the mouth to cheekbone	Elevates corner of mouth; smiling muscle
Chewing muscles		
Temporalis	Flat fan-shaped muscle over temporal bone	Closes jaw
Masseter	Covers the lateral part of the lower jaw	Closes jaw
Neck		
Sternocleidomastoid	Extends along the side of the neck; strong narrow muscle that extends obliquely from the sternum and clavicle to the mastoid process of the temporal bone	Flexes and rotates the head; praying muscle
Trapezius	Large, flat triangular muscle on the back of the neck and upper back to shoulders	Extends head so as to look at the sky; elevates shoulder and pulls it back; shrugs the shoulders
Trunk		
Muscles involved in breathing (thoracic muscles)		
External intercostals	Intercostal spaces (between ribs)	Breathing (enlarges thoracic cavity)
Internal intercostals	Intercostal spaces (between ribs)	Breathing (decreases thoracic cavity in forced expiration)
Diaphragm	Dome-shaped muscle that separates the thoracic and abdominal cavities	Breathing: chief muscle of inspiration (enlarges thoracic cavity)
Muscles of abdominal wall External oblique Internal oblique Transversus abdominis Rectus abdominis	The muscles are arranged vertically, horizontally, and obliquely so as to strengthen the abdominal wall	As a group, the abdominal wall muscles compress the abdomen; the rectus abdominis also flexes the vertebral column
Muscles of the vertebral column	Muscles attached to the vertebrae	Movement of vertebral column
Muscles of the pelvic floor	Flat muscle sheets	Support pelvic viscera; assist in the function of the genitalia
Muscles That Move the Shoulder and Upper Arm		
Trapezius	Broad muscle on posterior neck and shoulder	Extends the head; looks at the sky Elevates shoulder and pulls it back; shrugs the shoulders
Serratus anterior	Forms the upper sides of the chest wall below the axilla	Pulls scapula forward; aids in raising arms
Pectoralis major	Large muscle that covers upper anterior chest	Adducts and flexes upper arm across chest Pulls shoulder forward and downward
Latissimus dorsi	Large broad flat muscle on mid and lower back	Adducts and rotates arm behind the back; "swimmer's muscle"

Table 8 • 1

MUSCLES OF THE BODY Continued

MUSCLE	DESCRIPTION	FUNCTION
Deltoid	Thick muscle that covers the shoulder joint	Abducts arm as in "scarecrow" position

Rotator cuff muscles
  Supraspinatus
  Subscapularis
  Infraspinatus
  Teres minor
	A group of four muscles that attaches the humerus to the scapula; forms a cuff over the proximal humerus	Rotate the arm at the shoulder joint

Muscles That Move the Forearm and Hand

MUSCLE	DESCRIPTION	FUNCTION
Biceps brachii	Major muscle on anterior surface of upper arm	Flexes and supinates forearm; muscle used to "make a muscle"; acts synergistically with brachialis and brachioradialis
Triceps brachii	Posterior surface of upper arm	Extends forearm; "boxer's muscle"
Brachialis	Deep to biceps	Flexes forearm
Brachioradialis	Muscles of forearm	Flexes forearm
Flexor and extensor carpi groups	Anterior and posterior forearm to hand	Flex and extend hand
Flexor and extensor digitorum groups	Anterior and posterior forearm to fingers	Flex and extend fingers

Muscles That Move the Thigh

MUSCLE	DESCRIPTION	FUNCTION
Gluteus maximus	Largest and most superficial of the gluteal muscles; located on posterior surface of the buttocks	Forms the buttocks; extends the thigh; muscle for sitting and climbing stairs
Gluteus medius	Thick muscle partly behind and superior to the gluteus maximus	Abducts and rotates thigh; Common site of intramuscular injections
Gluteus minimus	Smallest and deepest of the gluteal muscles	Abducts and rotates the thigh
Iliopsoas	Located on anterior surface of groin; crosses over hip joint to the femur	Flexes the thigh; antagonist to gluteus maximus

Adductor group
  Adductor longus
  Adductor brevis
  Adductor magnus
  Gracilis
	Medial inner thigh region	Adducts thigh; muscles used by horseback riders to stay on horse

Muscles That Move the Leg

MUSCLE	DESCRIPTION	FUNCTION

Quadriceps femoris
  Rectus femoris
  Vastus lateralis
  Vastus medialis
  Vastus intermedius
	Located on anterior and lateral surface of thigh; form a common tendon that inserts in tibia	Group used to extend the leg (eg, kicking) Rectus femoris can flex thigh at the hip joint Vastus lateralis is the common site for intramuscular injections in children

Sartorius	Long muscle that crosses obliquely over the anterior thigh	Allows you to sit in the crossed leg or lotus position

Hamstrings
  Biceps femoris
  Semitendinosus
  Semimembranosus
	Located on posterior surface of thigh; as a group they attach to the tibia and fibula	Flex leg; extend thigh; antagonistic to quadriceps femoris

Muscles That Move the Ankle and Foot

MUSCLE	DESCRIPTION	FUNCTION
Tibialis anterior	Anterior leg	Dorsiflexes foot; inversion of foot
Peroneus	Lateral surface of leg	Plantar flexion; eversion of foot; supports arch
Gastrocnemius	Posterior surface of leg; large two-headed muscle that forms the calf	Plantar flexion of foot; toe-dancer muscle
Soleus	Posterior surface of leg	Plantar flexion of foot

Muscles of the Head

The muscles of the head are grouped into two categories: the facial muscles and the chewing muscles (Fig. 8–9).

Facial Muscles

Many of the facial muscles are inserted directly into the soft tissue of the skin and other muscles of the face. When the facial muscles contract, they pull on the soft tissue. This kind of muscular activity is responsible for our facial expressions like smiling and frowning.

The facial muscles include

- *Frontalis:* The **frontalis** is a flat muscle that covers the frontal bone. It extends from the cranial aponeurosis to the skin of the eyebrows. Contraction of the muscle raises the eyebrows, giving you a surprised look. It also wrinkles your forehead.
- *Orbicularis oculi:* The **orbicularis oculi** is a sphincter muscle that encircles the eyes. A **sphincter** is a ring-shaped muscle that controls the size of an opening. Contraction of the muscle closes the eye and assists in winking, blinking, and squinting.
- *Orbicularis oris:* The **orbicularis oris** is a sphincter muscle that encircles the mouth. Contraction of this muscle assists in closing the mouth, forming words, and pursing the lips. It is sometimes called the kissing muscle.
- *Buccinator:* The **buccinator** is a muscle that inserts into the orbicularis oris and flattens the cheek when contracted. The buccinator is used in whistling and playing the trumpet. It is sometimes called the trumpeter's muscle. The buccinator is also classified as a chewing muscle because, upon contraction, it helps position the food between the teeth for chewing.
- *Zygomaticus:* The **zygomaticus** is the smiling muscle, which extends from the corners of the mouth to the cheekbone.

Chewing Muscles

The chewing muscles are also called the muscles of **mastication** (chewing). All of them are inserted on the mandible, the lower jaw bone, and

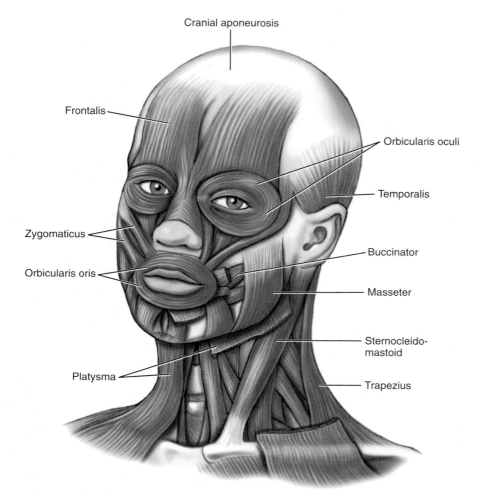

Cranial aponeurosis

Frontalis

Orbicularis oculi

Temporalis

Zygomaticus

Buccinator

Orbicularis oris

Masseter

Sternocleidomastoid

Platysma

Trapezius

FIGURE 8–9 • Muscles of the head (facial and chewing muscles) and neck.

are considered some of the strongest muscles of the body (see Table 8–1). Chewing muscles include

- *Masseter:* The **masseter** is a muscle that extends from the zygomatic process of the temporal bone in the skull to the mandible. Contraction of this muscle closes the jaw. It acts synergistically (ie, works with) the temporalis muscle to close the jaw.
- *Temporalis:* The **temporalis** is a fan-shaped muscle that extends from the flat portion of the temporal bone to the mandible. It works synergistically with the other chewing muscles.

Muscles of the Neck

Many muscles are involved in the movement of the head and shoulders and participate in movements within the throat.

Sternocleidomastoid

As the name implies, the **sternocleidomastoid** muscle extends from the sternum and clavicle to the mastoid process of the temporal bone in the skull. Contraction of both muscles on either side of the neck causes flexion of the head. Because the head bows as if in prayer, the muscle is called the praying muscle. Contraction of only one of the sternocleidomastoid muscles causes the head to rotate.

A spasm of this muscle can cause **torticollis,** or wryneck. This condition is characterized by the twisting of the neck and rotation of the head to one side.

Trapezius

The **trapezius** muscle attaches to the base of the occipital bone in the skull and to the spines of the upper vertebral column (see Fig. 8–8B). Contraction of the trapezius extends the head; the head tilts back so that the face looks at the sky. The trapezius works antagonistically with the sternocleidomastoid muscle, which flexes and bows the head. The trapezius is also attached to the shoulder.

Muscles of the Trunk

The muscles of the trunk are involved in breathing, form the abdominal wall, move the vertebral column, and form the pelvic region.

Muscles Involved in Breathing

The chest, or thoracic, muscles include the intercostal muscles and the diaphragm. These muscles are primarily responsible for breathing (Fig. 8–10). The **intercostal muscles** are located between the ribs and are responsible for raising and lowering the rib cage during breathing. There are external and internal intercostal muscles. (The ribs you barbeque are the intercostals.)

The **diaphragm** is a dome-shaped muscle that separates the thoracic cavity from the abdominal cavity. The diaphragm is the chief muscle of inhalation, the breathing-in phase of respiration. Without the contraction and relaxation of the intercostal muscles and the diaphragm, breathing could not occur.

FIGURE 8–10 ● Breathing muscles. The intercostal muscles and the diaphragm.

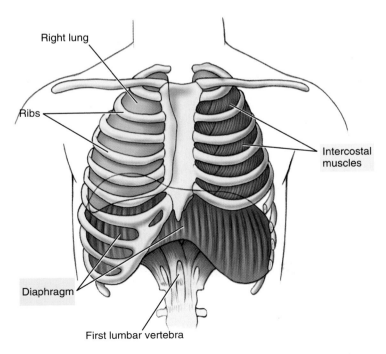

Right lung

Ribs

Intercostal muscles

Diaphragm

First lumbar vertebra

Muscles That Form the Abdominal Wall

The abdominal wall consists of four muscles (see Fig. 8–8) in an arrangement that provides considerable strength. The muscles are layered so that the fibers of each of the four muscles run in four different directions. This arrangement enables the muscles to contain, support, and protect the abdominal organs. Contraction of the abdominal muscles performs other functions. It causes flexion of the vertebral column and compression of the abdominal organs during urination, defecation, and childbirth.

The four abdominal muscles include

- *Rectus abdominis.* As the name implies, the fibers of the **rectus abdominis** run in an up-and-down, or longitudinal, direction. They extend from the sternum to the pubic bone. Contraction of this muscle flexes, or bends, the vertebral column.
- *External oblique.* Abdominal muscles called the **external obliques** make up the lateral walls of the abdomen. The fibers run obliquely (ie, they are slanted).
- *Internal oblique.* The **internal oblique** muscles are a part of the lateral walls of the abdomen. They add to the strength provided by the external oblique muscles, as the fibers of the oblique muscles form a criss-cross pattern.
- *Transversus abdominis.* The **transversus abdominis** muscles form the innermost layer of the abdominal muscles. The fibers run horizontally across the abdomen.

The abdominal muscles are surrounded by fascia that forms a large aponeurosis along the midline of the abdominal wall. The aponeuroses of the abdominal muscles on opposite sides of the midline of the abdomen form a white line called the **linea alba.** The linea alba extends from the sternum to the pubic bone.

Muscles That Move the Vertebral Column

A group of muscles is attached to the vertebrae. These muscles assist in the movement of the vertebral column.

Muscles That Form the Pelvic Floor

The pelvic floor consists primarily of two flat muscle sheets and the surrounding fascia. These structures support the pelvic viscera and play a role in expelling the contents of the urinary bladder and rectum.

Muscles of the Shoulder and Upper Arm

Many muscles move the shoulder and the upper arm. The most important are the trapezius, serratus anterior, pectoralis major, latissimus dorsi, deltoid muscles, and a group of muscles called the rotator cuff muscles (see Fig 8–8B).

- *Trapezius.* The trapezius attaches to the thoracic vertebrae and scapula (the wing bone). When contracted, the trapezius shrugs the shoulders. It also moves the head. The muscle gets its name because the right and left trapezius form the shape of a trapezoid.
- *Serratus anterior.* The **serratus anterior** is located on the sides of the chest and extends from the ribs to the scapula. The serratus muscle has a jagged shape, much like the jagged edge of a serrated knife blade. When the serratus anterior contracts, the shoulders are lowered, and the upper arm moves forward as if pushing a cart. The trapezius and the serratus anterior attach the scapula to the axial skeleton.
- *Pectoralis major.* The **pectoralis major** is a large, broad muscle that helps to form the anterior chest wall. It connects the humerus (upper arm) with the clavicle (collarbone) and structures in the anterior chest. Contraction of this muscle moves the upper arm across the front of the chest.
- *Latissimus dorsi.* The **latissimus dorsi** is a large, broad muscle located in the middle and lower back region. It extends from the back structures to the humerus. Contraction of this muscle lowers the shoulders and brings the arm back as in swimming and rowing. The pectoralis major and the latissimus dorsi attach the humerus to the axial skeleton.
- *Deltoid.* The **deltoid** forms the rounded portion of the shoulder. It is the muscle under your shoulder pad. The deltoid extends from the clavicle and scapula to the humerus. Contraction of the deltoid muscle extends the arm, raising it to a horizontal position (the scarecrow position). Because of its size, location, and good blood supply, the deltoid is a common site of intramuscular injection.
- *Rotator cuff muscles.* The **rotator cuff muscles** are a group of four muscles that attach the humerus to the scapula. These muscles form a cap, or a cuff, over the proximal humerus. The muscles help to rotate the arm at the shoulder joint. The names of the individual muscles making up the rotator cuff are listed in Table 8–1.

Muscles That Move the Lower Arm

The primary muscles involved in the movement of the lower arm (forearm) are located along the humerus. They are the triceps brachii, biceps brachii, brachialis, and brachioradialis.

The **triceps brachii** lies along the posterior surface of the humerus. When contracted, it extends the forearm. The triceps brachii is the muscle that supports the weight of the body when someone walks with crutches. It is also the muscle that packs the greatest punch for a boxer and is called the boxer's muscle (see Fig. 8–8).

The **biceps brachii** is located along the anterior surface of the humerus. The biceps brachii acts synergistically with the **brachialis** and **brachioradialis** to flex the forearm. When someone is asked to "make a muscle," the biceps brachii becomes most visible.

Muscles That Move the Hand and Fingers

More than 20 muscles move the hand and fingers. The muscles are numerous but small, making the hand and fingers capable of delicate movements. The muscles are generally located along the forearm and consist of **flexors** and **extensors.** The flexors are located on the anterior surface while the extensors are located on the posterior surface. The flexors of the fingers are stronger than the extensors, so that in a relaxed hand, the fingers are slightly flexed.

If a person is unconscious for an extended period, the fingers remain in a flexed position. In response to inactivity, the tendons of the fingers shorten, thereby preventing extension of the fingers. This gives a claw-like appearance to the hand. This problem can be prevented by an exercise program that includes passive exercises of the hands and fingers.

Muscles That Move the Thigh, Leg, and Foot

The muscles that move the thigh, leg, and foot are some of the largest and strongest muscles in the body.

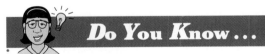

Do You Know...

What is the difference between isometric contraction and isotonic contraction?

An **isotonic muscle contraction** is a muscle contraction that causes movement. Examples include jogging, swimming, and weight lifting. An isometric muscle contraction is a muscle contraction that does not cause movement. For example, if you try to lift a 1000-pound object, your muscles contract but do not move the object (it is too heavy).

As you sit reading this text, you can do isometric exercises. Tighten the muscle in your thigh. Hold the tension for 30 seconds and then relax the muscle. Repetition of this type of exercise can provide you with a mini-workout without leaving your desk.

Muscles That Move the Thigh

The muscles that move the thigh all attach to some part of the pelvic girdle and the femur (thigh bone). These muscles include the gluteal muscles, the iliopsoas, and a group of adductor muscles. Contraction of these muscles moves the hip joint (see Fig. 8–8).

The **gluteal muscles** are located on the posterior surface and include the **gluteus maximus, gluteus medius,** and **gluteus minimus.** The gluteal muscles abduct the thigh (ie, they raise the thigh sideways to a horizontal position). The gluteus maximus is the largest muscle in the body and forms the area of the buttocks; it is the muscle you sit on.

In addition to abducting the thigh, the gluteus maximus also straightens, or extends, the thigh at the hip, as you do while climbing stairs. The gluteus medius lies partly behind and superior to the gluteus maximus. Both gluteal muscles are commonly used sites for intramuscular injections.

The **iliopsoas** is located on the anterior surface of the groin. Contraction of this muscle flexes the thigh, making it antagonist to the gluteus maximus.

The **adductor muscles** are located on the medial (inner) surface of the thigh. These muscles adduct the thighs, pressing them together. These are the muscles a horse rider uses to stay on the horse. The adductor muscles include the **adductor longus, adductor brevis, adductor magnus,** and **adductor gracilis.**

Muscles That Move the Leg

The muscles that move the leg are located in the thigh. They include the quadriceps femoris group, the sartorius, and the hamstring group.

The **quadriceps femoris group** consists of four muscles located on the anterior and lateral surface of the thigh. All four muscles insert into the tibial tuberosity by the patellar tendon. As a group, they extend, or straighten, the leg at the knee. You would use them when kicking a football.

The muscles that make up this group include the **vastus lateralis,** the **vastus intermedius,** the **vastus medialis,** and the **rectus femoris.** The vastus lateralis is a frequently used injection site for children because it is more developed than the gluteal muscles. Because the rectus femoris originates on a pelvic bone, this muscle can also flex the thigh at the hip joint.

The **sartorius** is the longest muscle in the body. It is a strap-like muscle located on the anterior surface of the thigh. The sartorius passes over the quadriceps in an oblique direction and allows the legs to rotate so that you can sit cross-legged. At one time tailors used to sit cross-legged as they worked. The Latin word for tailor is *sartor,* so this muscle was named the sartorius.

The **hamstrings** are a group of muscles located on the posterior surface of the thigh. All the muscles extend from the ischium (pelvic bone) to the tibia. They flex the leg at the knee and are therefore antagonistic to the quadriceps femoris. Because these muscles also span the hip joint, they extend the thigh. The strong tendons of these muscles can be felt behind the knee. These same tendons are found in hogs. Butchers used to use these tendons to hang the hams for smoking and curing, hence the name *hamstrings*. The hamstring muscles include the **biceps femoris,** the **semimembranosus,** and the **semitendinosus.**

Frequently, an athlete pulls a hamstring or experiences a groin injury. These injuries involve

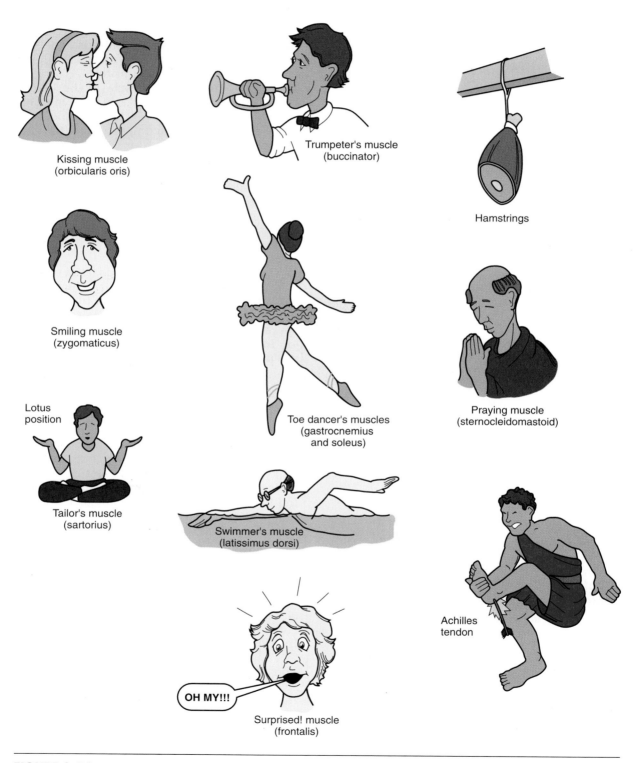

Kissing muscle (orbicularis oris)

Trumpeter's muscle (buccinator)

Hamstrings

Smiling muscle (zygomaticus)

Lotus position

Tailor's muscle (sartorius)

Toe dancer's muscles (gastrocnemius and soleus)

Praying muscle (sternocleidomastoid)

Swimmer's muscle (latissimus dorsi)

Achilles tendon

OH MY!!!

Surprised! muscle (frontalis)

FIGURE 8–11 ● A medley of special muscles. These muscles are named for their common use.

one or more of the hamstring muscles or their tendons.

Muscles That Move the Foot

The muscles that move the foot are located on the anterior, lateral, and posterior surfaces of the leg. The **tibialis anterior** is located on the anterior surface. It causes dorsiflexion of the foot. The **peroneus longus muscle** is on the lateral surface. It everts (turns outward) the foot, supports the arch of the foot, and assists in plantar flexion. The **gastrocnemius** and the **soleus** are the major muscles on the posterior surface of the leg and form the calf of the leg. They attach to the calcaneus (heel bone) by the **calcaneal tendon,** or **Achilles tendon.** Contraction of these muscles causes plantar flexion. The gastrocnemius is sometimes called the toe dancer's muscle because it allows you to stand on tiptoe.

Runners, especially sprinters, occasionally tear or rupture the Achilles tendon. Because the heel then cannot be lifted, this injury severely impedes the ability of the runner to perform.

Some muscles have acquired rather interesting names. In Figure 8–11, note how many interesting movements we are able to make.

✳ **SUM IT UP!** The skeleton is stabilized and covered with muscle. The ability of the muscles to contract and relax allows the skeleton to move about and to engage in all the activities that make life so enjoyable. The location and function of the major muscles of the body are summarized in Table 8–1.

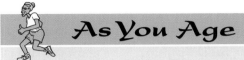

As You Age

1. At about the age of 40, the number and diameter of muscle fibers decrease. Muscles become smaller, dehydrated, and weaker. Muscle fibers are gradually replaced by connective tissue, especially adipose or fat cells. By the age of 80, 50% of the muscle mass has been lost.
2. Mitochondrial function in muscles decreases, especially in muscles that are not exercised regularly.
3. Motor neurons are gradually lost, resulting in muscle atrophy.
4. These changes lead to decreased muscle strength and slowing of muscle reflexes.

Disorders of the Muscular System

Atrophy (muscle)	Wasting of muscle tissue. The muscles become smaller. Disuse atrophy refers to muscle wasting due to lack of use in a muscle that has an intact nerve supply. Disuse atrophy is often seen in a casted extremity. Denervation atrophy refers to muscle wasting due to the lack of stimulation by the motor neurons that normally supply the muscle. It is seen in patients who have experienced spinal cord injury.
Cramp	A painful, involuntary skeletal muscle contraction.
Fibromyositis	Also called a charleyhorse. Fibromyositis refers to pain and tenderness in the fibromuscular tissue of the thighs usually due to muscle strain or tear.
Flatfoot	Abnormal flatness of the sole and the arch of the foot.
Frozen shoulder	Frozen shoulder is a condition in which the shoulder becomes stiff and painful, making normal movement difficult. It is often caused by disuse of the shoulder because of an injury or the pain associated with bursitis or tendonitis.
Hypertonia	Increased muscle tone causing spasticity or rigidity.
Hypotonia	Decrease in or absence of muscle tone, causing loose, flaccid muscles.
Myalgia	Pain or tenderness in the muscles. Fibromyalgia is a group of common rheumatic disorders characterized by chronic pain in muscles and soft tissues surrounding joints (affects the fibrous connective tissue portions of muscles, tendons, and ligaments).

continued

Disorders of the Muscular System *continued*

Myopathy	Any disease of the muscles that is not associated with the nervous system. A dystrophy is a myopathy that is characterized by muscle degeneration. Muscular dystrophy refers to a group of diseases, usually inherited, in which there is progressive degeneration and weakening of the skeletal muscles. Deterioration of the muscle fibers causes decreased muscle function, atrophy, and motor disability.
Plantar fasciitis	Inflammation at the heel bone caused when the inflexible fascia in the heel is repeatedly stretched (as in running). The inflammatory response can produce spike-like projections of new bone called spurs (calcaneal spurs).
Shin splints	An exercise-related inflammatory condition involving the extensor muscles and surrounding tissues in the lower leg. Pain is generally experienced along the inner aspect of the tibia.
Torticollis	Also called wryneck. Torticollis refers to the twisting of the neck into an unusual position. It is caused by prolonged contraction of the neck muscles.

Summary Outline

The purpose of muscle is to contract and to cause movement.

I. Muscle Function: Overview

A. Types and Functions of Muscles
1. Skeletal muscle is striated and voluntary; it functions to produce movement, maintain body posture, stabilize joints, and maintain body temperature.
2. Smooth muscle is nonstriated and involuntary; it is called visceral muscle because it is found in the viscera and helps the organs perform their functions.
3. Cardiac muscle is striated and involuntary; it is found only in the heart and allows the heart to function as a pump.

B. Structure of the Whole Muscle
1. A large muscle consists of thousands of single muscle fibers (muscle cells). Muscle cells are the contractile units.
2. Connective tissue binds the muscle fibers (cells) together and attaches muscle to bone and other tissue.
3. Muscles attach to other structures directly, by tendons, and by aponeuroses.

C. Structure and Function of a Single Muscle Fiber
1. The muscle fiber (cell) is surrounded by a cell membrane (sarcolemma). The cell membrane penetrates to the interior of the muscle as the transverse tubule (T tubule).
2. An extensive sarcoplasmic reticulum (SR) stores calcium.
3. Each muscle fiber consists of a series of sarcomeres. Each sarcomere contains the contractile proteins actin and myosin.

D. How Muscles Contract
1. Muscles shorten or contract as the actin and myosin (in the presence of calcium and ATP) interact through crossbridge formation according to the sliding filament hypothesis.
2. For skeletal muscle to contract, it must be stimulated by a motor nerve. The nerve impulse causes the release of neurotransmitter (ACh) from the nerve terminal into the neuromuscular junction (NMJ). The ACh diffuses across the NMJ and binds to the postjunctional (muscle) membrane. The binding of the ACh causes an electrical signal to form in the muscle membrane. The ACh is inactivated by an enzyme called acetylcholinesterase found near the muscle membrane.
3. The electrical signal runs along the muscle membrane and the T-tubular system.
4. The electrical signal stimulates the SR to release calcium into the sarcomere area (actin and myosin).
5. Actin, myosin, and ATP interact to form crossbridges, which cause the filaments to slide past each other (cause the muscle to contract or shorten).
6. Calcium is pumped back into the SR and the muscles relax.

E. Responses of a Whole Muscle
1. A single muscle fiber contracts in an all-or-nothing response; a whole muscle can contract partially (ie, not all-or-nothing).
2. A whole muscle increases its force of contraction by recruitment of additional muscle fibers.
3. Three terms describe the contractile activity of a whole muscle: twitch, summation, and tetanus. A twitch occurs when a single stimulus is delivered to a muscle; the muscle contracts and fully relaxes. Summation refers to the inability of a muscle to relax fully when the electrical stimuli are delivered in rapid

Summary Outline, continued

I. Muscle Function: Overview, *continued*

E. Responses of a Whole Muscle, *continued*
succession. Tetanus refers to a sustained muscle contraction.

4. Energy for muscle contraction can be obtained from three sources: burning fuel aerobically, burning fuel anaerobically, and metabolizing creatine phosphate.

F. Terms That Describe Muscle Movement
1. Origin: the origin of the muscle attaches to the stationary bone.
2. Insertion: the insertion of the muscle attaches to the more movable bone.
3. Prime mover: the chief muscle (the muscle generally responsible for most of the movement).
4. Synergist: the helper muscle (helps the prime mover).
5. Antagonist: the muscle that opposes the action of another muscle.

II. Muscles from Head to Toe

A. Skeletal muscles are named according to size, shape, direction of fibers, location, number of origins, place of origin and insertion, and muscle action.

B. See Table 8–1 for a list of the body's muscles.

Review Your Knowledge

1. What are the three types of muscles?

2. State three ways in which muscles form attachments to other structures, such as bones and other muscles.

3. What gives skeletal muscle its striped appearance?

4. What is the relationship of the sliding filament hypothesis of muscle contraction to the shortening of muscles? How is the shortening of sarcomeres related to a trombone?

5. What three structures make up the neuromuscular junction (NMJ)? What is the role of acetylcholine in the transfer of information from nerve to muscle at the NMJ?

6. How do calcium, actin, myosin, and ATP play a role in muscle contraction?

7. What is thought to cause muscle weakness in myasthenia gravis?

8. How does curare promote muscular relaxation?

9. How does botulism (a serious form of food poisoning) cause muscle paralysis?

10. List the steps involved in the contraction and relaxation of skeletal muscle.

11. What is the difference between twitch, summation, and tetanus?

12. Name the origin and insertion of the biceps brachii. What is the antagonist of the biceps brachii?

13. How is a contracture related to immobility?

14. Name seven ways in which muscles are named or classified.

15. State the basis on which the following muscles are named:
    a. Gluteus maximus
    b. Trapezius
    c. Rectus abdominis
    d. Pectoralis major
    e. Triceps brachii
    f. Sternocleidomastoid
    g. Adductor magnus

16. Name the muscles responsible for the following movements:
    a. Wrinkling the forehead
    b. Winking the eye
    c. Kissing
    d. Whistling
    e. Smiling
    f. Praying
    g. Looking at the sky

17. Which two muscles are important for breathing?

18. Which four muscles are commonly used for intramuscular injections?

19. Name the major muscle found in the following areas:
    a. Neck
    b. Back
    c. Chest
    d. Buttocks
    e. Thigh

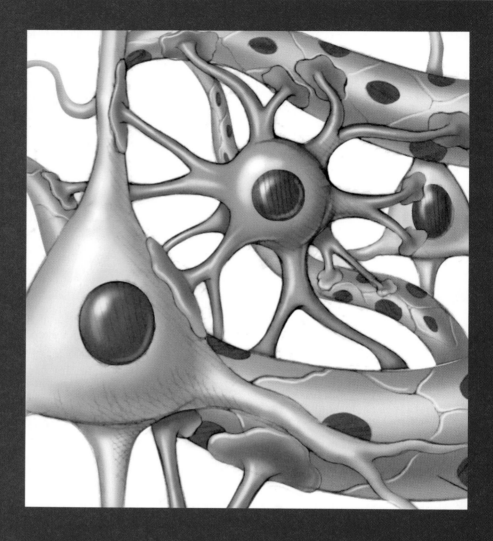

9 NERVOUS SYSTEM: NERVOUS TISSUE AND BRAIN

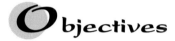
Objectives

1. Define the two divisions of the nervous system.

2. List three general functions of the nervous system.

3. Compare the structure and functions of the neuroglia and neuron.

4. Explain the importance of the myelin sheath.

5. Define the three types of neurons.

6. Explain how a neuron transmits information.

7. Describe what happens at the synapse.

8. Describe the functions of the four major areas of the brain.

9. Describe the functions of the four lobes of the cerebrum.

10. Identify common neurotransmitters.

11. Describe how the skull, meninges, cerebrospinal fluid, and blood-brain barrier protect the central nervous system.

If you have ever listened to an orchestra warming up before a performance, you know something about the need for its conductor. Without the conductor, the sound is more like noise than music. It takes the conductor to coordinate, interpret, and direct the sound into the beautiful strains of a symphony. So it is with the nervous system; the various organ systems of the body need an interpreter to coordinate and direct them. This role is performed magnificently by the nervous system. The music of the body is every bit as beautiful as the strains of a symphony!

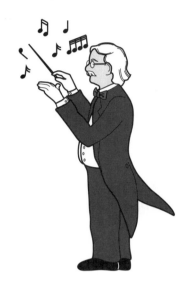

THE NERVOUS SYSTEM: STRUCTURE AND FUNCTION

Divisions of the Nervous System

The structures of the nervous system are divided into two parts: the central nervous system and the peripheral nervous system. The **central nervous system (CNS)** includes the brain and the spinal cord. The CNS is located in the dorsal cavity. The brain is located in the cranium; the spinal cord is enclosed in the spinal cavity. The **peripheral nervous system** is located outside the CNS and consists of the nerves that connect the CNS with the rest of the body (Fig. 9–1).

Functions of the Nervous System

As conductor, the nervous system performs three general functions: a sensory function, an integrative function, and a motor function. The three functions are illustrated in Figure 9–2.

Sensory Function

Sensory nerves gather information from inside the body and from the outside environment. The nerves then carry the information to the CNS. For instance, information about the cat is picked up by special cells in the eye.

Integrative Function

Sensory information brought to the CNS is processed or interpreted. The brain not only sees the cat but also does much more. It recalls very quickly how a cat behaves. It may determine that the cat is acting hungry or is distressed and ready to attack. The brain integrates, or puts together, everything it knows about cats and then makes its plan.

Motor Function

Motor nerves convey information from the CNS toward the muscles and glands of the body. Motor nerves carry out the plans made by the CNS. For instance, the person may decide to feed the hungry cat. Information must travel along the motor nerves from the CNS to all of the skeletal muscles needed to feed the cat. The motor nerve converts the plan into action.

CELLS THAT MAKE UP THE NERVOUS SYSTEM

Nervous tissue is composed of two types of cells: the neuroglia and the neurons.

Neuroglia

Neuroglia (noo-rŏg′lē-ə), or glial cells, is the nerve glue. Neuroglia is the most abundant of the nerve cells and is located in the CNS. Glial cells support, protect, insulate, nourish, and generally care for the delicate neurons. Some of the glial cells participate in phagocytosis; others assist in the secretion of cerebrospinal fluid. Glial cells, however, do not conduct nerve impulses.

Two of the more common glial cells are the astrocytes and the ependymal cells (Fig. 9–3). The star-shaped **astrocytes** are the most abundant of the glial cells; they support the neurons and also form a protective barrier around the neurons of the CNS. This barrier helps to prevent toxic substances in the blood from entering the nervous tissue of the brain and spinal cord. A second glial cell is the **ependymal cell.** These cells line the inside

FIGURE 9–1 ● Divisions of the nervous system: the central nervous system, consisting of the brain and the spinal cord, and the peripheral nervous system.

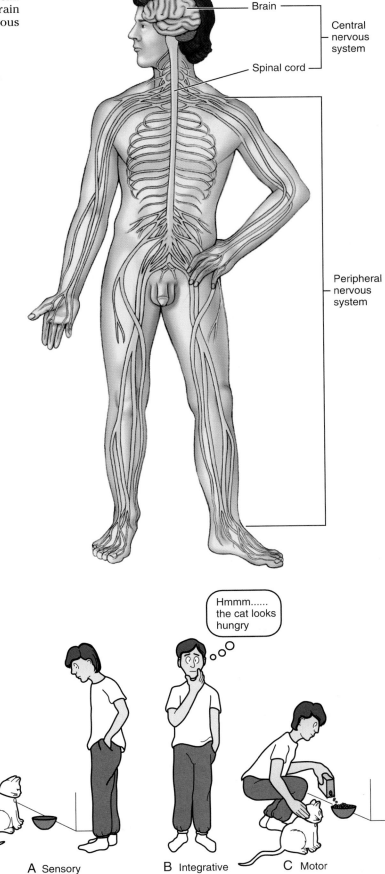

Brain

Central nervous system

Spinal cord

Peripheral nervous system

FIGURE 9–2 ● Three functions of the nervous system. A, Sensory function: the information (light) is "sensed" by the eyes and carried to the brain. B, Integrative function: the brain identifies the object as a hungry cat. C, Motor function: the brain sends a command by the motor nerves to feed the cat.

Hmmm...... the cat looks hungry

A Sensory   B Integrative   C Motor

A

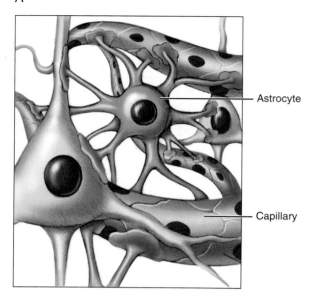

B

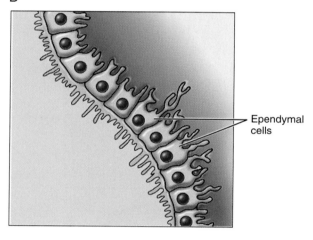

FIGURE 9–3 ● Neuroglia, or glia. There are four types of glial tissue. The two shown here are the astrocytes and the ependymal cells.

cavities of the brain and assist in the formation of cerebrospinal fluid. Other glial cells are listed in Table 9–1.

Neuron

The second type of nerve cell is the neuron. Of the two types of nerve cells, the **neuron** (nŏŏr'ŏn) is most important in the transmission of information. The neuron enables the nervous system to act as a vast communication network. Neurons have many shapes and sizes. Some neurons are extremely short; others are very long, some measuring 4 feet in length.

Parts of a Neuron

The three parts of the neuron are identified in Figure 9–4. They include the **dendrites,** tree-like structures that receive information from other neurons and then transmit the information toward the cell body. One neuron may have thousands of dendrites. Another part of the neuron is the **cell body,** which contains the nucleus and is essential for the life of the cell. The third part of the neuron is the **axon,** a long extension that transmits information away from the cell body. The end of the axon undergoes extensive branching to form hundreds to thousands of **axon terminals;** it is within the axon terminals that the chemical neurotransmitters are stored. Information travels from the dendrite to the cell body to the axon. The arrow in Figure 9–4 indicates the direction in which information travels over the neuron.

The Axon: A Special Structure

What is so special about the axon? An enlarged view of the axon shows several unique structures: the myelin sheath, the neurilemma, and the nodes of Ranvier (see Fig. 9–4). Most long nerve fibers of both the CNS and the peripheral

Table 9 ● 1	TYPES OF NEUROGLIA
CELL NAME	**FUNCTION**
Astrocytes	Star-shaped cells present in blood-brain barrier; also anchor or bind blood vessels to nerves for support
Ependymal cells	Line the ventricles as part of the choroid plexus; involved in the formation and circulation of cerebrospinal fluid
Microglia	Protective role: phagocytosis of pathogens and damaged tissue
Oligodendrocytes	Produce myelin sheath for neurons in the central nervous system (The myelin sheath of neurons in the peripheral nervous system is produced by Schwann cells.)

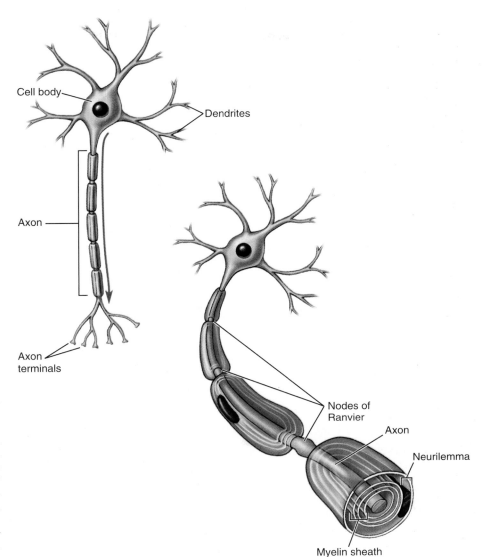

FIGURE 9–4 • Structure of a neuron: dendrites, the cell body, the axon, and axon terminals. The structure surrounding the axon is the myelin sheath. The nodes of Ranvier are the spaces between the myelin. Neurilemma surrounds the myelin sheath. The arrow indicates the direction in which the information moves along the axon.

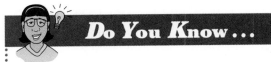

Why do some nerves "short circuit"?

The importance of myelin is evident when a person has multiple sclerosis (MS). MS is a demyelinating disease. The myelin, which encases many nerves, is gradually replaced by scar tissue. The scar tissue is unable to transmit the electrical signals and so interferes with neuron function. As a result, the person experiences episodes of numbness, tingling, muscle weakness, and double vision. While the symptoms may first appear to be mild and vague, the progressive nature of MS may eventually lead to paralysis and generalized severe impairment.

nervous system are encased by a layer of white fatty material called the **myelin sheath. Myelin** (mī′ə-lĭn) protects and insulates the axon. Nerve fibers covered by myelin are said to be myelinated. (Some neurons are not encased in myelin and are called unmyelinated neurons.)

The formation of myelin sheath differs in the peripheral and central nervous systems. Surrounding the axon of a neuron in the peripheral nervous system is a layer of special cells called **Schwann cells.** The Schwann cells form the myelin sheath that surrounds the axon. The nuclei and cytoplasm of the Schwann cells lie outside the myelin sheath and are called the **neurilemma.** The neurilemma is important in the event that the nerve is accidentally cut. Specifically, the neurilemma is responsible, in part, for nerve regeneration. Thus, the nerves in a severed limb that is surgically reattached may eventually reestablish proper connections, and the person may regain sensation and movement.

In the CNS, the myelin sheath is formed not by Schwann cells but by **oligodendrocytes,** a type of glial cell (see Table 9–1). Without Schwann cells, there is no neurilemma. The lack of the neurilemma surrounding the axons accounts, in part, for the inability of the CNS neurons to regenerate. This is why a spinal cord injury is so serious; nerve damage and the resulting paralysis are permanent.

The **nodes of Ranvier** appear regularly along the axon. The nodes are areas of the axon not covered by myelin.

Three Types of Neurons

Three types of neurons are the sensory neuron, the motor neuron, and the interneuron. A **sensory neuron** carries information from the periphery toward the CNS. Sensory neurons are also called **afferent neurons.** A **motor neuron** carries information from the CNS toward the periphery. Motor neurons are also called **efferent neurons.** Sensory and motor neurons are found in both the CNS and the peripheral nervous system.

Do You Know...

How does the brain "grow" in light of the fact that the number of neurons does not increase?

Although the neurons do not increase in number after birth, their size and degree of myelination increase. In addition to the growth of the neurons, the glial cells increase in number and size after birth. Consequently, the adult brain is three times as heavy as the infant brain.

The third type of neuron is the **interneuron;** it is found only in the CNS. Interneurons form connections between sensory and motor neurons. In the brain, interneurons play a role in thinking, learning, and memory.

White Matter Versus Gray Matter

The tissue of the CNS is white and gray. **White matter** is white because of the myelin. Myelinated fibers are gathered together in the CNS, according to function, in **tracts.** The **gray matter** is composed primarily of cell bodies, interneurons, and unmyelinated fibers.

Sometimes cell bodies appear in small clusters and are given special names. Clusters of cell bodies located in the CNS are generally referred to as **nuclei** (singular, nucleus). Small clusters of cell bodies are located in the peripheral nervous system and are called **ganglia** (singular, ganglion). For instance, patches of gray called the **basal nuclei** are located in the brain. (Sometimes, these patches of gray are called basal ganglia, despite their location within the CNS.)

Do You Know...

Why can brain tumors develop even though neurons do not divide?

Tumor formation is associated with an increase in the number of cells. Neurons in the CNS do not increase in number. Thus primary malignant tumors of the brain are tumors of glial cells rather than neurons. These tumors are called **gliomas.** Because gliomas have extensive roots, they are difficult to remove surgically without damaging large amounts of nontumorous tissue.

✳ **SUM IT UP!** The nervous system plays a crucial role in allowing us to interact with our environment, both internal and external. Information is constantly brought to the CNS for evaluation. The CNS, particularly the brain, receives, interprets, and makes decisions about this information. Finally, the brain directs the body to respond or act. The rapid communication demanded of this system is due primarily to the neuron. The three parts of the neuron are dendrites, cell body, and axon.

THE NEURON CARRYING INFORMATION

How do neurons carry information? Neurons allow the nervous system to convey information rapidly from one part of the body to the next. A stubbed toe makes itself known almost immediately. Think of how fast the information travels from your toe, where the injury occurred, to your brain, where the injury is interpreted as pain. Information is carried along the neuron in the form of an electrical signal, or **nerve impulse.**

The Nerve Impulse: What It Is

The nerve impulse is an electrical signal that conveys information along a neuron. A series of events causes the electrical charge inside the cell to move from its resting state (negative, −) to its depolarized state (positive, +) and back to its resting state (−). These events are the **action potential** (ăk'shən pə-tĕn'shəl) or nerve impulse. The action potential is a process of polarization, depolarization, and repolarization. Follow Figure 9–5 through the events of the action potential.

Polarization

Polarization characterizes the resting state of the neuron. When the neuron is polarized, the inside of the neuron is more negative than the outside. As long as the neuron is polarized, no nerve impulse is being transmitted. The cell is quiet, or resting.

Depolarization

When the neuron is stimulated, a change occurs in the cell's electrical state. In the resting (polarized) state, the inside of the cell is negative. When the cell is stimulated, the inside becomes positive. As the inside of the cell changes from negative to positive, it is said to **depolarize** (**depolarization,** dē-pō"lər-ĭ-zā'shən).

Repolarization

Very quickly, however, the inside of the cell again becomes negative; in other words, it returns to its resting state. This return to the resting state is called **repolarization** (rē"pō-lər-ĭ-zā'shən). Unless the cell repolarizes, it cannot be stimulated again. The cell's inability to accept another stimulus until it repolarizes is called its **refractory period.** The refractory period is its unresponsive period.

Nerve Impulse: What Causes It

The changes associated with the action potential, or nerve impulse, are due to the movement of specific ions across the cell membrane of the neuron (Fig. 9–6). Remember that the nerve impulse includes polarization, depolarization, and repolarization.

FIGURE 9–5 ● Nerve impulse (action potential): polarization, depolarization, and repolarization. The series of electrical changes in the neuron is the basis of the nerve impulse, or action potential. A, The unstimulated, or resting, neuron has a negative (−) charge on the inside. This is a state of polarization. B, When stimulated, the inside of the neuron becomes positive (+) for a brief period. This is a state of depolarization. C, The cell very quickly returns to its resting state with a negative (−) charge inside the cell. The return to resting state is called repolarization.

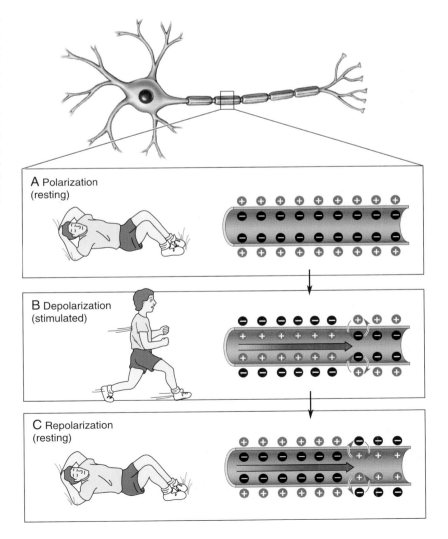

A Polarization (resting)

B Depolarization (stimulated)

C Repolarization (resting)

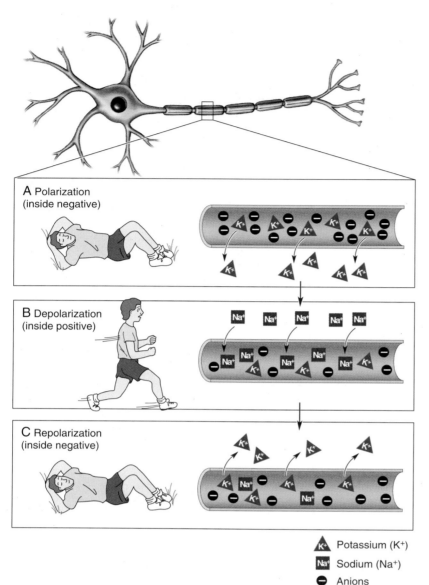

A Polarization
(inside negative)

B Depolarization
(inside positive)

C Repolarization
(inside negative)

K⁺ Potassium (K⁺)

Na⁺ Sodium (Na⁺)

⊖ Anions

FIGURE 9–6 ● What causes the nerve impulse? The electrical changes associated with the nerve impulse are caused by the movement of ions across the membrane. A, Polarization: the resting or polarized cell has an internal negativity. This phase is caused by the outward diffusion of potassium ions (K⁺). B, Depolarization occurs when the cell is stimulated. The inside of the cell becomes positive because of an inward diffusion of sodium ions (Na⁺). C, Repolarization is caused by the outward diffusion of potassium ions (K⁺); this process causes the inside of the cell to become negative again.

Polarization (Resting State)

What makes the inside of the cell negative (−) in the resting state? The resting state is due to the numbers and types of ions located inside the neuron. The chief intracellular ions include the positively charged potassium ions (K⁺) and several anions (negatively charged ions). How do these ions get into the cell in such high concentrations? They are pumped in by an ATP-driven pump in the cell membrane. In the resting state, the K⁺ ions tend to leak out of the cell, taking with them the positive charge. The positive charge lost from the inside of the cell and the excess anions trapped in the cell make the inside of the cell negative (−).

Depolarization (Stimulated State)

Why does the interior of the cell become positive (+) when stimulated? When the neuron is stimulated, the neuronal membrane changes in a way that allows sodium ions (Na⁺) to cross the membrane into the cell. Sodium ion (Na⁺) is the chief extracellular cation. With much more Na⁺ outside the cell than inside, Na⁺ diffuses into the cell, carrying with it a positive charge. This process makes the inside of the cell positive. Thus, it is the inward diffusion of Na⁺ that causes depolarization.

Repolarization (Return to Resting)

Why does the inside of the cell quickly return to its resting, negative state? Soon after the cell depolarizes, the neuronal membrane undergoes a second change. The change in the membrane does two things: it stops additional diffusion of Na⁺ *into* the cell, and it allows K⁺ to diffuse *out of* the cell. The outward movement of K⁺ removes positive charge from the inside of the cell, leaving behind the negatively (−) charged anions. Thus the outward movement of K⁺ causes repolarization.

Eventually, the sodium will be removed from the neuron by pumps located in the neuronal membrane. (The pumps are ATP-driven pumps that help to maintain the sodium and potassium concentrations.) Note that the repolarizing phase of the nerve impulse is *not* due to the removal of sodium (Na^+) by the pump. Repolarization is due to the outward diffusion of potassium (K^+).

Nerve Impulse: What Causes It to Move

To convey information, a nerve impulse must move the length of the neuron. The nerve impulse moves along the neuron toward the axon at the neuron's terminal end. Figure 9–7 shows that when nerve impulse #1 forms at point A, it also depolarizes the next segment of the membrane (point B), causing nerve impulse #2 to form. Nerve impulse #2 then depolarizes the next segment of membrane at point C, causing the formation of nerve impulse #3.

Because of the ability of each nerve impulse to depolarize the adjacent membrane, the nerve impulse moves toward the axon terminal much like a wave. In addition to showing the movement of the nerve impulse, Figure 9–7 also shows that each nerve impulse fires in an all-or-nothing manner. The all-or-nothing firing means that the height of each nerve impulse is the same. This point is important because it ensures that the nerve impulse does not weaken as it travels the length of a long axon.

FIGURE 9–7 ● What causes the nerve impulse to move from the cell body to the axon terminals? A, In response to a stimulus, nerve impulse #1 (NI #1) forms at the beginning of the axon (point A). The formation of nerve impulse #1 depolarizes point B. B, The membrane at point B forms a second nerve impulse. As nerve impulse #2 (NI #2) forms, it depolarizes point C. C, Nerve impulse #3 (NI #3) forms and depolarizes point D. This series of events continues until the nerve impulse makes it to the axon terminals.

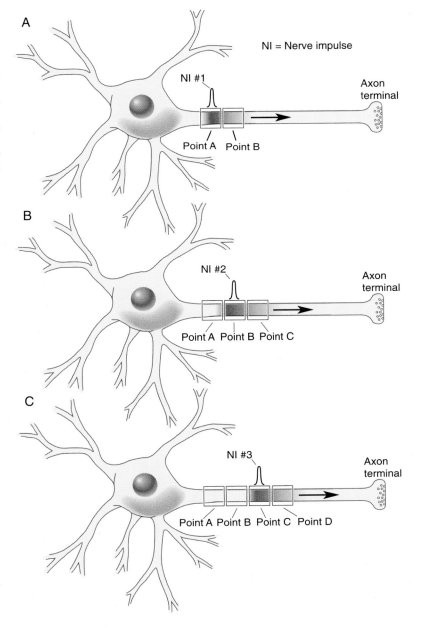

Myelination and Speed

How does **myelination** affect the movement of the nerve impulse along the axonal membrane? Recall that the axons of most nerve fibers are myelinated; that is, they are wrapped in a fatty myelin material. At intervals called the nodes of Ranvier, the axonal membrane is bare, or exposed, so that it is not covered with myelin.

How does the lack of myelin affect the nerve impulse? The nerve impulse enters the axon region but cannot develop on any part of the membrane covered with myelin. The nerve impulse can, however, develop at the nodes of Ranvier (the exposed axonal membrane). Thus in a myelinated fiber, the nerve impulse jumps from node to node, much like a kangaroo, to the end of the axon (Fig. 9–8). This "jumping" from node to node is called **saltatory conduction** (from Latin *saltare,* meaning to dance or leap). Saltatory conduction allows the nerve impulse to travel long distances in a short period. Thus saltatory conduction increases the speed with which the nerve impulse travels along

the nerve fiber. For this reason, myelinated fibers are considered fast-conducting nerve fibers.

Synapse Across Neurons

A synapse helps information move from one neuron to the next. A **synapse** (sĭn′ăps) is a junction, or space, between two neurons. Information is transmitted from one neuron to the next across the synapse (Fig. 9–9). The big question is how.

PARTS OF A SYNAPSE

Synaptic Cleft. The synapse (from the Greek meaning to join or clasp) is a space. The space exists because the axon terminal of neuron A does not physically touch the dendrite of neuron B. The space is called the **synaptic cleft.**

Neurotransmitters. The axon terminal of neuron A contains thousands of tiny vesicles that store chemical substances called **neurotransmitters** (nōōr″ŏ-trăns′mĭt-ərz). The most common neurotransmitters are acetylcholine (ACh) and

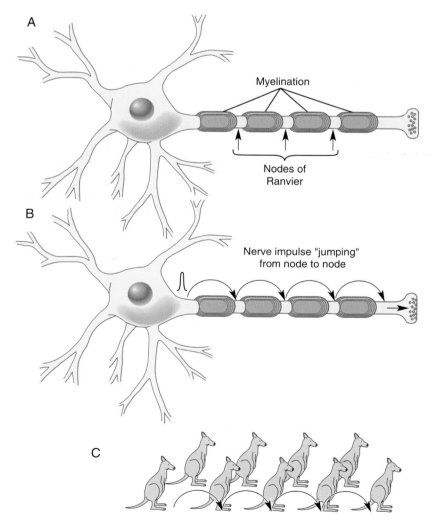

FIGURE 9–8 • Jumping from node to node. A, A myelinated axon showing the exposed axonal membrane at the nodes of Ranvier. B, The nerve impulse jumps from node to node toward the axon terminal. The jumping allows the nerve impulse to travel the length of the axon very fast. C, The jumping of the nerve impulse resembles the jumping or hopping of a kangaroo. Think of how fast a kangaroo can move by jumping rather than walking!

Myelination

Nodes of Ranvier

Nerve impulse "jumping" from node to node

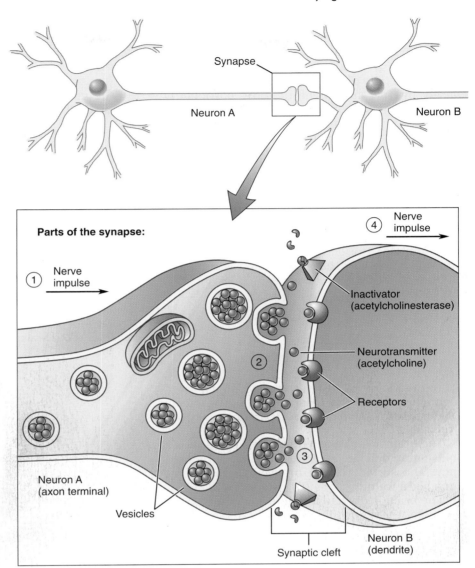

FIGURE 9–9 ● The synapse. The synapse is located in the space between neuron A and neuron B. Parts of the synapse include the neurotransmitters, inactivators, and receptors. The neurotransmitters are located in the vesicles of neuron A. The inactivators are located on the membrane of neuron B. The receptors are located on the membrane of neuron B.

norepinephrine. Other CNS transmitters include epinephrine, serotonin, GABA, and endorphins.

Inactivators. Inactivators are substances that inactivate, or terminate, the activity of the neurotransmitters when they have completed their task. For instance, the neurotransmitter ACh is terminated by acetylcholinesterase. Acetylcholinesterase, the inactivator substance, is an enzyme located in the same area as the receptor sites on dendrite B. Once ACh has completed its task, it is inactivated by acetylcholinesterase.

Receptors. The dendrite of neuron B contains receptor sites. **Receptor sites** are places on the membrane to which the neurotransmitters attach, or bind. For instance, ACh binds to the receptors on dendrite B. Each receptor site has a specific shape and accepts only those neurotransmitters that "fit" its shape.

Events at the Synapse (see Fig. 9–9).

1. The nerve impulse travels along neuron A to its axon terminal.

2. The nerve impulse causes the vesicles to merge, or fuse, with the membrane of the axon terminal. The vesicles open and release neurotransmitter into the synaptic cleft.

3. The neurotransmitter diffuses across the synaptic cleft and binds to the receptor sites. The binding of the neurotransmitter to the receptor sites causes a change in the membrane of the dendrite of neuron B. The membrane change is responsible for the formation of a new nerve impulse in the dendrite of neuron B.

4. This nerve impulse travels toward the cell body and axon of neuron B. What has happened at the synapse? Information from neuron A has been transmitted by chemicals (ACh) to neuron B.

✳ **SUM IT UP!** The electrical signal that travels along the neuron is called the nerve impulse or action potential. The nerve impulse has three phases: polarization, depolarization, and repolarization. The phases of the nerve impulse are caused by the movement of ions, particularly sodium (Na^+) and potassium (K^+). Once the axon membrane is stimulated, the nerve impulse travels the length of the axon. Many of the axons are myelinated to increase the speed of the nerve impulse. The nerve impulse travels along the neuron from the dendrite to the end of the axon (axon terminal). The nerve impulse stimulates the release of neurotransmitter stored in the axon terminal into the synaptic cleft. The transmitter diffuses across the synaptic cleft, binds to the receptor, and stimulates the dendrites of the second neuron. This is the way that information is transmitted from one neuron to the next.

BRAIN: STRUCTURE AND FUNCTION

You read a book, listen to music, sing a song, laugh, rage, remember, learn, feel, move, sleep, awaken, and so much more. All these are functions of the brain!

The brain is located in the cranial cavity. It is a pinkish-gray delicate structure with a soft consistency. The surface of the brain appears bumpy, much like a walnut.

The brain is divided into four major areas: the cerebrum, the diencephalon, the brain stem, and the cerebellum (Fig. 9–10).

Cerebrum

The **cerebrum** (sĕr′ə-brəm) is the largest part of the brain. It is divided into the **right** and **left cerebral hemispheres.** The cerebral hemispheres are joined together by bands of white matter that form a large fiber tract called the **corpus callosum.** Each cerebral hemisphere has four major lobes: a frontal lobe, parietal lobe, temporal lobe, and occipital lobe (Fig. 9–11). These four lobes are named for the overlying cranial bones.

Gray on the Outside, White on the Inside

The cerebrum contains both gray and white matter. A thin layer of gray matter forms the outermost portion of the cerebrum. This is called the **cerebral cortex.** The cerebral cortex is composed primarily of cell bodies and interneurons. The gray matter of the cerebral cortex allows us to perform higher mental tasks such as learning, reasoning, language, and memory.

Do You Know...

Are you a left-brain or a right-brain person?

Some years ago a surgeon severed the corpus callosum in the brain of a patient with severe epilepsy. This surgical procedure eliminated all communication between the left and right cerebral hemispheres. From these and other experiments, neuroscientists learned that there is a left and right brain and that these two brains have different abilities. The left brain is more concerned with language and mathematical abilities; it is the reasoning and analytical side of the brain. The right side of the brain is far superior with regard to spatial relationships, art, music, and the expression of emotions. The right brain is intuitive; it is the poet and the artist. Many of us are predominantly left-brain or right-brain persons. How much richer our lives are when we access both sides of our brains!

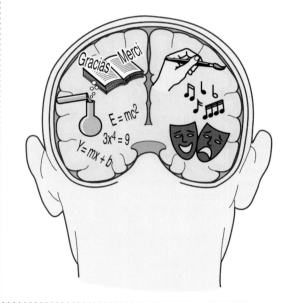

The bulk of the cerebrum is composed of **white matter** located directly below the cortex. The white matter is composed primarily of myelinated axons that form connections between the parts of the brain and spinal cord. Scattered throughout the white matter are patches of gray matter called nuclei.

Markings of the Cerebrum

The surface of the cerebrum has numerous markings, or structures, with special names. The surface of the cerebrum is folded into elevations that resemble speed bumps on a road. The elevations are called **convolutions,** or **gyri** (singular, gyrus).

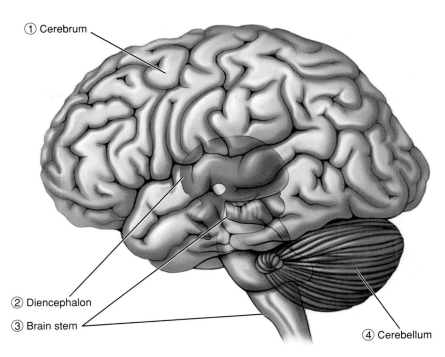

FIGURE 9–10 ● The brain's four major areas: cerebrum, diencephalon, brain stem, and cerebellum.

① Cerebrum

② Diencephalon

③ Brain stem

④ Cerebellum

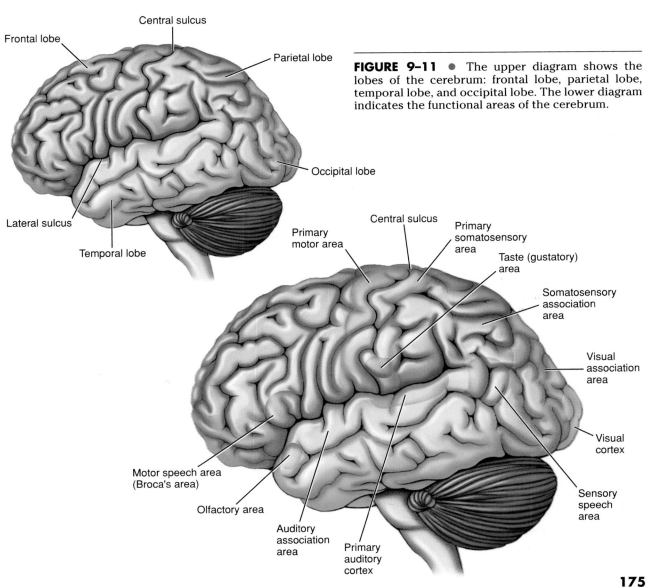

FIGURE 9–11 ● The upper diagram shows the lobes of the cerebrum: frontal lobe, parietal lobe, temporal lobe, and occipital lobe. The lower diagram indicates the functional areas of the cerebrum.

Central sulcus

Frontal lobe

Parietal lobe

Lateral sulcus

Occipital lobe

Temporal lobe

Primary motor area

Central sulcus

Primary somatosensory area

Taste (gustatory) area

Somatosensory association area

Visual association area

Visual cortex

Sensory speech area

Motor speech area (Broca's area)

Olfactory area

Auditory association area

Primary auditory cortex

This extensive folding arrangement increases the amount of cerebral cortex, or thinking tissue. It is thought that intelligence is related to the amount of cerebral cortex and therefore to the numbers of convolutions or gyri. The greater the numbers of convolutions in the brain, the more intelligent is the species. For instance, the cerebral cortex of the human brain has many more convolutions than does the brain of an elephant.

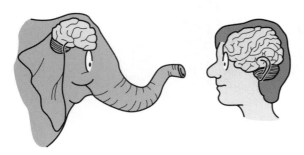

Gyri are separated by grooves called **sulci** (singular, sulcus). A deep sulcus is called a **fissure**. Sulci and fissures separate the cerebrum into lobes. Figure 9–11 illustrates two of the numerous sulci and fissures: the central sulcus and the lateral sulcus. (Identify each structure on the diagram as it is described in the text.)

The **central sulcus** separates the frontal lobe from the parietal lobe. The central sulcus is an important landmark. For instance, it separates the precentral and postcentral gyri. The **precentral gyrus** is located in the frontal lobe, directly in front of the central sulcus, and the **postcentral gyrus** is located in the parietal lobe, directly behind the central sulcus. The **lateral fissure** separates the temporal lobe from the frontal and the parietal lobes. The **longitudinal fissure** separates the left and right cerebral hemispheres (not shown).

Division Into Cerebral Lobes

What does each cerebral lobe do? The cerebral cortex is associated with specific functions (Table 9–2).

FRONTAL LOBE. The **frontal lobe** (frŭn′tl lōb) is located in the front of the cranium under the frontal bone (see Fig. 9–11). The frontal lobe plays a key role in voluntary motor activity, personality development, emotional and behavioral expression, and the performance of high-level tasks such

Table 9 • 2	BRAIN STRUCTURE AND FUNCTION
STRUCTURE	**FUNCTIONS**
Cerebrum	
Frontal lobe	Motor area, personality; behavior; emotional expression; intellectual functions; memory storage
Parietal lobe	Somatosensory area (especially from skin and muscle; taste; speech; reading)
Occipital lobe	Vision; vision-related reflexes and functions (reading, judging distances, seeing in three dimensions)
Temporal lobe	Hearing (auditory area); smell (olfactory area); taste; memory storage; part of speech area
Diencephalon	
Thalamus	Relay structure and processing center for most sensory information going to the cerebrum
Hypothalamus	Integrating system for the autonomic nervous system; regulation of temperature, water balance, sex, thirst, appetite, and some emotions (pleasure and fear); regulates the pituitary gland and controls endocrine function
Brain Stem	
Midbrain	Relays information (sensory and motor); associated with visual reflexes
Pons	Relays information (sensory and motor); plays a role in respiration
Medulla	Vital function (regulation of heart rate, blood flow, blood pressure, respiratory centers); reflex center for coughing, sneezing, swallowing, and vomiting
Cerebellum	Smooths out and coordinates voluntary muscle activity; helps in the maintenance of balance and muscle tone
Other Structures	
Limbic system	Experience of emotion and behavior (emotional brain)
Reticular formation	Mediates wakefulness and sleep
Basal nuclei	Smooths out and coordinates skeletal muscle activity

Patches of Gray

Scattered throughout the cerebral white matter are patches of gray matter called *basal nuclei* (sometimes called basal ganglia). The basal nuclei help regulate body movement and facial expression. The neurotransmitter dopamine is largely responsible for the activity of the basal nuclei.

A deficiency of dopamine within the basal nuclei is called **Parkinson's disease.** It is characterized by problems with movement: a shuffling and uncoordinated gait (walk), rigidity, slowness of speech, drooling, and a mask-like facial expression. Because of the characteristic shaking (called tremors), Parkinson's disease is sometimes called shaking palsy. Dopamine or dopamine-like drugs are usually prescribed for the parkinsonian patient.

Diencephalon

The **diencephalon** is the second main area of the brain. It is located beneath the cerebrum and above the brain stem. The diencephalon includes the thalamus and the hypothalamus (Fig. 9–13).

The **thalamus** serves as a relay station for most of the sensory fibers traveling from the lower brain and spinal cord region to the sensory areas of the cerebrum. The thalamus sorts out the sensory information, gives us a "hint" of the sensation we are to experience, and then directs the information to the specific cerebral areas for more precise interpretation.

For instance, pain fibers coming from the body to the brain pass through the thalamus. At the level of the thalamus, we become aware of pain, but we are not yet aware of the kind of pain or the exact location of the pain. Fibers that transmit pain information from the thalamus to the cortex provide us with that additional information.

The **hypothalamus** (hī″pō-thăl′ə-məs) is the second structure in the diencephalon. It is situated directly below the thalamus and helps regulate many body processes: body temperature, water balance, and metabolism. Because the hypothalamus helps regulate the function of the autonomic (involuntary) nerves, it exerts an effect on heart rate, blood pressure, and respiration.

Located under the hypothalamus is the pituitary gland. The pituitary gland directly or indirectly affects almost every hormone in the body. Because the hypothalamus controls pituitary function, the widespread effects of the hypothalamus are obvious. (Endocrine function is discussed further in Chapter 12.)

Brain Stem

The **brain stem** (brān′stĕm) connects the spinal cord with higher brain structures. It is composed of the midbrain, pons, and medulla oblongata (see Fig. 9–13). The white matter of the brain stem includes **tracts** that relay both sensory and motor information to and from the cerebrum. Scattered throughout the white matter of the brain stem are patches of gray matter called nuclei. These nuclei exert profound effects on functions such as blood pressure and respiration.

The **midbrain** extends from the lower diencephalon to the pons. Like the rest of the brain

FIGURE 9–13 • Diencephalon and brain stem. The diencephalon consists of the thalamus and hypothalamus. Note the relationship between the hypothalamus and the pituitary gland. The brain stem is composed of the midbrain, pons, and medulla.

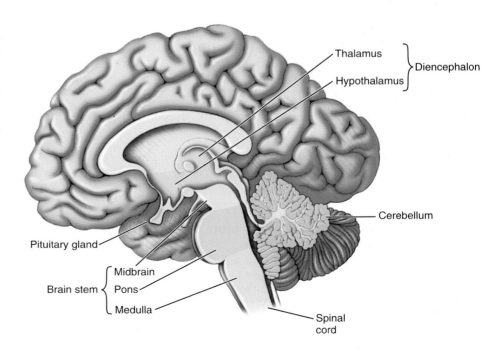

stem structures, the midbrain relays sensory and motor information. The midbrain also contains nuclei that function as reflex centers for vision and hearing.

The **pons** (bridge) extends from the midbrain to the medulla oblongata. It is composed primarily of tracts that act as a bridge for information traveling to and from several important brain structures. The pons also plays an important role in the regulation of breathing rate and rhythm. Damage to the pons can cause severe disturbances in rhythmic breathing.

The **medulla oblongata** connects the spinal cord with the pons. The medulla contains many tracts and therefore acts as a relay for sensory and motor information. Several important nuclei within the medulla control heart rate, blood pressure, and respiration. Because of its importance with regard to vital functions, the medulla oblongata is often called the vital center. Because these functions are vital to the body, you can understand the seriousness of a fracture at the base of the skull. The medulla is also extremely sensitive to certain drugs, especially the narcotics.

An overdose of a narcotic causes depression of the medulla oblongata and death because the person stops breathing. This danger is the reason for counting the respiratory rate before giving a narcotic. If the respiratory rate is less than 10 respirations per minute, the drug cannot be safely administered.

Cerebellum

The **cerebellum** (sĕr″ə-bĕl′əm), the fourth major area, is the structure that protrudes from under the occipital lobe at the base of the skull (see Figs. 9–10 and 9–13). The cerebellum is concerned primarily with the coordination of voluntary muscle activity. Information is sent to the cerebellum from many areas throughout the body, including the eyes, ears, and skeletal muscles. The cerebellum integrates all of the incoming information to produce a smooth coordinated muscle response.

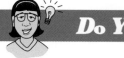

Do You Know...

Why does the physician ask you to place a finger on the tip of your nose?

Placing a finger on your nose is a diagnostic test for cerebellar function. The cerebellum normally coordinates and smoothes out skeletal muscle activity. In attempting to touch an object, a patient with cerebellar dysfunction may overshoot, first to one side and then the next.

Damage to the cerebellum produces jerky muscle movements, staggering gait, and difficulty maintaining balance or equilibrium. The person with cerebellar dysfunction may appear intoxicated.

Structures Across Divisions of the Brain

Two important structures are not confined to any of the four divisions of the brain because they "overlap" several structures. The two structures are the limbic system and the reticular system.

Limbic System: The Emotional Brain

Parts of the cerebrum and the diencephalon form a wishbone-shaped group of structures called the limbic system. The **limbic system** (lĭm′bĭk sĭs′təm) functions in emotional states and behavior. It also contributes to memory. For instance, when the limbic system is stimulated by microelectrodes, states of extreme pleasure or rage can be induced. Because of these responses, the limbic system is called the emotional brain.

Reticular Formation: Wake Up!

What keeps us awake? Why don't we slip into a coma when we go to sleep? Extending through the entire brain stem, with numerous connections to the cerebral cortex, is a special mass of gray matter called the **reticular formation** (rĭ-tĭk′yə-lər fôr-mā′shən). The reticular formation is concerned with sleep/awake cycle and consciousness. Signals passing up to the cerebral cortex from the reticular formation stimulate us, keeping us awake and tuned in.

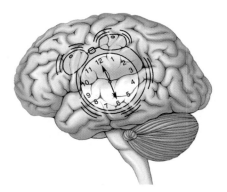

The reticular formation is very sensitive to the effects of certain drugs and alcohol. For example, the dangerous combination of benzodiazepines (tranquilizers) and alcohol can damage the reticular formation, causing permanent unconsciousness.

CONSCIOUSNESS, SLEEP, AND COMA. **Consciousness** is a state of wakefulness. Consciousness depends on the reticular activating system (RAS).

The RAS continuously samples sensory information from all over the body and then selects and presents essential, unusual, and threatening information to the higher structures in the cerebral cortex. There are different levels of consciousness, such as attentiveness, alertness, relaxation, and inattentiveness. **Sleep** occurs when the RAS is inhibited, or slowed. The precise cause of RAS inhibition (ie, sleep) is unknown. **Coma** is a sleep-like state with several stages, ranging from light to deep coma. In the lightest stages of coma, some reflexes are intact; the patient may respond to light, sound, touch, and painful stimuli. As the coma deepens, however, these reflexes are gradually lost, and the patient eventually becomes unresponsive to all stimuli. Damage to the reticular formation is associated with a state of deep coma, which can be permanent.

Many clinical conditions affect level of consciousness (LOC), often leading to coma. These include brain tumors, brain injury, drugs, toxins, hypoxia, hyperglycemia, acid-base imbalance, and electrolyte imbalance. As a clinician, you must be able to assess the patient's LOC.

Do You Know . . .

What happens when the brain is deprived of oxygen?

The brain depends on a constant supply of oxygen-rich blood. If the brain is deprived of oxygen, even for a brief period, undesirable effects occur. Loss of consciousness occurs when the brain is deprived of oxygen for longer than 5 seconds. Convulsions occur with oxygen deprivation of 15–20 seconds. After 9 minutes without oxygen, the brain suffers irreversible damage.

STAGES OF SLEEP. The two types of sleep are **non-rapid eye movement (NREM) sleep** and **rapid eye movement (REM) sleep.** The four stages of NREM sleep progress from light to deep. In a typical 8-hour sleep period, a person regularly cycles through the various stages of sleep, descending from light to deep sleep and then ascending from deeper sleep to lighter sleep. The person then ascends from NREM deep sleep to stage 2 (NREM) sleep to REM sleep. After a short period of REM sleep, the person descends again through the stages of NREM sleep. REM sleep totals 90 to 120 minutes per night.

REM sleep is characterized by fluctuating blood pressure, respiratory rate and rhythm, and pulse rate. The most obvious characteristic of REM sleep is rapid eye movements, for which the sleep segment is named. Most dreaming occurs during REM sleep. For unknown reasons, REM sleep deprivation is associated with mental and physical distress. Most sedatives and CNS depressants adversely affect REM sleep, perhaps accounting for a "hung-over" feeling that often follows their use.

Protecting the Central Nervous System

The tissue of the CNS (brain and spinal cord) is very delicate. Injury to CNS neuronal tissue cannot be repaired. Thus the CNS has an elaborate protective system that consists of four structures: bone, meninges, cerebrospinal fluid, and the blood-brain barrier.

Bone: First Layer of Protection

The CNS is protected by bone. The brain is encased in the skull, while the spinal cord is encased in the vertebral column. These structures protect the delicate brain and spinal cord. (The skull and vertebral column were described in Chapter 7.)

Do You Know . . .

Why may an infant develop water on the brain?

Occasionally, a newborn infant is born with a block in the ventricular system of the brain. Cerebrospinal fluid (CSF) is formed at a normal rate but cannot be drained because of the block. The fluid accumulates within the ventricles, thereby increasing intracranial pressure and causing the skull to enlarge. This condition is called **hydrocephalus** (water on the brain). Head expansion in the infant is possible because the suture lines of the skull bones have not yet fused. If a block (eg, tumor) were to occur in an older child or adult, the intracranial pressure would increase. The skull, however, could not expand because of the fused sutures. Without surgical intervention, the increased pressure would result in death.

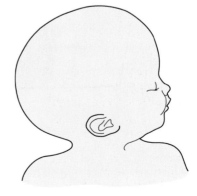

Meninges: Second Layer of Protection

Three layers of connective tissue surround the brain and spinal cord (Fig. 9–14). These tissues are called the **meninges** (mə-nĭn′jēz). The outermost layer is a thick, tough, connective tissue called the **dura mater,** literally meaning "hard mother." Inside the skull, the dural membrane splits to form the dural sinuses. These sinuses are filled with blood. Beneath the dura mater is a small space called the subdural space. The middle layer is the **arachnoid (meaning spider-like) layer,** so named because the membrane looks like a spider web.

The **pia mater** is the innermost layer and literally means soft, or gentle, mother. The pia mater is a very thin membrane that contains many blood vessels and lies delicately over the brain and spinal cord. These blood vessels supply the brain with much of its blood. Between the arachnoid layer and the pia mater is a space called the **subarachnoid space.** A fluid called the **cerebrospinal fluid** (sĕr″ə-brō-spī′nəl flōō′ĭd) circulates within this space and forms a cushion around the brain and spinal cord. If the head is jarred sud-

Do You Know...

Why is mannitol used to decrease intracranial pressure?

After head injury, the brain may swell because of an accumulation of fluid in the interstitial space. This condition is called cerebral edema. Cerebral edema is serious because it can increase pressure in the skull (increased intracranial pressure). An increase in intracranial pressure can cause serious brain damage and other life-threatening effects such as respiratory arrest, profound hypertension, and severe elevation in body temperature. Mannitol is a polysaccharide administered intravenously. Mannitol increases the osmolarity of the blood, thereby pulling water from the interstitial space of the brain into the blood vessels. The blood carries the excess fluid from the brain to the kidneys for elimination as urine. The mannitol-induced diuresis decreases cerebral edema and results in decreased intracranial pressure and the relief of life-threatening symptoms.

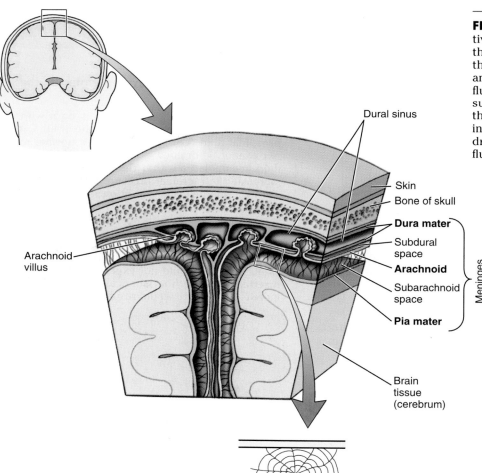

FIGURE 9–14 ● Protective layers of the CNS. The three layers of meninges are the dura mater, arachnoid, and pia mater. Cerebrospinal fluid circulates within the subarachnoid space. Note the arachnoid villi projecting into the dural sinus for drainage of cerebrospinal fluid.

denly, the brain first bumps into this soft cushion of fluid. Specialized projections of the arachnoid membrane, called the **arachnoid villi** (singular, villus), protrude up into the blood-filled dural sinuses.

The meninges can become inflamed or infected, causing meningitis. **Meningitis** is serious because the infection can spread to the brain, sometimes causing serious irreversible brain damage. The bacterial or viral organism causing the meningitis can often be found in a sample of cerebrospinal fluid obtained by lumbar puncture.

Cerebrospinal Fluid: Third Layer of Protection

The cerebrospinal fluid (CSF) forms a third protective layer of the CNS. CSF is formed from the blood within the brain. It is a clear fluid similar in composition to plasma. The CSF is composed of water, glucose, protein, and several ions, especially sodium ion (Na^+) and chloride ion (Cl^-). An adult circulates about ½ cup of CSF.

Where is cerebrospinal fluid formed? CSF is formed within the ventricles of the brain by a structure called the choroid plexus (Fig. 9–15A). There are four ventricles: two lateral ventricles, and a third and a fourth ventricle. The **choroid plexus,** a grape-like collection of blood vessels and neuroglial ependymal cells (see Table 9–1), is suspended from the roof of each ventricle. Water and dissolved substances are transported from the blood across the walls of the choroid plexus into the ventricles (Fig. 9–15B).

Where does the CSF flow? As CSF leaves the ventricles, it follows two paths. Some of the CSF flows through a hole in the center of the spinal cord called the **central canal.** The central canal

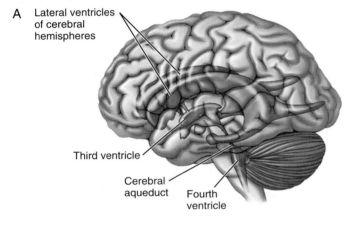

A Lateral ventricles of cerebral hemispheres

Third ventricle

Cerebral aqueduct   Fourth ventricle

FIGURE 9–15 ● Cerebrospinal fluid (CSF): formation, circulation, and drainage. A, CSF forms within the ventricles of the brain (lateral, third, and fourth ventricles). B, Cerebrospinal fluid flows down through the central canal to the base of the spinal cord. CSF also flows from the fourth ventricle into the subarachnoid space surrounding the brain. CSF flows into the arachnoid villus, which protrudes into the dural sinuses. CSF diffuses across the membrane of the villus into the dural sinuses, where it mixes with venous blood. The blood in the sinuses drains the CSF away from the brain, into the veins.

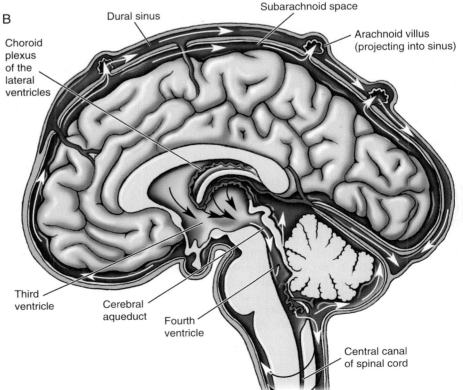

B

Choroid plexus of the lateral ventricles

Dural sinus

Subarachnoid space

Arachnoid villus (projecting into sinus)

Third ventricle

Cerebral aqueduct

Fourth ventricle

Central canal of spinal cord

eventually drains into the subarachnoid space at the base of the spinal cord. The rest of the CSF flows from the fourth ventricles laterally through tiny holes, or **foramina** (singular, foramen), into the subarachnoid space that encircles the brain.

Do You Know...

What is meant by a blood clot on the brain?

Although the brain is well protected, a head injury may cause bleeding. Boxers, for instance, are often hit in the head. As the head snaps in response to the blow, blood vessels rupture, and bleeding occurs. Blood often accumulates under the dural membrane, forming a subdural hematoma (also called a blood clot). The blood clot continues to expand and exerts pressure on the surrounding brain tissue. Increasing pressure may lead to a loss of consciousness, paralysis, and the possibility of death.

How does the CSF leave the subarachnoid space? Eventually, CSF flows into the arachnoid villi and drains into the blood within the dural sinuses. Blood flows from the dural sinuses into the cerebral veins and back to the heart. Remember that the CSF is formed across the walls of the choroid plexus within the ventricles, circulates throughout the subarachnoid space around the brain and spinal cord, and then drains into the dural sinuses. The rate at which CSF is formed must equal the rate at which it is drained. If either excess CSF is formed or drainage is impaired, CSF will accumulate in the ventricles of the brain, increasing the pressure within the skull. The resulting increase in intracranial pressure can cause brain damage and death.

Blood-Brain Barrier: Fourth Layer of Protection

The **blood-brain barrier** is an arrangement of cells associated with the blood vessels that supply the brain and spinal cord. These cells select the substances allowed to enter the CNS from the blood. In other words, if a potentially harmful substance is present in the blood, the cells of the blood-brain barrier prevent that substance from entering the brain and the spinal cord. Brain capillaries are constructed of densely packed cells with a continuous basement membrane. This cell layer prevents most unwanted substances from entering the brain.

While the blood-brain barrier is successful in screening many harmful substances, not all toxic substances are blocked. Alcohol, for instance, crosses the blood-brain barrier and affects (and in some cases destroys) brain tissue. Glial cells, particularly the astrocytes, play an important role in the formation of the blood-brain barrier.

The blood-brain barrier may present a problem in the pharmacologic treatment of infections within the CNS. Some antibiotics, for instance, cannot cross the blood-brain barrier and therefore cannot reach the site of infection. Given this problem, how is an infection of the CNS treated? There are two options: (1) select an antibiotic that does cross the blood-brain barrier or (2) inject the antibiotic directly into the subarachnoid space. (This procedure is an intrathecal injection.)

✳ **SUM IT UP!** The CNS, especially the brain, performs eloquently as a conductor. It coordinates the various organ systems of the body efficiently, with fine precision. The brain makes us humans—thinking, caring, feeling, remembering persons. The brain is divided into four regions: cerebrum, diencephalon, brain stem, and cerebellum. The cerebrum is the largest part of the brain and consists of two hemispheres. The four lobes of the cerebrum are frontal lobe (motor activity, analysis, thinking), parietal lobe (sensory), temporal lobe (hearing), and occipital lobe (vision). The diencephalon is composed of the thalamus and the hypothalamus. The brain stem is composed of the midbrain, pons, and medulla oblongata. The medulla is considered a vital structure in that it affects basic functions such as respirations, cardiac function, and blood vessel tone. Two other areas are the reticular formation, which keeps us awake, and the limbic system, or the emotional brain. Because of the crucial role played by the CNS, it is afforded excellent protection: tough bone, three layers of meninges, a soft cushion of fluid, and a blood-brain barrier.

As You Age

1. Beginning at the age of 30, the number of neurons decreases. The number lost, however, is only a small percentage of the total number of brain cells and does not cause mental impairment. While a decrease in short-term memory may cause some forgetfulness, most memory, alertness, intellectual functioning, and creativity remain intact. Severe alteration of mental functioning is generally due to age-related diseases such as arteriosclerosis.

2. Impulse conduction speed decreases along an axon; amounts of neurotransmitter are reduced; and the number of receptor sites decreases at the synapses. These changes result in progressive slowing of responses and reflexes.

Disorders of the Nervous Tissue and the Brain

Alcohol-induced neurotoxicity
Chronic and excessive ingestion of alcohol causing irreversible injury to the nervous system. The result is mental deterioration, loss of memory, inability to concentrate, irritability, and uncoordinated movement. Wernicke-Korsakoff syndrome is an alcohol-related type of encephalopathy.

Alzheimer's disease
A degenerative disease of the brain usually occurring in older persons. Alzheimer's disease is characterized by progressive loss of memory and impaired intellectual function. Evidence suggests brain atrophy, especially of the frontal and temporal lobes.

Cerebral palsy (CP)
A group of neuromuscular disorders that result from injury to an infant before, during, or shortly after birth. All forms of CP cause impairment of skeletal muscle activity. Mental retardation and speech difficulties may accompany the disorder.

Cerebrovascular accident (CVA)
Commonly called a stroke. A CVA is due to a sudden lack of blood, causing oxygen deprivation and brain damage. Depending on the location and severity of the brain damage, a CVA results in loss of sensory and motor function (causing paralysis) and speech impairment. The major causes of CVA are thrombosis and cerebral hemorrhage. The hemorrhage may be due to a ruptured aneurysm, such as a Berry aneurysm (a congenital aneurysm of the circle of Willis).

Concussion
A transient loss of consciousness, usually following head trauma.

Contusion
A bruise of the brain involving a torn cerebral or meningeal blood vessel.

Epilepsy
From the Greek word meaning to seize upon. Epilepsy refers to a group of symptoms that have many causes (brain tumor, toxins, trauma, fever). Neurons in the brain fire suddenly and unpredictably. Grand mal (big illness) seizures occur when the motor areas fire repetitively, causing convulsive seizures and loss of consciousness. Petit mal (small illness) seizures occur when sensory areas are affected. While there is a brief period of altered consciousness, petit mal seizures are not accompanied by convulsions or prolonged unconsciousness.

Headache (migraine)
Severe, recurring headaches that usually affect only one side of the head. (The word *migraine* comes from the Latin *hemicranium*, meaning one side of the head.) A migraine may be preceded and accompanied by fatigue, nausea, vomiting, and a visual sensation of zigzag lines. Not all headaches are migraines. A simple tension headache may develop when a person is anxious or tense. Headaches may also develop in response to increased intracranial pressure, irritation of the meninges, and spasm of the cerebral blood vessels.

Hematomas
Refers to blood clots and generally caused by trauma. An epidural hematoma forms between the dura and the skull. A subdural hematoma forms under the dura mater. As the hematoma enlarges, it compresses the brain, elevates intracranial pressure, and can cause death unless the pressure is relieved.

Inflammations
Encephalitis, meningitis. Encephalitis is an inflammation of the brain usually caused by a virus. Meningitis is an inflammation of the meninges, caused by viruses and bacteria.

Phenylketonuria (PKU)
A disease caused by a hereditary deficiency of phenylalanine hydroxylase, an enzyme needed to metabolize the amino acid phenylalanine. In the absence of the enzyme, the unmetabolized phenylalanine is excreted in the urine; hence the name phenylketonuria. Unless treated promptly, PKU causes severe mental retardation. Routine screening for PKU occurs in all newborn nurseries in the United States.

Tumors
Malignant and benign tumors in nervous tissue. The tumors can destroy nervous tissue, exert pressure on surrounding structures, and cause a life-threatening increase in intracranial pressure. Examples of tumors include gliomas (malignant tumors arising from glial tissue such as an astrocytoma), meningiomas (tumors arising from the meninges), and neuromas (tumors arising from the nerves).

Summary Outline

The purpose of the nervous system is to bring information to the central nervous system, interpret the information, and enable the body to respond to the information.

I. The Nervous System: Overview

A. Divisions of the Nervous System
1. The central nervous system (CNS) includes the brain and the spinal cord.
2. The peripheral nervous system includes the nerves that connect the CNS with the rest of the body.

B. Cells That Make Up the Nervous System
1. Neuroglia (glia) support, protect, nourish, and generally take care of the neurons. Glial cells do not conduct nerve impulses.
2. Neurons conduct the nerve impulse. The three parts of a neuron are dendrites (tree-like structures that conduct the nerve impulse toward the cell body), the cell body, and the axon (conducts the nerve impulse away from the cell body).

C. Types of Neurons
1. Sensory, or afferent, neurons carry information toward the CNS.
2. Interneurons are located in the CNS and make connections between sensory and motor neurons.
3. Motor, or efferent, neurons carry information away from the CNS toward the periphery.

D. White Matter and Gray Matter
1. White matter is due to myelinated fibers.
2. Gray matter is composed primarily of cell bodies, interneurons, and unmyelinated fibers.
3. Clusters of cell bodies (gray matter) dispersed throughout white matter are called ganglia or nuclei.

II. The Neuron Carrying Information

A. Nerve Impulse
1. The electrical signal is called the action potential or nerve impulse.
2. The nerve impulse is due to changes in the neuron: during polarization the inside of the cell is negative; during depolarization the inside of the cell is positive; during repolarization the inside of the cell is negative.
3. The nerve impulse is due to flows, or fluxes, of ions. The resting membrane potential (polarization) is due to the outward flux of K^+; depolarization is due to the influx of Na^+; and repolarization is due to the outward flux of K^+.
4. The refractory period is the unresponsive period of the neuron; it is the inability of a cell to receive a depolarizing stimulus.
5. The nerve impulse moves along a myelinated axon by saltatory, or leaping, conduction. The myelin sheath increases the speed of the nerve impulse as it travels along the axon.
6. The nerve impulse causes the release of the neurotransmitter from the axon terminal.

B. Synapse
1. The synapse is a space between two neurons.
2. The parts of the synapse include the axon terminal, synaptic cleft, neurotransmitters, inactivators, and receptors.
3. The nerve impulse of the first (presynaptic) neuron causes the release of neurotransmitter into the synaptic cleft. The neurotransmitter diffuses across the synaptic cleft and binds to the receptors on the second (postsynaptic) membrane. The activation of the receptors stimulates a nerve impulse in the second neuron.

III. Brain: Structure and Function

A. Cerebrum
1. The right and left hemispheres are joined by the corpus callosum.
2. The outer layers are gray; the inner layers are white.
3. The gray matter is arranged in convolutions (gyri); the gyri are separated by sulci or fissures.
4. The four main cerebral lobes are the frontal, parietal, temporal, and occipital lobes. Functions of each lobe are summarized in Table 9–2.
5. Large areas of the cerebrum, called association areas, are concerned with interpreting, integrating, and analyzing information.
6. Patches of gray (nuclei) are scattered throughout the cerebrum and other parts of the brain.

B. Diencephalon
1. The thalamus is a relay station for most sensory tracts traveling to the cerebrum.
2. The hypothalamus controls many body functions, such as water balance, temperature, and the secretion of hormones from the pituitary gland; it exerts an effect on the autonomic nervous system.

C. Brain Stem
1. The brain stem is formed by the midbrain, pons, and medulla oblongata.
2. The medulla oblongata is called the vital center because it controls the heart rate, blood pressure, and respirations (the vital functions).

D. Cerebellum
1. The cerebellum is called the little brain.
2. The cerebellum is concerned primarily with the coordination of voluntary muscle activity.

E. Structures Involving More Than One Lobe
1. The limbic system is the emotional brain.
2. The reticular formation is concerned with the sleep/awake cycle. It keeps us conscious and prevents us from slipping into a coma state.

Summary Outline, continued

III. Brain: Structure and Function, *continued*

F. Protection of the CNS

1. The cranium and vertebral column, composed of hard bone, house the brain and spinal cord.
2. Three layers of meninges (pia mater, arachnoid, and dura mater) surround the CNS.
3. Cerebrospinal fluid is secreted across the ependymal cells of the choroid plexus within the cerebral ventricles. CSF circulates through the subarachnoid space, surrounding the brain and spinal cord.
4. The blood-brain barrier refers to the selectivity of the capillary cells in the brain. The barrier prevents toxic substances from entering the CNS from the blood.

Review Your Knowledge

1. How is the central nervous system different from the peripheral nervous system?

2. What is the difference between neuroglia and neurons? Name the functions of astrocytes and ependymal cells.

3. What are the three parts of a neuron? What is the difference between a sensory neuron and a motor neuron?

4. On what structure would you find the myelin sheath, the neurilemma, and the nodes of Ranvier?

5. How is the formation of the myelin sheath different in the peripheral and central nervous systems? Where are Schwann cells found? Where are oligodendrocytes found?

6. What is a nerve impulse? What three events take place with the action potential or nerve impulse? What term refers to the inability of the cell to accept another stimulus until it repolarizes? Which ions are involved with changes associated with the action potential or nerve impulse?

7. How does myelination affect the movement of the nerve impulse along the axonal membrane? What happens if there is a lack of myelin surrounding the axon? What does saltatory conduction mean?

8. How is information transmitted from one neuron to the next across the synapse? What are the two most common neurotransmitters?

9. List the four major areas of the brain.

10. What is the function of the four lobes of the brain? How is a sulcus different from a gyrus? What part of the brain is concerned with motor speech?

11. Why does damage to the left side of the brain cause paralysis of the right side of the body? What does decussation mean? What disease is caused by a deficiency of dopamine within the basal nuclei?

12. What are the two parts of the diencephalon? What are the three parts of the brain stem?

13. An overdose of a narcotic may cause death because the person stops breathing; what part of the brain is depressed by narcotics?

14. What symptoms are present in a person with cerebellar dysfunction?

15. What part of the brain is known as the emotional brain? Which part of the brain keeps us awake and keeps us from slipping into a coma when we go to sleep?

16. Name four structures that protect the brain. What are the layers of the meninges, going from the inside to the outside layer?

17. Where is cerebrospinal fluid (CSF) formed? Where does CSF flow?

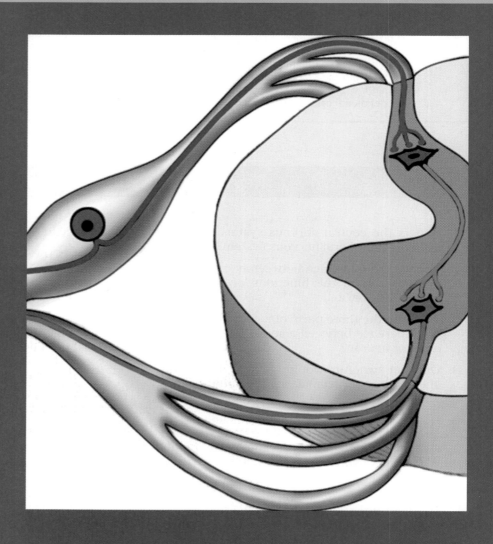

Key Terms

Afferent neuron (ăf′ər-ənt nŏŏr′ŏn)
Autonomic nervous system
  (ô″tə-nŏm′ĭk nûr′vəs sĭs′təm)
Cranial nerves (krā′nē-əl nûrvz)
Dermatome (dûr′mə-tōm″)
Dorsal root (dôr′səl rōōt)
Efferent neuron (ĕf′ər-ənt nŏŏr′ŏn)
Gray matter (grā măt′ər)
Interneuron (ĭn″tər-nŏŏ′rŏn)
Mixed nerve (mĭkst nûrv)
Motor nerve (mō′tər nûrv)
Nerve (nûrv)
Nerve tract (nûrv trăkt)

Parasympathetic nervous system
  (păr″ə-sĭm″pə-thĕt′ĭk nûr′vəs sĭs′təm)
Peripheral nervous system
  (pə-rĭf′ər-əl nûr′vəs sĭs′təm)
Plexuses (plĕk′səs-ĭz)
Reflex arc (rē′flĕks ärk)
Sensory nerve (sĕn′sə-rē nûrv)
Spinal nerves (spī′nəl nûrvz)
Sympathetic nervous system
  (sĭm″pə-thĕt′ĭk nûr′vəs sĭs′təm)
Ventral root (vĕn′trəl rōōt)
White matter (wīt măt′ər)

• • • Selected terms in bold type in this chapter are defined in the Glossary.

10 NERVOUS SYSTEM: SPINAL CORD AND PERIPHERAL NERVES

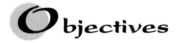

Objectives

1. Describe three functions of the spinal cord.

2. List four components of the reflex arc.

3. Describe the functions of the 12 pairs of cranial nerves.

4. Identify the classification of spinal nerves.

5. List the functions of the three major plexuses.

6. Explain the structure and function of the autonomic nervous system.

7. Compare the structure and function of the sympathetic and parasympathetic nervous systems.

The brain, spinal cord, and peripheral nervous system work together as a vast communication system. The spinal cord continuously carries information to and from the brain. In the absence of spinal cord function, there is no sensory activity, so that the person cannot feel. The person also lacks voluntary motor activity and so cannot move.

WHAT THE SPINAL CORD IS

The spinal cord is a continuation of the brain stem. It is a tube-like structure located within the spinal cavity. The diameter, or thickness, of the spinal cord is similar to the thickness of your thumb. The spinal cord is about 17 inches (43 cm) long and extends from the foramen magnum of the occipital bone to the level of L1, just below the bottom rib. Like the brain, the spinal cord is well protected by bone, the meninges, and cerebrospinal fluid (CSF) (Fig. 10–1).

Do You Know...

How is epidural anesthesia used in childbirth?

During the last, uncomfortable phase of childbirth, anesthetic agents are continuously infused into the epidural space. The nerves that are deadened by the anesthesia supply the lower pelvic region of the body, thereby relieving the pain of childbirth.

An infant's spinal cord extends the full length of the spinal cavity. As the infant grows, however, the spinal cavity grows faster than the cord. Because of the different rates of growth, the spinal cavity eventually becomes longer than the spinal cord, with the spinal cord extending only to L1 in the adult. The meningeal membranes, however, extend the length of the spinal cavity.

This anatomical arrangement forms the basis for the site of a **lumbar puncture** (Fig. 10–1B,C). In this procedure, a hollow needle is inserted into the subarachnoid space, between L3 and L4, at about the level of the top of the hip bone. A sample of CSF is withdrawn from the subarachnoid space. The CSF is then examined for pathogens, blood, or other abnormal signs. Because the spinal cord ends at L1, there is no danger of injuring the cord with the needle.

Do You Know...

Why does a ruptured disc cause pain?

A ruptured disc is the herniation, or protrusion, of the central portion of the intervertebral disc into the spinal cavity. The herniated disc presses on a spinal nerve root, causing severe pain.

Gray on the Inside, White on the Outside

Gray Matter

A cross section of the spinal cord shows an area of gray matter and an area of white matter (Fig. 10–2). The **gray matter** (grā măt′ər) is located centrally and is shaped like a butterfly. It is composed primarily of cell bodies and **interneurons** (ĭn″tər-noo′rŏn). Two projections of the gray matter are the **dorsal,** or **posterior, horn** and the **ventral,** or **anterior, horn.** In the middle of the gray matter is the central canal. The **central canal** is an opening, or hole, that extends the entire length of the spinal cord. It is open to the ventricular system in the brain and to the subarachnoid space at the bottom of the spinal cord. CSF flows from the ventricles in the brain down through the central canal into the subarachnoid space at the base of the spinal cord. The CSF then circulates throughout the subarachnoid space surrounding the spinal cord and brain.

White Matter

The **white matter** (wīt măt′ər) of the spinal cord is composed primarily of myelinated axons. These neuronal axons are grouped together into **nerve tracts** (nûrv trăkts). For instance, the pain fibers are grouped together in a particular tract while the motor fibers are grouped in other tracts.

Sensory tracts carry information from the periphery up the spinal cord, toward the brain (see Fig. 10–2). They are therefore called **ascending tracts.** The spinothalamic tract is an example of an ascending tract. It carries sensory information for touch, pressure, and pain from the spinal cord to the thalamus, in the brain. Note that the name of the tract (spinothalamic) often indicates its origin (spinal cord) and destination (thalamus).

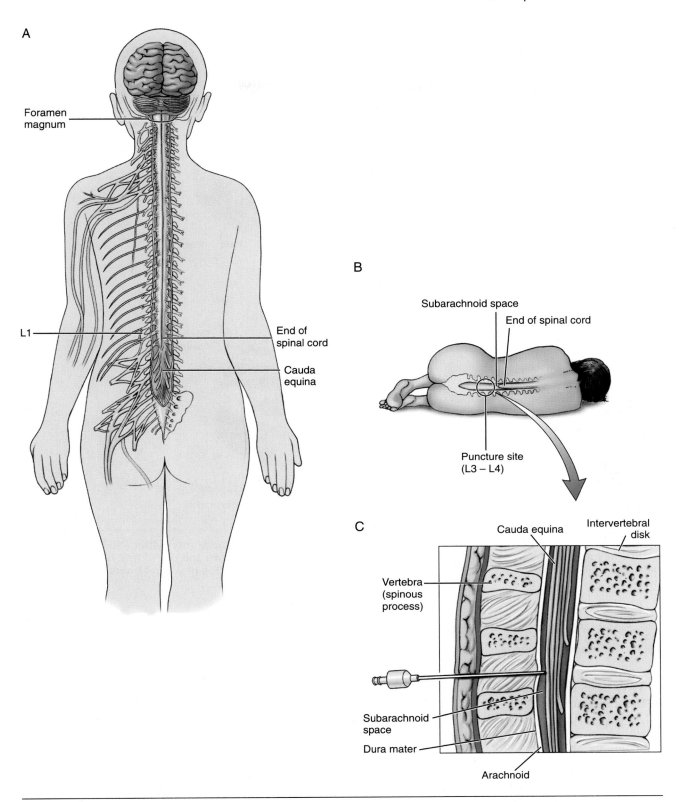

FIGURE 10–1 ● A, Location of the spinal cord. It extends from the foramen magnum of the occipital bone to L1. The cauda equina descends from the base of the spinal cord (L1) to the bottom of the spinal cavity. B, Note that the spinal cord is shorter than the spinal cavity. C, The telescoped area shows a lumbar puncture (spinal tap). A needle is inserted into the subarachnoid space between the L3 and L4 vertebrae. Note that the person is lying so that the vertebral column is flexed. This position separates the vertebrae and facilitates the insertion of the needle.

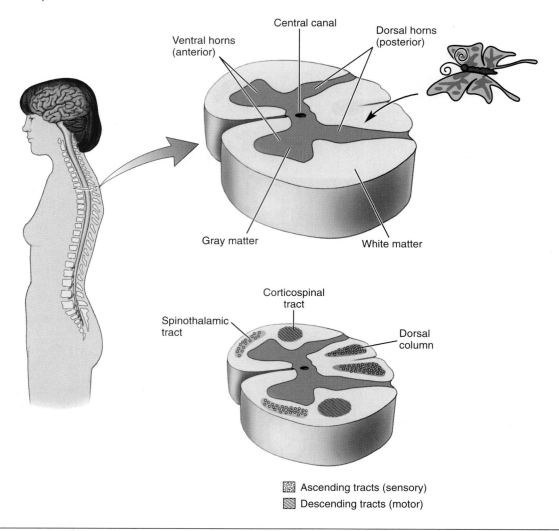

FIGURE 10–2 ● Spinal cord. The cross section of the spinal cord shows the inner gray matter ("butterfly") and the outer white matter. The butterfly wings (gray matter) have names: the dorsal horn and the ventral horn. The central canal is a hole in the middle of the spinal cord. The white matter shows the location of several tracts.

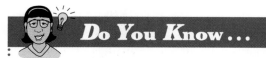

Do You Know...

Why does the polio virus cause skeletal muscle paralysis?

The polio virus attacks and destroys the motor neurons (particularly the anterior horn cells) that supply the skeletal muscles. This neural destruction causes a flaccid paralysis of the involved muscles. Because the polio virus generally attacks children and causes paralysis, the condition is frequently called infantile paralysis.

Motor tracts carry information from the brain down the spinal cord, toward the periphery. They are called **descending tracts.** The major descend-

ing tracts are the pyramidal and extrapyramidal tracts. The pyramidal tract, also called the corticospinal tract, is the major motor tract, originating in the frontal lobe of the cerebrum. As its name (corticospinal) implies, motor information is carried from the cortical region of the brain toward the spinal cord. Additional information concerning tracts and their functions is found in Table 10–1.

If injured, the neurons of the brain and spinal cord do not regenerate. If, for instance, the neck is broken, the spinal cord might be severed or crushed. Automobile accidents, falls, and diving accidents are common causes of spinal cord injuries (Fig. 10–3).

If the spinal cord is severed at the neck region, the trunk and all four extremities are paralyzed. This condition is called **quadriplegia.** This type of spinal cord injury is common in automobile acci-

Table 10 • 1	MAJOR SPINAL CORD TRACTS

TRACTS	FUNCTIONS
Ascending	
Spinothalamic	Temperature; pressure; pain; light touch
Dorsal column	Proprioception; deep pressure; vibration
Spinocerebellar	Proprioception
Descending	
Pyramidal (corticospinal)	Skeletal muscle tone; voluntary muscle movement
Extrapyramidal	Skeletal muscle activity (balance and posture)

Spinal Nerves Attached to the Spinal Cord

Attached to the spinal cord are the **spinal nerves** (spī′nəl nûrvz). Each nerve is attached to the spinal cord by two roots, the dorsal root and the ventral root (Fig. 10–4). *Sensory* nerve fibers travel to the cord through the **dorsal root** (dôr′səl rōōt). The cell bodies of the sensory fibers are gathered together in the **dorsal root ganglia.** Note that the ganglia are located outside the spinal cord. The **ventral root** (vĕn′trəl rōōt) is composed of *motor* fibers. These motor fibers are distributed to voluntary muscles, involuntary muscles, and glands. The cell bodies of the motor fibers are located in the gray matter of the spinal cord in the ventral horns. The dorsal and ventral roots are "packaged" together to form a spinal nerve. Because spinal nerves contain both sensory and motor fibers, all spinal nerves are **mixed nerves** (mĭkst nûrvz).

WHAT THE SPINAL CORD DOES

The spinal cord serves three major functions: sensory pathway, motor pathway, and reflex center.

dents and diving accidents in which the head is either compressed or bent excessively (see Fig. 10–3). If the spinal cord injury is lower, involving only the lumbar region of the spinal cord, the person has full use of the upper extremities but is paralyzed from the waist down. Paralysis of the lower extremities is called **paraplegia.**

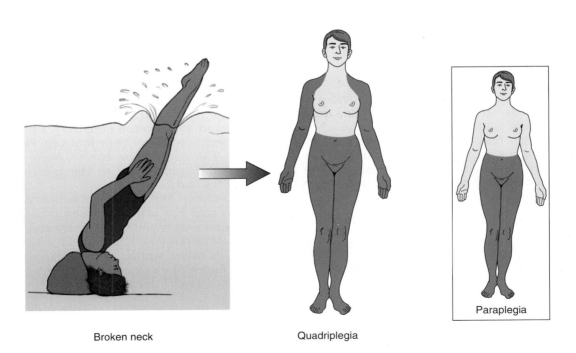

Broken neck   Quadriplegia   Paraplegia

FIGURE 10–3 ● Spinal cord injuries. Diving into a shallow pool can result in a damaged spinal cord. A higher spinal cord injury, such as a broken neck, causes paralysis of all four extremities (quadriplegia). A lower spinal cord injury causes paralysis of the lower extremities (paraplegia).

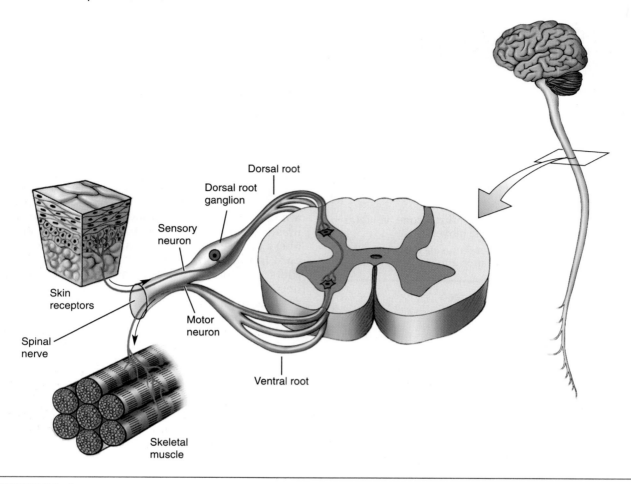

FIGURE 10–4 ● Attachment of the spinal nerves to the spinal cord. Spinal nerves contain both sensory and motor fibers. The sensory neurons attach to the spinal cord at the dorsal root; the motor neurons attach to the spinal cord at the ventral root.

● *Sensory pathway:* The spinal cord provides a pathway for *sensory* information traveling from the periphery to the brain. For instance, when you stick your finger with a sharp tack, sensory information travels from the finger toward the spinal cord. The information then ascends the spinal cord to the brain, where you experience the information as pain.

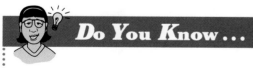

How is spinal anesthesia achieved?

Anesthetic agents such as novocaine may be injected into the subarachnoid space to achieve **spinal anesthesia.** When injected into the subarachnoid space, these drugs deaden, or anesthetize, the lumbar and sacral sensory nerves. Feelings of pain from the areas innervated by these deadened nerves are temporarily lost.

● *Motor pathway:* The spinal cord provides a pathway for *motor* information coming from the brain and going to the periphery. For instance, you decide to move your foot (eg, kick a football). The information travels from the brain down the spinal cord to the muscles of the lower leg and foot.
● *Reflex center:* The spinal cord acts as a major reflex center. For instance, when you stick your finger on a tack, you very quickly and automatically withdraw your finger from the source of injury. In other words, you reflexively remove your finger. The spinal cord, not the brain, performs this reflex act for you.

What Reflexes Are

What is a reflex? Many of the activities that we engage in every day occur very rapidly and without any conscious control. In other words, they happen reflexively. Many of the reflexes occur at the level of the spinal cord. A **reflex** is an involuntary response to a stimulus. If you touch a hot surface, for instance, you very quickly remove your hand. Your hand is safely away from the source of injury long before you consciously say, "This is hot. I must remove my hand!" Similarly, your ability to walk and maintain your balance requires hundreds of reflex movements.

A typical reflex response is demonstrated by the **patellar,** or **knee-jerk reflex** (Fig. 10–5). During a physical examination, the doctor taps the tendon below your kneecap. In response to the tap, your lower leg quickly and involuntarily pops up. The physician has elicited the patellar, or knee-jerk, reflex. How does this reflex help you? If you are standing erect and your knee bends, even slightly, the patellar reflex is stimulated. In response to the bending, the quadriceps muscle in the thigh contracts, thereby straightening the lower leg and helping you to maintain an upright position.

The Reflex Arc

The knee-jerk reflex illustrates the four basic components of the reflex arc (see Fig. 10–5). The **reflex arc** (rē′flĕks ärk) is the nerve pathway involved in a reflex. The four basic components of the reflex arc include

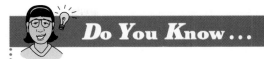

What is Lou Gehrig's disease?

Lou Gehrig was a famous New York Yankee baseball player who developed amyotrophic lateral sclerosis (ALS). ALS is a devastating neurologic disorder that destroys motor function while leaving sensory function intact. Over a long period, motor nerves gradually deteriorate. There is also a loss of nerve fibers and a sclerosing, or hardening, of the lateral columns of the white matter of the spinal cord, causing lateral sclerosis. The skeletal muscles supplied by these nerves wither away (the meaning of *amyotrophic*). The person with ALS gradually becomes completely paralyzed. ALS is frequently called Lou Gehrig's disease.

1. A **sensory receptor.** By tapping the tendon, the hammer stimulates sensory receptors in muscles of the leg.
2. An **afferent,** or **sensory, neuron** (ăf′ər-ənt nŏŏr′ŏn). The nerve impulse is carried by the sensory neuron to the spinal cord.
3. An **efferent,** or **motor, neuron** (ĕf′ər-ənt nŏŏr′ŏn). The nerve impulse is carried by the motor nerve to the muscles of the leg.

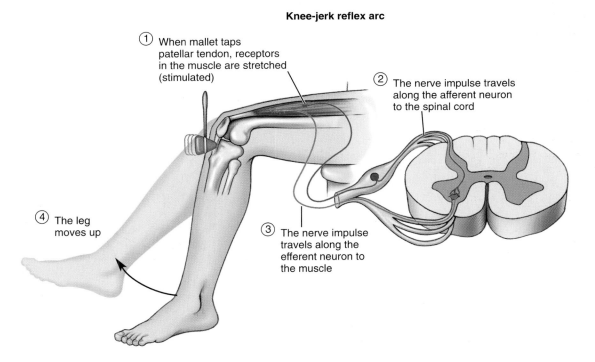

FIGURE 10–5 ● Reflex arc. The knee-jerk reflex illustrates the four components of the reflex arc. (1) Stimulation of the receptor. (2) Transmission of the signal (sensory) toward the spinal cord along the afferent neuron. (3) Transmission of the signal away from the cord (motor) along the efferent neuron. (4) The motor response of the effector organ (eg, contraction of the skeletal muscle, which jerks the leg upward).

4. An **effector organ.** The muscles of the leg, specifically the quadriceps femoris, are the effector organs. In response to the nerve impulse, the muscles contract and move the lower leg in an upward movement.

Ouch! The Withdrawal Reflex

The **withdrawal reflex** (Fig. 10–6A) helps protect you from injury. For instance, this reflex quickly moves your finger away from a hot iron, thereby preventing a severe burn. The "ouch" occurs after your finger is safely away from the hot iron.

Many, Many Reflexes

Reflexes also help regulate organ function. Figure 10–6 illustrates some of the reflexes that regulate body function. The **pupillary reflex,** for instance, regulates the amount of light that enters the eye. When a bright light is directed at the eye, the muscles that control pupillary size constrict. The size of the pupil diminishes, thereby restricting the amount of additional light entering the eye.

Blood pressure is also under reflex control. When blood pressure declines, the **baroreceptor reflex** causes the heart and blood vessels to respond in a way that restores blood pressure to normal.

In addition to performing important physiologic functions, these reflexes are used diagnostically to assess nerve function. Abnormal findings may indicate central nervous system (CNS) lesions, tumors, and other neurologic diseases such as multiple sclerosis. You may have observed a physician elicit the Babinski reflex (see Fig. 10–6) by stroking the lateral sole of the foot in the direction of heel to toe with a hard blunt object. In the adult, the Babinski reflex is normal, or negative, if the response to the stroking is plantar flexion, a curling of the toes. An abnormal, or positive, Babinski reflex is dorsiflexion of the big toe, sometimes with fanning, the spreading of the other toes. An infant responds differently to this stimulus; up to the age of 2 years, an infant's Babinski reflex is normally positive and reflects the immaturity of the infant's nervous system. Some clinically significant reflexes and their functions are listed in Table 10–2.

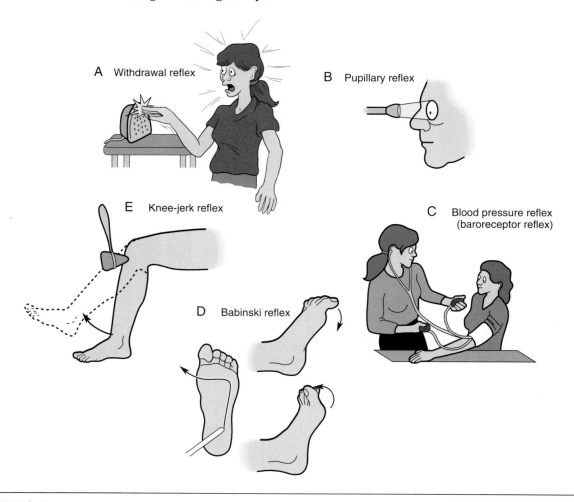

FIGURE 10–6 • Many reflexes. A, Withdrawal reflex. B, Pupillary reflex. C, Blood pressure, or baroreceptor, reflex. D, Babinski reflex. E, Knee-jerk reflex.

Table 10•2 CLINICALLY SIGNIFICANT REFLEXES

REFLEX	DESCRIPTION	MEANING
Patellar (knee-jerk reflex)	A stretch reflex; the hammer strikes the patellar tendon below the knee—in response, the lower leg kicks up.	Impaired in damage to nerves involved in the reflex Impaired in damage to lumbar region of spinal cord Impaired in patients with diseases that affect the nerves and spinal cord (diabetes mellitus, neurosyphilis, and chronic alcoholism)
Achilles tendon (ankle-jerk reflex)	A stretch reflex; the hammer strikes the Achilles tendon, causing plantar flexion.	Impaired in damage to nerves involved in the reflex Impaired in damage to lower spinal cord (L5 to S2)
Abdominal	With stroking of the lateral abdominal wall, the abdominal wall contracts and moves the umbilicus toward the stimulus.	Impaired in lesions of peripheral nerves Impaired in lesions of spinal cord (thoracic) and in patients with multiple sclerosis
Babinski	With stroking of the lateral sole of the foot from heel to toe, the toes curl under with slight inversion of the foot. The response is called a negative Babinski reflex. A positive or abnormal reflex results in dorsiflexion of the big toe and spreading of the other toes.	Impaired in lesions/damage of the spinal cord In children less than 2 years of age, the Babinski reflex is positive.

✳ **SUM IT UP!** The spinal cord and the peripheral nervous system allow the brain to communicate with the body and external environment. The spinal cord transmits information up and down the cord. Sensory information is brought to the brain from the lower cord region, while motor information is transmitted away from the brain, down the cord toward the periphery. In addition to providing pathways for the flow of information, the spinal cord acts as a center of reflex activity. Many functions, such as maintaining balance and the regulation of blood pressure, are achieved by the spinal cord.

PERIPHERAL NERVOUS SYSTEM

The **peripheral nervous system** (pə-rĭf′ər-əl nūr′vəs sĭs′təm) consists of the nerves and ganglia located outside the central nervous system (brain and spinal cord).

What a Nerve Is

Before classifying the nerves, you need to differentiate between a nerve and a neuron (see Chapter 9). A neuron is a single nerve cell; a **nerve** (nûrv) contains the fibers of many neurons. The nerve contains many fibers bundled together with blood vessels and then wrapped in connective tissue (Fig. 10–7). Nerves are located outside the CNS. (Within the CNS, bundles of

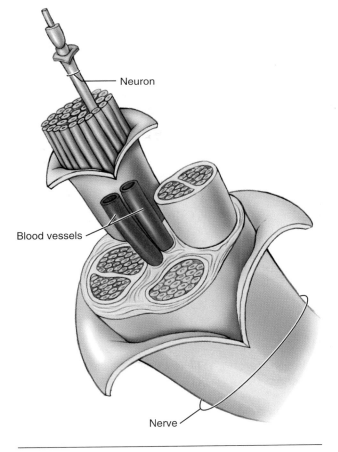

FIGURE 10–7 ● Difference between a neuron and nerve. A neuron is a single nerve cell. A nerve consists of many neurons bundled together by connective tissue. The nerve also contains blood vessels.

nerve fibers are called tracts.) Nerves are classified as

- **Sensory nerves** (sĕn′sə-rē nûrvz), composed only of sensory neurons.
- **Motor nerves** (mō′tər nûrvz), composed only of motor neurons.
- **Mixed nerves,** containing both sensory and motor neurons. Most nerves are mixed.

Classifying the Peripheral Nervous System

The peripheral nervous system can be classified in two ways, structurally (by the parts) or functionally (according to what they do).

Structural Classification of the Peripheral Nervous System

The structural, or anatomical, classification of the peripheral nervous system divides the nerves into cranial and spinal nerves. The classification is based on the origin of the fiber (where it comes from, or originates).

CRANIAL NERVES
Names and Numbers of Cranial Nerves. Twelve pairs of **cranial nerves** (krā′nē-əl nûrvz) are shown in Figure 10–8. Each cranial nerve has a specific number, always designated by a Roman numeral, and a name. The numbers indicate the order in which the nerves exit the brain from front to back. For instance, the second cranial nerve (CN II) is the optic nerve.

In general, the name of the nerve indicates the specific anatomical area served by the nerve. The optic nerve serves the eye. While the cranial nerves primarily serve the head, face, and neck region, one pair, the vagus, branches extensively and extends throughout the thoracic and abdominal cavities.

A common mnemonic used to memorize the cranial nerves in proper order is shown in Table 10–3: *On Old Olympus Towering Tops A Finn Viewed Germans Vaulting And Hopping.* The first letter of each word is the same as the first letter of each cranial nerve. You may want to develop your own mnemonic.

Functions of Cranial Nerves. Cranial nerves perform four general functions. First, they carry sensory information for the special senses—smell, taste, vision, and hearing. Second, they carry general sensory information regarding touch, pressure, pain, temperature, and vibration. Third, they carry motor information that results in voluntary control of skeletal muscle. Fourth, they carry motor information that results in the secretion of glands and the contraction of cardiac and smooth muscle. Cranial nerve function is summarized in Table 10–3. Locate each nerve on Figure 10–8.

Table 10 • 3 CRANIAL NERVES

MNEMONIC	NERVE	TYPE	FUNCTION
On	I Olfactory	Sensory	Sense of smell
Old	II Optic	Sensory	Sense of sight
Olympus	III Oculomotor	Mixed (mostly motor)	Movement of eyeball, raising of eyelid; change in pupil size
Towering	IV Trochlear	Mixed (mostly motor)	Movement of eyeball
Tops	V Trigeminal	Mixed	Chewing of food; sensations in face, scalp, and teeth
A	VI Abducens	Mixed (mostly motor)	Movement of eyeball
Finn	VII Facial	Mixed	Facial expressions; secretion of saliva and tears; taste
Viewed	VIII Vestibulocochlear	Sensory	Sense of hearing and balance
Germans	IX Glossopharyngeal	Mixed	Swallowing, secretion of saliva; taste; sensory for the reflex regulation of blood pressure
Vaulting	X Vagus	Mixed	Visceral muscle movement and sensations; sensory for reflex regulation of blood pressure
And	XI Accessory	Mixed (mostly motor)	Swallowing; head and shoulder movement; speaking
Hopping	XII Hypoglossal	Mixed (mostly motor)	Speech and swallowing

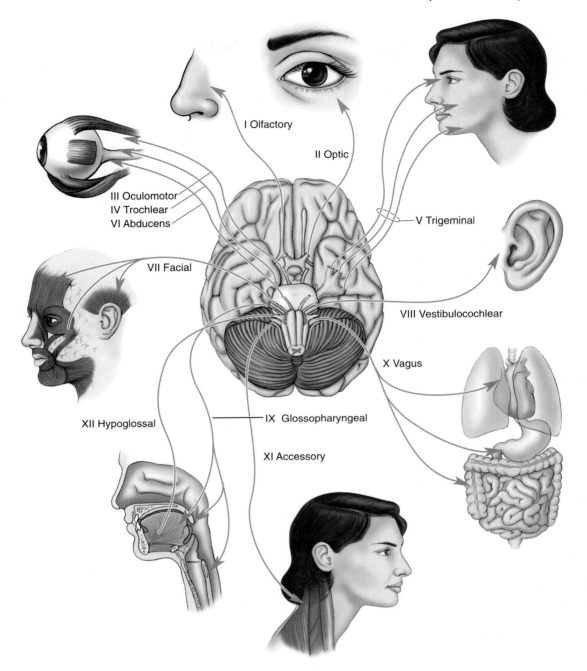

FIGURE 10–8 • Twelve pairs of cranial nerves. The cranial nerves are numbered according to the order in which they leave the brain.

CN I, Olfactory Nerve. A sensory nerve that carries information from the nose to the brain. The olfactory nerve is concerned with the sense of smell. A person who damages the olfactory nerve may lose the sense of smell. In addition, the person may complain of loss of taste for food because the appeal of food is determined by both taste and smell.

CN II, Optic Nerve. A sensory nerve that carries visual information from the eye to the brain,

specifically the occipital lobe of the cerebrum. Damage to the optic nerve causes diminished vision or blindness in the affected eye.

CN III, Oculomotor Nerve. Primarily a motor nerve that causes contraction of the extrinsic eye muscles, thereby moving the eyeball in the socket. The oculomotor nerve also raises the eyelid and constricts the pupil of the eye.

An increase in intracranial pressure can press on the oculomotor nerve, thereby interfering with the ability of the pupil of the eye to respond to light. When this occurs, the pupil is said to be dilated and fixed.

CN IV, Trochlear Nerve. Primarily a motor nerve that contracts one of the extrinsic muscles of the eyeball, thereby helping to move the eyeball.

CN V, Trigeminal Nerve. A mixed nerve with three branches supplying the facial region. The two sensory branches carry information regarding touch, pressure, and pain from the face, scalp, and teeth to the brain. The motor branch innervates the muscles of mastication (ie, chewing).

A person may experience a neuralgia of the trigeminal nerve. This condition is called **trigeminal neuralgia,** or **tic douloureux.** It is characterized by bouts of severe facial pain. The pain may be triggered by such events as eating, shaving, and exposure to cold temperatures. In an effort to avoid these triggers, the patient often becomes a prisoner of the disease, refusing to eat, shave, or leave the house in cold weather.

CN VI, Abducens Nerve. Primarily a motor nerve that, like the trochlear, controls eye movement by innervating only one of the extrinsic eye muscles.

CN VII, Facial Nerve. A mixed nerve that performs mostly motor functions. Its sensory function is taste. Facial expression and the secretion of saliva and tears are largely due to the facial nerve.

If the facial nerve is damaged, facial expression is absent on the affected side of the face. This condition is called Bell's palsy. Cosmetically, this condition is very distressing because one side of the face may smile and look alive while the other side of the face is expressionless, or blank.

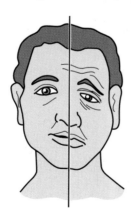

CN VIII, Vestibulocochlear Nerve (Auditory Nerve). A sensory nerve that carries information for hearing and balance from the ear to the brain. The vestibular branch of this nerve is responsible for equilibrium, or balance, and the cochlear branch is responsible for hearing. Damage to this nerve may cause loss of hearing or balance or both. (This function is further discussed under hearing in Chapter 11.)

CN IX, Glossopharyngeal Nerve. A mixed nerve that carries taste sensation from the posterior tongue to the brain. A second sensory function involves the regulation of blood pressure. Motor fibers stimulate the secretion of salivary glands in the mouth. Other motor fibers innervate the throat and aid in swallowing. The glossopharyngeal nerve is also associated with the gag reflex. The gag reflex plays an important role in preventing food and water from entering the respiratory passages. Normally, when something goes down the wrong way, you gag and cough until the airway is cleared. Loss of the gag reflex places you at risk for choking.

CN X, Vagus Nerve. A mixed nerve that carries fibers to and from most of the organs in the thoracic and abdominal cavities (eg, lungs, stomach, intestines). The sensory fibers of the vagus nerve participate in the regulation of blood pressure. The motor fibers of the vagus nerve also supply the voicebox in the throat (pharynx) and the glands that line the entire digestive tract. The word *vagus* literally means wanderer; the name refers to the far-reaching distribution of this nerve.

CN XI, Accessory Nerve. Primarily a motor nerve that supplies the sternocleidomastoid and the trapezius muscles, thereby controlling movement of the head and shoulder regions. This nerve and associated muscles allow you to shrug your shoulders.

CN XII, Hypoglossal Nerve. Primarily a motor nerve that controls movement of the tongue, thereby affecting speaking and swallowing activities.

A neurologic assessment includes simple procedures that test the ability of each cranial nerve to perform these functions. Table 10–4 illustrates simple methods used to test cranial nerve function. The table also includes common disorders and abnormal findings involving the cranial nerves.

SPINAL NERVES

Names and Numbers of Spinal Nerves. Thirty-one pairs of spinal nerves emerge from the spinal cord (Fig. 10–9). Each pair is numbered according to the level of the spinal cord from which it arises. The 31 pairs are grouped as follows: 8 pairs of cervical nerves, 12 pairs of thoracic nerves, 5 pairs of lumbar nerves, 5 pairs of sacral nerves, and 1 pair of coccygeal nerves. The lumbar and sacral nerves at the bottom of the cord extend the length of the spinal cavity before exiting from the vertebral column. These nerves are called **cauda equina** because they look like a horse's tail. The nerves exit from the bony vertebral column through tiny holes in the vertebrae called **foramina.**

Spinal Nerve Plexuses. As the spinal nerves exit from the vertebral column, they divide into

Table 10•4	CRANIAL NERVES: ASSESSMENT AND DISORDERS	
NERVE	**ASSESSMENT**	**SOME DISORDERS**
I Olfactory	Person is asked to sniff and identify various odors (eg, vanilla).	Inability to smell (anosmia); consequently, food tastes flat
II Optic	Examination of the interior of the eye by ophthalmoscopic visualization. Use of eye charts and tests of peripheral vision (eg, testing the point at which the person can first see an object moving into the visual field).	Loss of vision
III Oculomotor	Test the ability of the eyes to follow a moving object. Examination of pupils for size, shape, and size equality. Pupillary reflex is tested with a penlight (the pupils should constrict, ie, become smaller, in response to light). Test the ability of the eyes to converge (eg, have the patient follow an object as it is moved closer to the eyes).	Drooping upper eyelid (ptosis) Absence of pupillary reflex (eg, dilated and fixed pupils that may indicate an increase in intracranial pressure) Difficulty in focusing eyes on an object (diplopia/double vision and strabismus/ crossed eyes)
IV Trochlear	Test ability of the eyes to follow a moving object.	Inability to move eyeball in a particular direction
V Trigeminal	Sensations (pain/touch/temperature) are tested with sharp pin and hot/cold objects. Corneal reflex is tested with a cotton wisp. Motor function is tested by asking the person to open the mouth (against resistance) and to move the jaw from side to side.	Loss of sensation (pain/touch) Paresthesias (abnormal tingling, itching, and numbness) Difficulty in chewing Deviation of jaw to side of lesion when opened Severe spasms in sensory branches cause pain (trigeminal neuralgia or tic douloureux)
VI Abducens	Test ability of the eyes to follow a moving object.	Inability to move eyes laterally (eye cocked in) Diplopia, strabismus
VII Facial	Test anterior two thirds of tongue for sweet, salty, sour, and bitter taste. Person is asked to cause facial muscle movement (eg, smile, close eyes, wrinkle forehead, whistle). Ability to secrete tears is tested by asking person to sniff ammonia fumes.	Bell's palsy (expressionless face, drooping mouth and drooling, inability to close eyes) Loss of taste on anterior two thirds of tongue on side of lesion
VIII Vestibulocochlear (auditory)	Hearing is checked by air and bone conduction (use of tuning fork).	Loss of hearing, noises in ear (tinnitus) Loss of balance (vertigo)
IX Glossopharyngeal	Check gag and swallowing reflex. Person is asked to speak and cough. Test posterior two thirds of tongue for taste.	Loss of gag reflex Difficulty in swallowing (dysphagia) Loss of taste on posterior two thirds of tongue Decreased salivation
X Vagus	Similar to testing for CN IX (because they both innervate throat).	Sagging of soft palate Hoarseness of voice due to paralysis of vocal fold
XI Accessory	Ask person to rotate head from side to side and to shrug shoulders (against resistance).	Drooping shoulders Inability or difficulty in rotating head (wryneck)
XII Hypoglossal	Person is asked to stick out tongue— note any deviation in position of the protruded tongue.	Some difficulty in speaking (dysarthria), chewing, and swallowing (dysphagia)

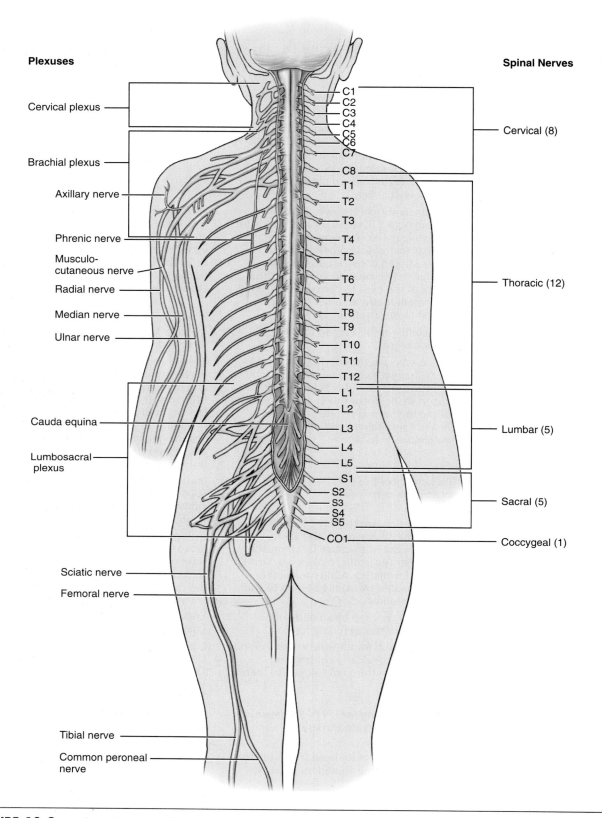

FIGURE 10–9 • Spinal nerves (31 pairs): eight cervical, 12 thoracic, five lumbar, five sacral, and one coccygeal. The spinal cord ends at L1; the cauda equina (extension of the lumbar and sacral nerves) extends the length of the spinal cavity. Three major nerve plexuses (networks): cervical plexus, brachial plexus, and lumbosacral plexus.

Table 10•5	SPINAL NERVE PLEXUSES		
PLEXUS	**SPINAL NERVE ORIGIN**	**REGION INNERVATED**	**MAJOR NERVES EMERGING FROM PLEXUS**
Cervical	C1–C4	Skin and muscles of the neck and shoulder; diaphragm	Phrenic
Brachial	C5–C8, T1	Skin and muscles of the upper extremities	Axillary Radial Median Musculocutaneous Ulnar
Lumbosacral	T12, L1–L5 S1–S4	Skin and muscle of lower torso and lower extremities	Femoral Obturator Sciatic Pudendal

many fibers. At various points, these nerve fibers converge, or come together again, into nerve **plexuses** (plĕk′sǝs-ĭz), or networks. The three major nerve plexuses are the cervical plexus, the brachial plexus, and the lumbosacral plexus (see Fig. 10–9). Each plexus sorts out the many fibers and sends nerve fibers to a specific part of the body. The three plexuses and the major nerves that emerge from each plexus are listed in Table 10–5. The results of damage to major peripheral nerves are listed in Table 10–6.

Cervical Plexus (C1–C4). Fibers from the cervical plexus supply the muscles and skin of the neck. Motor fibers (C3, C4, and C5) from this

plexus also pass into the phrenic nerve. The phrenic nerve stimulates the contraction of the diaphragm, a major breathing muscle (Fig. 10–10 and see Fig. 10–9).

If the spinal cord is severed below the C5 level, the person is paralyzed but can breathe. If the level of injury is higher (eg, C2) and the phrenic nerve is injured, motor impulses to the diaphragm are interrupted, and the person cannot breathe normally. To breathe, the person generally needs the assistance of a ventilator.

Brachial Plexus (C5–C8, T1). The nerves that emerge from the brachial plexus supply the muscles and skin of the shoulder, arm, forearm, wrist,

Table 10•6	MAJOR PERIPHERAL NERVES: RESULTS OF DAMAGE	
NERVE	**BODY AREA SERVED**	**RESULTS OF NERVE DAMAGE**
Phrenic	Diaphragm	Impaired breathing
Axillary	Muscles of shoulder	Crutch palsy
Radial	Posterior arm, forearm, hand; thumbs and first two fingers	Wristdrop (inability to lift or extend hand at wrist)
Median	Forearm and some muscles of the hand	Inability to pick up small objects
Ulnar	Wrist and many muscles in hand	Clawhand—inability to spread fingers apart
Intercostal	Rib cage	Impaired breathing
Femoral	Lower abdomen, anterior thigh, medial leg, foot	Inability to extend leg and flex hip
Sciatic	Lower trunk; posterior thigh and leg	Inability to extend hip and flex knee
Common peroneal	Lateral area of leg and foot	Footdrop—inability to dorsiflex foot
Tibial	Posterior area of leg and foot	Shuffling gait due to inability to invert and dorsiflex foot

CERVICAL PLEXUS   BRACHIAL PLEXUS   LUMBOSACRAL PLEXUS

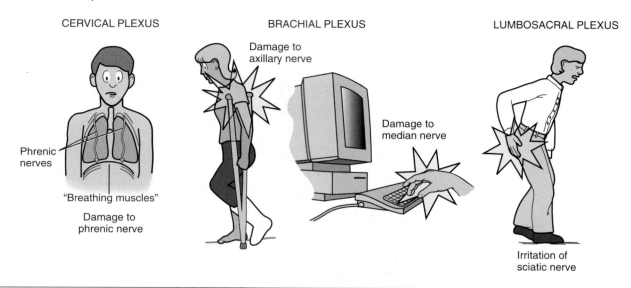

FIGURE 10–10 ● Damage to nerves: phrenic nerve damage, axillary nerve damage, median nerve damage, and sciatic nerve damage.

and hand. The axillary nerve emerges from this plexus and travels through the shoulder into the arm.

The axillary nerve in the shoulder region is susceptible to damage. For instance, a person using crutches is taught to bear the weight of the body on the hands and not on the armpit, or axillary region. The weight of the body can damage the axillary nerve, causing crutch palsy.

The radial and ulnar nerves, which serve the lower arm, wrist, and hand, also emerge from the brachial plexus. Damage to the radial nerve can cause a wristdrop, while injury to the ulnar nerve causes the hand to appear claw-like; the person is unable to spread the fingers apart.

Lumbosacral Plexus (T12, L1–L5, S1 to end). The lumbosacral plexus gives rise to nerves that supply the muscles and skin of the lower abdominal wall, external genitalia, buttocks, and lower extremities. The sciatic nerve, the longest nerve in the body, arises from this plexus. The sciatic nerve supplies the entire musculature of the leg

and foot. The sciatic nerve can become inflamed and cause intense pain in the buttock and posterior thigh region. A common cause of sciatica is a ruptured or herniated vertebral disc (see Fig. 10–10).

What a Dermatome Is. Each spinal nerve innervates a particular area of the skin; this distribution of nerves is called a **dermatome** (dûr′mə-tōm). Figure 10–11 illustrates the dermatomes for the entire body. Each dermatome is named for the particular nerve that serves it. For instance, the C4 dermatome is innervated by the C4 spinal nerve. Dermatomes are useful clinically. For instance, if the skin of the shoulder region is stimulated with the tip of a pin and the person cannot feel the stick sensation, the clinician has reason to believe the C4 nerve is impaired.

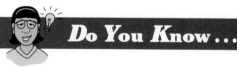

What do chickenpox and shingles have in common?

Chickenpox and shingles (herpes zoster) are caused by the same virus. In shingles, clusters of vesicles develop along cranial or spinal dermatomes. The lesions evolve into crusts on the skin.

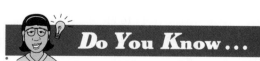

How do you avoid hitting the sciatic nerve when giving an intramuscular (IM) injection into the buttock?

The buttock is divided into quadrants. The sciatic nerve runs in the inner quadrants. By administering IM injections into the gluteus medius, in the center of the upper outer quadrant, a clinician can avoid injury to the sciatic nerve.

✳ **SUM IT UP!** The peripheral nervous system consists of the nerves and ganglia located outside the central nervous system. Nerves are sensory, motor, and mixed. Mixed nerves carry both sensory and motor neurons. The peripheral nervous system can be classified structurally and functionally. The structural classification divides the nerves into cranial and spinal nerves. There are 12 pairs of cranial nerves; their fibers originate in the brain (see Fig. 10–8 and Table 10–3). With the exception of the vagus nerve, the cranial nerves innervate structures in the head and neck region. There are 31 pairs of spinal nerves; their fibers originate in the spinal cord (see Fig. 10–9 and Tables 10–5 and 10–6). The spinal nerve fibers converge into nerve plexuses, or networks. The three major nerve plexuses are the cervical plexus, the brachial plexus, and the lumbosacral plexus. When the nerves exit the plexuses, they are distributed throughout the body. Each spinal nerve innervates a particular area of the body. This distribution of nerves is called a dermatome.

Functional Classification of the Peripheral Nervous System

The functional classification explains where the nerves go and what they do. The functional classification for the peripheral nervous system includes

- The somatic afferent nerves, which bring sensory information from the different parts of the body, particularly the skin and muscles, to the CNS. (The somatic afferent nerves are discussed further in Chapter 11.)

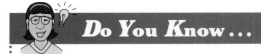

Do You Know...

How does the dentist deaden your jaw before a tooth extraction?

To eliminate the pain associated with dental work, the dentist injects an anesthetic agent into an area of the jaw that contains the sensory nerves of the painful tooth. By eliminating the transmission of stimuli along the sensory nerves, the dentist eliminates the sensation.

- The somatic efferent nerves, which bring motor information from the CNS to the skeletal muscles throughout the body. (The events that oc-

---

FIGURE 10–11 • Major nerves of the body: dermatomes. Each dermatome (segment) is named for the spinal nerve that serves it.

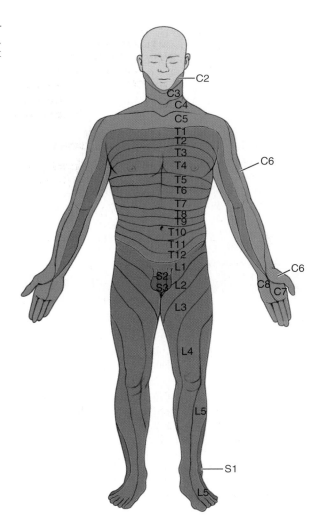

cur at the neuromuscular junction, which links somatic nerve and skeletal muscle, are described in Chapter 8.)

- The **autonomic nervous system** (ŏ″tə-nŏm′ĭk nûr′vəs sĭs′təm) (ANS) is composed of nerves that supply the organs (viscera) and glands. The ANS is further divided into the **sympathetic** (sĭm″pə-thĕt′ĭk) and **parasympathetic** (păr″ə-sĭm″pə-thĕt′ĭk) **nervous systems.**

AUTONOMIC NERVOUS SYSTEM

Autonomic/Automatic. Throughout the day you are busy doing things. You walk across a room, run up the stairs, write, type, and chew your food. You perform all of these activities voluntarily and consciously. Your body, however, performs many more activities unconsciously and automatically. For instance, when you eat, you do not consciously think, "I am eating, so I should increase the flow of my digestive enzymes and then increase the rate of contraction of my intestinal muscles to enhance the digestive process." Instead, your body automatically and unconsciously makes these decisions and carries them out for you. This automatic response is the function of the autonomic nervous system.

Structure: Dual Innervation. The ANS is the part of the peripheral nervous system that supplies motor activity to the glands, the smooth muscle of the hollow organs, and the heart. It works automatically and unconsciously.

The two divisions of the ANS are the sympathetic nervous system and the parasympathetic nervous system. A single organ generally receives fibers from both divisions of the ANS. In most instances, stimulation of one division causes a specific effect, while stimulation of the other division causes an opposing effect. For instance, the cells of the heart that determine heart rate receive both sympathetic and parasympathetic fibers. Stimulation of the sympathetic fibers causes the heart rate to increase, while stimulation of the parasympathetic fibers causes the heart rate to decrease. Table 10–7 indicates the effects of sympathetic and parasympathetic stimulation on some major organs of the body.

Functions of the Autonomic Nervous System: Fight or Flight and Feed and Breed. In general, the sympathetic nervous system is activated during periods of stress or times when the person feels threatened in some way (Fig. 10–12). For this reason, the sympathetic nervous system is also called the **fight-or-flight** system. In other words, the sympathetic nervous system causes you to be prepared either to confront the situation (fight) or remove yourself from the threatening situation (flight). Recall a time when you were frightened. Your heart raced and pounded in your chest. The pupils of your eyes opened wide. You began to breathe more quickly and more deeply. The palms of your hands became wet with perspiration, and your mouth became so dry that you could hardly speak. These are the effects of the sympathetic nervous system.

The parasympathetic nervous system is most active during quiet, nonstressful conditions. The parasympathetic nervous system plays an important role in the regulation of the digestive system and in reproductive function. For this reason, it is sometimes referred to as the **feed-and-breed** division of the autonomic nervous system. Another descriptive term for the parasympathetic nervous system is resting and digesting.

The sympathetic nervous system is activated during periods of stress. These periods are normally short-lived. If you keep yourself stressed out, however, the sympathetic nervous system keeps the body in a state of high alert. Over time, this state takes its toll on the body through stress-induced illnesses. Laughter, play, rest, and relaxation diminish sympathetic outflow and are good buffers against the effects of stress.

Table 10•7	AUTONOMIC NERVOUS SYSTEM: ORGAN RESPONSES	
ORGAN	**SYMPATHETIC RESPONSE**	**PARASYMPATHETIC RESPONSE**
Heart	Increases rate and strength of contraction	Decreases rate: no direct effect on strength of contraction
Bronchial tubes	Dilates	Constricts
Iris of eye	Dilates (pupil enlarges)	Constricts (pupil becomes smaller)
Blood vessels	Constricts (usually)	No innervation
Sweat glands	Stimulates	No innervation
Intestine	Inhibits motility	Stimulates motility and secretion
Adrenal medulla	Stimulates secretion of epinephrine and norepinephrine	No effect
Salivary glands	Stimulates thick secretion	Stimulates profuse, watery secretions

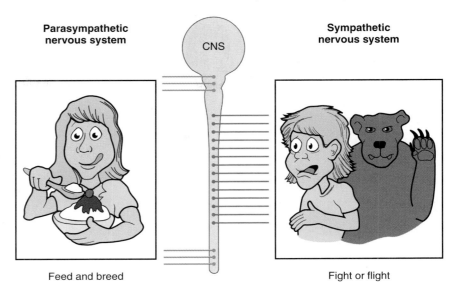

Parasympathetic nervous system

CNS

Sympathetic nervous system

Feed and breed

Fight or flight

FIGURE 10–12 • Autonomic nervous system: The parasympathetic nervous system is called the craniosacral outflow. It is the feed-and-breed system. The sympathetic nervous system is called the thoracolumbar outflow. It is the fight-or-flight system.

AUTONOMIC NERVE FIBERS: HOW THEY ARE ARRANGED. The motor pathways of the ANS use two neurons with one ganglion between each neuron (Fig. 10–13A). The cell body of neuron #1 is located in the CNS, in either the brain or the spinal cord. The axon of neuron #1 leaves the CNS and extends to the ganglion (the cell body of neuron #2). The axon of neuron #1 is called the **preganglionic fiber.** The axon of neuron #2 leaves the ganglion and extends to the organ. This axon is called the **postganglionic fiber.** The postganglionic fibers of the sympathetic and parasympathetic nervous system secrete different neurotransmitters. These neurotransmitters account for the different effects that the sympathetic and parasympathetic nerves have on the organs.

Parts of the Sympathetic Nervous System. The fibers of the sympathetic nervous system exit the spinal cord at the thoracic and lumbar levels (Fig. 10–13B). The sympathetic nervous system is therefore called the **thoracolumbar outflow.** The sympathetic fibers travel for a short distance and then form a synapse within ganglia located close to the cord. The sympathetic ganglia form a chain that runs alongside, or parallel to, the vertebral column. This chain is called the **paravertebral ganglia** or **sympathetic chain ganglia.**

Postganglionic fibers leave the ganglia and extend to the various organs. The neurotransmitter secreted by the postganglionic fibers of the sympathetic nervous system is **norepinephrine.** (Another name for norepinephrine is **noradrenalin.**) The fibers are named after the neurotransmitter, nor*adrenalin,* and are therefore called **adrenergic fibers.**

Parts of the Parasympathetic Nervous System. The fibers of the parasympathetic nerves exit the CNS at the level of the brain stem and the sacrum (Fig. 10–13C). The parasympathetic nervous system is therefore called the **craniosacral outflow.** The preganglionic fibers are long because the ganglia of the parasympathetic nervous system are located away from the spinal cord and near or within the organs.

Because the ganglia are located close to the organs, the parasympathetic nerves do not have a chain of ganglia running alongside the spinal cord. The short postganglionic fibers extend from the ganglia to the smooth muscle or glands within the organ. The neurotransmitter secreted by the postganglionic fibers of the parasympathetic nerves is **acetylcholine.** These postganglionic fibers are named after acetylcholine and are therefore called **cholinergic fibers.** Table 10–8 compares the sympathetic and parasympathetic nervous systems.

✳ **SUM IT UP!** The functional classification of the peripheral nerves identifies three roles: (1) the somatic afferent nerves bring information from the periphery to the CNS, (2) the somatic efferent nerves bring information from the CNS to the skeletal muscles, and (3) the autonomic (or automatic) nervous system supplies the organs or viscera).

The autonomic nervous system has two parts: the sympathetic nervous system and the parasympathetic nervous system. The sympathetic nervous system, also called the thoracolumbar outflow, has adrenergic postganglionic fibers and secretes norepinephrine as the neurotransmitter. The sympathetic nervous system is activated in periods of stress for its fight or flight responses. The parasympathetic nervous system, also called the craniosacral outflow, has cholinergic postganglionic fibers and secretes acetylcholine as its neurotransmitter. The parasympathetic nervous system is concerned with feeding or breeding activity.

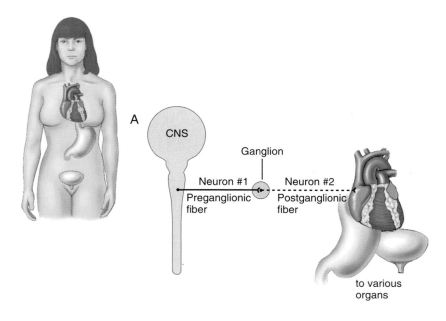

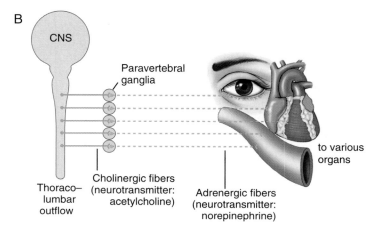

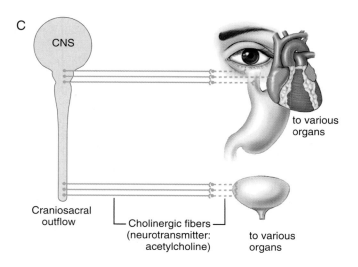

FIGURE 10–13 ● A, Arrangement of autonomic fibers. The motor pathways of the autonomic nervous system use two neurons. Neuron #1 extends from the CNS to the ganglion and is called the preganglionic fiber. Neuron #2 extends from the ganglion to the organ and is called the postganglionic fiber. B, Sympathetic nervous system (SNS). The fibers of the SNS leave the spinal cord at the thoracolumbar region, hence the name *thoracolumbar outflow*. After they synapse with the ganglia in the paravertebral ganglia, the postganglionic fibers extend to various organs. C, Parasympathetic nervous system. The fibers of the parasympathetic nervous system leave the spinal cord at the level of the cranium and the sacrum, hence the name *craniosacral outflow*. Long preganglionic fibers extend to the organ and synapse with the ganglia located in the organ. Short postganglionic fibers penetrate the organ.

Table 10•8	AUTONOMIC NERVOUS SYSTEM: CHARACTERISTICS	
CHARACTERISTIC	**SYMPATHETIC**	**PARASYMPATHETIC**
Origin of fibers	Thoracolumbar	Craniosacral
General effect	Fight or flight (expends energy)	Feed and breed
Ganglia	Paravertebral ganglia	Located near/within organ
Neurotransmitter (postganglionic)	Norepinephrine; adrenergic fibers	Acetylcholine; cholinergic fibers

As You Age

1. Aging causes an increase in synaptic delay and a 5% to 10% decrease in the speed of nerve conduction. Consequently, nervous reflexes slow.

2. Aging causes a loss of the sense of vibration at the ankle after the age of 65. This change is accompanied by a decrease of the ankle-jerk reflex and may affect balance, increasing the chance of falling.

3. An aging autonomic nervous system causes many changes. For instance, a less efficient sympathetic nervous system may cause transient hypotension and fainting. Fainting spells in the elderly often result in skeletal injuries, such as a broken hip.

4. Decreased autonomic nerve activity supplying the eyes causes changes in pupil size and pupillary reactivity. There is some decline in function of cranial nerves mediating taste and smell.

Disorders of the Spinal Cord and Peripheral Nerves

Multiple sclerosis	A progressive demyelination of the neurons and destruction of the oligodendrocytes. This degeneration impairs sensory and motor activity.
Peripheral neuropathy	Loss of sensation due to nerve damage. The loss is most severe in the hands and feet. While neuropathy can be caused by a number of conditions, diabetes mellitus is a common cause.
Poliomyelitis	A contagious infection that affects the brain and the spinal cord. Specifically, the polio virus destroys the lower motor neurons in the brain stem and the spinal cord. As motor neurons are destroyed, paralysis occurs.
Sciatica	A form of neuritis characterized by sharp pains along the sciatic nerve and its branches. Pain usually radiates from the buttocks into the hip and thigh areas.
Shingles	Also called herpes zoster. Shingles is an acute inflammation of the dorsal root ganglia. Shingles develops when the dormant virus that caused childhood chickenpox becomes activated and attacks the root ganglia. Pain and rash progress along the course of one or more spinal nerves, usually the intercostal nerves (sometimes the trigeminal nerve). Painful lesions eventually develop along the affected nerves.
Spina bifida	A congenital defect in the wall of the spinal cavity. Spina bifida is generally accompanied by a meningocele (protrusion of meninges) or myelomeningocele (protrusion of the spinal cord and meninges).
Spinal cord injury	Any condition or event that damages the neurons of the spinal cord. Complete transection of the cord produces quadriplegia or paraplegia, depending on the level of injury. Immediately after the injury, the person experiences spinal shock that may last from several hours to several weeks.

Summary Outline

The brain, spinal cord, and peripheral nervous system act as a vast communication system. The spinal cord transmits information to and from the brain. The peripheral nervous system brings information to the CNS (its sensory role) and delivers information from the CNS to the periphery (its motor role).

I. Spinal Cord

Composed of nervous tissue, the spinal cord is a tube-like structure located in the spinal cavity, extending from the foramen magnum (occipital bone) to L1.

A. Arrangement of Nervous Tissue
1. The gray matter is a butterfly-shaped area located centrally.
2. The white matter is composed of myelinated fibers arranged in tracts. Ascending tracts are sensory tracts. Descending tracts are motor tracts.
3. Spinal nerves are attached to the spinal cord. All spinal nerves are mixed (they contain sensory and motor fibers).
4. Sensory nerve fibers travel to the cord through the dorsal root. Motor nerve fibers travel in the ventral root.

B. Functions of the Spinal Cord
1. The spinal cord relays sensory information from the periphery to the brain and relays motor information from the brain to the periphery.
2. The spinal cord acts as a major reflex center.

C. Reflexes
1. A reflex is an involuntary response to a stimulus.
2. The four components to a reflex are a sensory receptor, an afferent (sensory) neuron, an efferent (motor) neuron, and an effector organ.
3. Examples of reflexes include the patellar (knee-jerk) reflex, the withdrawal reflex, and the baroreceptor reflex.

II. Peripheral Nervous System

A. Nerve
1. A nerve is a group of neurons.
2. There are sensory nerves, motor nerves, and mixed nerves.

B. Cranial and Spinal Nerves
1. A classification of nerves on the basis of structure divides nerves into cranial nerves and spinal nerves. There are 12 pairs of cranial nerves and 31 pairs of spinal nerves.
2. Spinal nerves are sorted out at nerve plexuses. The three major plexuses are the cervical plexus, the brachial plexus, and the lumbosacral plexus.
3. A dermatome is the area of skin innervated by each spinal nerve.

C. Somatic and Autonomic Nerves
1. A classification of nerves based on function divides the nerves into somatic afferent nerves (which bring sensory information to the CNS), somatic efferent nerves (which bring motor information from the CNS to the skeletal muscles), and the autonomic nervous system.
2. The autonomic nervous system is composed of the sympathetic and parasympathetic nervous systems.
3. The sympathetic nervous system is the fight-or-flight system; it is also called the thoracolumbar outflow. The sympathetic nerves have paravertebral ganglia (sympathetic chain ganglia).
4. The postganglionic fiber of a sympathetic nerve is adrenergic (secretes norepinephrine).
5. The parasympathetic nervous system is the feed-or-breed system; it is also called the craniosacral outflow.
6. The postganglionic fiber of a parasympathetic nerve is cholinergic (secretes acetylcholine).

Review Your Knowledge

1. During a lumbar puncture, a hollow needle is inserted into the subarachnoid space between L3 and L4. Why is there no danger of injuring the spinal cord with the needle during this procedure?

2. In which space surrounding the spinal cord and brain does CSF flow?

3. How are sensory and motor tracts different in function?

4. If the spinal cord is severed at the neck region, the trunk and all four extremities are paralyzed. What is this condition called?

5. Which nerve fibers travel to the spinal cord through the dorsal root? Which nerve fibers are found in the ventral root?

6. Describe three major functions of the spinal cord.

7. What is a reflex?

8. Describe four basic components of the reflex arc.

9. Name the reflexes described below:
  a. Occurs when you move your finger away from a hot iron
  b. Regulates the amount of light that enters the eye
  c. When blood pressure declines, the heart and blood vessels respond in a way that restores blood pressure to normal

10. What is the difference between a nerve and a neuron?

11. Describe the 12 pairs of cranial nerves.

12. Which cranial nerve extends throughout the thoracic and abdominal cavities?

13. Name four general functions of cranial nerves.

14. Which cranial nerve is responsible for equilibrium and hearing?

15. How many pairs of spinal nerves are there?

16. What is the longest nerve in the body?

17. What is the difference between afferent and efferent nerves?

18. What is the difference between the sympathetic and parasympathetic nervous systems?

19. Which neurotransmitter is secreted by the postganglionic fibers of the sympathetic nervous system? Which neurotransmitter is secreted by the postganglionic fibers of the parasympathetic nervous system?

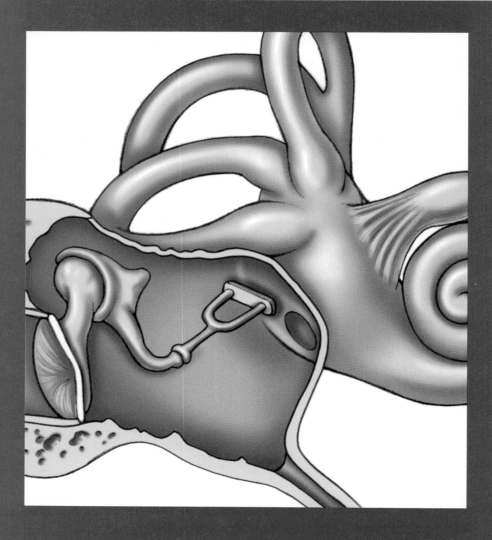

11 SENSORY SYSTEM

*O*bjectives

1. State the functions of the sensory system.

2. Define the five types of sensory receptors.

3. Describe the four components involved in the perception of a sensation.

4. Differentiate general senses from special senses.

5. Describe the five general senses: pain, touch, pressure, temperature, and proprioception.

6. Describe five special senses: smell, taste, sight, hearing, and balance.

7. Describe the visual accessory organs.

8. Describe the structure of the eye.

9. Explain the movement of the eyes.

10. Describe how the size of the pupils changes.

11. Describe the three divisions of the ear.

12. Describe the functions of the parts of the ear involved in hearing.

13. Explain the role of the ear in maintaining the body's equilibrium.

The sensory system allows us to experience the world. Senses allow us to see the trees, hear the voices of our friends, feel the heat of the sun, and taste our favorite foods. When the environment becomes threatening, the sensory system also acts as a warning system. For instance, if you place your hand on a hot surface, the sensory system experiences the episode as pain. The pain is a danger signal indicating that the body must make an adjustment to remove the harmful stimulus.

In addition to sensing outside information, the sensory system also allows us to keep track of what is happening within our bodies. For instance, when the stomach fills with food, sensory information is carried to the central nervous system (CNS). In response to this information, the stomach is told to digest the food.

RECEPTORS AND SENSATION

Cells That Detect Stimuli

Sensory neurons transmit information to the CNS (Table 11–1). A **receptor** is a specialized area of a sensory neuron that detects a specific stimulus. For instance, the receptors in the eye respond to light, while the receptors on the tongue respond to chemicals in food. Five types of sensory receptors are

- **Chemoreceptors** (kē″mō-rǐ-sĕp′tərz): sensory receptors stimulated by changes in the chemical concentration of substances.
- **Pain receptors** (pān rǐ-sĕp′tərz), or **nociceptors:** sensory receptors stimulated by tissue damage.
- **Thermoreceptors:** sensory receptors stimulated by changes in temperature.
- **Mechanoreceptors** (mĕk″ə-nō-rǐ-sĕp′tərz): sensory receptors stimulated by changes in pressure or movement of body fluids.
- **Photoreceptors** (fō″tō-rǐ-sĕp′tərz): sensory receptors stimulated by light.

What Sensation Is

A **sensation** is the conscious awareness of incoming sensory information. "Ouch," for example, indicates that you have become aware of a painful stimulus. Remember that the sensation, or feeling, is experienced by the brain and not by the receptor or sensory neuron. For instance, you see an object, hear a voice, or feel pain because the sensory information has stimulated a part of the brain (see Chapters 9 and 10).

Experiencing a Sensation

Four Components

Four components are involved in the perception of a sensation. Using the sense of sight as an example, these four components are illustrated in Figure 11–1.

- **Stimulus:** Light is the stimulus for the sense of sight. In the absence of light you cannot see.
- **Receptor:** Light waves stimulate the photoreceptors in the eye, producing a nerve impulse.
- **Sensory nerve:** The nerve impulse is conducted by a sensory nerve to the occipital lobe of the brain.
- **Special area of the brain:** The sensory information is interpreted as sight in the occipital lobe of the brain.

As you study each sensation, identify the stimulus, the type of receptor, the name of the sensory nerve, and the specific area of the brain that interprets the sensation.

Ouch! and Pew!

Two important characteristics of sensation are projection and adaptation. **Projection** (prō-jĕk′shən) describes the process by which the brain, after receiving a sensation, refers that sensation back to its source. You see with your eyes, hear with your ears, and feel pain in your injured

Table 11 ● 1	TYPES OF SENSORY RECEPTORS		
RECEPTOR	**STIMULUS**		**EXAMPLE**
Chemoreceptors	Changes in chemical concentrations of substances		Taste and smell
Pain receptors (nociceptors)	Tissue damage		Pain
Thermoreceptors	Changes in temperature		Heat and cold
Mechanoreceptors	Changes in pressure or movement of fluids		Hearing and equilibrium
Photoreceptors	Light energy		Sight

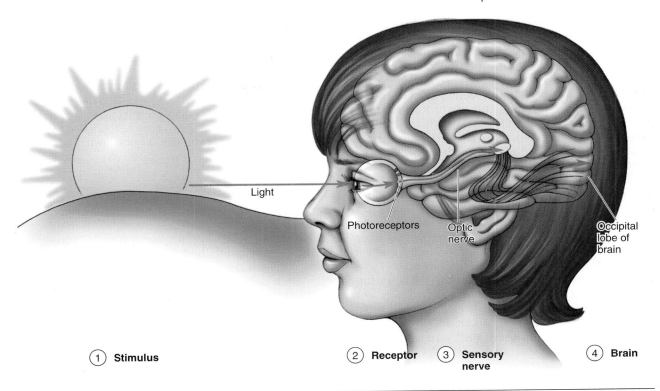

FIGURE 11–1 ● Four components of sensation: (1) stimulus (light), (2) receptor (photoreceptors), (3) sensory nerve (optic nerve), and (4) CNS (occipital lobe of the brain). The light stimulates the photoreceptors in the eyes. The photoreceptors convert the stimulus to a nerve impulse. The nerve impulse is transmitted by the optic nerve to the occipital lobe of the brain, where the information is interpreted as sight.

finger because the cortex of your brain receives the sensation and projects it back to its source. Projection answers the question "If pain is experienced by the brain, why is it that my injured finger hurts" (Fig. 11–2). Although the brain experiences the sensation, the brain makes the feeling seem to come from the receptors as they are stimulated.

The experience of phantom limb pain is another example of projection. If a leg is amputated, the person may still feel pain in the amputated leg

FIGURE 11–2 ● Projection. A, The sense of pain is interpreted in the brain but "felt" in the thumb. B, Phantom limb. When a limb is amputated, the person still feels the missing limb as if it is still there. The dashed line represents the amputated part.

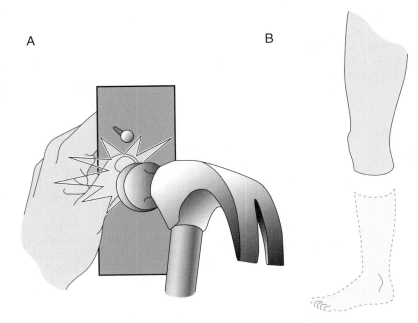

(see Fig. 11–2). The missing leg often throbs with pain. What is the cause of phantom limb pain? The severed nerve endings of the amputated leg continue to send sensory information to the parietal lobe of the brain. The brain interprets the information as pain and projects the feeling back to the leg area. For most amputees the phantom limb pain diminishes as the severed nerves heal, but the person often experiences a phantom limb presence. The leg still feels as though it is attached. This sensation may help a patient learn to use an artificial limb.

Sensory **adaptation** (ăd″ăp-tā′shən) is another characteristic of sensation. It is illustrated by the sense of smell. Pew! When you enter a room with a strong odor, the odor at first seems overwhelmingly strong. After a short period, however, the odor becomes less noticeable. The sensory receptors in the nose have adapted. When continuously stimulated, these receptors send fewer and fewer signals to the area of the brain that interprets sensory information as smell.

Receptors vary in their ability to adapt. Pain receptors, for instance, do not adapt, while receptors for pressure and touch adapt rapidly. Receptors that determine body position and detect blood chemistries adapt very slowly because they are important in maintaining homeostasis.

Two groups of senses are general and special senses. **General senses** are called general, or somatic, because their receptors are widely distributed throughout the body. The **special senses** are localized within a particular organ in the head. The special senses include taste, smell, sight, hearing, and balance.

THE GENERAL SENSES

General senses include pain, touch, pressure, temperature, and proprioception (Fig. 11–3). Receptors for the general senses are distributed widely throughout the body. They are found in the skin, muscles, joints, and visceral organs.

Pain

The receptors for pain consist of free nerve endings that are stimulated by tissue damage. Pain receptors do not adapt and may continue to send signals after the stimulus is removed. Pain receptors are widely distributed throughout the skin, the visceral organs, and other internal tissues. Oddly enough, the nervous tissue of the brain lacks pain receptors. Tissues surrounding the brain, like the meninges and the blood vessels, however, do contain pain receptors. You can feel a headache.

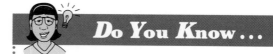

Do You Know...

What is an itch?

An itch is a mild pain sensation that may be experienced as real pain if not scratched. How scratching relieves an itch is not known.

Pain serves a protective function. Being unpleasant, pain motivates the person to remove its cause. The failure of the pain receptors to adapt is also protective. If pain receptors adapted, we would be less inclined to investigate the underlying cause of the pain. Ignoring pain, in turn, might cause a delay in diagnosis and implementation of proper treatment. For instance, a cancerous tumor may exert pressure on a surrounding structure, causing pain. If the pain diminished through adaptation of the pain receptors, the person might delay seeking medical attention and the cancer would have additional time to spread, thereby lessening the chance of a successful outcome. Although unpleasant and undesirable, pain serves the body well.

What stimulates the pain receptors? The specific signals that stimulate pain are not well understood. Three pain triggers have been identified. First, tissue injury promotes the release of certain chemicals that stimulate pain receptors. Second, a deficiency of oxygen is thought to stimulate pain receptors. For instance, if the blood supply to a visceral organ is diminished (a condition called ischemia), the tissue is deprived of oxygen, and the person experiences pain. The severe crushing pain of a heart attack is thought to be due in part to the oxygen deprivation experienced by the cardiac muscle. The administration of oxygen helps to relieve pain. Third, pain may be experienced when tissues are stretched or deformed. It appears that the stimulus is mechanical (distention, distortion) rather than chemical. For instance, if the intestine becomes distended, the person will often experience a severe cramping pain.

Why is pain originating in the heart often experienced in the shoulder and left arm? When pain feels as if it is coming from an area other than the site where it originates, it is called **referred pain** (rĭ-fûrd′ pān). Patients with heart disease often complain of pain or an aching sensation that starts in the shoulder region and moves down the left arm into the fourth and fifth fingers. In other words, stimulation of pain receptors in the heart causes pain that is experienced as being outside the heart. Areas of referred pain generated by the heart and other organs are illustrated in Figure 11–4.

What is the explanation for referred pain? The occurrence of referred pain is due to shared sen-

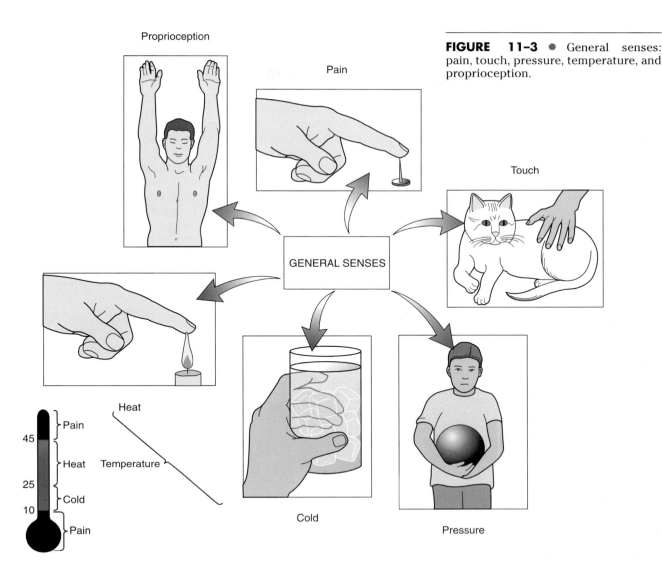

Proprioception

Pain

Touch

GENERAL SENSES

Heat

45 ⎱Pain

Heat   Temperature

25

10 ⎱Cold

⎱Pain

Cold

Pressure

sory nerve pathways. The nerve pathways that carry information from the heart are the same pathways that carry information from the shoulder and left arm. As a result, the brain interprets heart pain as shoulder and arm pain.

Once the pain receptors are stimulated, where does the information go? Pain impulses for most of the body travel up the spinal cord in a sensory nerve tract called the spinothalamic tract. The information is then transmitted to the thalamus, where the person first becomes aware of the pain, and then to the cerebral cortex of the parietal lobe. The cerebral cortex can identify the source of the pain and judge its intensity and other characteristics. In other words, the parietal lobe will determine the origin of pain and if the pain is sharp or dull, deep or superficial.

Touch and Pressure

The receptors for touch and pressure are mechanoreceptors; they respond to forces that press, move, or deform tissue. Touch receptors

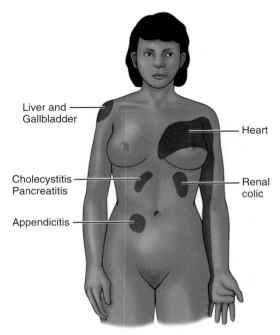

Liver and Gallbladder

Heart

Cholecystitis Pancreatitis

Renal colic

Appendicitis

FIGURE 11–4 ● Sites of referred pain.

217

are also called **tactile receptors** and are found mostly in the skin and allow us to feel a cat's soft fur (see Fig. 11–3). They are particularly numerous in the lips and the tips of the fingers, toes, tongue, penis, and clitoris. Receptors for heavy pressure are located in the skin, subcutaneous tissue and in the deep tissue. Pressure receptors are stimulated by the heavy ball in the boy's arms (see Fig. 11–3).

Temperature

The two types of thermoreceptors are heat and cold receptors. Thermoreceptors are found in free nerve endings and in other specialized sensory cells beneath the skin and are scattered widely throughout the body. Note the temperature scale in Figure 11–3. The **cold receptors** are stimulated at between 10° and 25°C. **Heat receptors** are stimulated at between 25° and 45°C. At both ends (extremes) of the temperature scale, pain receptors are stimulated. In other words, below 10°C, pain receptors are stimulated, producing a freezing sensation. Above 45°C, pain receptors are stimulated, producing a burning sensation. Both heat and cold thermoreceptors display adaptation, so that the sensation of heat or cold fades rapidly.

Immerse your hand in warm water and note how quickly the feeling of warmth disappears, even though the temperature of the water has not decreased. Your heat receptors have adapted. Remember that pain receptors do not adapt. If you place your hand in boiling water, you will feel intense continuous pain. Sensory information regarding temperature is sent to the parietal lobe.

Proprioception

Proprioception (prō″prē-ō-sĕp′shən) is the sense of orientation, or position. This sense allows you to locate a body part without looking at it. In other words, if you close your eyes, you can still locate your arm in space; you do not have to see your arm to know that it is raised over your head (see Fig. 11–3). Proprioception plays an important role in maintaining posture and coordinating body movement.

The receptors for proprioception (proprioreceptors) are the muscle spindles and Golgi tendon organs. These receptors are located in muscles, tendons, and joints. Proprioceptive receptors are also found in the inner ear, where they function in equilibrium. The cerebellum, which plays a major role in coordinating skeletal muscle activity, receives sensory information from these receptors. Sensory information regarding movement and position is also sent to the parietal lobe.

✳ **SUM IT UP!** The sensory system is designed to detect information from within and outside the body and to convey that information to the CNS for interpretation. Receptors located on sensory neurons respond to specific stimuli. Senses are classified as either general or special. The general senses include pain, touch, pressure, temperature, and proprioception.

THE SPECIAL SENSES

The five special senses are smell, taste, sight, hearing, and balance (Table 11–2). The organs of the special senses are located in organs of the head.

Sense of Smell: The Nose

The sense of smell, the **olfactory sense,** is associated with sensory structures located in the upper nose (Fig. 11–5). These **olfactory receptors** (ŏl-făk′tə-rē rĭ-sĕp′tərz) are classified as chemoreceptors, meaning that they are stimulated by chemicals that dissolve in the moisture of

Table 11 ● 2	**SPECIAL SENSES**			
SENSE	**ORGAN**	**SPECIFIC RECEPTOR**	**STIMULUS**	**TYPE OF RECEPTOR**
Smell	Nose	Olfactory cell	Changes in chemical concentrations of substances	Chemoreceptor
Taste	Tongue	Gustatory cell	Changes in chemical concentrations of substances	Chemoreceptor
Sight	Eye	Rods and cones	Light energy	Photoreceptor
Hearing	Inner ear: cochlea	Organ of Corti (hair cells)	Movement of fluids	Mechanoreceptor
Balance	Inner ear: vestibular apparatus	Hair cells	Movement of fluids	Mechanoreceptor

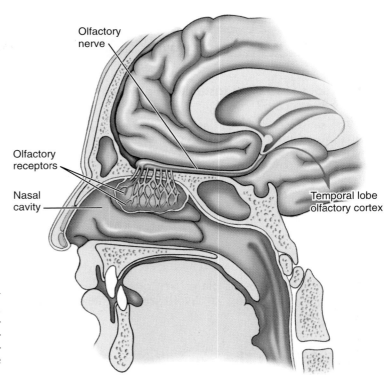

FIGURE 11–5 ● Sense of smell: the nose. The olfactory (smell) receptors are chemoreceptors and are located in the upper nose. Sensory information is transmitted through the olfactory nerve to the temporal lobe of the cerebrum.

the nasal tissue. Once the olfactory receptors have been stimulated, the sensory impulses travel along the olfactory nerve (cranial nerve I). The sensory information is eventually interpreted as smell within the olfactory cortex of the temporal lobe (as Chapter 9 describes). Olfactory receptors adapt quickly.

Sense of Taste: The Tongue

The sense of taste is also called the **gustatory sense. Taste buds** are the special organs of taste. The taste receptors are located on the tongue and are classified as chemoreceptors, meaning that they are sensitive to the chemicals in our food. The four basic taste sensations are salty, sweet, sour, and bitter. Each sensation is concentrated on a particular area of the tongue, as illustrated in Figure 11–6. The tip of the tongue is most sensitive to sweet and salty substances. Sour sensations are found primarily on the sides of the tongue, while bitter substances are most strongly tasted on the back part of the tongue. When the taste receptors are stimulated, the taste impulses travel along two cranial nerves (the facial and glossopharyngeal nerves) to various parts of the brain, eventually arriving in the gustatory cortex in the parietal lobe (see Chapter 9).

Taste receptors adapt. They also seem especially sensitive to bitter-tasting substances. This sensitivity serves a protective role because the

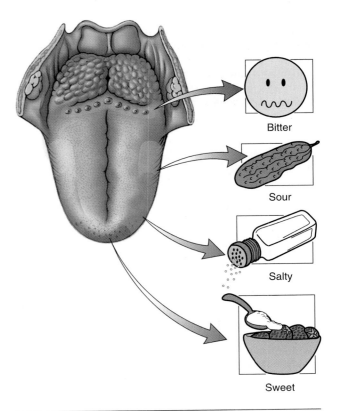

FIGURE 11–6 ● The sense of taste in the tongue (gustatory sense). Taste buds located on specific areas of the tongue identify four taste sensations: bitter, sour, salty, and sweet.

Do You Know...

Why does food often taste different when you have a cold?

The senses of taste and smell are closely related. When interpreted in the cerebral cortex, information from both senses may combine to produce a different taste sensation. This process implies that a taste is related to a smell. Therefore, food often tastes different when you have a cold and stuffy nose. Your sense of smell is disturbed and alters the taste of your food.

poisonous substances in plants are often bitter. Bitterness is a warning to avoid eating these plants.

Sense of Sight: The Eye

The sense of sight is one of our most cherished senses. Think of all that you see that brings so much joy to your life—the smiles of your children, the faces of your friends, and the beautiful colors of the trees and flowers. The eyes are the organs of vision; they contain the visual receptors. Assisting the eyes in their function and protecting them from injury are the visual accessory organs.

Visual Accessory Organs

The visual accessory organs include the eyebrows, eyelids, eyelashes, lacrimal apparatus, and extrinsic eye muscles (Fig. 11–7).

EYEBROWS. The eyebrows, patches of hair located above the eyes, perform a protective role. They keep the perspiration out of the eyes and shade the eyes from glaring sunlight.

EYELIDS. Anteriorly, the **eyelids** protect the eyes. The upper and lower eyelids meet at the corners of the eyes. The corners are called the **medial (inner) canthus** and **lateral (outer) canthus.** The eyelids are composed of four layers: skin, skeletal muscle, connective tissue, and conjunctiva. The skeletal muscles open and close the eyelids. The levator muscle (levator meaning to raise, like an elevator) opens the eye, while the orbicularis oculi muscle closes it. Sometimes the patient is unable to lift the eyelid completely, so the eye looks half closed. The person has a sleepy look. This condition is called **ptosis** of the eyelid.

The **conjunctiva** is a thin mucous membrane that lines the inner surface of the eyelid. The conjunctiva also folds back to cover a portion of the anterior surface of the eyeball, called the white of the eye. The anterior surface of the eye must be

kept moist. Failure to keep the eye moist may cause ulceration and scarring. The surface of the eye is normally kept moist by blinking the eyelids. Blinking stimulates the secretion of tears and then moves the tears across the anterior surface of the eye.

EYELASHES. Eyelashes line the edges of the eyelid and help trap dust and other foreign objects.

Occasionally, the area around a hair follicle at the edge of the lid becomes infected, usually by *Staphylococcus* bacteria. This infection is called a **sty** or **hordeolum;** it is red, swollen, and painful.

LACRIMAL APPARATUS. The lacrimal apparatus is composed of the lacrimal gland and a series of ducts called tear ducts (see Fig. 11–7). The lacrimal gland is located in the upper lateral part

Do You Know...

What is meant by 20/20 vision?

The ability of the eye to focus an image on the retina is assessed by use of the **Snellen chart.** This chart is composed of lines of letters arranged in decreasing size. The person is placed at a distance 20 feet away from the chart and is asked to cover one eye and read a line of letters. A score of 20/20 means that the person is able to see at 20 feet what a person with normal eye function can see. Thus, 20/20 vision is considered normal. A score of 20/40 means that a person can see at 20 feet what a person with normal vision can see at 40 feet. Thus, 20/40 vision is less perfect than 20/20 vision. A score of 20/200 indicates severely impaired vision, and the person is considered legally blind.

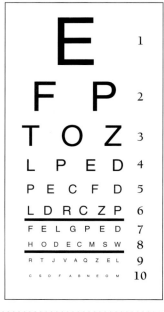

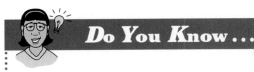
of the orbit. The lacrimal gland secretes tears, which flow across the surface of the eye toward the nose. The tears drain through small openings called **lacrimal puncta** and from there into the **lacrimal sac** and **nasolacrimal ducts.** The nasolacrimal ducts eventually empty into the nasal cavity. If the secretion of tears increases, as in crying, the nose begins to run. The excess tears may overwhelm the drainage system and spill onto the cheeks.

Tears perform several important functions. They moisten, lubricate, and cleanse the surface of the eye. Tears, which are composed primarily of

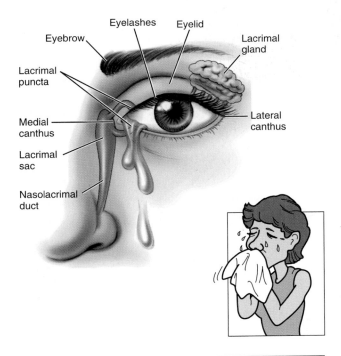

FIGURE 11–7 ● Visual accessory organs: the eyebrows, eyelids, eyelashes, and the lacrimal apparatus. Tears are secreted by the lacrimal gland, wash over the surface of the eye, and drain into the lacrimal sac and finally into the nasolacrimal duct. Crying floods the system, causing tears to flow over the cheeks.

water, also contain an enzyme called **lysozyme,** which helps to destroy bacteria and prevents infection. Routine use of eyewashes may do more harm than good by washing away natural antibacterial secretions, which help to prevent infection.

EXTRINSIC EYE MUSCLES. Extrinsic eye muscles also function as visual accessory organs (see later discussion under Muscles of the Eye).

The Eyeball

The eyeball has a spherical shape and is approximately ¾ to 1 inch (2 to 3 cm) in diameter (Fig. 11–8A). Most of the eyeball sits within the bony orbital cavity of the skull and is therefore well protected. The eyeball is composed of three layers, or tunics: the sclera (outer layer), the choroid (middle layer), and the retina (inner layer).

SCLERA. The outermost layer is called the **sclera** (sklē′rə). The sclera is a thick fibrous connective tissue that covers about five sixths of the posterior eyeball. The sclera helps to contain the contents of the eye; it also shapes the eye and is the site of attachment for the extrinsic eye muscles. The sclera extends toward the front of the eye and is called the **cornea** (kôr′nēə).

The cornea is the most anterior portion of the sclera. The cornea is avascular (contains no blood vessels) and transparent, meaning that light rays can go through, or penetrate, this structure. Because light enters the eye first through the cornea, it is called the window of the eye. The cornea has a rich supply of sensory nerve fibers and is therefore sensitive to touch. If the surface of the cornea is touched lightly, the eye blinks to remove the source of irritation. This response is called the **corneal reflex.** It serves a protective function. Think of how your eye responds to a piece of dust—blinking, tearing, pain.

CHOROID. The middle layer of the eye is the **choroid.** The choroid layer is highly vascular (has many blood vessels) and is attached to the innermost layer (the retina). The choroid layer provides the retina with a rich supply of blood. Dark

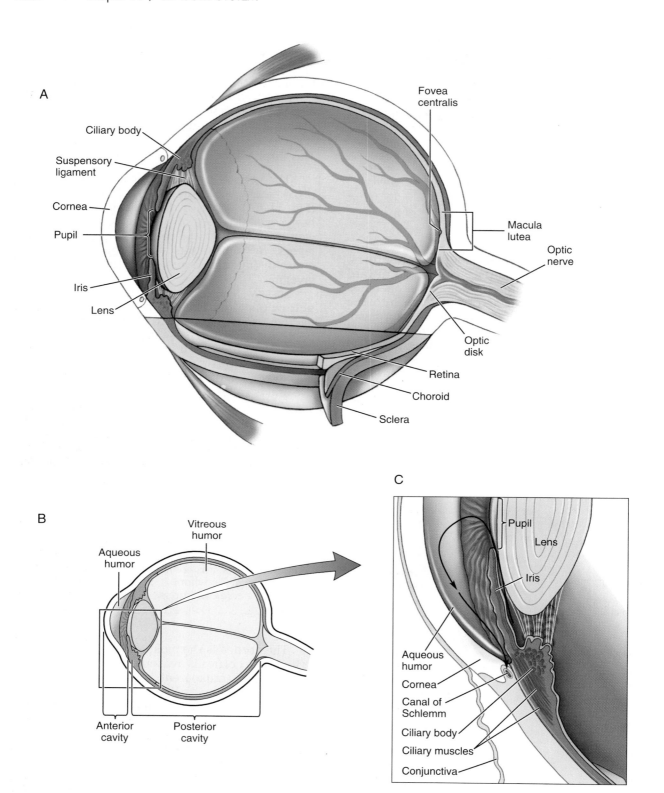

FIGURE 11-8 • A, Structure of the eyeball. B, Cavities and fluids. The posterior cavity lies between the retina and the lens; it is filled with vitreous humor. The anterior cavity lies between the lens and the cornea. C, Note the flow of aqueous humor from the ciliary body to the canal of Schlemm (see *arrow*).

pigments located in the choroid absorb any excess light to prevent glare.

The choroid extends toward the front of the eyeball to form the ciliary body and the iris. The **ciliary body** is located toward the front of the eye and performs two functions: it secretes a fluid called aqueous humor, and it gives rise to a set of intrinsic eye muscles, called the **ciliary muscles.** The most anterior portion of the choroid is the **iris,** the colored portion of the anterior eye. The song "Beautiful Brown Eyes" is a serenade to the iris.

The opening, or hole, in the middle of the iris is called the **pupil.** The size of the pupil is determined by two sets of intrinsic eye muscles located in the iris. The iris regulates the amount of light entering the eye. When the light is very bright, the circular muscles of the iris contract, and the pupil becomes smaller, or constricts. When the light is dim, the radial muscles of the iris contract, and the pupil dilates, or grows larger.

RETINA. The innermost layer of the eyeball is the **retina** (rĕt'ĭ-nə). It lines the posterior two thirds of the eyeball. The retina is the nervous layer. It is the only area of the body where the blood vessels may be directly examined. With an ophthalmoscope, an ophthalmologist can detect vascular changes caused by high blood pressure, diabetes, and hardening of the arteries.

The retina contains the visual receptors, which are sensitive to light and are therefore called photoreceptors. The two kinds of photoreceptors are rods and cones. The **rods** are scattered throughout the retina but are more abundant along its periphery. The **cones** are most abundant in the central portion of the retina. The area of the retina that contains the highest concentration of cones is called the **fovea centralis,** an area in the center of a yellow spot called the **macula lutea** (Fig. 11–8A). Because the fovea centralis contains so many cones, it is considered the area of most acute vision.

A second small circular area of the retina is in the back of the eye. The neurons of the retina converge there to form the optic nerve; it contains no rods or cones. This area is called the **optic disc.** Because there are no photoreceptors on the optic disc, images that focus on the blind spot are not seen. The optic disc is therefore called the blind spot.

A head-injured person may develop increased intracranial pressure. This increased pressure pushes the optic disc forward. The bulging optic disc seen on ophthalmic examination is described as a choked disc.

CAVITIES AND FLUIDS. The two cavities in the eyeball are the posterior and anterior cavities (Fig. 11–8B). The **posterior cavity** is larger and is located between the lens and the retina. The posterior cavity is filled with a gel-like substance called the vitreous humor. The **vitreous humor** gently pushes the retina against the choroid layer, thereby ensuring that the retina receives a good supply of blood.

The **anterior cavity** is located between the lens and the cornea. The anterior cavity is filled with a watery fluid called **aqueous humor.** Aqueous humor is produced by the ciliary body and circulates through the pupil into the space behind the cornea (see Fig. 11–8B). The aqueous humor performs two functions: it maintains the shape of the anterior portion of the eye, and it provides nourishment for the cornea. The aqueous humor leaves, or exits, from the anterior cavity by way of tiny canals located at the junction of the sclera and the cornea. These outlet canals are called **venous sinuses** or the **canals of Schlemm** (Fig. 11–8C).

Do You Know...

Why do we sometimes see spots in front of our eyes?

The spots are called **floaters** or **muscae volitantes,** meaning flying flies. They are either particles or red blood cells that have escaped from the capillaries in the eye. These substances float through the vitreous humor, occasionally getting in our line of vision. The presence of these substances is considered normal and harmless.

Under certain conditions, drainage of aqueous humor through the canal of Schlemm is impaired. Aqueous humor accumulates in the eye and elevates the pressure in the eye (the intraocular pressure). An elevated intraocular pressure is called **glaucoma.** Glaucoma is serious because the elevated pressure compresses the choroid, thereby choking off the blood supply to the retina. Retinal damage causes blindness.

Muscles of the Eye

The two groups of muscles associated with the eye are the extrinsic eye muscles and the intrinsic eye muscles. The extrinsic eye muscles move the eyeball in its bony orbit. The intrinsic eye muscles move structures in the eyeball.

EXTRINSIC EYE MUSCLES. How do you move your eyes? The extrinsic eye muscles are skeletal muscles located outside the eye (Fig. 11–9A). The six extrinsic eye muscles attach to the bone of the eye orbit and to the sclera, the tough outer connective tissue layer of the eyeball. There are four rectus muscles and two oblique muscles.

A

B

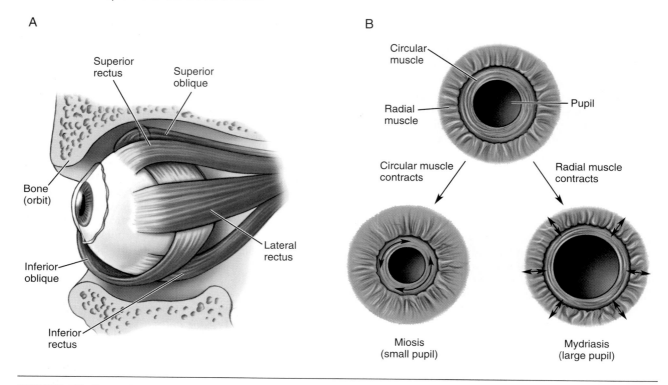

FIGURE 11–9 ● A, Extrinsic muscles of the eyeball. There are six extrinsic eye muscles (only five are shown). There are four rectus muscles and two oblique muscles. B, Intrinsic eye muscles control the size of the pupils. Contraction of the circular muscle causes the pupil to constrict (the process of miosis). Contraction of the radial muscle causes the pupil to dilate (process of mydriasis).

The extrinsic eye muscles move the eyeball in various directions. You can move your eyes up, down, and sideways because of the rectus muscles. You can also roll your eyes because of the oblique muscles. The extrinsic eye muscles are innervated by three cranial nerves, the most important being the oculomotor nerve (cranial nerve III).

Occasionally, the movement of the eyeballs is not coordinated; one eye appears to be looking in one direction and the second eye in another direction. The eyes do not work together. This condition is called **strabismus** (Fig. 11–10). See also ptosis, hordeolum (sty), and conjunctivitis in Figure 11–10. If the eye deviates medially toward the nasal side, the eyes look crossed. Hence, the term crosseyed. This condition is called convergent strabismus. Eyes can also deviate laterally so that one eye appears to be looking off to the side. This condition is called divergent strabismus. If uncorrected, strabismus not only presents a serious cosmetic problem but can also lead to loss of vision.

INTRINSIC EYE MUSCLES. How and why do the size of your pupils change? The intrinsic muscles are smooth muscles located in the eyeball, specifically in the iris and the ciliary body. There are three intrinsic eye muscles. The iris contains two eye muscles, the radial muscle and the circular muscle (see Fig. 11–9B). These muscles control

the size of the pupil and therefore regulate the amount of light that enters the eye. The muscle fibers of the radial muscle are arranged like the spokes of a wheel. Just as the spokes radiate from the center of the wheel, the radial muscle fibers radiate from the area of the pupil. Contraction of the radial muscle causes the pupil to dilate, thereby increasing the amount of light entering the eye. Sympathetic nerve fibers supply the radial muscles. Thus, sympathetic nerve stimulation causes pupillary dilation, or **mydriasis.** Drugs that dilate the pupil are called mydriatic agents.

The second muscle located in the iris is the circular muscle. Its fibers are arranged in a circular fashion. Contraction of the circular muscles causes the pupil to constrict, thereby decreasing the amount of light entering the eye. The circular muscle is supplied by parasympathetic nerve fibers in the oculomotor nerve (cranial nerve III). Parasympathetic nerve stimulation causes pupillary constriction, or **miosis** (see Fig. 11–9B). Drugs that constrict the pupils are called miotic agents. Some drugs, such as narcotics, constrict the pupils so intensely that the pupils are described as pinpoint. (Hint: an easy way to remember the difference between mydriasis and miosis is that the words **dilate** and **mydriasis** both contain the letter **d.**)

Do You Know...

Why do people with diabetes frequently experience vision loss?

A person with diabetes often experiences severe damage of the retinal blood vessels. The blood vessels develop microaneurysms. The aneurysms rupture, causing bleeding and scar formation throughout the retina. Over time, retinal damage results in loss of vision and even blindness.

When the eyes are suddenly exposed to bright light, the pupils immediately constrict, thereby restricting the amount of light entering the eye. This response is called the **pupillary reflex.** The clinician assesses this reflex by shining a penlight at the pupil of the eye.

The third intrinsic eye muscle is the **ciliary muscle.** The ciliary muscles arise from the ciliary process. The ciliary muscles attach to the lens and help focus the light waves on the retina.

How You See

For us to see, the light waves must enter the eye, focus on the retina, and stimulate the photoreceptors. Then the stimulated photoreceptors send a nerve impulse to the brain, where it is interpreted as sight (see Fig. 11–1).

LIGHT ENTERING THE EYE. To stimulate the photoreceptors, the light must enter the eye and pass through the following structures: cornea, aqueous humor, lens, and vitreous humor (see Fig. 11–8A).

LIGHT FOCUSING ON THE RETINA. Before you can see a sharp image, the light waves must bend, and they must focus on a particular spot (X) on the retina. The bending of light waves is called **refraction** (rĭ-frăk′shən). The cornea, aqueous humor, and lens are all capable of refracting light. Refraction by the lens is illustrated in Figure 11–11. In the top panel, the light waves are shown traveling in a straight line toward the retina. Unless light waves #1 and #3 are bent, they will not focus on point X. In the middle panel, the light wave #1 is bent to focus on the retina.

Do You Know...

What is night blindness?

Stimulation of the rods (night vision photoreceptors) by light waves causes the breakdown of a chemical substance called rhodopsin. This breakdown, in turn, stimulates nerve impulses. As nerve impulses are formed, the amount of rhodopsin is used up and must be replaced. The synthesis of additional rhodopsin requires vitamin A. Because night vision depends on an adequate supply of rhodopsin, a deficiency of vitamin A causes night blindness.

FIGURE 11–10 ● A, Ptosis of the eyelid, droopy eyelid. B, Hordeolum, or sty. C, Conjunctivitis, or pink eye. D, Strabismus. Note that the eyeball deviates from the midline.

HERE'S LOOKING AT YOU!

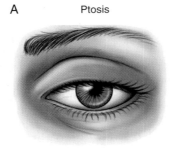
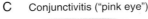
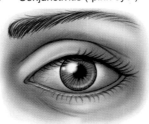
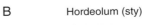
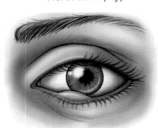
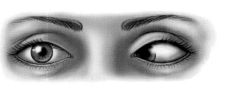

A Ptosis
B Hordeolum (sty)
C Conjunctivitis ("pink eye")
D Strabismus

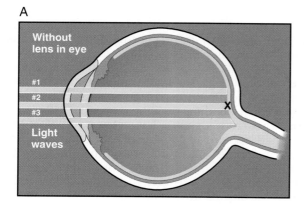

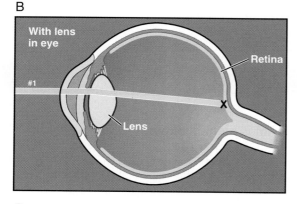

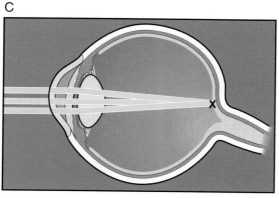

FIGURE 11-11 ● Refraction, the bending of light waves. Light waves must focus on a particular area of the retina (X). A, Path that the light waves are traveling. The first and third wave will not focus on point X on the retina unless they are bent. B, Bending of the first light wave by the lens. The bottom of the light wave hits the lens before the top of the light wave does so and is slowed down. Because the top and bottom of the light wave travel at different speeds, the wave is bent. C, Bending, or refraction, of the first and third light waves so as to focus on point X.

How does the lens bend light waves? The bottom part of the light wave hits the lens first and is slowed before penetrating it. The top of the light wave continues to travel until it hits the lens. For a split second, the top of the light wave travels faster than the bottom. The light wave therefore bends. The bottom panel illustrates how the lens bends several light waves. For sharp vision, light waves must be refracted to focus on one particular area of the retina.

Why and how does the lens change its shape? Although light waves are refracted by the cornea, aqueous humor, and lens, it is the lens that adjusts the amount of refraction. The lens can change its shape, becoming fatter or thinner. The lens is an elastic structure held in place by the suspensory ligaments attached to ciliary muscles (see Fig. 11–8A). When the ciliary muscles contract and relax, the tension on the lens causes the changes in the shape of the lens. The lens either flattens out or becomes rounder. The change in shape affects how much the light is bent. For instance, if the lens becomes rounder or fatter, the light wave is bent at a sharper angle. If the lens flattens, the degree of refraction lessens and the light wave is not bent as much.

The ability of the lens to change its shape allows the eye to focus objects close up or at a distance. For instance, if you hold a pencil 6 inches in front of your eyes, you will be able to see it clearly. The focusing of the close-up object (pencil) on the retina is due primarily to the lens. The lens becomes rounder and can bend the light waves more acutely so as to focus them on the retina. This ability of the lens to change its shape to focus on a close object is called **accommodation** (ə-kŏm″ə-dā′-shən).

With advancing age, the lens loses some of its ability to change shape, thereby diminishing the ability to accommodate for close objects. This condition, which is often evident after age 40, is called **presbyopia** (a presbyter is an elderly person). Persons with presbyopia have difficulty adjusting to close objects. Presbyopia accounts for the tendency of older persons to hold the newspaper at arm's length. You may have heard elderly persons good naturedly comment on how their arms have shortened with age.

LIGHT STIMULATING THE PHOTORECEPTORS. Once the light penetrates the various eye structures, it must stimulate the photoreceptors, the rods and cones.

Why do you see black and white at night and color during daylight? The rods are widely scattered throughout the retina but are more abundant in the periphery. Rods are sensitive to dim light and provide us with black and white vision. The image produced by the stimulation of rods is somewhat fuzzy. Because rods respond to dim light, stimulation of rods is often called **night vision.**

Cones are the photoreceptors for **color vision.** Cones are most abundant in the central portion of the retina, especially in the macula lutea, which contains all cones and is considered an area of acute vision. The image produced by the stimulation of cones is sharp. There are three types of cones, each with a different visual pigment (a light-sensitive chemical). One type of cone produces a green color; another produces blue; and a third produces red. Stimulation of combinations of these cones produces the many different colors and shades of colors we enjoy.

Do You Know...

How do you locate your blind spot?

The blind spot is the area on the retina that has no rods or cones. Therefore, any image that focuses on the blind spot cannot be seen. You can locate your own blind spot. Draw a rectangle with an X on the left side and a dot on the right. Using only one eye (cover the second eye), look at the X as you move it closer to your eye. At some point you will not be able to see the dot on the right when it focuses on your blind spot.

STIMULATED PHOTORECEPTORS INFORMING THE BRAIN. Nerve impulses that arise from the photoreceptors leave the eye by way of the optic nerve (cranial nerve II) (see Fig. 11–1). The nerve impulses travel along the fibers of the optic nerve to the occipital lobe of the brain. (Chapter 9 describes the different lobes of the brain.) This pathway from the eye to the brain is called the visual pathway.

Figure 11–12 illustrates the pathways of the optic nerves as each leaves the eye. Note that half the fibers from the left eye cross over and travel to the right side of the brain. Half the fibers from the right eye cross over and travel to the left side of the brain. The crossing over of the fibers allows the occipital lobe to integrate the information from both eyes and produce only one image. The point at which the fibers from the left and right eyes criss-cross is called the **optic chiasm** (ŏp′tĭk kī′ăz-əm). The optic chiasm is located directly in front of the pituitary gland.

Putting It All Together: Making You See

When all of the parts of the eye are working correctly, you can see. Light waves enter your eye, are refracted, and focus on the photoreceptors of the retina. The photoreceptors translate the light signal to a nerve impulse, which is then transmitted from the retina, along the optic nerve, to the occipital lobe of the brain, where you experience vision.

When the parts of the eye do not work normally, the person may experience diminished vision or blindness. Any defect along this pathway from the cornea to the brain can interfere with vi-

Do You Know...

Why might a person with a tumor of the pituitary gland experience visual disturbances?

A patient with a tumor of the pituitary gland often experiences visual disturbances because the enlarged gland presses on the optic chiasm and interferes with the transmission of the nerve impulse to the occipital lobe.

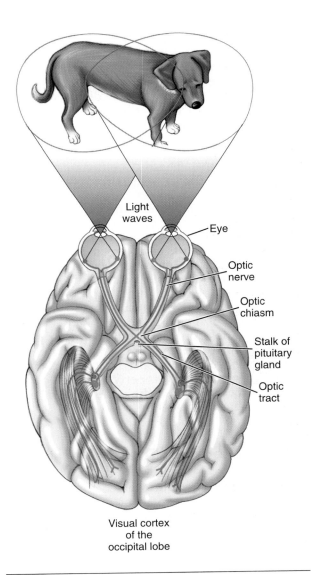

FIGURE 11–12 ● Visual pathway. The nervous route that the nerve impulses follow as they travel from the retina to the occipital lobe of the brain. Note that half of the fibers of the optic nerve of each eye cross over to the opposite side of the brain, forming the optic chiasm. Note the location of the pituitary gland behind the optic chiasm.

sion. Certain conditions may prevent the entrance of light into the eye. For instance, a scarred cornea or a cloudy lens (a cataract) may block the entrance of light, thereby preventing the stimulation of the rods and cones. Certain conditions can damage the retina. For instance, increased intraocular pressure (glaucoma) may squeeze the blood vessels of the choroid, thereby depriving the retina of an adequate blood supply. The cells of the retina then die and blindness results. Or, for unknown reasons, the photoreceptors of the macula lutea can degenerate, causing macular degeneration and a loss of vision. Certain conditions can destroy the optic nerve. For instance, a tumor on the optic nerve or at the optic chiasm can interfere with the transmission of the nerve impulse along the nerve to the brain. Finally, tumors, blood clots, or trauma can damage the occipital lobe of the brain, causing cortical blindness (a blindness due to the loss of cortical brain tissue).

What happens when light does not focus on the retina? This problem may be due to errors in refraction. An **error of refraction** refers to the inability of the refracting structures of the eye (particularly the cornea and lens) to focus the light waves on the retina. Errors of refraction are common eye problems. These conditions cause vast numbers of persons to wear corrective lenses in eyeglasses or contact lenses.

Figure 11–13A illustrates the improper focusing of the image in front of the retina. This condition is called **myopia,** or **nearsightedness,** because only near objects can be seen clearly. Figure 11–13B illustrates the improper focusing of the object behind the retina. This is called **hyperopia,** or **farsightedness,** because only distant objects can be seen clearly. An **astigmatism** refers to an abnormal curvature of the cornea or lens (Fig. 11–13C). With astigmatism, one part of the cornea is generally flatter than another part. This variation results in an uneven refraction of light waves, so that the image cannot be properly focused on the retina. Corrective lenses refract the light waves so that they focus on the retina.

Sense of Hearing: The Ear

For the next 2 minutes listen to the sounds around you. Perhaps some of it is background noise that you mostly ignore. Other sounds provide you with information. Most importantly, you hear sounds that you enjoy, such as the voices of friends and sounds of music. The ear is the organ of the sense of hearing.

Structure of the Ear

The ear is divided into three parts: the external ear, the middle ear, and the inner ear (Fig. 11–14).

ERRORS OF REFRACTION

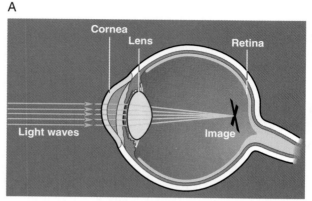

Myopia (nearsightedness)

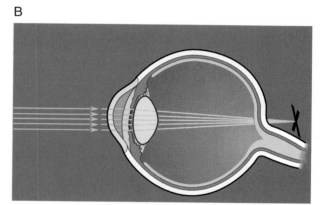

Hyperopia (farsightedness)

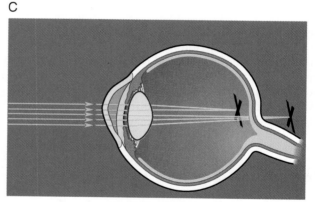

Astigmatism

FIGURE 11–13 ● A, Light waves are refracted too acutely, so that they focus in front of the retina. This condition is called myopia, or nearsightedness. B, Light waves are not refracted enough, so that they focus at a point behind the retina. This condition is called hyperopia, or farsightedness. C, Light waves may be focused both in front of and behind the retina because the refracting structures, usually the cornea, have uneven or flattened surfaces that refract the light waves unevenly. This condition is called astigmatism.

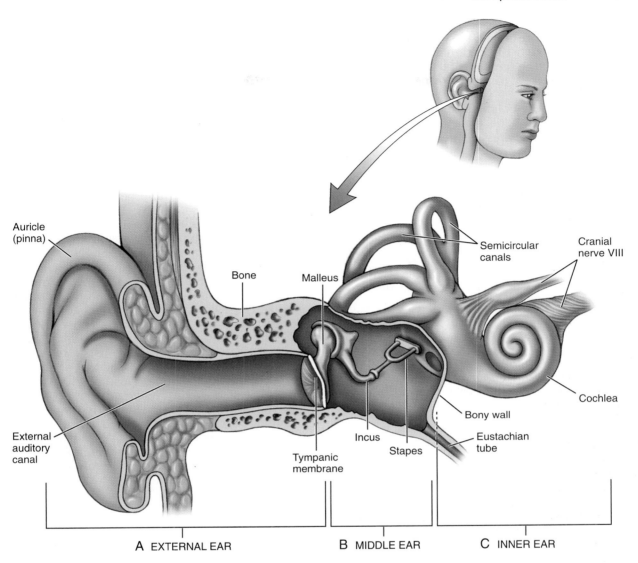

FIGURE 11-14 • Structure of the ear: the three divisions.

EXTERNAL EAR. The external ear is the part of the ear you can see. It is composed of the auricle and the external auditory canal. The **auricle,** or the **pinna** (Latin for wing), is composed of cartilage covered by a layer of loose-fitting skin. The auricle opens into the **external auditory canal.** This canal provides a passageway for sound waves to enter the ear. The external auditory canal is hollowed out of the temporal bone. It is about 1 inch long (2.5 cm) and ½ inch (1.25 cm) wide and extends to the **tympanic membrane,** or eardrum. The tympanic membrane separates the external ear from the middle ear.

The external auditory canal is lined with tiny hairs and glands that secrete **cerumen,** a yellowish waxy substance we call earwax. The hairs and cerumen help prevent dust and other foreign objects from entering the ear. Cerumen tends to be a victim of our cleanliness fetish. We insert hairpins, toothpicks, and other sharp objects into the canal in an attempt to dig out the wax. These objects may damage the tympanic membrane. Cotton-tipped applicators, while appearing safer, actually remove very little wax and usually push any accumulated wax up against the eardrum. The wax can be safely washed out, but only by a trained medical person. It is best not to insert any objects into the ear canal.

MIDDLE EAR. The middle ear is a small air-filled chamber located between the tympanic membrane (eardrum) at one end and a bony wall at the other end (see Fig. 11-14). The middle ear contains several structures: the tympanic membrane, three tiny bones, and the eustachian tube.

The tympanic membrane is composed primarily of connective tissue and has a rich supply of nerves and blood vessels. The tympanic membrane vibrates in response to sound waves entering the ear through the external auditory canal. The vibration of the tympanic membrane is transmitted, or passed on, to the tiny bones in the middle ear.

The middle ear contains three tiny bones, or **ossicles** (ŏs′ĭ-kəlz). These are the tiniest bones in the body. The bones are arranged so that they ex-

Do You Know...

Why do children tend to outgrow ear infections?

The size and position of the eustachian tube in a child are different than in an adult. The eustachian tube of a child (A) is shorter and lies in a more horizontal position than the adult (B) eustachian tube. The child who develops a cold will often sniff, thereby forcing the nasal drainage from the throat region into the eustachian tubes and middle ear. This drainage results in a middle ear infection called **otitis media.**

As the child grows, the eustachian tube grows longer and becomes less horizontal. There is less chance for bacteria to enter the middle ear from the throat. In this sense, children are said to outgrow ear infections.

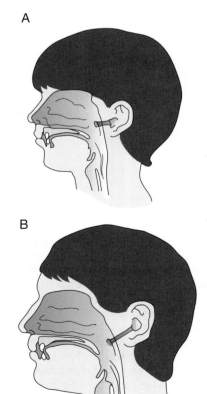

A

B

tend from the tympanic membrane to the **oval window,** a membranous structure in the bony wall that separates the middle ear from the inner ear. The names of the bones are the **malleus** (hammer), **incus** (anvil), and **stapes** (stirrup). The malleus makes contact with the inner surface of the tympanic membrane, while the stapes is seated within the oval window. The ossicles transmit vibration from the tympanic membrane to the oval window.

The middle ear has a passageway connecting it to the pharynx, or throat. This passageway is called the **auditory tube,** or the **eustachian tube** (yōo″stā′kē-ən tōob). The purpose of the tube is to equalize the pressure on both sides of the tympanic membrane by permitting air to pass from the area of the throat into the middle ear. If the pressures across the membrane become unequal, the tympanic membrane bulges. As the tympanic membrane is stretched, pain receptors are stimulated. Pain caused by stretched tympanic membranes is the reason your ears hurt when you take off and land in an airplane.

INNER EAR. The inner ear consists of an intricate system of tubes, or passageways, hollowed out of the temporal bone. This coiled network of tubes is called a **bony labyrinth** (Fig. 11–15). Inside the bony labyrinth is a similarly shaped **membranous labyrinth.** The bony labyrinth is filled with a fluid called **perilymph.** The membranous labyrinth is surrounded by perilymph and is itself filled with a thick fluid called **endolymph.** The perilymph and the endolymph form the fluid of the inner ear. The inner ear has three parts: the vestibule, the semicircular canals, and the cochlea. The cochlea is concerned with hearing. The vestibule and the semicircular canals are concerned with balance.

The **cochlea** (kŏk′lē-ə) is a snail-shaped part of the bony labyrinth. Sitting on a membrane within the cochlea and immersed in endolymph are the receptors for hearing. The receptors are cells that contain tiny hairs and are called the **organ of Corti.** When the hairs on the receptor cells are bent, a nerve impulse is sent by the cochlear branch of the vestibulocochlear nerve (cranial nerve VIII) to the temporal lobe of the brain, where the sensation is interpreted as hearing. Note that the receptors are stimulated by the bending of the hairs; hence, the receptors are classified as mechanoreceptors.

Putting It All Together: Making You Hear

Hearing is accomplished by structures within the external, middle, and inner ears. How do we hear the sounds of music? As Figure 11–16 illustrates, the vibrating guitar strings disturb the air, causing sound waves. The sound waves travel through the external auditory canal and hit the tympanic membrane, causing the tympanic mem-

Receptors for Balance

Receptors for Hearing

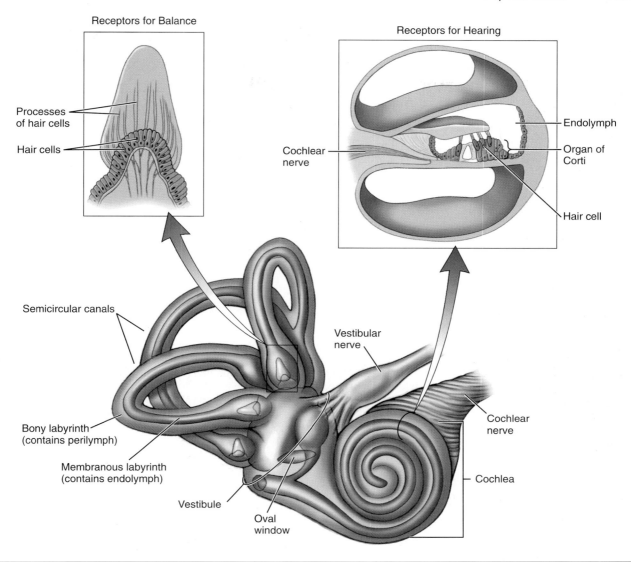

Processes
of hair cells

Hair cells

Cochlear
nerve

Endolymph

Organ of
Corti

Hair cell

Semicircular canals

Vestibular
nerve

Bony labyrinth
(contains perilymph)

Membranous labyrinth
(contains endolymph)

Vestibule

Oval
window

Cochlear
nerve

Cochlea

FIGURE 11–15 ● Inner ear. The hearing part of the inner ear is composed of the cochlea. The receptors for hearing (organ of Corti) are located within the cochlea. The cochlear division of cranial nerve VIII carries information to the temporal lobe of the brain. The balance part of the inner ear is the vestibule and the semicircular canals. The receptors for balance are cells containing hair-like projections. As the head changes position, the hairs of the receptor cells bend, thereby stimulating a nerve impulse. The nerve impulse travels through the vestibular branch of the vestibulocochlear nerve (cranial nerve VIII) to various parts of the brain.

brane to vibrate. This vibration, in turn, causes the middle ear bones (malleus, incus, and stapes) to vibrate. The stapes, sitting within the oval window, then causes the fluid in the inner ear to move. Because the hairs (organ of Corti) are sitting within the fluid, movement of the fluid causes the hairs to bend. The bending of the hairs triggers a nerve impulse carried by the cochlear branch of the vestibulocochlear nerve (cranial nerve VIII) to the brain. The temporal lobe of the cerebrum interprets the impulses as sound.

What happens when the parts do not work? Following the steps listed in Figure 11–16, consider the number of ways our hearing may become impaired. For example, the vibration of the tym-

panic membrane may become dampened or blunted if a plug of cerumen (earwax) becomes lodged against the tympanic membrane. The sound waves may then be unable to vibrate the eardrum. The tiny ossicles may also become fused or attached to one another. This condition diminishes the ability of the bones to transmit vibration from the tympanic membrane to the oval window. This problem often develops in children who have experienced repeated ear infections.

Another problem is that the stapes may become glued, or fixed, to the oval window. This condition diminishes the transmission of vibration to the inner ear. The temporal lobe that interprets the nerve impulse as hearing may be damaged.

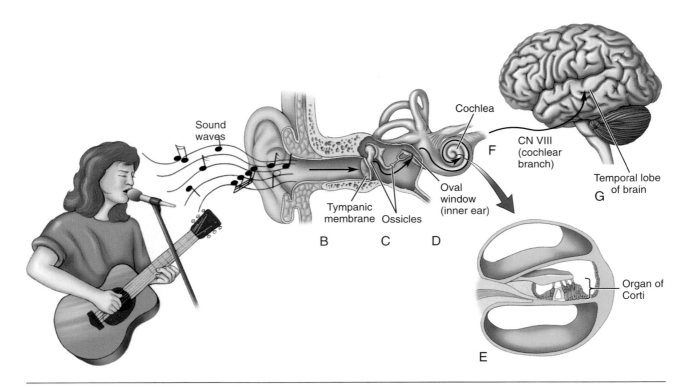

FIGURE 11-16 ● Steps in hearing. A, The guitar creates sound waves that enter the external ear. B, The sound waves cause the tympanic membrane to vibrate. C, The tympanic membrane causes the tiny bones (ossicles) within the middle ear to vibrate. D, The stapes, which sits in the oval window, causes the fluid within the cochlea of the inner ear to move. E, The movement of the fluid bends the hairs (organ of Corti), generating a nerve impulse. F, The nerve impulse travels along the cochlear branch of the vestibulocochlear nerve (cranial nerve VIII) to the temporal lobe of the brain. G, The temporal lobe interprets the information as sound.

The person will then experience a cortical deafness. Or the cochlear branch of cranial nerve VIII may be damaged. The damaged nerve cannot conduct nerve impulses from the ear to the brain. This condition develops in persons exposed to prolonged periods of loud noise. For example, "rock and roll deafness" is hearing loss associated with loud music. Nerve damage also occurs in response to certain drugs, especially antibiotics. Drugs that cause damage to the vestibulocochlear nerve are called ototoxic agents.

Sense of Balance: The Ear

While we all appreciate our ears as organs of hearing, we may not realize that our ears play an important role in **equilibrium** (ē″kwə-lĭb′rē-əm), or balance. Damage to certain parts of the ear, for instance, may make it impossible for us to stand without losing balance.

The receptors for balance are mechanoreceptors. These cells contain hair-like projections immersed in the fluid of the inner ear. The receptors are located within the vestibule and the semicircular canals of the inner ear (see Fig. 11–15). The **vestibule** (vĕs′tə-byool) contains the receptors

that provide information about the position of the head at rest. The receptors in the semicircular canals provide information about the position of the body as it moves about. These receptors sense the changing positions of the head. When the positions change, the hairs are bent, and the receptor cells send nerve impulses through the vestibular branch of the vestibulocochlear nerve (cranial nerve VIII) to several parts of the brain, including the cerebellum, midbrain, and temporal lobe.

Because the vestibulocochlear nerve carries sensory information concerning both hearing and balance, the person with an ear infection may complain of feeling dizzy. The person should be assured that as the ear infection clears, the dizzy feeling will also disappear.

⁎ **SUM IT UP!** The special senses include smell, taste, sight, hearing, and balance. The nose and tongue are the organs of smell and taste, respectively. The eye, the organ of sight, includes a number of visual accessory organs. Sight requires light, which focuses on the retina, stimulating the photoreceptors and causing nerve impulses. The nerve impulses go to the occipital lobe of the brain and are interpreted as vision. The ear is an organ containing structures that stimulate nerve impulses that the brain perceives as sound. The ear is also the organ that senses balance.

As You Age

1. In general, the senses diminish with age. There is a decrease in the number and sensitivity of sensory receptors, dermatomes, and neurons, resulting in dulling of pain, touch, and tactile sensation.

2. There is a gradual loss in taste and smell beginning around the age of 50 years.

3. There is cumulative damage to hair cells in the organ of Corti after the age of 60. Older adults lose the ability to hear high-pitched sounds and the consonants ch, f, g, s, sh, t, th, and z. Twenty-five percent of older adults are hearing impaired.

4. Vision diminishes by the age of 70, primarily because of a decrease in the amount of light that reaches the retina and impaired focusing of the light on the retina.

5. The muscles of the iris become less efficient, so the pupils remain somewhat constricted most of the time.

6. The lacrimal glands become less active, and the eyes become dry and more susceptible to bacterial infection and irritation.

Disorders of the Sensory System

Amblyopia	Also called lazy eye. Amblyopia is the loss of vision in an eye that is not used.
Corneal abrasion	A scratching of the cornea causing pain and tearing and commonly caused by a speck of dust or contact lenses.
Deafness	Loss of hearing. Conduction deafness is due to impaired conduction of sound caused by impacted ear wax or fused middle ear ossicles. Sensorineural deafness is due to damage of the nervous structures associated with hearing.
Detached retina	Retina detached from the choroid, its nutritive supply. The result is retinal damage and blindness.
Keratitis	Inflammation of the cornea.
Macular degeneration	Deterioration of the macula lutea of the retina, causing loss of central vision.
Meniere's disease	A disorder of the inner ear resulting in vertigo (dizziness), tinnitus (ringing or buzzing in the ear), and hearing loss.
Motion sickness	Also called car sickness and sea sickness. Motion sickness is characterized by vertigo, nausea, vomiting, and drowsiness that occurs in response to excessive stimulation of the equilibrium receptors in the inner ear.
Retinopathy	Irreversible damage to the retina usually caused by hypertension or diabetes mellitus. Retinopathy causes loss of vision and even blindness.
Ruptured ear drum	Ear drum rupture as a result of direct injury with a sharp object (including the use of a hairpin to remove ear wax), trauma, or infection such as otitis media (middle ear infection). Repeated infection and tearing of the ear drum may cause hearing loss. Sometimes tubes are placed through the ear drum so as to drain fluid from the middle ear, thereby preventing rupture of the ear drum. This procedure is called a myringotomy.

Summary Outline

The sensory system allows us to experience the world through a variety of sensations: touch, pressure, pain, proprioception, temperature, taste, smell, vision, hearing, and equilibrium.

I. Receptors and Sensation

A. Receptor
1. A receptor is a specialized area of a sensory neuron that detects a specific stimulus.
2. The five types of receptors are chemoreceptors, pain receptors (nociceptors), thermoceptors, mechanoreceptors, and photoreceptors.

B. Sensation
1. A sensation is a conscious awareness of incoming sensory information.
2. The four components of a sensation are a stimulus, a receptor, a sensory nerve, and a special area of the brain.
3. The two characteristics of sensation are projection and adaptation.

II. General Senses

A. Pain
1. Pain receptors are free nerve endings.
2. The stimulus for pain is tissue damage caused by chemicals produced by the injured tissue, lack of oxygen, and stretching or distortion of tissue.

B. Touch and Pressure
1. Receptors for touch and pressure are mechanoreceptors and respond to forces that press, move, or deform tissue.
2. The receptors for pressure are located in the skin, subcutaneous tissue, and the deep tissue.

C. Temperature
1. There are thermoreceptors for heat and cold.
2. Thermoreceptors are found in free nerve endings and in other specialized sensory cells beneath the skin.

D. Proprioception
1. Proprioreceptors are located primarily in the muscles, tendons, and joints.
2. Proprioreceptors sense orientation or position; the sense of proprioception plays an important role in maintaining posture and coordinating body movement.

III. Special Senses

A. Sense of Smell: the Nose
1. Olfactory receptors are chemoreceptors.
2. Sensory information travels along cranial nerve I (olfactory nerve) to the temporal lobe.

B. Sense of Taste: the Tongue
1. Taste buds on the tongue are the special organs of taste (gustatory sense); these receptors are classified as chemoreceptors.
2. There are four basic taste sensations: sweet, salty, sour, and bitter.
3. Sensory information travels along the facial (VII) and glossopharyngeal (IX) cranial nerves to various parts of the brain, eventually arriving at the gustatory cortex in the parietal lobe.

C. Sense of Sight: the Eye
1. The visual accessory organs include the eyebrows, eyelids, eyelashes, lacrimal apparatus, and extrinsic eye muscles (which move the eyeball in its socket).
2. The eyeball has three layers: the sclera (outermost layer, which extends anteriorly to form the cornea), the choroid (middle layer, which has a rich supply of blood vessels), and the retina (innermost nervous layer, which contains the photoreceptors, the rods and cones).
3. The eyeball has two cavities. One is a posterior cavity located between the lens and the retina. The posterior cavity is filled with vitreous humor. The other is an anterior cavity located between the lens and the cornea. The anterior cavity is filled with aqueous humor.
4. There are two sets of eye muscles: the extrinsic eye muscles and the intrinsic eye muscles.
5. The extrinsic eye muscles are external to the eyeball and control the movement of the eyeball.
6. The intrinsic eye muscles control the size of the pupil and the shape of the lens.
7. To make you see, light enters the eye and stimulates the photoreceptors. The nerve impulse carries the information from the photoreceptors along the optic nerve (cranial nerve II) to the occipital lobe of the cerebrum.

D. Sense of Hearing: the Ear
1. There are three parts of the ear: the external ear, the middle ear (which contains the three ossicles: malleus, incus, and stapes), and the inner ear.
2. The inner ear structure concerned with hearing is the cochlea. It contains the hearing receptors, organ of Corti (hair-like projections on the cells are mechanoreceptors).
3. You hear as sound waves enter the external ear and cause the tympanic membrane to vibrate. The vibrating tympanic membrane causes the ossicles in the middle ear to vibrate. The vibrating stapes causes the fluid in the inner ear to move. The moving inner ear fluid bends the hair-like projections. Activation of the organ of Corti creates nerve impulses that travel along the cochlear branch of cranial nerve VIII to the temporal lobe.

E. Sense of Balance: the Ear
1. The receptors are mechanoreceptors (hair-like projections) located in the vestibule and the semicircular canals of the inner ear.
2. The receptors are activated when the head changes position.
3. Activation of the receptors creates nerve impulses that travel along the vestibular branch of cranial nerve VIII to many areas of the brain, including the cerebellum, midbrain, and temporal lobe.

Review Your Knowledge

1. What are five types of sensory receptors?

2. What organ in the body experiences sensation? What are four components involved in the perception of a sensation?

3. Which characteristic of sensation answers the question: "If pain is experienced by the brain, why is it that my injured finger hurts?" Which characteristic of sensation answers the question: "When I enter a room with a strong odor, the odor at first seems overwhelmingly strong; why does it become less noticeable after a short period?"

4. What are the five general senses? Name three pain triggers, or signals that stimulate pain. Why is pain originating in the heart often experienced in the shoulder and left arm?

5. If you close your eyes, you can still locate your arm in space; what sense allows you to experience this?

6. Which part of the brain receives sensory information from proprioreceptors and plays a major role in coordinating skeletal muscle activity?

7. What are the five special senses?

8. When we cry, why do our noses run? How do tears help fight infection?

9. What are the names of the following structures?

a. Outermost coat of the posterior eye
b. Most anterior portion of the sclera
c. Middle layer of the eye
d. Colored portion of the eye
e. Opening in the middle of the iris
f. Innermost layer of the eyeball

10. Why do we not see images that focus on the blind spot? What is the difference between the vitreous humor and the aqueous humor?

11. What is the most important cranial nerve that innervates the extrinsic eye muscles? How do sympathetic nerve fibers relate to mydriasis? How do refraction and accommodation help us to see clearly?

12. What happens to the eye in persons with presbyopia?

13. How are rods and cones different?

14. Name the parts of the external, middle, and inner ear. What is the waxy substance produced by glands in the external auditory canal?

15. What is the function of the eustachian tube?

16. Where are the receptors for hearing and equilibrium located? Why may a person with an ear infection complain of being dizzy?

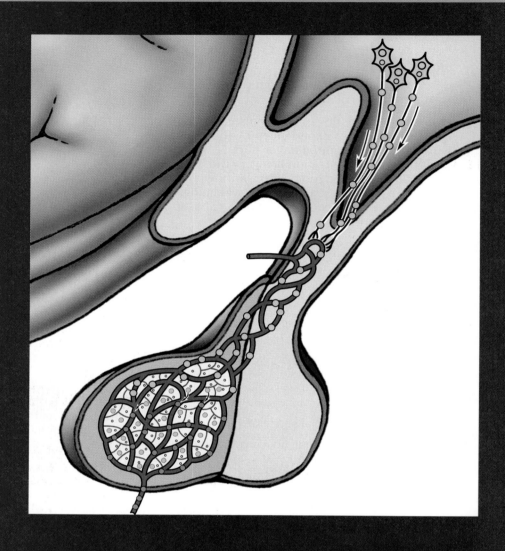

● ● ● Selected terms in bold type in this chapter are defined in the Glossary.

12 ENDOCRINE SYSTEM

$\mathbf{\mathcal{O}}$bjectives

1. List the functions of the endocrine system.

2. Differentiate between protein hormones and steroid hormones.

3. Explain negative feedback control as a control for hormone levels.

4. Describe the relationship of the hypothalamus to the anterior and posterior pituitary glands.

5. Describe the structure and function of the pituitary gland.

6. List the six major hormones secreted by the anterior pituitary gland.

7. Describe the two major hormones of the posterior pituitary gland.

8. Identify the major endocrine glands of the body.

9. Describe the actions of the hormones secreted by the major endocrine glands.

10. Explain the effects of hyposecretion and hypersecretion of the following hormones: insulin, growth hormone, T_3, T_4, cortisol, PTH, and ADH.

While performing his mating ritual, Rooster is dancing out the meaning of the word *hormone,* the main focus of the endocrine system. The word comes from the Greek and literally means to arouse or to set into motion. Rooster's testosterone has truly set him in motion. It has him prancing and dancing his mating ritual and has both him and Hen aroused.

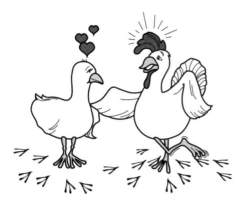

The nervous system and the endocrine system are the two chief communicating and coordinating mechanisms in the body. They regulate nearly all organ systems. Although the nervous and endocrine systems work together closely, they have several differences. The nervous system communicates through electrical signals called nerve impulses. Nerve impulses communicate information rapidly and generally achieve short-term effects. The endocrine system, in contrast, communicates through chemical signals called hormones. The endocrine system responds more slowly and generally exerts longer-lasting effects.

GLANDS AND HORMONES

The endocrine system is composed of endocrine glands, which are widely distributed throughout the body (Fig. 12–1). **Endocrine glands** (ĕn′də-krĭn glăndz) secrete the chemical substances called hormones. Endocrine glands are ductless glands; that is, they secrete the hormones directly into the capillaries (bloodstream) and not into ducts. For instance, the hormone insulin is secreted by the pancreas into the blood. The blood delivers the insulin throughout the body.

Exocrine glands, on the other hand, empty their secretions into ducts, which transport the secretions to a body surface such as the skin or the inside of the digestive tract. For instance, the secretions of the salivary glands are emptied into ducts that transport them to the mouth.

In general, the endocrine system and its hormones help regulate metabolic processes involving carbohydrates, proteins, and fats. Hormones also play an important role in growth and repro-

duction and help regulate water and electrolyte balance. When you become hungry, thirsty, hot, or cold, your body's response includes secretion of hormones. Lastly, hormones help your body to meet the demands of infection, trauma, and stress.

HORMONES

The endocrine system achieves its effects through the secretion of hormones. A **hormone** (hôr′mōn) is a chemical messenger that influences or controls the activities of other tissues or organs. A few hormones are secreted into the extracellular space surrounding the hormone-secreting cell and exert effects locally on nearby cells. Most hormones, however, are transported through the blood to other parts of the body, and they exert effects on more distant tissues.

Classification of Hormones

Chemically, hormones are classified as either proteins (or protein-related substances) or steroids (Table 12–1). With the exception of secretions from the adrenal cortex and the sex glands (testes and ovaries), all hormones are protein or protein-related. The adrenal cortex and the sex glands secrete steroids.

Targets

Each hormone binds to a specific tissue, called its **target tissue** (tär′gĭt tĭsh′oo) (Fig. 12–2A). (Sometimes the term **target organ** is used instead of target tissue.) The target tissue may be located close to or at a distance from the endocrine gland. Some hormones, such as thyroid hormone and insulin, have many target tissues and therefore exert more widespread, or generalized, effects. Other hormones, such as parathyroid hormone, have fewer target tissues and therefore exert fewer effects. In fact, adrenocorticotropic hormone (ACTH) has only one target organ, the adrenal cortex.

Hormone Receptors

Hormones interact with the receptor sites of the cells of their target tissues. The two types of **receptors** (rĭ-sĕp′tərz) are those located on the outer surface of the cell membrane (membrane receptors) and those located within the cell (intracellular receptors).

How do hormones recognize their target tissues? The hormone and its receptor (located on

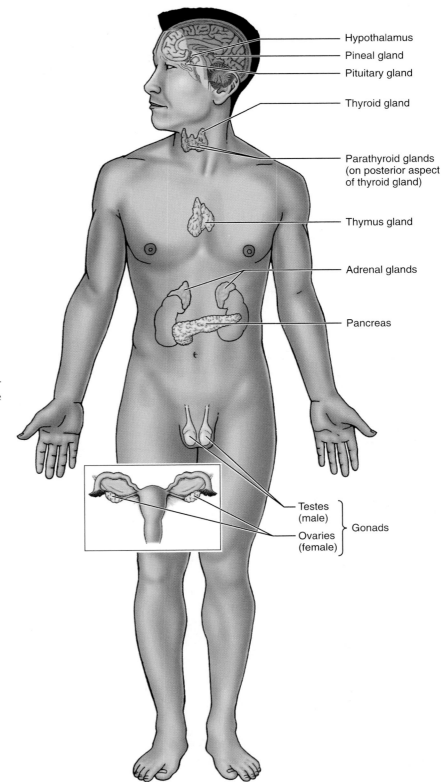

FIGURE 12–1 ● Major endocrine glands of the body.

Hypothalamus
Pineal gland
Pituitary gland
Thyroid gland
Parathyroid glands (on posterior aspect of thyroid gland)
Thymus gland
Adrenal glands
Pancreas
Testes (male)
Ovaries (female)
Gonads

the target cell) can be likened to a lock and key. The key must fit the lock. The same is true for the hormone and receptor; a part of the hormone (key) "fits into" its receptor (lock) on the target. Unless the match is perfect, the hormone cannot lock into, or stimulate, the receptor. For example, the hormone insulin circulates throughout the body in the blood and is therefore delivered to every cell in the body. Insulin, however, can only stimulate the cells that have insulin receptors. The lock-and-key theory guarantees that a particular hormone affects only certain cells.

Table 12 • 1 — EXAMPLES OF HORMONES

HORMONE TYPE	FORMED FROM	NAME OF HORMONE
Protein/protein-related substances		
Amines	Amino acids	Catecholamines (epinephrine and norepinephrine)
Peptides	Amino acids	Thyroid-releasing hormone (TRH)
		Thyroxin (T$_4$)
		Triiodothyronine (T$_3$)
		Antidiuretic hormone (ADH)
		Oxytocin
Proteins	Amino acids	Growth hormone (GH)
		Prolactin (PRL)
		Thyroid-stimulating hormone (TSH)
		Follicle-stimulating hormone (FSH)
		Luteinizing hormone (LH)
		Parathyroid hormone (PTH)
		Calcitonin
		Insulin
Steroids	Cholesterol	Cortisol
		Aldosterone
		Testosterone
		Estrogens
		Progesterone

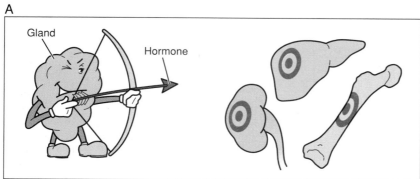

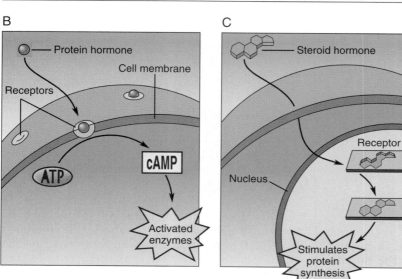

FIGURE 12–2 ● What hormones do. A, Hormones are aimed at target tissues or target organs. B, Protein and protein-related hormones bind to receptors located on the outer surface of the cell membrane. The hormone-receptor interaction stimulates the formation of cAMP, thereby activating the cell. C, The steroid hormones penetrate the cell membrane and interact with intracellular receptors. The hormone-receptor complex activates the cell by stimulating protein synthesis.

Protein hormones generally combine with the receptor sites located on the cell membrane (Fig. 12–2B). The interaction of the hormone with its receptor stimulates the production of a **second messenger** (sĕk′ənd mĕs′ən-jər) such as cyclic adenosine monophosphate (cAMP). The cAMP, in turn, helps to activate the enzymes in the cell. For instance, when epinephrine stimulates its receptors on the heart, cAMP forms and stimulates the heart to increase its rate and force of contraction. A liver cell stimulated by insulin burns, or uses up, glucose as fuel. When the hormone glucagon stimulates a liver cell, the cell makes glucose.

The second type of receptor is located intracellularly (Fig. 12–2C). Steroid hormones, which are lipid-soluble, pass through the plasma membrane of the target cell and bind to receptors in the nucleus. The steroid-receptor complex then stimulates protein synthesis.

Control of Hormone Secretion

Three mechanisms control the secretion of hormones. They are negative feedback control, biorhythms, and control by the central nervous system.

Negative Feedback, or "Enough Is Enough"

Normal endocrine function depends on normal plasma levels of hormones. Life-threatening complications develop when the glands either hypersecrete or hyposecrete hormones. For instance, if too much insulin is secreted, amounts of

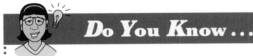

Do You Know...

Why do you not die of hypoglycemia between meals?

After you eat a meal, the blood level of glucose rises as the food products are absorbed from the digestive tract into the blood. The increased blood glucose level signals the release of insulin from the pancreas. The insulin then causes the blood glucose level to decrease by moving the glucose from the blood into the cells and stimulating the cells to burn the glucose as fuel. As the blood glucose levels decrease, however, other hormones such as growth hormone, epinephrine, and cortisol are secreted. These other hormones antagonize insulin by increasing blood glucose and preventing fatal hypoglycemia. Thus, you can fast for weeks and not become hypoglycemic! Chances are that you will not die from fasting—it will only feel as if you are dying.

blood glucose decrease to dangerous levels. On the other hand, if the secretion of insulin is inadequate, the blood glucose levels increase and cause serious problems. So how does the pancreas, the insulin-secreting gland, know when it has secreted enough insulin?

Many of the endocrine glands maintain normal plasma levels of their hormones through a mechanism called **negative feedback** (nĕg′ə-tĭv fēd′băk) (Fig. 12–3). With negative feedback, information about the hormone or the effects of that hormone are fed back to the gland that secretes the hormone. The pattern of insulin secretion is one example of negative feedback. When plasma levels of glucose increase after eating, insulin is released from the pancreas; in other words, glucose is the stimulus for insulin release. Insulin causes glucose to move from the extracellular fluid into the cell. As the glucose enters the cells, the plasma levels of glucose decrease. As plasma glucose levels decrease, the stimulus for insulin secretion also decreases.

What information was fed back to the gland? It was the decrease in plasma glucose. What was the gland's response? The gland decreased its secretion of insulin. Negative feedback is a common means of control within the endocrine system. Various hormones operate through negative feedback.

Biorhythms

Plasma levels of some hormones are also controlled by less-understood mechanisms called biorhythms. A **biorhythm** is a rhythmic alteration in a hormone's rate of secretion. Some hormones, such as cortisol, are secreted in a circadian rhythm. A **circadian rhythm** (*circa* means around; *dian* means day) is a 24-hour rhythm; its pattern repeats every 24 hours. Because of its circadian rhythm, cortisol secretion is highest in the morning hours (peak at about 8 AM) and lowest in the evening hours (lowest at midnight). The female reproductive hormones represent another biorhythm. They are secreted in a monthly pattern, hence the monthly menstrual cycle.

Unfortunately, biorhythms can be disturbed by travel and alterations in sleep patterns. For instance, jet lag and the symptoms of fatigue experienced by persons who work the night shift are thought to be related to alterations of biorhythms. The problem has become so acute that some hospitals have developed staffing schedules based on biorhythms.

Sometimes drugs are administered on a schedule that mimics normal biorhythms. For instance, steroids are administered in the morning, when natural steroid levels are highest. Cooperating with the natural rhythms increases the effectiveness of the drug and causes fewer side effects.

A

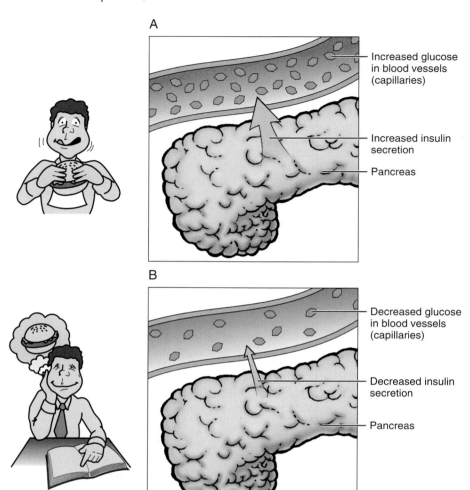

Increased glucose
in blood vessels
(capillaries)

Increased insulin
secretion

Pancreas

B

Decreased glucose
in blood vessels
(capillaries)

Decreased insulin
secretion

Pancreas

FIGURE 12–3 ● Negative feedback control. A, Increased blood glucose levels trigger the release of insulin from the pancreas. The effect of insulin is to lower blood glucose. B, Decreased blood glucose levels cause the pancreas to decrease its secretion of insulin.

Control by the Central Nervous System

The central nervous system (CNS) helps to control the secretion of hormones in two ways: activation of the hypothalamus and stimulation of the sympathetic nervous system. Think about this! The CNS exerts a powerful influence over the endocrine system. Because the CNS is also the center for our emotional life, it is not surprising that our emotions, in turn, affect the endocrine system.

For instance, when we are stressed out, the CNS causes several of the endocrine glands to secrete stress hormones, thereby alerting every cell in the body to the threat. Moreover, many women can attest to the effect of stress on the menstrual cycle. Stress can cause the menstrual period to occur early or late; it may even cause the cycle to skip a month. These effects illustrate the power of emotions on our body. In fact, the functions of the nervous system and the endocrine system are so closely related that the word neuroendocrinology is commonly used.

✳ **SUM IT UP!** The endocrine system is composed of endocrine glands widely distributed throughout the body. The endocrine glands secrete hormones, chemical substances released into the blood and distributed throughout the body. Hormones stimulate target tissues by binding to cell receptors. The receptors are located either on the outer surface of the cell membrane or within the cell. By binding with the receptor, the hormone activates the cell to perform a particular function. Three control mechanisms regulate the secretion of hormones: negative feedback, biorhythms, and CNS activity.

THE PITUITARY GLAND

The Pituitary Gland and the Hypothalamus

The pituitary gland is a small, pea-sized gland, also called the **hypophysis.** The pituitary is located under the hypothalamus near the brain in the saddle-like depression of the sphenoid bone, just behind the optic chiasm. The pituitary is attached to the undersurface of the hypothalamus by a short slender stalk called the **infundibulum.** The pituitary contains two main parts: the anterior pituitary gland and the posterior pituitary gland. The major endocrine glands and hormones are summarized in Table 12–2.

The secretion of the anterior pituitary gland is controlled by the hypothalamus (Fig. 12–4). Although it is part of the brain, the hypothalamus secretes several hormones and so is also considered to be an endocrine gland. The hypothalamus secretes hormones called **releasing hormones** and **release-inhibiting hormones.** These hormones either stimulate or inhibit the secretion of a specific anterior pituitary hormone. For instance, prolactin-releasing hormone, secreted by the hypothalamus, stimulates the pituitary gland to secrete prolactin (PRL). Prolactin-inhibiting hormone (PIH), secreted by the hypothalamus, inhibits the secretion of prolactin by the anterior pituitary gland.

How do the hypothalamic hormones reach the anterior pituitary gland? The hypothalamus secretes its hormones into a network of capillaries (tiny blood vessels) that connect the hypothalamus with the anterior pituitary gland (see Fig. 12–4A). These connecting capillaries are called the **hypothalamic-hypophyseal portal system.** Thus, hormones secreted by the hypothalamus flow through the portal capillaries to the anterior

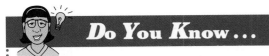

Do You Know...

Why can a tumor of the pituitary gland cause disturbances in vision?

Why is the pituitary gland called the "master gland"? The pituitary gland is called the master gland because it controls the activity of many other endocrine glands. It secretes eight hormones and therefore affects almost every body function.

pituitary. The hypothalamic hormones control the secretion of anterior pituitary hormones.

Anterior Pituitary

The anterior pituitary gland is composed of glandular epithelial tissue. The anterior pituitary is also called the **adenohypophysis** (ăd″ə-nō-hī-pŏf′ĭ-sĭs) (*adeno* means glandular; *hypophysis* means pituitary). The anterior pituitary secretes six major hormones (see Fig. 12–4A and Table 12–2). These control other glands and affect many

organ systems. In fact, the anterior pituitary affects so many other glands that it is often called the master gland. The hormones of the anterior pituitary include thyroid-stimulating hormone (TSH), adrenocorticotropic hormone (ACTH), growth hormone (GH), the gonadotropins (FSH and LH), and prolactin (PRL).

Growth Hormone

Growth hormone (GH) is also called **somatotropin** or **somatotropic hormone (STH).** Its primary effects are on the growth of skeletal muscles and the long bones of the body, thereby determining a person's size and height. GH also exerts powerful metabolic effects. It causes amino acids to be built into proteins and fats to be broken down and used for energy. It also stimulates the conversion of protein to glucose. GH thus causes blood glucose levels to rise.

As its name implies, GH exerts a profound effect on growth. A person who hypersecretes GH as a child develops **gigantism** and will grow very tall, often achieving a height of 8 or 9 feet. If hypersecretion of GH occurs in an adult after the epiphyseal discs of the long bones have sealed, only the bones of the jaw, the eyebrow ridges, the nose, the hands, and the feet enlarge. This condition is called **acromegaly.** GH deficiency in childhood causes the opposite effect, a **pituitary dwarfism.** With this condition, body proportions are normal, but the person's height is short (usually no taller than 4 feet).

If GH is concerned with growth, why is it secreted in an adult? In addition to playing an important role in growth and development, GH performs other functions. It is necessary for cell repair, protein synthesis, and the maintenance of blood glucose levels, especially during periods of fasting between meals. Hence GH, named for its function in the child, also plays an important role in the adult. GH is secreted during periods of exercise, sleep, and hypoglycemia.

Prolactin

Prolactin (PRL) is also called **lactogenic hormone.** As its name suggests (*pro* means for; *lact* means milk), PRL promotes milk production in women. Its primary target organ is the breasts. PRL causes the mammary glands in the breasts to produce milk after childbirth but does not cause the milk to be ejected from the breasts. A hormone from the posterior pituitary gland and other neural influences are responsible for the ejection of milk. If the lactating mother continues to breastfeed, PRL levels remain high. (PRL is discussed in more detail in Chapter 23.) The role of PRL in males is not known.

Text continued on page 247

Table 12·2 MAJOR ENDOCRINE GLANDS AND HORMONES

ENDOCRINE GLAND	HORMONE	TARGET TISSUES/ORGANS	PRIMARY EFFECT OF HORMONE
Hypothalamus	Releasing and release-inhibiting hormones	Anterior pituitary gland	Releasing hormones stimulate the secretion of hormones. Release-inhibiting hormones inhibit the secretion of hormones.
Anterior pituitary gland (adenohypophysis)	Growth hormone (GH) (somatotropin)	Bones and soft tissue	Promotes growth of all tissues.
	Prolactin (PRL)	Mammary glands (breasts)	Stimulates milk production.
	Thyroid-stimulating hormone (TSH, thyrotropin)	Thyroid gland	Stimulates the thyroid gland to produce thyroid hormones (T_3 and T_4).
	Adrenocorticotropic hormone (ACTH)	Adrenal cortex	Stimulates the adrenal cortex to secrete cortical hormones, especially cortisol.
	Gonadotropic hormones		
	Follicle-stimulating hormone (FSH)	Gonads (ovaries and testes)	Stimulates the development of ova and sperm; also stimulates the secretion of estrogen in women.
	Luteinizing hormone (LH) (called interstitial cell–stimulating hormone in men; ICSH)	Gonads (ovaries and testes)	Causes ovulation; stimulates the secretion of progesterone in women and testosterone in men.
Posterior pituitary gland (neurohypophysis)	Antidiuretic hormone (ADH)	Kidneys, blood vessels	Stimulates water reabsorption by the kidney; also constricts blood vessels.
	Oxytocin	Uterus, mammary glands (breasts)	Contracts uterine muscle during labor; releases or ejects milk from the mammary glands.
Thyroid gland	Thyroid hormones (T_3 and T_4)	All tissues	Stimulates metabolic rate; regulates growth and development.
	Calcitonin	Bones, kidneys	Favors bone formation; lowers blood calcium.
Parathyroid gland	Parathyroid hormone (PTH)	Bones, kidneys, and intestine	Causes bone resorption; raises blood calcium. Stimulates the absorption of calcium by the kidneys and intestine; stimulates the excretion of phosphate by the kidneys.

Table 12 • 2   MAJOR ENDOCRINE GLANDS AND HORMONES *Continued*

ENDOCRINE GLAND	HORMONE	TARGET TISSUES/ORGANS	PRIMARY EFFECT OF HORMONE
Adrenal gland			
Medulla	Epinephrine (small amount of norepinephrine)	Many tissues, especially heart and blood vessels	Stimulates fight-or-flight response; helps to increase blood glucose levels. Part of the stress response.
Cortex	Glucocorticoids (cortisol)	All tissues	Helps regulate carbohydrate, protein, and fat metabolism; raises blood glucose. Part of the stress response.
	Mineralocorticoids (aldosterone)	Kidneys	Stimulates the kidneys to reabsorb sodium and to excrete potassium; helps to regulate fluid and electrolyte balance.
	Sex hormones	Sex organs, bones, muscle, and skin	Stimulates the development of secondary sex characteristics in the male and female.
Pancreas			
Islets of Langerhans (alpha cells)	Glucagon	Liver, muscles, and adipose tissues	Raises blood glucose.
Islets of Langerhans (beta cells)	Insulin	Liver, muscles, and adipose tissues	Regulates metabolism of carbohydrates, fats, and proteins. Lowers blood glucose.
Gonads			
Ovaries	Estrogens and progesterone	Sex organs, skin, bones, and muscle	Stimulates the development of ova (eggs); stimulates the development of female sex characteristics.
Testes	Androgens (testosterone)	Sex organs, skin, and muscle	Stimulates the development of sperm; stimulates the development of male sex characteristics.
Thymus gland	Thymosin	T-lymphocytes	Stimulates the maturation of T-lymphocytes.
Pineal gland	Melatonin	Various tissues	Helps set biorhythms; thought to be the "biologic clock."

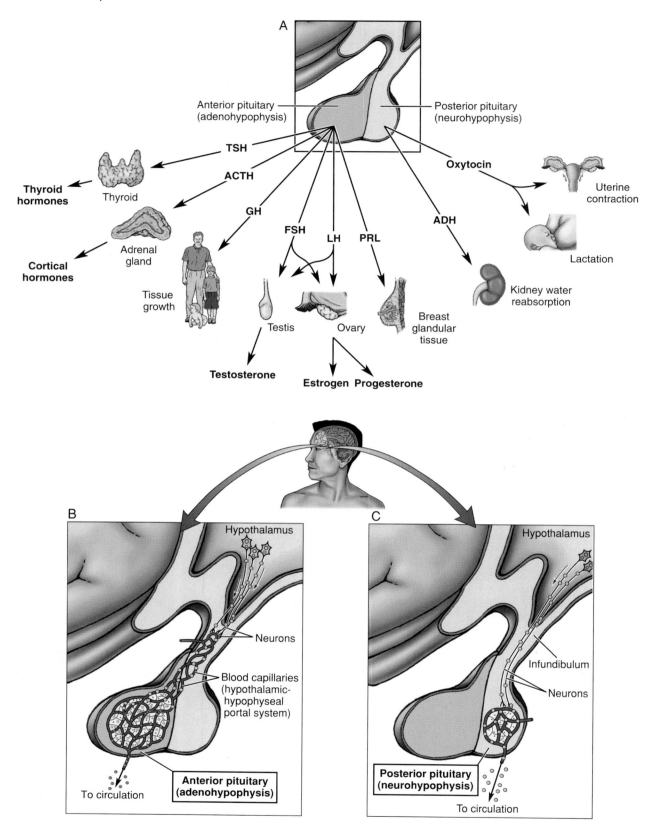

FIGURE 12–4 ● Pituitary gland. A, Hormones secreted by the anterior and posterior pituitary glands; also shows the target organs. B, Relationship of the hypothalamus to the anterior pituitary gland (hypothalamic-hypophyseal portal system). C, Relationship of the hypothalamus to the posterior pituitary gland.

Tropic Hormones

The remaining hormones of the anterior pituitary gland are **tropic hormones.** Tropic hormones are aimed at and control other glands. The names of tropic hormones usually end in *tropin,* or *tropic,* as in thyro*tropin* or adrenocortico*tropic* hormone. The tropic hormones include

- **Thyrotropin, or thyroid-stimulating hormone:** The target gland for **thyroid-stimulating hormone (TSH)** is the thyroid gland. TSH stimulates the thyroid gland to secrete two thyroid hormones. The secretion of TSH is controlled by the releasing hormone, thyrotropin-releasing hormone (TRH), secreted by the hypothalamus.
- **Adrenocorticotropic hormone:** The target gland for **adrenocorticotropic hormone (ACTH)** is the adrenal cortex. ACTH stimulates the adrenal cortex to secrete three steroids, particularly cortisol.
- **Gonadotropic hormones:** The target glands for the **gonadotropic hormones** are the gonads, or sex glands (the ovaries in the female and the testes in the male). The two gonadotropins are **follicle-stimulating hormone (FSH)** and **luteinizing hormone (LH).** FSH stimulates the development of ova (eggs) in the female and sperm in the male. LH causes ovulation in the female and causes the secretion of sex hormones in both the male and the female. LH in the male is also called **interstitial cell–stimulating hormone (ICSH)** because it stimulates the interstitial cells in the testes to synthesize and secrete testosterone. (These hormones are described further in Chapters 22 and 23.)

Posterior Pituitary

The **posterior pituitary gland** is an extension of the hypothalamus (see Fig. 12–4C). The posterior pituitary is composed of nervous tissue and is therefore called the **neurohypophysis** (noŏr″ō-hī-pŏf′ĭ-sĭs). The two hormones of the posterior pituitary gland are produced in the hypothalamus, transported down the stalk, or infundibulum, and stored in the gland until needed. Nerve impulses from the hypothalamus stimulate release of posterior pituitary hormones. The two hormones are **antidiuretic hormone** and **oxytocin.**

Antidiuretic Hormone

Antidiuretic hormone (ADH) is released from the posterior pituitary gland in response to many conditions: concentrated plasma (as occurs in dehydration), pain, stress, trauma, and drugs such as morphine and nicotine. Alcohol, in contrast, inhibits ADH secretion. The primary target organ for ADH is the kidney. ADH causes the kidney to reab-

sorb water and return it to the blood. By the kidney's reabsorbing water, the amount of urine it excretes decreases; hence the name antidiuretic hormone (*anti* means against; *diuresis* means urine production).

In the absence of ADH, a profound diuresis occurs, and the person may excrete up to 25 liters of urine per day. This ADH-deficiency disease is called **diabetes insipidus** and should not be confused with the more common diabetes mellitus (a deficiency of insulin). (The effect of ADH on the kidney is described in Chapter 20.)

Antidiuretic hormone has a second target organ: the blood vessels. ADH causes the muscles of the blood vessels to contract, thereby elevating blood pressure. Because of this blood pressure–elevating effect, ADH is also called **vasopressin.** (A pressor agent is one that elevates blood pressure.)

Oxytocin

The target organs of **oxytocin** are the uterus and the mammary glands (breasts). Oxytocin stimulates the muscles of the uterus to contract and plays a role in the initiation of labor and the delivery of a baby. Oxytocin also plays a role in breastfeeding. When the baby suckles, or nurses, at the breast, sensory information is sent from the breast to the hypothalamus. The hypothalamus responds by sending nerve impulses to the posterior pituitary gland, causing the release of oxytocin. The oxytocin then stimulates contraction of the smooth muscles around the mammary ducts within the breasts, thereby releasing breast milk. The release of milk in response to suckling is called the **milk let-down reflex.** (Note that oxytocin only stimulates the milk to be released. It is the PRL that stimulates the mammary glands to produce the milk.)

✳ **SUM IT UP!** The pituitary gland is called the master gland because it controls the activity of many other endocrine glands. The two main divisions of the pituitary gland are the anterior pituitary and the posterior pituitary. The anterior pituitary gland (adenohypophysis) is controlled by the hypothalamic hormones, called releasing hormones. These hormones are secreted into the hypothalamic portal system, the tiny blood vessels that connect the hypothalamus with the anterior pituitary gland. The anterior pituitary gland secretes six major hormones: growth hormone (GH), prolactin (PRL), thyroid-stimulating hormone (TSH), adrenocorticotropic hormone (ACTH), and two gonadotropic hormones called follicle-stimulating hormone (FSH) and luteinizing hormone (LH). The posterior pituitary gland is an extension of the hypothalamus and is called the neurohypophysis. The posterior pituitary gland secretes two hormones, antidiuretic hormone (ADH) and oxytocin.

THYROID GLAND

The **thyroid gland** (thī'roid glănd) is located in the anterior neck; it is situated on the front and sides of the trachea, just below the larynx (Fig. 12–5A). The thyroid has two lobes connected by a band of tissue called the **isthmus.** The gland is enclosed by a connective tissue capsule. The thyroid gland contains two types of cells: the **follicular cells,** located within the thyroid follicle,

and the **parafollicular cells,** located between the follicles. Each type of cell secretes a particular hormone.

Thyroid Follicle

The thyroid gland is composed of many secretory units called **follicles.** The cavity in each follicle is lined with cuboidal cells and filled with a

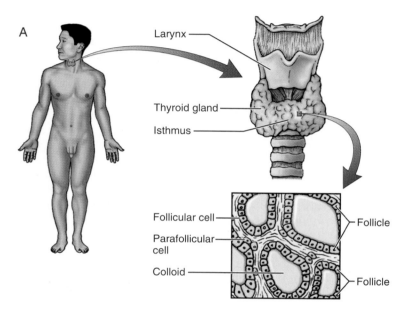

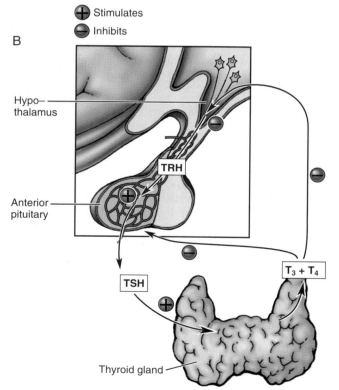

FIGURE 12–5 • Thyroid gland. A, Location in the anterior neck; the thyroid follicle. B, Control of the secretion of T_3 and T_4 from the thyroid gland. The hypothalamus secretes thyroid-releasing hormone (TRH), and the anterior pituitary gland secretes thyroid-stimulating hormone (TSH). The thyroid gland secretes T_3 and T_4, which feed back to decrease the secretion of TRH and TSH.

clear viscous substance called **colloid.** The follicular cells secrete hormones stored within them and attached to the colloid. Follicular cells secrete two thyroid hormones, **triiodothyronine (T₃)** and **tetraiodothyronine (T₄, or thyroxine).**

What Thyroid Hormones Do

The thyroid hormones T₃ and T₄ have similar functions, although T₃ is the more potent. In fact, T₄ is thought to exert its effect only after it has been converted to T₃. Thyroid hormones regulate the metabolism of carbohydrates, proteins, and fats. In general, thyroid hormones increase the rate of metabolism of most cells. They are also necessary for the normal maturation of the nervous system and for normal growth and development. If you were a tadpole, you would require adequate thyroid hormone before you could develop into a frog.

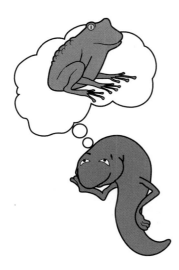

Perhaps the best way to demonstrate the importance of thyroid hormones is to observe the effects of thyroid hormone deficiency **(hypothyroidism)** and excess **(hyperthyroidism).** If an infant is born with no thyroid gland, a condition called **cretinism** develops. An infant with cretinism fails to develop both physically and mentally. The child will be short and stocky with abnormal skeletal development and severe mental retardation. Early diagnosis and prompt treatment with T₃, usually within 2 months after birth, can prevent further damage.

Hypothyroidism in an adult results in a condition called **myxedema.** Myxedema is a sloweddown metabolic state characterized by a slow heart rate, sluggish peristalsis resulting in constipation, a low body temperature, low energy, loss of hair, and weight gain. The skin becomes thick and puffy because of the accumulation of a thick

fluid under the skin; hence the name myxedema (*myx* means mucus; *edema* means swelling).

An excess of thyroid hormones produces hyperthyroidism, a speeded-up metabolic state. A common type of hyperthyroidism is **Graves' disease.** It is characterized by an increase in heart rate, an increase in peristalsis resulting in diarrhea, elevation in body temperature, hyperactivity, weight loss, and wide emotional swings. Note that the symptoms of hyperthyroidism are the opposite of those of the hypothyroid state. Hyperthyroidism is also characterized by bulging eyes, a condition known as **exophthalmia.** In exophthalmia, the eyes are thought to bulge forward because the fat pads behind the eyeballs enlarge in response to excess thyroid activity.

Regulation of Secretion

The regulation of the thyroid gland involves three structures: the hypothalamus, the anterior pituitary gland, and the thyroid gland (Fig. 12–5B). The hypothalamus secretes a releasing hormone (TRH), which stimulates the anterior pituitary to secrete TSH. TSH stimulates the thyroid gland to secrete T₃ and T₄. When the plasma levels of T₃ and T₄ increase sufficiently, negative feedback prevents further secretion of both TRH and TSH.

The Need for Iodine

The synthesis of T₃ and T₄ requires iodine. The iodine in the body comes from dietary sources. Most of the iodine in the blood is actively pumped into the follicular cells of the thyroid gland, where it is used in the synthesis of the thyroid hormones. Tetraiodothyronine, or thyroxine, contains four iodine atoms and therefore is called T₄. Triiodothyronine contains three iodine atoms and is called T₃. An iodine-deficient diet can result in low levels of T₃ and T₄ and can cause hypothyroidism.

Iodine Deficiency

Why does an iodine-deficient diet cause the thyroid gland to enlarge? In an iodine-deficient state, the amount of T₃ and T₄ production decreases because iodine is necessary for the synthesis of these thyroid hormones. The low plasma levels of T₃ and T₄ cause the secretion of TSH and the stimulation of the thyroid gland by TSH.

With insufficient iodine, thyroid hormones cannot be made in quantities great enough to shut off the secretion of TSH through negative feedback. A persistent secretion of TSH causes the thyroid gland to enlarge, producing a goiter. A **goiter** is an enlarged thyroid gland. A **simple goiter** secretes low levels of thyroid hormones. Other types of goiters hypersecrete thyroid hormones and are called **toxic goiters.**

Calcitonin

In addition to secreting T_3 and T_4, the thyroid gland also secretes a hormone called **calcitonin.** Calcitonin is secreted by the parafollicular cells found between the thyroid follicles. Calcitonin is a thyroid hormone, but it is very different from T_3 and T_4. It does not require iodine for synthesis, is not controlled by TRH and TSH, and has no effect on metabolic rate. Instead, calcitonin regulates plasma levels of calcium.

PARATHYROID GLANDS

Four tiny **parathyroid glands** (păr″ə-thī′roid glăndz) are embedded in the posterior wall of the thyroid gland (Fig. 12–6). The parathyroid glands secrete parathyroid hormone (PTH). The stimulus for the release of PTH is a low plasma level of calcium. PTH has three target organs: bone, digestive tract (intestine), and kidneys. The overall effect of PTH is to increase plasma calcium levels and to decrease plasma

phosphate levels. PTH elevates plasma calcium in three ways:

- PTH increases the release of calcium from bone tissue. It does so by stimulating osteoclastic (bone-breakdown) activity. In response, calcium moves from the bone to the blood.
- PTH stimulates the kidneys to reabsorb calcium from the urine. PTH also causes the kidneys to excrete phosphate. The excretion of phosphate by the kidneys is called a phosphaturic effect.
- Working with vitamin D, PTH increases the absorption of calcium by the digestive tract (intestine).

Plasma calcium concentration is also regulated by calcitonin and hydroxycholecalciferol, a vitamin D–related substance. The thyroid gland secretes calcitonin in response to elevated plasma levels of calcium. Calcitonin decreases blood calcium primarily by stimulating osteoblastic (bone-making) activity in the bones. This activity drives the calcium from the blood into the bone. Calcitonin also increases the excretion of calcium in the urine. Calcitonin acts as an antagonist to

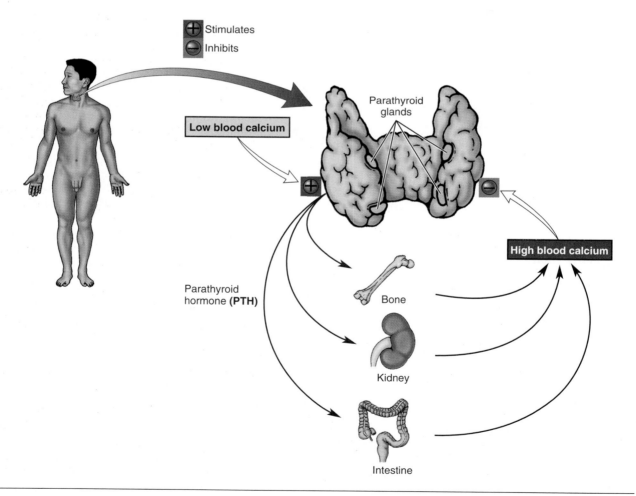

FIGURE 12–6 ● Parathyroid glands. The three target organs of parathyroid hormone (PTH): kidney, bone, and digestive tract (intestine). PTH increases blood calcium. The increased blood calcium, in turn, shuts off further secretion of PTH through negative feedback.

PTH. Blood calcium levels control the secretion of calcitonin and PTH. High blood calcium levels stimulate secretion of calcitonin and inhibit secretion of PTH. Low blood calcium levels inhibit secretion of calcitonin and stimulate secretion of PTH.

✻ **SUM IT UP!** The thyroid gland and the parathyroid glands are located in the anterior neck region. The thyroid gland secretes two iodine-containing hormones, T_3 and T_4. These hormones regulate the body's metabolic rate. Excess secretion of T_3 and T_4, called hyperthyroidism, or Graves' disease, increases the body's metabolic rate. Hypothyroidism (cretinism in infancy or myxedema in adults) causes a hypometabolic state. The secretion of T_3 and T_4 is regulated by TRH from the hypothalamus and TSH from the anterior pituitary gland. The thyroid gland also secretes calcitonin, which affects blood levels of calcium. Calcitonin decreases plasma levels of calcium by stimulating osteoblastic (bone-making) activity in the bone. The four parathyroid glands, embedded in the thyroid gland, secrete PTH. PTH increases plasma calcium levels through its effect on three target organs: bone, kidneys, and digestive tract. PTH stimulates osteoclastic (bone-breakdown) activity in the bone, calcium reabsorption by the kidneys, and increased absorption of dietary calcium from the digestive tract.

Do You Know...

Why may you be asked to tap the face of a patient who has just had a thyroidectomy?

The nurse should tap the area over the facial nerve. The face will twitch if the facial nerve is hyperirritable. This is called a positive (+) Cvostek's sign. Hyperirritability of the facial nerve occurs when the plasma levels of calcium decrease. Sometimes the parathyroid glands, which are embedded in the thyroid gland, are mistakenly removed during thyroid surgery. If the parathyroids are removed, plasma calcium levels decrease because there is no PTH. The nerves become so irritable that they fire continuously, causing continuous muscle contraction (tetany). Unless treated with intravenous calcium, the person may develop a fatal hypocalcemic tetany.

ADRENAL GLANDS

The two small glands located above the kidneys are called **adrenal glands** (ə-drē′nəl glăndz) (*ad* means near; *renal* means kidney), or the **suprarenal glands** (Fig. 12–7A). Their name comes from their location. An adrenal gland consists of two regions: an inner medulla and an outer cortex. The medulla and the cortex secrete different hormones. The adrenal cortex secretes hormones essential to life. The adrenal medullary hormones are not essential for life. The adrenal medulla may be removed without causing life-threatening effects.

Adrenal Medulla

The adrenal medulla is the inner region of the adrenal gland and is considered an extension of the sympathetic nervous system. Remember that the sympathetic nervous system is called the fight-or-flight system. The adrenal medulla secretes two hormones: **epinephrine (adrenalin)** and **norepinephrine.** Because these hormones exert effects similar to the effects of the sympathetic nervous system, they are called **sympathomimetic hormones** (hormones that mimic the sympathetic nervous system) or fight-or-flight hormones.

Epinephrine and norepinephrine are classified as amines (see Table 12–1). Because they contain a chemical group called a catechol group, they are called **catecholamines** (kăt″ĭ-kōl′ə-mēnz). These hormones are secreted in emergency or stress situations. You may have heard the expression "I can feel the adrenalin flowing"; it is another way of saying "I'm ready to meet the challenge." Epinephrine (adrenalin) and norepinephrine help the body respond to stress by causing the following effects:

- Elevating blood pressure
- Increasing heart rate
- Converting glycogen to glucose in the liver, thereby making more glucose available to the cells
- Increasing metabolic rate of most cells, thereby making more energy
- Causing bronchodilation (dilation of the breathing passages) to increase the flow of air into the lungs
- Changing blood flow patterns, causing dilation of the blood vessels to the heart and muscles and constriction of the blood vessels to the digestive tract

In general, epinephrine and norepinephrine increase blood pressure, increase the activity of the heart, and increase metabolism, thereby equipping the body to meet the challenges of stress. The hormones are released in response to the firing of the sympathetic nervous system.

Occasionally, a person develops a tumor of the adrenal medulla and displays signs and symptoms that resemble sympathetic nervous system excess. The tumor is called **pheochromocytoma.** It is characterized by very high blood pressure, increased heart rate, and elevated blood glucose.

A

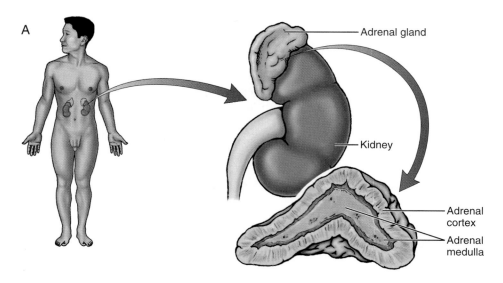

Adrenal gland

Kidney

Adrenal cortex

Adrenal medulla

B

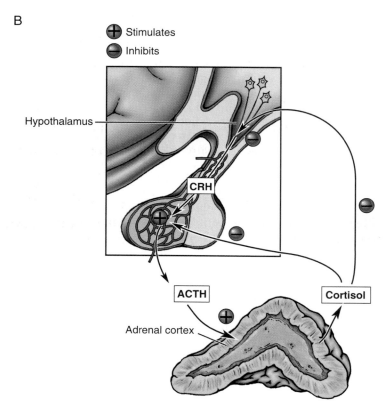

Stimulates

Inhibits

Hypothalamus

CRH

ACTH

Adrenal cortex

Cortisol

FIGURE 12–7 ● Adrenal glands. A, The adrenal glands are located on top of the kidneys. The two regions are the inner adrenal medulla and the outer adrenal cortex. B, Control of the adrenal cortex. The hypothalamus secretes corticotropin-releasing hormone (CRH), and the anterior pituitary gland secretes adrenocorticotropic hormone (ACTH). Cortisol is secreted by the adrenal cortex and feeds back to shut off the further secretion of CRH and ACTH.

Blood pressure is often high enough to be life-threatening. Treatment generally involves surgical removal of the tumor.

Adrenal Cortex

The adrenal cortex is the outer region of the adrenal gland (see Fig. 12–7A). It secretes hormones called steroids. **Steroids** (stĕr´oidz) are lipid-soluble compounds made from cholesterol.

The adrenal cortex secretes three steroids: glucocorticoids, mineralocorticoids, and sex hormones. An easy way to remember the functions of the adrenal cortical steroids is that they regulate sugar, salt, and sex.

Glucocorticoids

As their name implies, the glucocorticoids affect carbohydrates. They convert amino acids into glucose and help maintain blood glucose levels between meals. This action ensures a steady supply of glucose for the brain and other cells. Glucocorticoids also affect protein and fat metabolism, burning both substances as fuel to increase energy production. Glucocorticoids are essential for life. If the adrenal cortex is removed or its function is lost, death will occur unless steroids are administered.

The chief glucocorticoid is **cortisol** (also called **hydrocortisone**). Cortisol is a stress hormone in that it is secreted in greater amounts during times of stress. (By stress we mean physiologic stress such as disease, physical injury, hemorrhage, infection, pregnancy, extreme temperature, and emotional stress such as anger or rage.) Cortisol also has an anti-inflammatory effect. In other words it prevents injured tissues from responding with the classic signs of inflammation: redness, heat, swelling, and pain. For this reason cortisol is used as a drug to prevent inflammation in the treatment of arthritis, severe allergic responses, and the swelling associated with head trauma.

CONTROL OF CORTISOL SECRETION. The secretion of cortisol involves the hypothalamus, anterior pituitary, and adrenal gland (Fig. 12–7B). The hypothalamus secretes corticotropin-releasing hormone (CRH), which then stimulates the anterior pituitary gland to secrete adrenocorticotropic hormone (ACTH). ACTH, in turn, stimulates the adrenal cortex to secrete cortisol. Through negative feedback, the cortisol inhibits the further secretion of CRH and ACTH. This process, in turn, decreases the secretion of cortisol.

HYPOSECRETION AND HYPERSECRETION OF CORTICAL HORMONES. In some persons the adrenal gland fails to secrete adequate amounts of adrenal cortical hormones. This condition is called **adrenal insufficiency,** or **Addison's disease.** It is characterized by generalized weakness, muscle atrophy, a bronzing of the skin, and severe loss of fluids and electrolytes. Left untreated, adrenal insufficiency progresses to low blood volume, shock, and death. Adrenal insufficiency is life-threatening and must be treated with steroids and replacement of fluids and electrolytes.

In contrast, some persons have an excess of adrenal cortical hormones. This condition may be caused by an oversecretion of either ACTH by the anterior pituitary gland or cortisol by the adrenal cortex. Most often, however, elevated plasma levels of cortisol are due to the administration of steroids as drugs. Elevated plasma levels of steroids cause a condition called **Cushing's syndrome.** It is characterized by obesity, a rounded facial appearance (moon face), thin skin that bruises easily, bone loss, and muscle weakness. Salt and water retention cause blood volume and blood pressure to increase. Prolonged therapy with steroids causes many harmful effects, particularly in young athletes who take steroids to improve their athletic performance. The price of enhanced athletic performance is high. Severe and irreversible health problems, such as cancer, osteoporosis (bone softening), and mental illness are possible complications.

Mineralocorticoids

The chief mineralocorticoid is aldosterone. **Aldosterone** plays an important role in the regulation of blood volume and blood pressure and in the concentration of electrolytes in the blood. The primary target organ of aldosterone is the kidney. In general, aldosterone conserves sodium and water and eliminates potassium. Aldosterone release is controlled primarily through the renin-angiotensin-aldosterone system. The role and regulation of aldosterone is described in Chapter 20.

Sex Hormones

The sex hormones, secreted in small amounts, include the female hormones called estrogens and male hormones called **androgens.** The sex hormones of the ovaries usually mask the effects of the adrenal sex hormones. In females, the masculinizing effects of the adrenal androgens, such as increased body hair, may become evident after menopause, when levels of estrogens from the ovaries decrease.

The effects of steroid drugs on adrenal function provide a dramatic example of negative feedback control. Consider this situation: a patient is given cortisol as a drug for the treatment of arthritis. As plasma cortisol levels rise, the secretion of ACTH is inhibited by negative feedback. In the absence of ACTH, the adrenal gland becomes "lazy" and stops the production of cortisol. As long as the person continues to take the steroid drug, plasma cortisol levels remain high. If, however, the person suddenly discontinues the drug, the "lazy" adrenal gland no longer produces cortisol, and the person eventually dies from adrenal insufficiency. (Remember: cortisol is essential for life.) Because of lazy adrenal function, steroid drugs are never discontinued abruptly; dosage is tapered off over an extended period. This gradual reduction gives the "lazy" adrenal gland time to recover and regain its ability to respond to ACTH.

✳ **SUM IT UP!** The adrenal glands are located on top of the kidneys. The two regions of the adrenal glands are the adrenal medulla and the adrenal cortex. The adrenal medulla is an extension of the sympathetic nervous system and secretes two catecholamines called epinephrine (adrenalin) and norepinephrine. The catecholamines are stress hormones and produce effects similar to the fight-or-flight response of the sympathetic nervous system. The adrenal cortex secretes three steroids: the glucocorticoids (cortisol), the mineralocorticoids (aldosterone), and the sex hormones (estrogens and testosterone).

The adrenal cortex is controlled by corticotropin-releasing hormone (CRH) from the hypothalamus and ACTH from the anterior pituitary gland. The functions of the adrenal cortex are concerned with the regulation of sugar, salt, and sex. The adrenal cortex is essential to life. Hyposecretion of the adrenal cortex produces a life-threatening condition called Addison's disease. Treatment consists of replacement therapy with steroid drugs. A hypersecretion of adrenal cortical hormones produces Cushing's syndrome, which is also caused by the administration of steroids as drugs. Left untreated, Cushing's syndrome produces severe, long-term health complications.

PANCREAS

The **pancreas** (păn′krē-əs) is a long organ that lies transversely across the upper abdomen, extending from the curve of the duodenum to the spleen (Fig. 12–8 and see Fig. 12–1). The pancreas functions as both an exocrine gland and an endocrine gland. (Its exocrine function is concerned with the digestion of food and is discussed in Chapter 19.)

The pancreas secretes two hormones, insulin and glucagon. (Notice Ms. PIG in Figure 12–8. She will help remind you that the *p*ancreas secretes *in*-

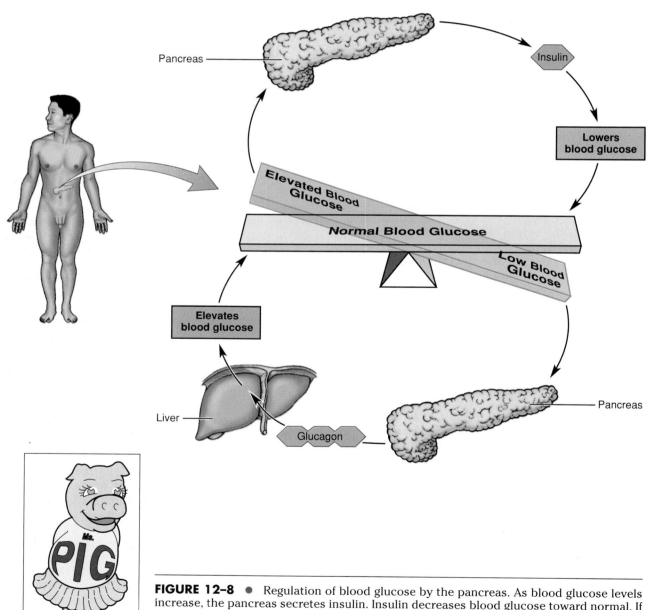

FIGURE 12–8 • Regulation of blood glucose by the pancreas. As blood glucose levels increase, the pancreas secretes insulin. Insulin decreases blood glucose toward normal. If blood glucose levels fall below normal, the pancreas secretes glucagon, which increases blood glucose toward normal. Ms. PIG reminds you that the *p*ancreas secretes *i*nsulin and *g*lucagon.

sulin and *glucagon*.) The hormone-secreting cells of the pancreas are called the **islets of Langerhans.** The islets of Langerhans have two types of cells: the alpha cells, which secrete glucagon, and the beta cells, which secrete insulin. Both insulin and glucagon help regulate blood glucose levels. The overall effect of insulin is to lower blood glucose. The overall effect of glucagon is to increase blood glucose.

Do You Know...

Why do some diabetic persons require insulin to control the disease while others do not?

Some diabetic persons require insulin injections, while others control their diabetes with a pill. The difference is that the pancreas of a person with severe diabetes produces no insulin, so this person must receive insulin injections. These people have insulin-dependent diabetes. In contrast, the pancreas of a person with another form of diabetes is still able to produce some insulin. This person may not require insulin injections but may benefit from oral medication. Some diabetic pills work by stimulating the person's pancreas to produce more insulin. Others work by preventing the hepatic (liver) synthesis of glucose. A diabetic person who does not require insulin injections is called a non–insulin-dependent diabetic.

Insulin

Figure 12–8 illustrates the regulation of insulin and glucagon secretion. Insulin is released in response to increased blood levels of glucose. The secretion of insulin decreases as blood levels of glucose decrease. Insulin has many target tissues and therefore exerts general effects. Insulin affects the liver, skeletal muscle, and adipose tissue with two main effects:

- Insulin helps to transport glucose into cells. Without insulin, glucose remains outside the cells, thereby depriving the cell of its fuel. The only tissue that does not require insulin for glucose transport is the brain. Glucose can enter the brain cells without insulin.
- Insulin helps to control carbohydrate, protein, and fat metabolism in the cell. Insulin stimulates the breakdown of glucose for energy. The liver and skeletal muscles store excess glucose as glycogen. Insulin also increases the transport of amino acids into cells and then stimulates the making, or synthesis, of protein from the amino acids. Lastly, insulin promotes the making of fats from fatty acids.

Do You Know...

What is the difference between diabetic coma and insulin shock?

Diabetic coma, also called diabetic ketoacidosis, develops in response to an insulin deficiency, elevated blood glucose (hyperglycemia), and overactive fatty acid metabolism. Unless treated with insulin, the person becomes comatose and dies. In contrast, insulin shock develops in response to excess insulin and decreased blood glucose (hypoglycemia). Because the brain depends on a constant supply of glucose, the insulin-induced hypoglycemia causes seizures and loss of consciousness. Unless the person is given glucose intravenously, the person will die. Note that both increased and decreased blood glucose levels can cause loss of consciousness. It is important to determine the cause of the unconsciousness before initiating treatment.

Insulin can decrease blood glucose levels for two reasons. First, insulin increases transport of glucose from the blood into the cells. Second, insulin stimulates the cells to burn glucose as fuel. Insulin is the only hormone that lowers blood glucose. All other hormones increase glucose levels (eg, growth hormone, epinephrine, glucagon, cortisol).

Because insulin plays such an important role in the metabolism of all types of foods (carbohydrates, proteins, and fats), a deficiency of insulin causes severe life-threatening metabolic disturbances. Insulin deficiency is called **diabetes mellitus.** It is characterized by the following signs:

- Hyperglycemia: Excess glucose in the blood is called **hyperglycemia.** This condition is due to two factors. The first is the inability of glucose to enter the cells, where it can be burned for energy. Failure to move the glucose into the cells causes the glucose to accumulate in the blood. The second is the making of additional glucose. In the absence of insulin, the body makes glucose from protein. The excess glucose cannot be used by the cells and therefore accumulates in the plasma. The diabetic person is said to be starving in the midst of plenty.
- Glucosuria or glycosuria: Glucose in the urine is called **glucosuria** or **glycosuria.** With glucosuria, the kidneys cannot reabsorb the excess glucose and therefore excrete it in the urine.
- Polyuria: Excretion of a large volume of urine is called **polyuria.** Whenever the kidney excretes a lot of glucose, it must also excrete a lot of water. Glucosuria therefore causes polyuria.

- Acidosis: An excess of acidic substances in the blood causes acidosis. Because the cells cannot burn glucose as fuel, they burn fatty acids instead. The rapid, incomplete breakdown of fatty acids produces strong acids called ketoacids. This process causes a condition called **diabetic ketoacidosis.**
- Fruity odor to the breath: Another ketone produced by fatty acid breakdown is acetone. Acetone smells like bananas and makes the patient's breath smell fruity. A fruity odor is a sign of ketoacidosis. Treatment of diabetic ketoacidosis requires the prompt administration of insulin and the correction of the fluid and electrolyte disturbances.

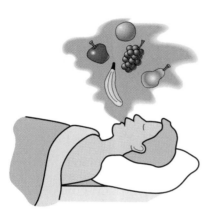

Glucagon

Glucagon is the second hormone secreted by the pancreas. The alpha cells of the islets of Langerhans secrete glucagon. Its primary action is to increase blood glucose levels (see Fig. 12–8). Glucagon raises blood glucose in two ways: by stimulating the conversion of glycogen to glucose in the liver and by stimulating the conversion of proteins into glucose. Both these processes ensure a ready supply of glucose for the busy cells. The stimulus that signals the need for glucagon is a decrease in plasma levels of glucose. Note that the pancreas secretes two hormones that affect blood glucose: insulin, which decreases blood glucose, and glucagon, which increases blood glucose.

✳ **SUM IT UP!** A number of hormones, particularly those secreted by the pancreas, regulate blood glucose levels. The hormone-secreting cells of the pancreas are called the islets of Langerhans. The alpha cells of the islets of Langerhans secrete glucagon, while the beta cells secrete insulin. Insulin works in two ways to decrease blood glucose levels: first, it increases the transport of glucose from the blood into the cells, and second, it stimulates the cells to burn glucose as fuel. Glucagon antagonizes (works against) the effects of insulin by increasing blood glucose levels. Other hormones, such as growth hormone, epinephrine, and cortisol assist glucagon in increasing blood glucose levels. Note that insulin is the only hormone that decreases blood glucose levels.

GONADS

The gonads are the sex glands and refer to the **ovaries** in the female and to the **testes** in the male. The gonads not only produce ova (eggs) and sperm but also secrete hormones. The gonads are therefore glands. (Reproductive anatomy and physiology are discussed in Chapters 22 and 23.)

Ovaries

There are two ovaries (see Fig. 12–1). They are located in the pelvic cavity on each side of the uterus. The ovaries secrete two female sex hormones: estrogens and progesterone. These hormones participate in the development and functioning of the female reproductive organs and in the expression of the female sex characteristics. The sex characteristics of the female develop primarily in response to estrogens. They include

- Development of breasts.
- Distribution of fat in the hips, thighs, and breasts.
- Distribution of hair in specific areas of the body. The different amounts and distribution of hair in the female and male are due to the sex hormones.
- Maturation of the reproductive organs.
- Closure of the epiphyseal discs of the long bones, thereby making females shorter than males.

Both estrogens and progesterone are controlled by releasing hormones from the hypothalamus and by the gonadotropins from the anterior pituitary gland. The effects of estrogens and progesterone on the maturation of the ovum (egg) and their effects on the uterus during the menstrual cycle are described in Chapter 22.

Testes

The testes are located in the scrotum of the male (see Fig. 12–1). The major hormone secreted by the testes is the male sex hormone **testosterone.** Testosterone is a steroid secreted by the interstitial cells of the testes. The stimulus for the secretion of testosterone is the anterior pituitary hormone called luteinizing hormone (LH).

Testosterone helps in the maturation of sperm and is responsible for the male sex characteristics. These include

- Growth and development of the male reproductive organs.
- Musculoskeletal growth.
- Growth and distribution of hair.
- Enlargement of the larynx, accompanied by voice changes.

Testosterone secretion is controlled by releasing hormones from the hypothalamus and by luteinizing hormone from the anterior pituitary gland.

✳ **SUM IT UP!** The gonads are glands and include the ovaries in the female and the testes in the male. The ovaries secrete estrogens and progesterone. The testes secrete testosterone. The gonads are regulated by releasing hormones from the hypothalamus and gonadotropins (FSH and LH) from the anterior pituitary gland. In addition to producing ova and sperm, the gonads secrete hormones responsible for the sex characteristics of the female and male.

THYMUS GLAND

The **thymus gland** (thī′məs glănd) lies in the upper part of the thoracic cavity. The thymus gland is much larger in a child than in an adult. The gland **involutes,** or becomes smaller, as the child enters puberty. The thymus gland secretes hormones called **thymosins,** which play a role in the immune system. (The thymus gland is described in Chapter 17.)

PINEAL GLAND

The **pineal gland** (pĭn′ē-əl glănd) is a cone-shaped gland located close to the thalamus in the brain. It has been called the body's biologic clock, controlling many of the biorhythms. The pineal gland secretes a hormone called melatonin. **Melatonin** affects the reproductive cycle by influencing the secretion of hypothalamic-releasing hormones. The amount of melatonin secreted is related to the amount of daylight. Longer daylight hours decrease the rate of melatonin secretion, whereas shorter daylight hours increase its rate of secretion.

Melatonin is also thought to play a role in the sleep/wake cycle. As melatonin levels increase, the person becomes sleepy. Melatonin is therefore said to have a tranquilizing effect. Persons who work night shifts and sleep during the day have a reversed cycle of melatonin production. The reversal of the melatonin cycle is related to the fatigue experienced by night-shift workers. Elevated melatonin levels have also been implicated in a type of depression called seasonal affective disorder (SAD). This condition occurs primarily in parts of the world where daylight hours are short in the winter, usually in areas far north and far south.

OTHER HORMONES

Hormones Associated With Specific Organ Systems

The glands identified in Figure 12–1 make up the endocrine system, but numerous hormone-secreting cells are scattered throughout the body. These hormones usually control the activities of a particular organ. For instance, hormone-secreting cells in the digestive tract secrete cholecystokinin, gastrin, and secretin. These hormones help to regulate digestion. The kidneys secrete erythropoietin, which helps regulate red blood cell production. The walls of the atria in the heart secrete atrial natriuretic factor (ANF), a hormone that stimulates the kidney to excrete sodium. (These hormones are described in the chapters concerned with those systems, namely the digestive system, the urinary system, and the cardiovascular system.)

Prostaglandins

The **prostaglandins** (prŏs″tə-glăn′dĭnz) are chemical substances (hormones) derived from the fatty acid arachidonic acid. The prostaglandins are produced by many tissues and generally act near their site of secretion. The prostaglandins play an important role in the regulation of smooth muscle contraction and the inflammatory response. Prostaglandins are also thought to increase the sensitivity of pain nerve endings. Drugs such as aspirin, ibuprofen, and acetaminophen block the synthesis of prostaglandins and are therefore useful in relieving the pain and inflammation of arthritis and other inflammatory conditions.

Melanin-Stimulating Hormone

The pituitary gland is divided into two main parts, the anterior and the posterior pituitary. A small third lobe of the pituitary secretes **melanin-stimulating hormone (MSH).** MSH stimulates the melanocytes. When stimulated, the melanocytes increase pigmentation of the skin. Excess secretion of MSH occurs with insufficient secretion of the adrenal cortical hormones (as in adrenal insufficiency, or Addison's disease) and causes bronzing of the skin.

Do You Know...

Why does a person with adrenal insufficiency appear to be bronzed?

A person with adrenal insufficiency secretes an increased amount of melanin-stimulating hormone (MSH). MSH stimulates the melanocytes to deposit dark pigment (melanin) in the skin. The increased pigmentation, in turn, makes the person appear bronzed.

✳ **SUM IT UP!** Other endocrine glands include the thymus and the pineal gland. The thymus gland secretes thymosins and plays an important role in the immune response. The pineal gland is thought to be the body's biologic clock, affecting reproduction and biorhythms. The pineal gland also secretes a hormone called melatonin. Secretion of melatonin is related to light/dark cycles (ie, the amount of light or daylight hours). Other hormone-secreting cells are scattered throughout the body. They secrete hormones such as cholecystokinin, erythropoietin, and ANF, which help regulate the activity of various organ systems. Prostaglandins are chemical substances that affect body functions near the organs that secrete them. Prostaglandins are chemical mediators of pain and inflammation. Drugs such as aspirin and ibuprofen block prostaglandins, thereby relieving pain and inhibiting the inflammatory response. Melanin-stimulating hormone (MSH) is se-creted by a small third lobe of the pituitary gland. MSH stimulates melanocytes to increase the pigmentation in the skin.

As You Age

1. In general, age-related endocrine changes include an alteration in the secretion of hormones, the circulating levels of hormones, the metabolism of hormones, and the biologic activity of hormones.

2. While most glands decrease their levels of secretion, normal aging does not lead to deficiency states. For instance, while adrenal cortical secretion of cortisol decreases, negative feedback mechanisms maintain normal plasma levels of the hormones, thereby preserving water and electrolyte homeostasis.

3. Changes in the thyroid gland cause a decrease in the secretion of thyroid hormones, thereby decreasing metabolic rate.

4. Decreased secretion of growth hormone causes a decrease in muscle mass and an increase in storage of fat.

5. There is a loss of circadian control of hormone secretion.

Disorders of the Endocrine System

Acromegaly	Excess secretion of growth hormone in the adult. Acromegaly is usually caused by a tumor.
Addison's disease	A deficiency of adrenal cortical hormones. If untreated, the patient may develop a life-threatening adrenal shock.
Cretinism	A deficiency of thyroid hormone during fetal development, causing profound physical and mental retardation.
Cushing's syndrome	Excess secretion of adrenal cortical hormones. Cushing's syndrome is also present in patients who take steroids as a medication (as in the treatment of arthritis).
Diabetes insipidus	A deficiency of antidiuretic hormone (ADH), causing the patient to urinate approximately 5 to 6 liters per day of pale dilute urine.
Diabetes mellitus	A deficiency of insulin. The deficiency affects carbohydrate, protein, and fat metabolism. If untreated, the patient develops diabetic ketoacidosis, profound dehydration, and shock. Diabetes mellitus is the most common endocrine disorder.

Disorders of the Endocrine System, *continued*

Gigantism	Excess secretion of growth hormone in a child, usually caused by a pituitary tumor. A deficiency of growth hormone in a child causes pituitary dwarfism.
Goiter	An enlargement of the thyroid gland. A toxic goiter is an enlargement that secretes excess thyroid hormones and produces symptoms of hyperthyroidism. A nontoxic goiter or iodine deficiency goiter does not produce excess thyroid hormones and therefore is not accompanied by symptoms of hyperthyroidism.
Graves' disease	Hypersecretion of thyroid hormone. The hyperthyroid state is characterized by an increase in metabolism. A severe episode of hyperthyroidism is called thyroid storm, a condition that can exhaust the body and cause the heart to fail.
Myxedema	A deficiency of thyroid hormone in adults. The deficiency causes a decrease in metabolism.
Tetany	A deficiency of parathyroid hormone (PTH) that results in low plasma levels of calcium. The hypocalcemia, in turn, causes neuromuscular hyperactivity and sustained muscle contraction (tetanus).

Summary Outline

The endocrine system and the nervous system are the two major communicating and coordinating systems in the body. The endocrine system communicates through chemical signals called hormones.

I. Hormones
  #### A. Classification of Hormones
  1. Hormones are chemical substances secreted by endocrine (ductless) glands directly into the blood.
  2. Hormones are classified as proteins (protein-related substances) and steroids.

  #### B. Hormone Receptors
  1. Hormones are aimed at receptors of target organs.
  2. Receptors are located on the outer surface of the membrane or inside the cell.
  3. The membrane receptors are usually stimulated by protein hormones and result in the activation of the second chemical messenger cyclic adenosine monophosphate (cAMP).
  4. Intracellular receptors are usually stimulated by steroids and result in increased protein synthesis.
  5. Hormone secretion is controlled by three mechanisms: negative feedback control, biorhythms, and control by the central nervous system.

II. Pituitary Gland
  #### A. Hypothalamic-Hypophyseal Portal System
  1. The hypothalamic-hypophyseal portal system is a system of capillaries that connects the hypothalamus and the anterior pituitary.
  2. The hypothalamus secretes releasing and release-inhibiting hormones through the portal system. These hormones control the secretion of hormones from the anterior pituitary gland.

  #### B. Hormones of the Anterior Pituitary Gland
  1. Growth hormone (GH) (somatotropic hormone) affects carbohydrate, protein, and fat metabolism. GH stimulates growth and maintains blood glucose during periods of fasting.
  2. Prolactin (lactogenic hormone) acts primarily on the breasts to stimulate milk production.
  3. Tropic hormones stimulate other glands to secrete hormones. These include thyrotropin, adrenocorticotropic hormone, and the gonadotropins.
  4. Thyrotropin (thyroid-stimulating hormone, or TSH) stimulates the thyroid gland.
  5. Adrenocorticotropic hormone (ACTH) stimulates the adrenal cortex.
  6. The gonadotropic hormones, follicle-stimulating hormone (FSH) and luteinizing hormone (LH), stimulate the gonads (ovaries and testes).

  #### C. Hormones of the Posterior Pituitary Gland
  1. Antidiuretic hormone (ADH) is released in response to low blood volume and increased osmolarity (concentration). ADH stimulates the kidney to reabsorb water.
  2. Oxytocin stimulates the uterine muscle (myometrium) to contract for labor. Oxytocin also stimulates the breast to release milk during suckling, through the milk let-down reflex.

continued

Summary Outline, continued

III. Glands

A. Thyroid Gland
1. The thyroid gland is composed of follicular cells and parafollicular cells.
2. The follicular cells, stimulated by TSH, synthesize triiodothyronine (T_3) and tetraiodothyronine (thyroxine, T_4). T_3 and T_4 regulate metabolic rate.
3. The parafollicular cells secrete calcitonin. Calcitonin stimulates osteoblastic activity and lowers blood calcium.

B. Parathyroid Glands
1. The parathyroid glands secrete parathyroid hormone (PTH).
2. PTH stimulates the bones, kidneys, and intestines to increase blood calcium levels.

C. Adrenal Gland
1. The adrenal medulla secretes the catecholamines epinephrine and norepinephrine. The catecholamines mimic the effects of the sympathetic nervous system and primarily affect the heart and blood vessels.
2. The adrenal cortex secretes the steroids: glucocorticoids (cortisol), mineralocorticoid (aldosterone), and sex hormones (estrogens and testosterone). The steroids affect metabolism and blood volume.

D. Pancreas
1. The pancreas secretes insulin and glucagon.
2. Insulin is secreted by the beta cells of the islets of Langerhans. Insulin lowers blood glucose.
3. Glucagon is secreted by the alpha cells of the islets of Langerhans. Glucagon increases blood glucose.

E. Gonads
1. The ovaries are stimulated by the gonadotropins FSH and LH. The ovaries secrete estrogens and progesterone. Estrogens stimulate the secondary sex characteristics in the female and affect reproduction.
2. The testes are stimulated by the gonadotropins FSH and LH. The testes secrete testosterone, which determines the secondary sex characteristics in the male. Testosterone is necessary for reproduction.

F. Thymus Gland
1. The thymus gland secretes thymosins.
2. The thymus plays an important role in the immune response.

G. Pineal Gland
1. The pineal gland houses the "biologic clock."
2. The pineal gland secretes melatonin.

H. Other Hormones
1. A number of hormones are associated with gastrointestinal function. These include cholecystokinin, secretin, and gastrin.
2. Other hormones include prostaglandins and melanin-stimulating hormone (MSH).

Review Your Knowledge

1. Name the two chief communicating and coordinating systems in the body.

2. How are endocrine and exocrine glands different in structure and function?

3. How does a second messenger such as cAMP help to activate enzymes within a cell?

4. What is the difference between the action of protein hormones and the action of steroid hormones?

5. How do negative feedback, biorhythms, and CNS action control hormone secretion?

6. Describe how the hypothalamic hormones reach the anterior pituitary glands.

7. What are the hormones produced by the anterior and posterior pituitary glands?

8. Name the target organs of the following hormones: growth hormone, prolactin, TSH, ACTH, FSH, LH, ADH, and oxytocin.

9. What are the effects of hypothyroidism and hyperthyroidism?

10. Name the hormones produced by the follicular and parafollicular cells of the thyroid gland.

11. Name three ways in which PTH elevates plasma calcium.

12. Name six effects of catecholamines (epinephrine and norepinephrine) as they help the body respond to stress.

13. How do the adrenal cortical steroids regulate sugar, salt, and sex?

14. What are the symptoms of hyposecretion and hypersecretion of the adrenal cortical hormones?

15. What is the relationship of insulin and glucagon to blood sugar levels?

16. Why does a person with diabetes mellitus have glycosuria, polyuria, acidosis, and a fruity odor to the breath?

17. What are the functions of the following hormones: thymosin, melatonin, estrogens, testosterone, erythropoietin, ANF, prostaglandins, and MSH?

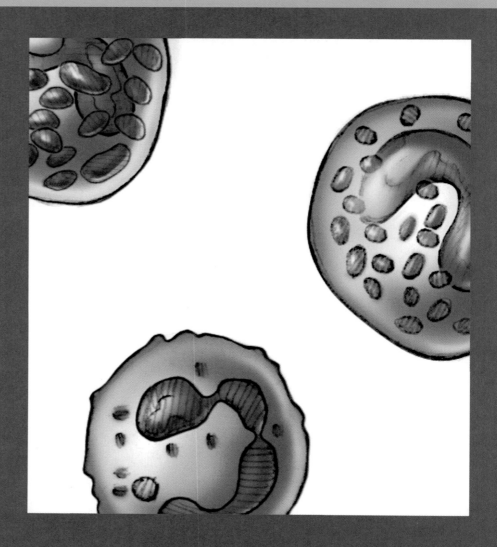

13 BLOOD

Objectives

1. Describe three functions of blood.
2. Describe the composition of blood.
3. Describe the three types of blood cells: erythrocytes, leukocytes, and thrombocytes.
4. Explain the formation of blood cells.
5. Explain the breakdown of red blood cells and the formation of bilirubin.
6. Identify the steps of hemostasis.
7. Describe the four blood types.
8. Describe the Rh factor.

Long before modern medicine, blood was viewed as the part of the body that possessed the life force. This belief arose from the observation that severe bleeding episodes often ended in death, suggesting that the life force flowed out of the body with the blood. Blood was also credited with determining personality traits and emotions. For instance, the wealthy were called bluebloods. Feuding groups often attributed the cause of the troubled relationship to bad blood. Anger was said to cause the blood to boil, while fear could generate blood-curdling screams. The qualities of blood seemed so magical that a sharing of a few drops of blood could make one's friend a blood brother. While we no longer speak of blood in such terms, we do recognize that an adequate blood supply is essential for life. Blood is a truly remarkable substance.

Blood flows through a closed system of blood vessels. The force that pushes the blood through the vessels is the pumping action of the heart (see Chapters 14 and 15).

WHAT BLOOD DOES

Blood performs three general functions: transport, regulation, and protection. First, the blood transports many substances around the body. For instance, blood delivers oxygen from the lungs to every cell in the body. Blood picks up waste material from the cells and delivers the waste to organs that eliminate it from the body. Nutrients, ions, hormones, and many other substances use blood as the vehicle for movement throughout the body. Second, blood participates in the regulation of fluid and electrolyte balance, acid-base balance, and body temperature. Third, blood helps protect the body from infection. Blood also contains clotting factors, which help protect the body from excessive blood loss.

COMPOSITION OF BLOOD

Blood is a type of connective tissue. The color of blood varies from a bright red to a darker blue-red. The difference in color is due to the amount of oxygen in the blood. Well-oxygenated blood is bright red, whereas oxygen-poor blood is blue-red. The quantity, or amount, of blood varies, depending on body size, gender, and age. The average adult has about 4 to 6 liters.

Other characteristics of blood include pH (7.35–7.45) and viscosity. Blood **viscosity** refers to the ease with which blood flows through the blood vessels. Viscosity is best demonstrated by comparing the flow of water and molasses. If water and molasses are poured out of a bottle, the molasses flows more slowly. Molasses is said to be more viscous, or thicker, than water. Blood is normally three to five times more viscous than water. While blood viscosity does not normally fluctuate widely, an increase in viscosity can thicken the blood so much that it puts an extra burden on the heart, thereby causing the heart to fail as a pump.

Blood is composed of two parts: the liquid portion, called the plasma, and the formed elements, called corpuscles, or blood cells.

The **plasma** (plăz′mə) is a pale yellow fluid composed mostly of water. The plasma also contains proteins, ions, nutrients, gases, and waste. The plasma proteins consist of **albumin** (ăl-byoo′mĭn), various clotting factors, antibodies, and complement. In general, the plasma proteins help regulate fluid volume, protect the body from pathogens, and prevent excessive blood loss in the event of injury. **Serum** (sîr′əm) is the plasma minus the clotting proteins, such as fibrinogen.

The formed elements are also called **corpuscles,** or blood cells. (Throughout the text we will refer to the formed elements as blood cells.) The blood cells include the following:

- **Red blood cells,** or **RBCs,** which are also called **erythrocytes** (ĕ-rĭth′rə-sīts) (from *erythro,* meaning red). RBCs are primarily involved in the transport of oxygen to all body tissues.
- **White blood cells,** or **WBCs,** which are also called **leukocytes** (loo′kə-sīts) (from *leuko,* meaning white). The several different types of WBCs protect the body from infection.
- **Platelets** (plāt′lĕts), which are also called **thrombocytes** (thrŏm′bə-sīts). They protect the body from bleeding.

The two parts, or phases, of blood (ie, plasma and blood cells) can be observed in a test tube. If a sample of blood is collected in a tube and spun at a high speed, two phases appear (Fig. 13–1). The heavier blood cells appear at the bottom of the tube, while the lighter plasma accumulates at the top.

The separation of blood into two phases forms the basis of a blood test called the **hematocrit** (hē-măt′ə-krĭt) (see Fig. 13–1). The hematocrit is the percentage of blood cells in a sample of blood. A sample of blood is normally composed of 45% blood cells and 55% plasma. The 45% (blood cells) is composed mainly of RBCs. A small layer of cells between the plasma and the RBCs is called the buffy coat and consists of WBCs and platelets. Because the buffy coat is so thin, any change in the hematocrit is generally interpreted as a change in the numbers of RBCs. For instance, a person with a low hematocrit is considered to be anemic, with a lower-than-normal number of RBCs.

Origin of Blood Cells

Where are the blood cells made? The three types of blood cells (RBCs, WBCs, and platelets) are made in hematopoietic tissue. The process of

BLOOD SAMPLE

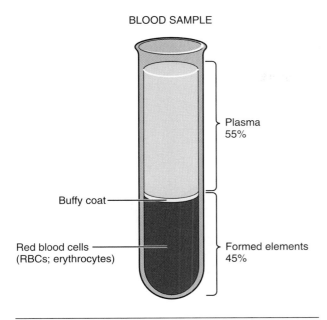

Plasma 55%

Buffy coat

Red blood cells (RBCs; erythrocytes)

Formed elements 45%

FIGURE 13-1 ● Hematocrit: the ratio of the blood cells to the total blood volume. Normally, 45% of the blood sample is composed of blood cells.

blood cell production is called **hematopoiesis** (hē″mə-tō-poi-ē′sĭs). The two types of hematopoietic tissue in the adult are the **red bone marrow,** which is found primarily in the flat and irregular bones, and the **lymphatic tissue,** which is found in the spleen, lymph nodes, and thymus gland.

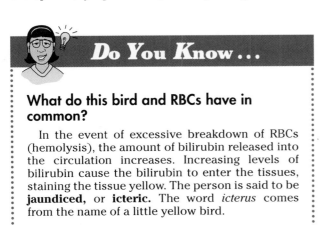

Do You Know...

What do this bird and RBCs have in common?

In the event of excessive breakdown of RBCs (hemolysis), the amount of bilirubin released into the circulation increases. Increasing levels of bilirubin cause the bilirubin to enter the tissues, staining the tissue yellow. The person is said to be **jaundiced,** or **icteric.** The word *icterus* comes from the name of a little yellow bird.

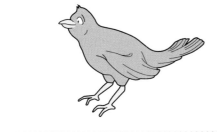

How does the red bone marrow produce three different kinds of blood cells? The three types of

blood cells are produced in the red bone marrow from the same cell. This cell is called a **stem cell.** Under the influence of specific growth factors, the stem cell changes, or differentiates, into an RBC, a WBC, or a platelet. Note the stem cell in Figure 13–2. In line 1, the stem cell differentiates into the RBC (erythrocyte). In lines 2, 3, and 4, the stem cells form five different WBCs (leukocytes). The **lymphocytes** (lĭm′fə-sīts) and **monocytes** (mŏn′ə-sīts) originate in the bone marrow but mature in the lymphatic tissue. In line 5, the stem cell differentiates into a **megakaryocyte,** a large blood cell that breaks up into tiny fragments. These are the platelets (thrombocytes). Note that the platelet is not a whole cell; it is a piece, or fragment, of the large megakaryocyte.

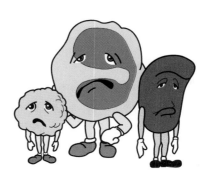

Bone Marrow Depression

Even bone marrow gets depressed! Under certain conditions, the bone marrow cannot produce sufficient numbers of blood cells. Bone marrow depression is called **myelosuppression** (from the Greek word *myelo,* meaning marrow). Depressed bone marrow can cause a severe deficiency of RBCs, causing a serious form of **anemia** (ə-nē′mē-ə) called **aplastic anemia.**

Myelosuppression can also cause a deficiency of WBCs (leukocytes) called **leukopenia.** The leukopenic person is defenseless against infection and may die from a common cold. Depressed bone marrow may also produce inadequate numbers of platelets, or thrombocytes. This condition is called **thrombocytopenia.** The thrombocytopenic person is at high risk for hemorrhage.

Why the concern for bone marrow depression? Because many drugs and certain procedures, such as radiation, depress the bone marrow, a person exposed to any of these therapies must be monitored for symptoms of myelosuppression.

Red Blood Cells (Erythrocytes)

The red blood cells (RBCs), or erythrocytes, are the most numerous of the blood cells. There are between 4.5 and 6.0 million RBCs in one microliter of

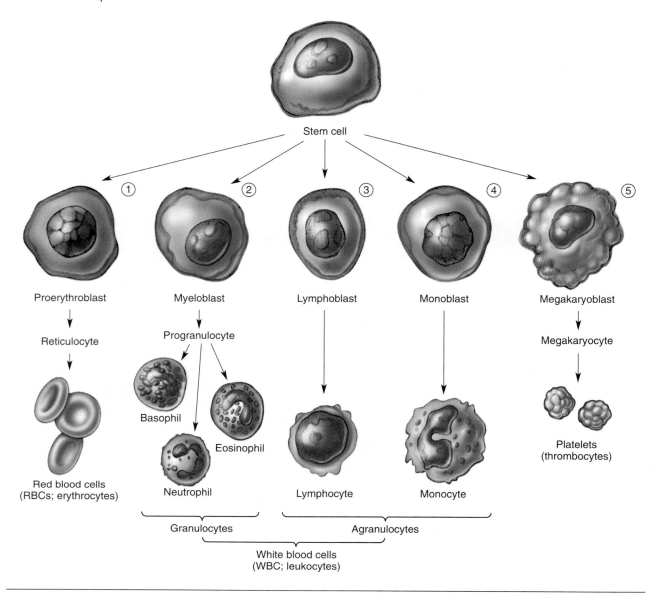

FIGURE 13–2 ● Differentiation of a stem cell. The stem cell differentiates into red blood cells (erythrocytes), white blood cells (leukocytes), and platelets (thrombocytes).

blood. The rate of production by the red bone marrow is several million RBCs per second. RBCs are primarily concerned with the transport of oxygen.

What do RBCs look like? They are tiny disc-shaped cells that have a thick outer rim and a thin center (Fig. 13–3). The RBC can bend and therefore squeeze its way through the tiniest blood vessels. This flexibility allows the RBC to deliver oxygen to every cell in the body. The RBC's ability to bend is important. If the RBC were not able to bend, it would not fit through the tiny blood vessels, and certain cells would be deprived of oxygen and die. Decreased oxygenation and cell death occur in a condition known as **sickle cell disease.** Instead of bending, the RBCs assume a C shape or sickle shape and actually block blood flow through the tiny blood vessels.

ROLE OF HEMOGLOBIN. Red blood cells are filled with a large protein molecule called **hemoglobin** (hē′mə-glō″bĭn) (Fig. 13–4). Hemoglobin consists of two parts, globin (protein) and heme, an iron-containing substance. Hemoglobin contains four globin chains, each globin with a heme group. The hemoglobin molecule is responsible for RBC function.

What is so important about heme? As the RBCs circulate through the blood vessels in the lungs, oxygen (O_2) attaches loosely to the iron atom in the heme. The oxygenated hemoglobin is referred to as **oxyhemoglobin.** Then, as the blood flows to the various tissues in the body, the oxygen detaches from the hemoglobin; it unloads. The unloaded oxygen diffuses from the blood to the cells, where it is used during cellular metabolism.

blue, or **cyanotic.** Cyanosis is a sign of **hypoxemia** (a deficiency of oxygen in the blood).

SUBSTANCES ESSENTIAL FOR HEMOGLOBIN PRODUCTION. What does the body need to make adequate amounts of hemoglobin? In addition to a healthy hematopoietic system, the body requires certain raw materials. Iron, vitamin B_{12}, folic acid, and protein are essential for hemoglobin synthesis. Recall that the heme, the oxygen-carrying component of hemoglobin, contains iron. A diet deficient in iron can result in inadequate hemoglobin synthesis and a condition called **iron-deficiency anemia.** As you might expect, young women are more prone to iron-deficiency anemia than are young men. Women not only are more apt to get caught up in rigorous and unhealthy dieting, but they also tend to lose more iron because of the blood loss associated with menstruation.

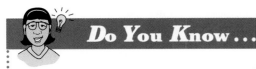

Do You Know...

Why is there a needle in this hip bone?

Because the red bone marrow is the site of blood cell production, certain abnormalities of blood cells can be detected through a bone marrow biopsy. In this procedure, a needle is inserted into the red bone marrow, usually at the iliac crest (hip bone) or the sternum (breast bone). A sample of bone marrow is withdrawn, or aspirated, and then microscopically studied. The analysis includes numbers and types of blood cells as well as the specific characteristics of each cell type.

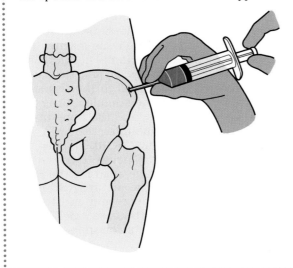

The globin portion of hemoglobin also plays a role in gas transport. Globin transports some of the carbon dioxide (CO_2) from its site of production (ie, the working, or metabolizing, cells) to the lungs, where it is excreted. The CO_2-hemoglobin complex is called **carbaminohemoglobin** (ie, carbon dioxide attaches to an amino acid portion of the globin chains).

Note: Hemoglobin is primarily concerned with the transport of *oxygen.* Hemoglobin transports only a small portion of the carbon dioxide. (Other more important means of CO2 transport are described in Chapter 18.)

WHY BLOOD CHANGES ITS COLOR. The color of blood changes from bright red to blue-red. When hemoglobin is oxygenated (ie, becomes oxyhemoglobin), blood appears bright red. When hemoglobin is unoxygenated, blood assumes a darker blue-red color. Thus, blood coming from the lungs is well oxygenated and appears red. Blood leaving the cells has given up its oxygen and appears blue-red. When a person is deprived of oxygen, the blood is a blue-red color, causing the skin to look

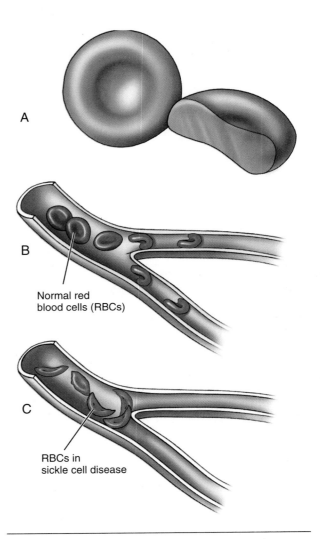

FIGURE 13–3 • Red blood cell: size and shape. A, The RBCs are large and donut-shaped. B, The RBCs must bend to fit through the capillary (a blood vessel). C, Sickled RBCs cannot bend and therefore block the flow of blood through the blood vessel.

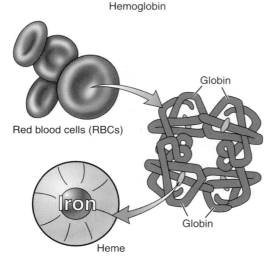

Hemoglobin

Globin

Red blood cells (RBCs)

Iron

Globin

Heme

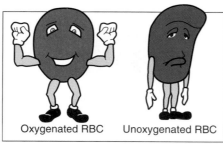

Oxygenated RBC   Unoxygenated RBC

FIGURE 13–4 ● Hemoglobin. Hemoglobin is composed of four globin (protein) chains and four iron-containing heme groups. The oxygen attaches to the iron molecules. Oxygenated hemoglobin (oxyhemoglobin) is red; unoxygenated hemoglobin is blue.

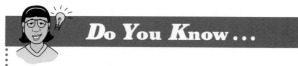

Do You Know...

How can a person be cherry red and hypoxic at the same time?

Blood is bright red when the hemoglobin is saturated with oxygen. In other words, oxyhemoglobin makes blood red. Carbon monoxide, like oxygen, binds to the iron and makes the blood bright cherry red. When carbon monoxide occupies the iron site, however, no oxygen can be carried by the hemoglobin. Therefore, the person with carbon monoxide poisoning can be both cherry red and hypoxic.

A deficiency of other raw materials can cause other specific anemias. A deficiency of folic acid, for instance, causes **folic acid–deficiency anemia.** Besides adequate dietary intake, raw materials must be absorbed from the digestive tract. Absorption of some of the raw materials requires

special transport proteins. Adequate absorption of vitamin B_{12}, for instance, requires a transport protein called **intrinsic factor.** Intrinsic factor is normally secreted by the lining of the stomach. The inability to secrete adequate intrinsic factor in some persons results in inadequate absorption of vitamin B_{12}. This condition results in a form of anemia called **pernicious anemia.**

REGULATION OF RBC PRODUCTION. New RBCs are constantly added to the circulation, while old, worn-out RBCs are constantly removed from the circulation. The steps for RBC release appear in Figure 13–5. When the oxygen in the body tissues starts to decrease, the kidneys (and liver, to a lesser extent) sense the need for additional oxygen and secrete a hormone called **erythropoietin** (ĕ-rĭth″rō-poi′ə-tĭn). Blood transports erythropoietin from the kidney to the bone marrow. The erythropoietin stimulates the bone marrow to release RBCs into the circulation. The increase in the number of RBCs causes an increase in the amount of oxygen transported to the tissues. As tissue oxygen increases, the stimulus for erythropoietin release diminishes, and the bone marrow slows its rate of RBC production.

REMOVAL AND BREAKDOWN OF RBCS. How does the body know when an RBC needs to be removed from the circulation? The life span for the RBC is about 120 days. Because the mature RBC has no nucleus, it cannot reproduce and must be replaced as it wears out. With time, as it performs its job, the RBC eventually gets misshapen, ragged around the edges, and fragile; the poor thing looks worn out. This change in the structure of the RBC is detected by the cells of the **tissue macrophage system** (the older term is the reticuloendothelial system, or RES). These macrophages, or big eaters, remove the RBCs from the circulation and phagocytose them. The macrophages of this system are found primarily in the spleen, the liver, and the red bone marrow.

Recycle! As the old, worn-out RBC is dismantled, its components are recycled. How is the RBC dismantled? The hemoglobin is broken down into globin and heme (Fig. 13–6). The globin is broken down into various amino acids, which are later used in the synthesis of other proteins. The heme is further broken down into iron and bile pigments. The iron returns to the bone marrow, where it is reused in the synthesis of new hemoglobin. Excess iron is stored in the liver. The liver removes bile pigments, especially bilirubin, from the blood and excretes them into the bile. Bile eventually flows into the intestines and is excreted from the body in the feces.

✳ **SUM IT UP!** The RBC is formed in the red bone marrow. Normal RBCs are formed only in the presence of adequate raw materials, normal genetic information that directs hemoglobin synthesis, and a healthy bone marrow. RBC production is regulated by erythropoietin, which, in turn, responds to tissue levels of oxygen. Hemoglobin is broken down into globin and bilirubin. The bilirubin is excreted in the bile.

White Blood Cells (Leukocytes)

White blood cells (WBCs), or leukocytes, are large round cells that contain nuclei. Because they lack hemoglobin, WBCs appear white. WBCs are

less numerous than RBCs. Normally, a microliter of blood contains between 5000 and 10,000 WBCs. WBCs function primarily to protect the body by destroying disease-producing microorganisms (pathogens) and to remove dead tissue and other cellular debris by **phagocytosis.** (Phagocytosis is a process by which a cell surrounds and digests substances.) When an infection is present in the body, the numbers of WBCs generally increase. This increase in the number of WBCs is called **leukocytosis.**

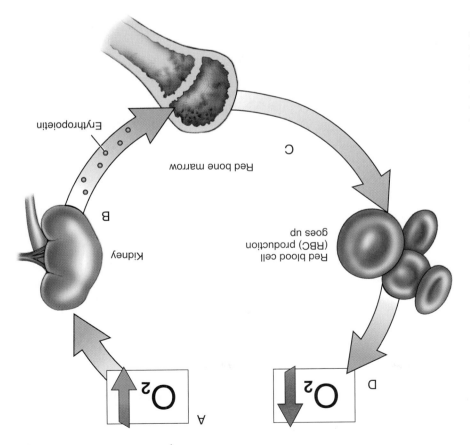

FIGURE 13–5 ● Regulation of RBC production by erythropoietin. A, The kidney senses low O_2 concentration in the blood. B, The kidney releases erythropoietin into the blood. C, Erythropoietin stimulates the bone marrow to produce more RBCs. D, As the numbers of RBCs increase, the amount of O_2 in the blood also increases. This process shuts off the stimulus for the release of more erythropoietin.

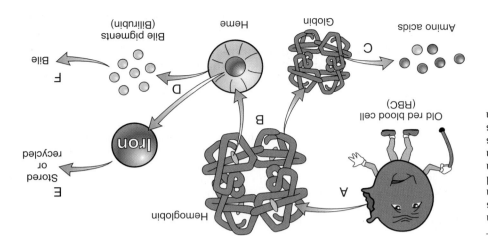

FIGURE 13–6 ● Breakdown of old RBCs. A, The RBC releases hemoglobin. B, The hemoglobin is broken down into globin and heme. C, The globin is broken down into amino acids, which are recycled. D, The heme is broken down into iron, which is recycled (E), and bilirubin, which is excreted into the bile (F).

Table 13 • 1

TYPES AND FUNCTIONS OF BLOOD CELLS*

CELL TYPE	NORMAL RANGE	PRIMARY FUNCTION
Red blood cells (RBCs)	4.5–6.0 million mm3†	Transports oxygen and carbon dioxide
Hemoglobin (Hgb)	12–18 g/dl	
Hematocrit (Hct)	38–54%	
Reticulocytes	0–1.5%	
White blood cells (WBCs)*	5000–10,000 mm3	Protects the body from infection
Platelets (thrombocytes)	150,000–350,000 mm3	Help control blood loss from injured blood vessels

*See Table 13–2 for the white blood cell differential count.
†mm3 = microliter.

Unlike RBCs, which normally circulate within the blood vessels, WBCs can leave the blood vessels. The WBCs squeeze through the cells of the blood vessel walls and move toward the site of infection, where they can destroy the pathogens and clean up by removing any cellular debris (Fig. 13–7).

KINDS OF WHITE BLOOD CELLS. Each of the five kinds of white blood cells (leukocytes) has a different name, appearance, and function (Table 13–2). How do we tell the difference? WBCs are classified according to granules in their cytoplasm. WBCs that contain granules are called **granulocytes.** Other WBCs do not have granules within their cytoplasm and are called **agranulocytes** (ie, without granules). Granulocytes are produced in the red bone marrow. Three types of granulocytes are neutrophils, basophils, and eosinophils.

The **neutrophil** (noo′tra-fil) is the most common granulocyte. Neutrophils account for 55% to 70% of the total WBC population and usually remain in the blood for a short period (about 10 to 12 hours). The neutrophil's most important role is phagocytosis. These cells quickly move to the site of infection where they phagocytose pathogens and remove tissue debris. The battle between the neutrophils and the pathogens at the site of infection leaves behind a collection of dead neutrophils, parts of cells, and fluid. This collection is called **pus.**

Sometimes the body can wall off the collection of pus from the surrounding tissue, forming an **abscess.** Abscess formation is one of the ways that the body has of containing or restricting the spread of infection. The neutrophil plays such an important role in the defense of the body that a deficiency of neutrophils (ie, **neutropenia** or **granulocytopenia**) is considered life-threatening. Unless resolved, the person may die from an overwhelming infection.

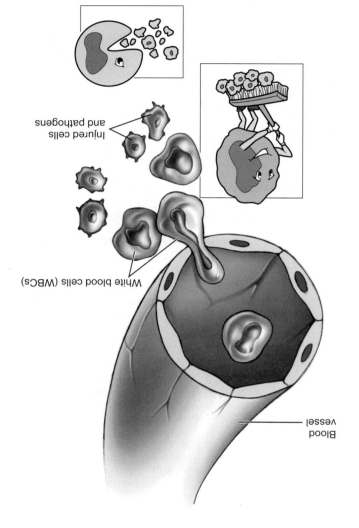

FIGURE 13-7 ● White blood cells. WBCs travel through the blood to the site of injury. They squeeze across the blood vessel wall and clean up the injured cells and pathogens.

Blood vessel

White blood cells (WBCs)

Injured cells and pathogens

Table 13•2 WHITE BLOOD CELLS (LEUKOCYTES)*

TYPE OF WBC	PERCENT OF TOTAL WBC COUNT	FUNCTION OF CELL
Granulocytes		
Neutrophils	55–70	Phagocytosis
Eosinophils	1–3	Inflammatory responses; parasitic infection; allergies
Basophils	0–1	Inflammatory responses; release heparin
Agranulocytes		
Lymphocytes	25–38	Immunity
Monocytes	3–8	Phagocytosis

*A differential white blood cell count indicates the percentage of each type of white blood cell.

NAMING THE NEUTROPHIL. Because it plays an important role in protecting the body from infection, the neutrophil is often the center of attention. Depending on its appearance and what it is doing at the moment, the neutrophil has many nicknames.

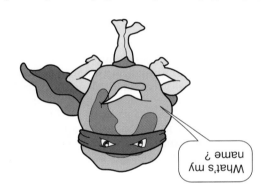

What's my name?

Polys, Polymorphs, or Polymorphonuclear Leukocytes. The neutrophil is a round cell that contains a nucleus. The nucleus can have many shapes (ie, it is a polymorph) and different sizes. Because of the many-shaped, or polymorphic, nucleus, neutrophils are called polymorphs (literally meaning many shapes). Sometimes they are simply called "polys." For the same reason, they are also called **polymorphonuclear leukocytes,** or **PMNs.**

Segs. The nucleus of the mature neutrophil appears segmented, or many-lobed, when viewed under a microscope. Neutrophils are therefore called segs.

Band Cells, Staff Cells, Stab Cells. The nucleus of the immature neutrophil looks like a thick, curved band, hence the name **band cells.** The band also resembles the shape of a staff, hence the name **staff cells.** Neutrophils are also called **stab cells,** a name that derives from a German word meaning to stab. The presence of many band cells indicates an active infection. As it tries to mount an attack against a pathogen, the body needs more neutrophils. The production of the neutrophils may be so rapid that the time for cells to mature is inadequate. A greater proportion of the neutrophils are therefore immature and appear banded.

BASOPHILS. The second type of granulocytic WBC, **basophils** (bā'sa-filz), are normally present in small numbers. Basophils make up less than 1% of the WBCs. Very little is known about the basophil. It plays a role in the inflammatory response, primarily through its release of histamine. The basophil also releases **heparin,** an anticoagulant. Because basophils are found in abundance in areas with large amounts of blood (eg, lungs and liver), the release of heparin is thought to reduce the formation of tiny blood clots.

EOSINOPHILS. The third type of granulocytic WBC is the **eosinophil** (e"o-sin'o-fil). Like the basophil, little is known about the eosinophil.

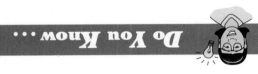

Do You Know . . .

What is a shift to the left?

When immature granulocytes (neutrophils) become prominent in the differential white blood cell count, the condition is called a **shift to the left.** The term derives from early studies that used tabular headings to report the numbers of each cell type. The cell types were listed across the top of the page, starting with blasts (immature WBCs) on the left and placing more mature neutrophils on the right. Large numbers of immature cells (as seen with severe infection) are listed to the left-hand column of the form. Thus, a shift to the left indicates an infection.

Eosinophils are present in small numbers, constituting only 1% to 3% of the WBCs. They are involved in the inflammatory response, secreting chemicals that destroy certain parasites, and become elevated in persons with allergies. A person with a parasitic infection or allergic reaction generally has an elevated eosinophil count.

DIFFERENT-COLORED GRANULOCYTES. The three granulocytes stain different colors. The three different colors are used to name the granulocytes. Neutrophils do not stain deeply; they are relatively neutral with regard to staining characteristics. For this reason they are called neutrophils. When stained and viewed under the microscope, the granules of the neutrophils appear a light lavender color. The other two granulocytes stain deeply and are named for the color stain each absorbs. The eosinophil stains a bright pink, while the basophil stains a dark blue.

AGRANULOCYTES. The two kinds of agranulocytes are the lymphocytes and the monocytes. These agranular WBCs are produced in the red bone marrow and also in the lymphoid tissue of the spleen, lymph nodes, and thymus gland. Lymphocytes constitute 25% to 38% of the WBCs and perform an important role in the body's immune response. (Immunity will be discussed further in Chapter 17.) Monocytes are the second type of agranulocyte. Like the neutrophil, the monocyte is phagocytotic. Although the neutrophils are more abundant (55-70% of the WBCs), the monocytes (3-8% of the WBCs) are more efficient phagocytes.

Monocytes differentiate, or change, into macrophages. These macrophages become either wandering or fixed. Wandering macrophages travel, or wander, about the body patrolling for pathogens and cleaning up debris. Wandering macrophages are particularly abundant under the mucous membrane and the skin. There they destroy pathogens that enter through breaks in the mucous membrane or skin. In contrast, fixed macrophages remain or become fixed in a particular organ, such as the liver, spleen, lymph nodes, or red bone marrow. (These are organs of the tissue macrophage system.) As blood or lymph flows through these organs, the fixed macrophages phagocytose any microorganisms in the blood, thereby helping to cleanse the blood of pathogens. These same macrophages also phagocytose worn-out RBCs, thereby helping remove them from circulation.

Platelets (Thrombocytes)

Platelets, or thrombocytes, are the tiniest formed elements of the blood. Normally, each microliter of blood contains between 150,000 and 450,000 platelets. They are produced in the red bone marrow from the large megakaryocyte (see Fig. 13-2). The platelet is not a whole cell; it is actually only a fragment of the megakaryocyte. Although it does not contain DNA or a nucleus, each platelet does contain cytoplasm with mitochondria and various enzymes surrounded by a cell membrane. Platelets have a life span of 5 to 9 days. Platelets prevent blood loss. Failure of the bone marrow to replace platelets at an adequate rate results in a deficiency called thrombocytopenia, a deficiency of thrombocytes in the blood. Thrombocytopenia is characterized by petechiae, little pinpoint hemorrhages under the skin, and abnormal bleeding episodes.

Complete Blood Count

A complete blood count (CBC) is a laboratory test that provides information about the constituents of the blood (see Table 13-1). A CBC provides the normal range of the numbers of RBCs, WBCs, and platelets. In addition to the numbers of blood cells, the CBC provides information specific to each cell type. Relative to the RBC, the CBC indicates the normal hemoglobin (Hgb) content of the RBC, the normal hematocrit (Hct), and the percentage of the reticulocytes (the immature RBCs). With regard to information concerning the WBCs, a CBC indicates the percentage of each type of WBC.

The percentage of each of the five types of WBCs is called the differential count (see Table 13-2). The differential count provides valuable diagnostic information because it indicates which WBC is involved. For instance, one infection may cause an elevation primarily in the numbers of neutrophils, but a different infection may cause an elevation in the monocytes. The differential count may therefore offer a clue in diagnosing infection.

✳ SUM IT UP! The WBCs (leukocytes) protect the body by destroying pathogens and remove dead tissue and other cellular debris by phagocytosis. The five kinds of WBCs are granulocytes (neutrophils, basophils, and eosinophils) and agranulocytes (lymphocytes and monocytes). Platelets (thrombocytes) are produced in the red bone marrow and play a key role in hemostasis.

HEMOSTASIS: PREVENTION OF BLOOD LOSS

Injury to a blood vessel often causes bleeding. Bleeding usually stops spontaneously when the injury is minor. A more serious bleeding episode, however, can be life-threatening and often requires medical intervention.

What causes the bleeding to stop? The process that stops bleeding after injury is called hemostasis (he"ma-sta'sis). The word literally means that the blood (hemo) stands still (stasis). Hemostasis involves three events: blood vessel spasm, the formation of a platelet plug, and blood clotting (Fig. 13–8). (Do not confuse the words *hemostasis* and *homeostasis*.)

Blood Vessel Spasm

When a blood vessel is injured, the smooth muscle in the blood vessel wall responds by contracting, or constricting. This process is called **vascular spasm.** Vascular spasm causes the diameter of the blood vessel to decrease, thereby decreasing the amount of blood that flows through the vessel. In the tiniest of vessels, vascular spasm stops the bleeding completely. In the larger vessels, vascular spasm alone may slow bleeding but is generally insufficient to stop bleeding.

Formation of a Platelet Plug

When a blood vessel is torn, the inner lining of the vessel stimulates, or activates, the platelets.

The platelets become sticky, and the platelets stick, or adhere, to the inner lining of the injured vessel and to each other. By sticking together, they form a **platelet plug.** The plug diminishes bleeding at the injured site. Over several minutes, the plug will be invaded by activated blood-clotting factors and will eventually evolve into a stable, strong blood clot. In addition to forming a plug, the platelets also release chemicals that further stimulate vascular spasm and help to activate the blood-clotting factors. Thus, the platelets participate in all three phases of hemostasis.

Blood Clotting

Vascular spasm and a platelet plug alone are not sufficient to prevent the bleeding caused by a large tear in a blood vessel. With a more serious injury to the vessel wall, bleeding stops only if a blood clot forms. **Blood clotting,** or **coagulation** (kō-ăg″ya-lā′-shan), is the third step in the process of hemostasis. A blood clot is formed by a series of

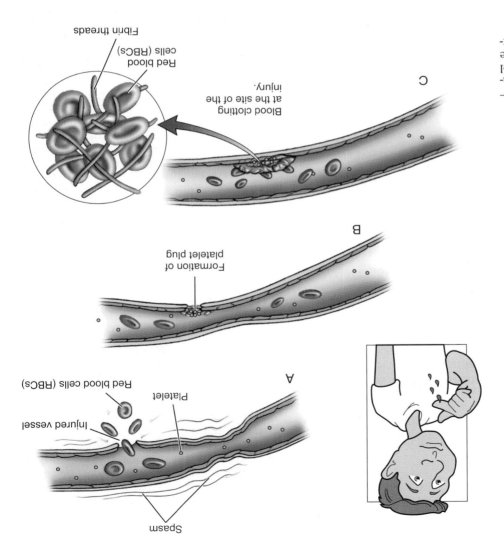

FIGURE 13-8 ● Hemostasis: steps. A, Blood vessel spasm. B, Formation of the platelet plug. C, Blood clotting (coagulation).

Spasm

Injured vessel

Platelet

Red blood cells (RBCs)

A

Formation of platelet plug

B

Blood clotting at the site of the injury.

C

Fibrin threads

Red blood cells (RBCs)

chemical reactions that result in the formation of a net-like structure. The net is composed of protein fibers called **fibrin** (fi'brin). As blood flows through the fibrin net, large particles in the blood, such as RBCs and platelets, become trapped within it. The structure formed by the fibrin net and the trapped elements is called a blood clot. The blood clot seals off the opening in the injured blood vessel and stops the bleeding.

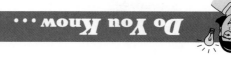

Why is exercise an anticoagulant?

Why is it so important to encourage your patient to walk? As blood circulates throughout the body, a certain amount of thrombin is continuously formed. If the amount of thrombin in any particular site accumulates, a blood clot is apt to develop. In patients who are confined to bed or who sit in a chair for long periods, the blood flow in the lower legs becomes very slow. The slow blood flow creates a condition in which thrombin accumulates and thrombin levels reach a critical concentration. This development ultimately causes a clot to form. By encouraging your patients to exercise, you diminish the chances of thrombosis. In this sense, exercise can be considered a form of anticoagulation.

Formation of the Blood Clot

How does the fibrin net form? The fibrin net is the result of a series of chemical reactions (stages)

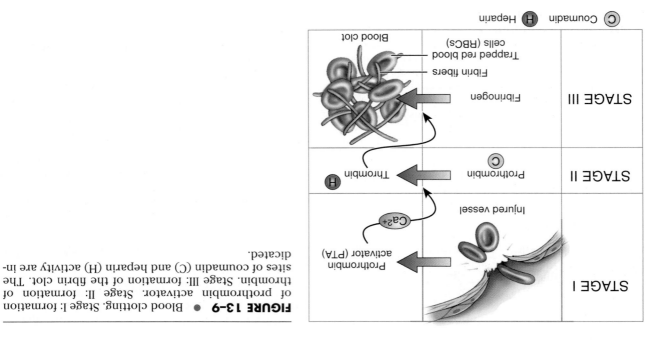

FIGURE 13-9 ● Blood clotting. Stage I: formation of prothrombin activator. Stage II: formation of thrombin. Stage III: formation of the fibrin clot. The sites of coumadin (C) and heparin (H) activity are indicated.

I–III) in which a number of clotting factors are activated. Follow the three stages of blood coagulation identified in Figure 13–9.

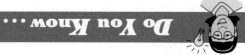

What do Queen Victoria, the "royal disease," and factor VIII have in common?

Hemophilia is a bleeding disorder caused by the deficiency of a clotting factor called **factor VIII**, or the hemophilic factor. Hemophilia was common in the royal families of Europe; hence it was called the "royal disease." Why was hemophilia so prevalent in the royal families? Hemophilia is genetically transmitted. Because of the tendency of the royals to intermarry (eg, cousin marrying cousin), the gene carrying hemophilia was kept in the family and expressed frequently in the royal offspring. Queen Victoria of England carried the gene for hemophilia. Queen Victoria, being both prolific and politically astute, placed a descendent on every throne in Europe. As each descendent married and intermarried, the incidence of hemophilia increased.

- Stage I: Injury to the blood vessel wall activates various clotting factors. These clotting factors normally circulate in the blood in their inactive form. When activated, the clotting factors produce a substance called **prothrombin activator (PTA)**.

- Stage II: In the presence of calcium, platelet chemicals, and PTA, **prothrombin** is activated to form **thrombin.**
- Stage III: Thrombin activates fibrinogen. Activated fibrinogen forms the fibrin fibers, or net. The net traps other blood cells and particles to form the clot. Other factors then stabilize and strengthen the clot.

Anticoagulants

While the body must be able to stop bleeding, it is equally essential for the body to prevent unnecessary clot formation. Several mechanisms prevent clot formation. Two of the most important mechanisms are a smooth inner lining (endothelium) of the blood vessels and the secretion of heparin, an anticoagulant.

ENDOTHELIUM. The inner lining (endothelium) of the blood vessels is smooth and shiny and allows blood to flow easily along its surface. If the surface of the endothelium becomes roughened, however, the platelets and the blood coagulation factors are activated, and blood clots are apt to form. A smooth, shiny endothelium therefore minimizes the risk of clot formation.

SECRETION OF HEPARIN. Heparin is secreted by the mast cells. (Mast cells are basophils that are located in the tissue.) Mast cells are concentrated in and around the liver and lungs. These are sites where the blood is rather stagnant and therefore apt to clot easily. Heparin acts as an anticoagulant by removing thrombin from the clotting process. Note in Figure 13-9 that the formation of thrombin in stage II is crucial for clot formation (the conversion of fibrinogen to fibrin).

ANTICOAGULANT MEDICATIONS. At times, the administration of anticoagulant drugs may be necessary. Anticoagulants are administered in an attempt to prevent the formation of a blood clot. The blood clot is called a **thrombus;** the process of blood clot formation is called **thrombosis.** A piece of the thrombus may break off and travel through the blood to the lungs. The traveling thrombus is called an **embolus.** The danger is that the embolus may lodge in the blood vessels of the lungs, causing a fatal **pulmonary embolus.**

Thrombosis may be prevented by the administration of two types of anticoagulants: heparin and Coumadin. Heparin, designated H in Figure 13-9, acts as an antithrombin agent. Another anticoagulant, called Coumadin, also prevents clot formation. Like heparin, Coumadin interferes with the clotting scheme but does so at a different step. Coumadin, designated C in Figure 13-9, decreases the hepatic (liver) synthesis of prothrombin, causing hypoprothrombinemia (a diminished amount of prothrombin in the blood), which means that less thrombin can be formed. Less thrombin means that blood clotting is diminished.

Clot Retraction

What happens to the clot after it forms? After the clot forms, it begins to condense, or pull itself together; the clot becomes smaller as water is squeezed out. This process is called **clot retraction.** As the clot retracts, the edges of the injured blood vessels are also pulled together. This pulling together slows bleeding and sets the stage for healing, or repair of the blood vessel.

Clot Busting, or Fibrinolysis

After the clot accomplishes its task, it is dissolved. Clots are dissolved by a process called **fibrinolysis** (Fig. 13-10). A substance called **plasmin** dissolves the clot. Plasmin is formed from its inactive form, **plasminogen,** which normally circulates within the blood. Several substances, one of which is **tissue plasminogen activator (TPA),** can activate plasminogen. Tissue plasminogen activator is formed by the tissue surrounding the injury. Recently, tPA has been administered as a drug to persons with life-threatening conditions caused by clots. tPA and related substances form a classification of drugs called clot busters. These drugs

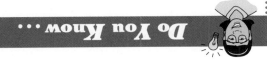

Do You Know...

Why does this toe need this leech?

This toe was accidentally severed from its owner. In reattaching the toe to the foot, the surgeon recognized that the toe graft would be successful only if the blood supply to the toe was good. Frequently after surgery of this type, blood clots develop at the graft site, resulting in a decrease in blood flow. Leeches, or bloodsuckers, may be applied to the site of the graft. As the leech attaches to the skin to feed, it injects a potent anticoagulant. The leech anticoagulant prevents blood clotting at the graft site, thereby maintaining a good blood flow and improving the chances for successful grafting.

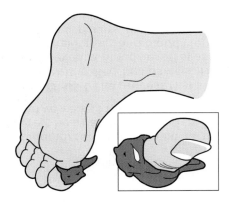

have revolutionized the treatment of myocardial infarction (eg, heart attacks caused by blood clots in the blood vessels of the heart).

✳ **SUM IT UP!** The process that stops bleeding after injury is called hemostasis. Hemostasis involves three events: blood vessel spasm, the formation of a platelet plug, and blood clotting (coagulation). Clotting occurs when thrombin causes the conversion of fibrinogen into the fibrin clot. The clot is dissolved by plasmin. After their job is done, blood clots are dissolved by plasmin.

BLOOD TYPES

Early in the history of medicine are accounts of attempted blood transfusions. Some were successful; others were medical disasters. The earliest physicians recognized that a severely wounded person was in need of blood. They did not realize, however, that blood from one person cannot always be mixed with the blood of another. These physicians unknowingly demonstrated the presence of different blood types.

Antigens and Blood Types

Blood is classified according to specific antigens on the surface of the RBC. An antigen is a genetically determined substance that the body recognizes as foreign. As a foreign substance, an antigen stimulates an antigen-antibody response. This response is designed to attack the antigen.

The **ABO grouping** contains four blood types: A, B, AB, and O. The letters A and B refer to the antigen on the RBC. What does it mean to be type A, B, AB, or O? Look at Table 13-3. A person with

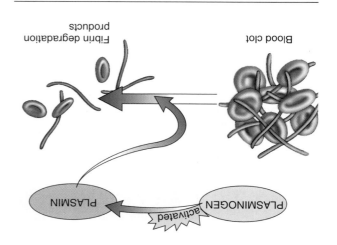

FIGURE 13-10 ● Fibrinolysis: "clot busting." Plasminogen is activated into plasmin, which dissolves the blood clot.

type A blood has the A antigen on the RBC. A person with type B blood has a B antigen on the RBC. A person with type AB blood has both A and B antigens on the RBC. A person with type O blood has neither A nor B antigens on the RBC. Remember: the antigen is located on the RBC membrane.

Antibodies and Blood Type

In addition to the antigens on the RBCs, specific **antibodies** are found in the plasma of each blood type (see Table 13-3). Antibodies bind to specific substances and inactivate them. A person with type A blood has anti-B antibodies in the plasma. A person with type B blood has anti-A antibodies in the plasma. A person with type AB blood has neither anti-A nor anti-B antibodies in the plasma. The person with type O blood has both anti-A and anti-B antibodies in the plasma.

Antigen-Antibody Interaction

Let's back up. Table 13-3 indicates that type A blood contains the A antigen (RBC) and anti-B antibodies (plasma). What would happen if a person had the A antigen on his RBCs and anti-A antibodies in his plasma? The A antigen and the anti-A antibody would cause a clumping reaction much like the curdling seen when milk and vinegar are mixed together.

This clumping of the antigen-antibody interaction is called **agglutination.** Agglutination reactions cause the RBCs to burst or lyse, a process called **hemolysis** (hē-mŏl'ĭ-sĭs). If rapid hemolysis were to occur within the circulation, hemoglobin would be liberated from the RBCs and would eventually clog the kidneys and possibly cause death.

Compatibility and Incompatibility of Blood Types

The curdling, or agglutination, reaction has important implications for blood transfusions. Some blood types mix without undergoing agglutination reactions; they are said to be **compatible blood groups.** Other blood groups agglutinate, causing severe hemolysis, kidney failure, and death. These blood groups are **incompatible.** To avoid giving a person incompatible blood, donor blood is first typed and cross-matched.

What do blood typing and cross-matching mean? First, the blood type (A, B, AB, or O) is determined. Then a sample of donor blood (blood from the person who donates it) is mixed (cross-matched) with a sample of recipient blood (blood from the person who is to receive the donated blood). Any evidence of agglutination indicates that the donor blood is incompatible with the recipient's blood.

Suppose a recipient of a blood transfusion has type A blood. She then can be given type A blood and type O blood (see Table 13–3). No antigen-antibody reaction (agglutination) would occur because type A donor blood has the A antigen and the recipient has only anti-B antibodies (plasma). The type O donor blood does not cause agglutination because that person's RBC has neither the A nor the B antigen. Type A and type O blood are therefore compatible with type A blood.

Note what happens, however, if the type A recipient receives type B blood (see Table 13–3). Type B donor blood has the B antigen on each RBC surface. The plasma antibodies of the recipient has anti-B and the anti-B antibodies cause agglutination. Thus, type B blood is incompatible with type A blood. What happens if the type A recipient is given type AB blood? In this case, the RBC contains both A and B antigens. The plasma of the recipient contains anti-B antibodies. Thus, when types A and AB are mixed, an agglutination reaction occurs; these blood groups are incompatible. The administration of incompatible blood groups forms the basis of blood transfusion reactions. The same line of reasoning is used to explain the compatibility/incompatibility characteristics of the four blood groups (see Table 13–3).

Note in Table 13–3 that type O blood can be given to all four blood groups. Type O blood is therefore called the **universal donor.** For this reason blood banks stock a large supply of type O blood. Note also that type AB blood can receive all four types of blood; it is called the **universal recipient.** Note that recipients can receive their own blood types. In other words, a type A recipient can receive type A blood. The type B recipient can re-

Table 13•3	ABO BLOOD GROUPS			
Blood Type	**Antigen** (RBC membrane)	**Antibody** (plasma)	**Can receive blood from**	**Can donate blood to**
A (40%)	A antigen	Anti-B antibodies	A, O	A, AB
B (10%)	B antigen	Anti-A antibodies	B, O	B, AB
AB* (4%)	A antigen, B antigen	No antibodies	A, B, AB, O	AB
O† (46%)	No antigen	Both Anti-A & Anti-B antibodies	O	O, A, B, AB

*Type AB: universal recipient.
†Type O: universal donor.

ceive type B blood. The same is true for types AB and O. Table 13–3 also indicates the prevalence of the four blood types. Type A blood occurs in 40% of the population. Ten percent of the population has type B. Four percent has type AB, and 46% has type O. Note that type O is the most common while type AB is the least common. What blood type are you?

Rh Classification System

Blood is also classified according to the Rh factor. The **Rh factor** is an antigen located on the surface of the RBC. The Rh factor was named for the Rhesus monkey, in which it was first detected. If an RBC contains the Rh factor, the blood is said to be **Rh-positive (+)**. If the RBC lacks the Rh factor, the blood is said to be **Rh-negative (−)**. Approximately 85% of the population is Rh-positive (+).

Plasma does not naturally carry anti-Rh antibodies. In two conditions however, the plasma of an Rh-negative (−) person can develop anti-Rh antibodies. The first condition involves the adminis-tration of Rh-positive (+) blood to an Rh-negative (−) person. If Rh-positive (+) blood (from a donor) is administered to an Rh-negative (−) per-son (the recipient), the Rh antigen of the donor stimulates the recipient to produce anti-Rh anti-bodies. The recipient is now said to be sensitized. If the Rh-negative (−) person is later given a sec-ond transfusion of Rh-positive (+) blood, the anti-Rh antibodies in the plasma of the recipient will at-tack the Rh antigen of the Rh-positive (+) donor blood, causing agglutination and hemolysis.

The Rh factor may cause a serious problem in a second condition, that of an Rh-negative (−) pregnant mother who is carrying an Rh-positive (+) fetus (Fig. 13–11). During this first pregnancy, the baby grows to term and is delivered unevent-fully. During childbirth, however, some of the baby's Rh-positive (+) blood crosses the placenta and enters the mother's circulation. The Rh anti-gen stimulates the mother's immune system to produce anti-Rh antibodies. In other words, the mother has become sensitized by her first baby. If the mother becomes pregnant for a second time with an Rh-positive (+) baby, the anti-Rh antibod-ies move from the mother's circulation into the baby's circulation. These anti-Rh antibodies attack

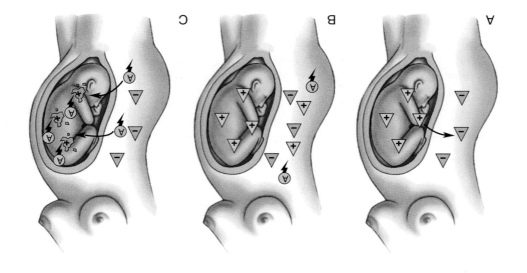

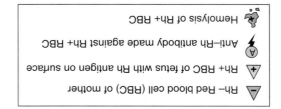

△ Rh− Red blood cell (RBC) of mother

⊕ Rh+ RBC of fetus with Rh antigen on surface

Ⓐ Anti−Rh antibody made against Rh+ RBC

✦ Hemolysis of Rh+ RBC

FIGURE 13–11 ● Hemolysis: erythroblastosis fetalis. The problem of the Rh-negative (−) mother carrying the Rh-positive (+) infant. A, During the first pregnancy, the mother is exposed to the Rh+ antigens from the infant. B, The mother produces anti-Rh antibodies to the Rh antigen. C, During a second pregnancy, the mother's anti-Rh antibodies attack the Rh antigen of the fetus, causing agglutination and hemolysis of red blood cells.

Disorders of the Blood

Anemia — A condition in which the number of red blood cells (RBCs) decreases or the amount of hemoglobin decreases. There are many types of anemia. Hemorrhagic anemia is due to loss of blood. Aplastic anemia is a decrease in RBCs because of impaired bone marrow activity. Hemolytic anemia develops in response to excess RBC destruction. Anemias may develop when necessary substances are not present. For instance, a dietary deficiency of iron causes iron-deficiency anemia. A dietary deficiency of folic acid causes folic acid–deficiency anemia. An inability to absorb vitamin B12 is called pernicious anemia.

Blood poisoning — Also called septicemia from the Greek word meaning rotten blood. Blood poisoning refers to the presence of harmful substances, such as bacteria and toxins, in the blood.

Ecchymosis — Also called a bruise. Blood leaks into the tissue following an injury. As the hemoglobin breaks down, it forms breakdown products, which color the skin black and blue and then dull yellow-brown.

Hemophilia — A hereditary deficiency of factor VIII, or the hemophilic factor, resulting in impaired ability to clot blood and severe bleeding episodes. There are many other hereditary bleeding disorders. Christmas disease is a deficiency of factor IX, and von Willebrand's disease is a deficiency of a protein that affects factor VIII function.

continued

As You Age

1. The volume and composition of blood remain constant with age, so most laboratory values remain normal. Alterations in laboratory values for blood usually indicate alterations in other organ systems. For instance, the fasting blood glucose level increases with aging. This alteration is not the result of changes in the blood, however. Rather, it is the result of age-related changes associated with insulin. The same is true regarding serum lipids. While serum lipids increase 25% to 50% after the age of 55, the increase is due to an altered metabolism and not to changes of the blood and blood-forming organs.

2. The amount of red bone marrow decreases with age. While the total number of blood cells remains normal, older persons take longer to form new blood cells and so recover more slowly from bleeding episodes (hemorrhages).

3. An age-related decline occurs in white blood cell (WBC) activity. Although WBC activity increases in response to infection, it does so more slowly.

---

the baby's RBCs, causing agglutination. In response, the baby becomes jaundiced and anemic as the RBCs undergo hemolysis.

This hemolytic condition is called **erythroblastosis fetalis.** The hemolysis causes a rapid rise in plasma levels of bilirubin. The hyperbilirubinemia (increased bilirubin in the blood), in turn, causes severe jaundice and a condition called kernicterus. **Kernicterus,** caused by the staining of a part of the brain with bilirubin, is characterized by severe retardation in mental development.

Erythroblastosis fetalis can be prevented by the administration of the drug RhoGam. RhoGam is administered to the mother during pregnancy and within 72 hours after delivery. The RhoGam surrounds, or coats, the baby's Rh-positive (+) antigens, thereby preventing them from stimulating the development of anti-Rh antibodies by the mother.

✳ **SUM IT UP!** Blood is classified according to the antigens on the surface of the RBC. The ABO grouping contains four blood types: A (A antigens), B (B antigens), AB (A and B antigens), and O (neither A nor B antigens). An antigen-antibody reaction, called agglutination, occurs when blood is mismatched. Type AB blood is the universal recipient blood. Type O blood is the universal donor blood. The Rh factor is another type of antigen on blood. Rh-positive blood has the Rh factor on the RBC, whereas Rh-negative blood does not contain the Rh factor.

Disorders of the Blood continued

Leukemia
Called cancer of the blood and characterized by uncontrolled leukocyte production. The abnormal leukocytes invade the bone marrow and impair normal blood cell production. As with other cancers, malignant cells metastasize through the body.

Polycythemia
Means many cells in the blood. Polycythemia vera (meaning true polycythemia) is due to the overproduction of blood cells (usually red blood cells) by the bone marrow. Secondary polycythemia refers to an increase in blood cell production in response to a condition that interferes with oxygenation, such as lung disease.

Summary Outline

Blood has three main functions: it delivers oxygen to all cells; it helps regulate body functions, such as body temperature; and it protects the body from infection and bleeding.

I. Blood

A. Composition of Blood
1. Blood is composed of plasma and formed elements.
2. Plasma contains water, electrolytes, nutrients, and plasma proteins.
3. The formed elements are called corpuscles, or blood cells.
4. There are three types of blood cells: red blood cells (RBCs, or erythrocytes), white blood cells (WBCs, or leukocytes), and platelets (thrombocytes).

B. Origin of the Blood Cells, Sites of Hematopoiesis
1. The red blood cells, white blood cells, and platelets are produced in the red bone marrow from a single stem cell.
2. Lymphocytes and monocytes originate in the red marrow but mature in the lymphatic tissue. Lymphocytes are also produced in lymphatic tissue.

C. Red Blood Cells (RBCs)
1. RBCs are tiny, disc-shaped cells that can bend.
2. RBCs are almost completely filled with hemoglobin; oxyhemoglobin transports oxygen, and carbaminohemoglobin transports carbon dioxide.
3. RBC synthesis requires many substances, including iron, vitamin B_{12}, and folic acid. A deficiency of these substances causes anemia.
4. RBC production is regulated by erythropoietin; this hormone is released by the kidneys in response to low tissue levels of oxygen.
5. RBCs are removed by the tissue macrophage system (macrophages found primarily in the liver, spleen, and red bone marrow).

D. White Blood Cells (WBCs)
1. WBCs are classified as granulocytes and agranulocytes.
2. The granulocytes include neutrophils (highly phagocytic), basophils, and eosinophils.
3. The nongranulocytes, or agranulocytes, are the lymphocytes (immunity) and the monocytes (phagocytic).

E. Platelets
1. Platelets are thrombocytes; they are fragments of megakaryocytes.
2. Platelets are involved in hemostasis.

II. Hemostasis

A. Stages of Hemostasis
1. The three stages of hemostasis are blood vessel spasm, formation of a platelet plug, and blood coagulation.
2. The three stages of blood coagulation are formation of prothrombin activator, conversion of prothrombin to thrombin, and conversion of fibrinogen into fibrin fibers (the clot).

B. Dissolving Clots and Preventing Clot Formation
1. Eventually the clot dissolves by a process called fibrinolysis; clot dissolution is achieved primarily by plasmin.
2. Natural anticoagulant mechanisms prevent clotting and include a smooth endothelial lining and heparin.

III. Blood Types

A. ABO Blood Types
1. Type A has A antigen on the RBC membrane and has anti-B antibodies in the plasma.
2. Type B has B antigen on the RBC membrane and has anti-A antibodies in the plasma.
3. Type AB has both A and B antigens on the RBC membrane and has neither anti-A nor anti-B antibodies in the plasma.

Summary Outline, continued

III. Blood Types, continued

4. Type O has neither A nor B antigen on the RBC membrane and has both anti-A and anti-B antibodies in the plasma.
5. Type O is the universal donor; type AB is the universal recipient.
6. Antigen-antibody reactions are the basis of transfusion reactions.

B. Rh Factor

1. An Rh-positive person has the Rh antigen on the RBC membrane; an Rh-positive person does not have anti-Rh antibodies in the plasma.
2. An Rh-negative person does not have the Rh antigen on the RBC membrane. An Rh-negative person may develop anti-Rh antibodies.
3. An Rh-negative mother carrying an Rh-positive baby may give birth to a baby with erythroblastosis fetalis. This condition is caused by an antigen-antibody reaction (Rh antigen–anti-Rh antibodies).

Review Your Knowledge

1. Name five substances that blood transports.
2. What are the two major ways blood aids the body in protection?
3. List words to describe the following characteristics of blood:
   a. Classification of tissue type
   b. Color
   c. Average amount of blood in body
   d. Consistency (thick or thin compared with water)
4. What are the two major parts of blood?
5. What are three functions of plasma proteins?
6. What is the major function of
   a. Red blood cells (erythrocytes)
   b. White blood cells (leukocytes)
   c. Platelets (thrombocytes)
7. What does the hematocrit measure? What is the significance of a low hematocrit?
8. How does the red bone marrow produce three different kinds of blood cells?
9. Name three conditions that develop when myelosuppression occurs.
10. State the normal blood counts for
    a. Red blood cells (erythrocytes)
    b. White blood cells (leukocytes)
    c. Platelets (thrombocytes)
11. Which four substances are necessary for the development of hemoglobin?
12. How does the body respond to a drop in the number of circulating red blood cells?
13. How are components of old red blood cells re-cycled?
14. What is the significance of an increased white blood cell count? What happens to the body if there are not enough white blood cells?
15. What is the function of macrophages?
16. What are the symptoms of a person with thrombocytopenia?
17. Why is a differential count often done with a white blood cell count?
18. What are the differences between hemostasis, coagulation, fibrinolysis, and hemorrhage?
19. Name the four blood types. Which type is the universal donor? Which type is the universal recipient?
20. What causes a blood transfusion reaction?
21. What happens if an Rh− mother has an Rh+ baby?

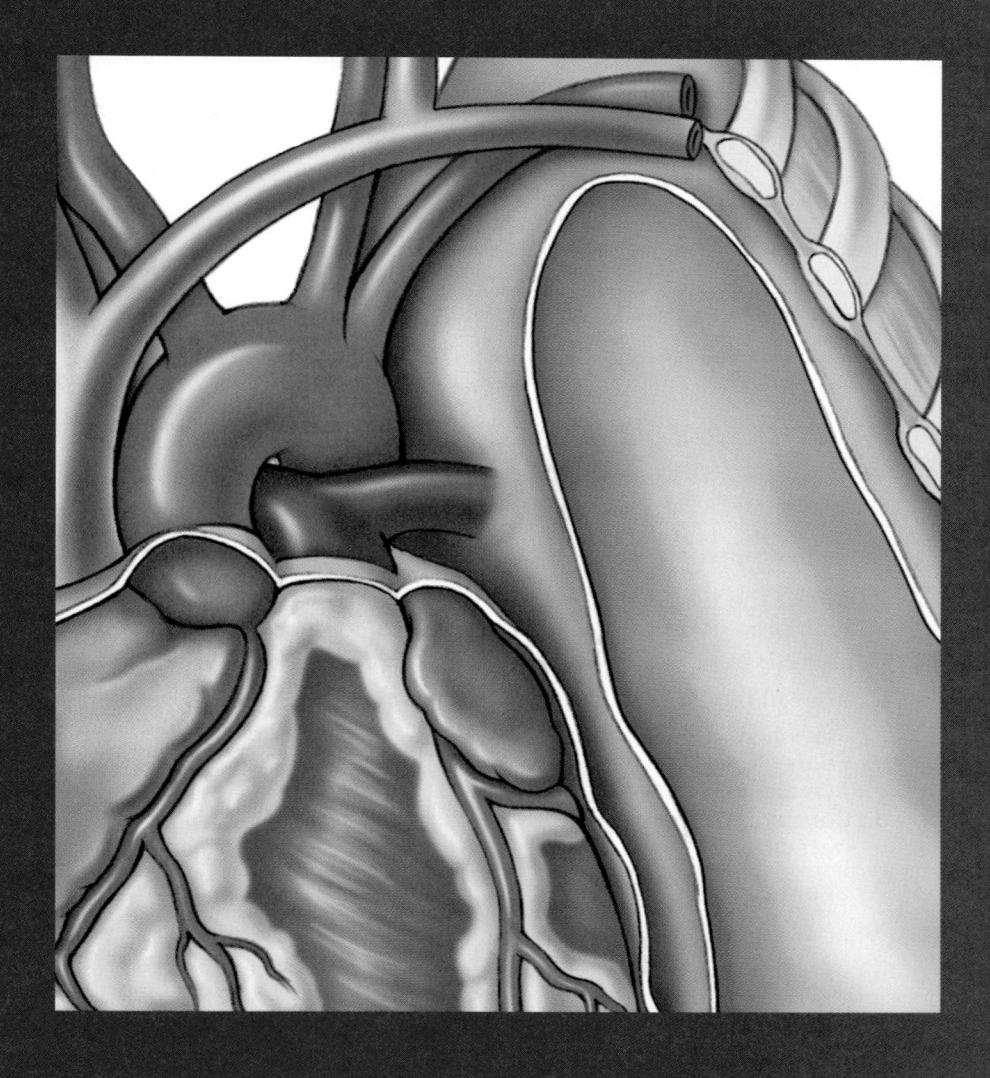

••• Key Terms

Atrium (ā'trē-əm)

Cardiac conduction system
(kär'dē-ăk kən-dŭk'shən sĭs'təm)

Cardiac cycle (kär'dē-ăk sī'kəl)

Cardiac output ((kär'dē-ăk out'poŏt)

Chordae tendineae (kôr'dē těn-dĭn'ē-ē)

Diastole (dī-ăs'tə-lē)

Electrocardiogram (ECG)
(ē-lěk"trō-kär'dē-ə-grăm")

Endocardium (ěn"dō-kär'dē-əm)

Epicardium (ěp'ĭ-kär'dē-əm)

Inotropic effect (ĭn"ə-trōp'ĭk ě-fěkt')

Mitral valve (bicuspid valve)
(mī'trəl vălv; bī-kŭs'pĭd vălv)

Myocardium (mī"ō-kär'dē-əm)

Pericardium (pěr"ĭ-kär'dē-əm)

Purkinje fibers (pûr-kĭn'jē fī'bûrz)

Semilunar valve (sěm"ē-loō'nər vălv)

Starling's law of the heart
(stär'lĭngz lô)

Stroke volume (strōk vŏl'yoōm)

Systole (sĭs'tə-lē)

Tricuspid valve (trī-kŭs'pĭd vălv)

Ventricle (věn'trĭ-kəl)

••• Selected terms in bold type in this chapter are defined in the Glossary.

14 HEART

*O*bjectives

1. Describe the location of the heart.
2. Name the three layers and covering of the heart.
3. Explain the function of the heart as two separate pumps.
4. Identify the four chambers of the heart.
5. Explain the functions of the four heart valves.
6. Describe the characteristics of the heart that affect the two main heart sounds.
7. Describe blood flow through the heart.
8. List the vessels that supply blood to the heart.
9. Identify the major components of the heart's conduction system.
10. Describe the events of the cardiac cycle.
11. Name five factors that affect heart rate.
12. List two ways in which stroke volume may be altered.

Throughout history, many functions have been attributed to the heart. Some philosophers have called it the seat of the soul. The ancient Egyptians, for instance, weighed the heart after a person's death because they believed that the weight of the heart equaled the weight of the soul. The heart has also been described as the seat of wisdom and understanding; accordingly, it thinks and makes plans. More often than not, however, history has portrayed the heart as the seat of the emotions. An overly compassionate person is described as soft-hearted. A generous person has a heart of gold. And a grief-stricken person is broken-hearted. Every Valentine's Day card displays hearts, hearts, and more hearts. These cards celebrate love. None ever mentions the heart as an efficient pump.

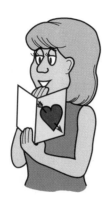

STRUCTURE OF THE HEART: WHAT IT IS

Location and Size

The heart is a hollow, muscular organ. Its primary function is to pump and force blood through the blood vessels of the body, providing every cell in the body with vital nutrients and oxygen. The heart pumps an average of 72 times each minute for your entire lifetime. If you live until you are 75, your heart will beat in excess of 3 billion times. What an amazing organ!

The adult heart is about the size of a closed fist. The heart sits in the chest within the mediastinum, between the two lungs (Fig. 14–1). It lies toward the left side of the body. Two thirds of the heart is located to the left of the midline of the sternum, and one third is located to the right. The upper flat portion of the heart is located at the level of the second rib. The other end of the heart is the **apex.** The apex is the lower and more pointed end of the heart and is located at the level of the fifth rib.

The heart lies within and is supported by a sling-like structure called the **pericardium** (pĕr″ĭ-kär′dē-əm). The pericardium attaches the heart to surrounding structures, such as the diaphragm. You need to know the precise location of the heart because you will be asked to evaluate different heart sounds, accurately position electrodes for electrocardiographic readings, and provide life-saving cardiopulmonary resuscitation (CPR).

The Heart's Layers and Coverings

The heart is made up of three layers of tissue: endocardium, myocardium, and epicardium (Fig. 14–2).

Endocardium

The **endocardium** (ĕn″dō-kär′dē-əm) is the heart's innermost layer. It is a thin layer of tissue composed of simple squamous epithelium overlying a layer of connective tissue. The smooth and shiny surface allows blood to flow over it easily. The endocardial lining also lines the valves and is continuous with the blood vessels that enter and leave the heart.

Myocardium

The **myocardium** (mī″ō-kär′dē-əm) is the thick middle layer of the heart. It is the thickest of the three layers. The myocardium is composed of cardiac muscle tissue. The cardiac muscle allows the heart to contract and therefore to propel blood, or force it forward, through the blood vessels.

The myocardium consists of bundles of muscle fibers twisted into a ring-like arrangement. This arrangement of muscle is reinforced by dense fibrous connective tissue, sometimes called the skeleton of the heart. This ring-like arrangement of myocardial tissue enables the heart to pump effectively.

Epicardium

The **epicardium** (ĕp″ĭ-kär′dē-əm) is the thin outermost layer of the heart (see Fig. 14–2). The epicardium is continuous at the apex of the heart with the inner lining of the pericardium, the loose-fitting, sling-like structure that protects and supports the heart. The outer side of the pericardium anchors the heart to surrounding structures such as the diaphragm and sternum.

Pericardium

Between the epicardium and the pericardium is a space called the **pericardial space,** or **pericardial cavity.** The pericardial membranes are serous membranes that secrete a small amount of slip-

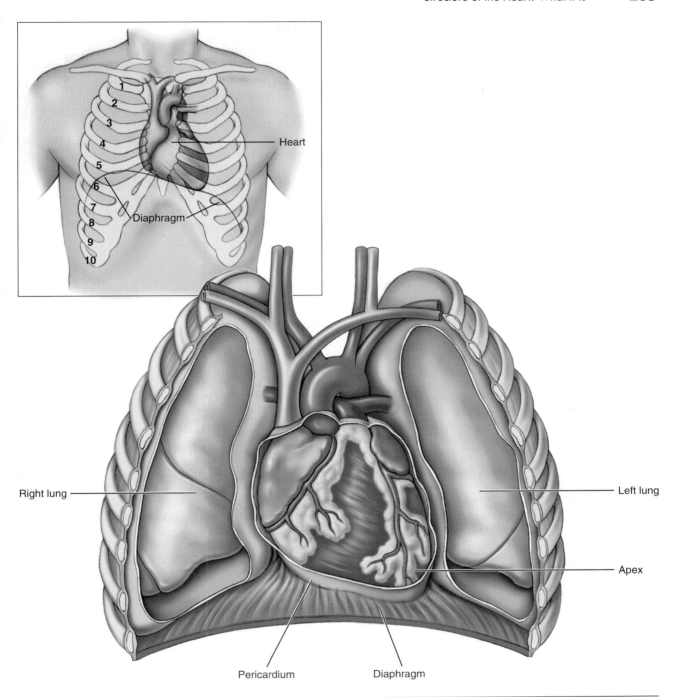

FIGURE 14-1 ● Location of the heart. The heart is located within the mediastinum, mostly left of the midline of the body. The heart is supported by a sling-like structure called the pericardium.

pery serous fluid into the pericardial space. The pericardial fluid lubricates the surfaces of the membranes and allows them to slide past one another with very little friction or rubbing.

At times, the pericardial membranes become inflamed and secrete excess serous fluid into the pericardial space. This collection of fluid in the pericardial space compresses the heart externally, making it difficult for the heart to relax and fill with blood. Consequently, the heart is unable to pump a sufficient amount of blood to the body. This life-threatening condition is called **cardiac tamponade.** The symptoms of cardiac tamponade may be relieved by inserting a long needle into the pericardial space and aspirating (sucking out) the serous fluid through the needle.

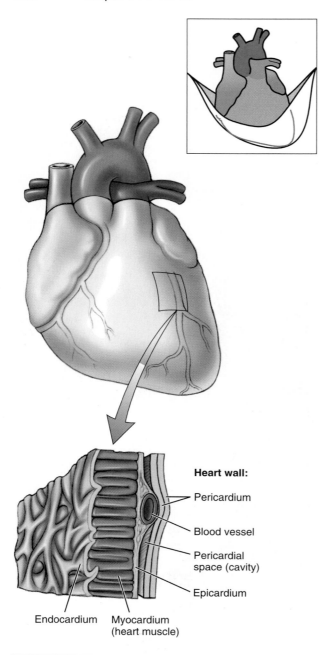

Heart wall:

Pericardium

Blood vessel

Pericardial
space (cavity)

Epicardium

Endocardium   Myocardium
(heart muscle)

FIGURE 14–2 ● Layers of the heart and the pericardium: endocardium, the inner layer; myocardium, the thick middle layer; epicardium, the outer layer. The heart is supported by a sling-like structure called the pericardium. Note the pericardial space (cavity) between the epicardium and the pericardium.

A Double Pump and Two Circulations

The myocardium enables the heart to pump blood. The heart is like a double pump, or two pumps that beat as one. The pumps are the **right heart** and the **left heart** (Fig. 14–3). The right

heart receives unoxygenated blood from the superior and inferior venae cavae, large veins that collect blood from all parts of the body. The right heart is colored blue because it contains unoxygenated blood. The right heart pumps blood to the lungs, where the blood is oxygenated.

The path that the blood follows from the right side of the heart to and through the lungs and back to the left side of the heart is called the **pulmonary circulation.** The only function of the pulmonary circulation is to circulate blood through the lungs so that oxygen can be loaded and carbon dioxide can be unloaded. Oxygen diffuses from the lungs into the blood, while carbon dioxide diffuses from the blood into the lungs for excretion.

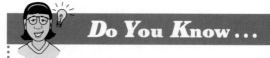

What is a failing heart?

A failing heart refers to the inability to pump enough blood out of the heart to supply the cells of the body with nutrients and oxygen. The failing heart is a sick pump. Heart failure is either right-sided (failing right ventricle) or left-sided (failing left ventricle).

The left heart receives the oxygenated blood from the lungs and pumps it to all the organs of the body. The left heart is colored red because it contains oxygenated blood. The path that the blood follows from the left heart to all the organs of the body and back to the right heart is called the **systemic circulation.** The systemic circulation is the larger of the two circulations.

The Heart's Chambers and Large Vessels

The heart has four chambers: two atria and two ventricles (Fig. 14–4). The **atria** (the upper chambers, singular **atrium** [ā'trē-əm]) receive the blood; the **ventricles** (věn'trĭ-kəlz) (lower chambers) pump the blood out of the heart. The right and left hearts are separated from one another by a septum. The **interatrial septum** separates the two atria; the **interventricular septum** separates the two ventricles.

Right Atrium

The right atrium is a thin-walled cavity that receives unoxygenated (blue) blood from the large veins called the superior and inferior venae cavae.

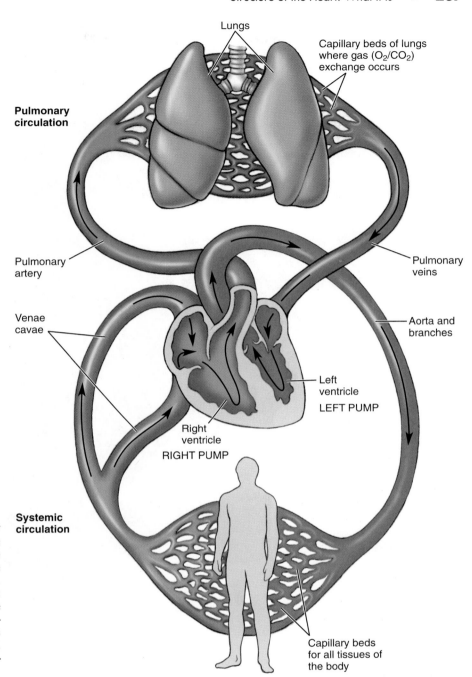

FIGURE 14-3 ● A double pump and two circulations. The heart is a double pump, the right heart and the left heart. The right heart (blue) pumps blood to the lungs. This is the pump for the pulmonary circulation. The left heart (red) pumps blood to all the cells of the body. This is the pump for the systemic circulation.

The **superior vena cava** collects blood from the head and the upper body region and delivers it to the right atrium. The **inferior vena cava** receives blood from the lower part of the body and delivers it to the right atrium.

Right Ventricle

The right ventricle receives unoxygenated blood from the right atrium and pumps it to the lungs through the pulmonary artery. The primary function of the right ventricle is to pump blood to the lungs. The main pulmonary artery divides into

right and left branches, which carry blood to both the right and left lungs.

Left Atrium

The left atrium is a thin-walled cavity that receives oxygenated (red) blood from the lungs through four pulmonary veins.

Left Ventricle

The left ventricle receives oxygenated blood from the left atrium. The primary function of the

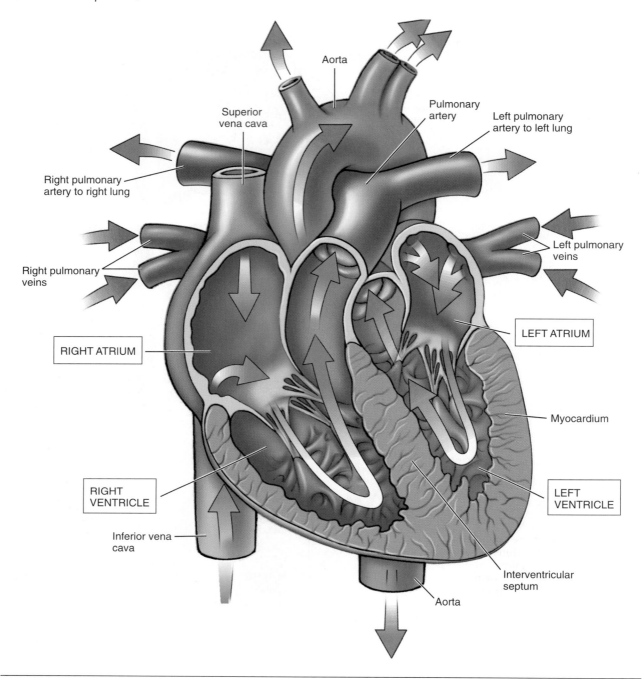

FIGURE 14–4 ● Chambers of the heart and the large vessels. There are four cardiac chambers: two atria (right and left) and two ventricles (right and left). The large vessels include the venae cavae, the pulmonary artery, and the aorta.

left ventricle is to pump blood into the systemic circulation. Blood leaves the left ventricle through the **aorta,** the largest artery of the body. Note the thickness of the myocardial layer of the ventricles. The thick muscle is needed to generate enough force to pump blood out of the heart. Note also that the left ventricular myocardium is thicker than the right ventricular myocardium. This difference is due to the greater amount of force required to pump blood into the systemic circulation.

Heart Valves

The purpose of the heart valves is to keep the blood flowing in a forward direction. The four valves in the heart lie at the entrance and exit of the ventricles (Fig. 14–5). Two of the valves are called **atrioventricular valves,** or **AV valves.** They are located between the atria and the ventricles. Blood flows from the atria through the atrioventricular valves into the ventricles.

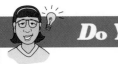

Why can an impaired left ventricle cause fluid to accumulate in the lungs?

Blood normally flows from the pulmonary capillaries into the left side of the heart. The left ventricle then pumps the blood out of the heart into the systemic circulation. If the left ventricle cannot pump effectively, blood accumulates in the left side of the heart and in the pulmonary veins and pulmonary capillaries. Fluid seeps out of the pulmonary capillaries into the lungs, causing severe difficulty in breathing and cyanosis. The inability of the left ventricle to pump effectively is called left-sided heart failure.

Atrioventricular valves are entrance valves because they allow blood to enter the ventricles. The other two valves are classified as **semilunar valves** (sĕm″ē-loo′nər vălvz), so named because the flaps of the valves resemble a half-moon (*semi* means half; *lunar* means moon). The semilunar valves help determine the outflow of blood from the right and left ventricles and are therefore exit valves.

Atrioventricular Valves

The AV valves are entrance valves. They are located between the atria and the ventricles on each side of the heart. The AV valves have cusps, or flaps (see Fig. 14–5). When the ventricles are relaxed, the cusps hang loosely within the ventricles; in this position the valves are open and permit the flow of blood from the atria into the ventricles.

What closes the AV valves? When the ventricles contract, the heart muscle compresses and squeezes the blood in the ventricles. The blood then pushes the cusps upward toward the atria, into a closed position. The closed AV valves prevent the backward flow of blood from the ventricles to the atria.

Why are the cusps not pushed completely through the openings, into the atria, as the pressures within the ventricles increase during muscle contraction? The cusps are attached to the ventricular wall by tough fibrous bands of tissue called **chordae tendineae** (kôr′dē tĕn-dĭn′ē-ē) (see Fig. 14–5). As blood pushes the cusps into a closed position, the chordae tendineae are

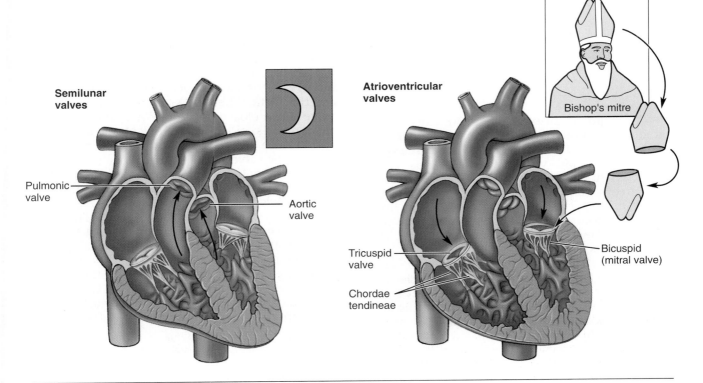

FIGURE 14–5 ● Valves of the heart. There are four valves: two atrioventricular (AV) valves and two semilunar (SL) valves. The SL valves are the pulmonic valve and the aortic valve. The AV valves are the tricuspid and bicuspid (mitral) valves. The cusps, or flaps, of the AV valves are attached to the walls of the ventricles by the chordae tendineae.

stretched to their full length. The stretched chordae tendineae hold onto the cusps and prevent them from "blowing" through into the atria.

Do You Know...

What do this umbrella and the chordae tendineae have in common?

This unfortunate umbrella has been turned inside out by the wind. The chordae tendineae attach to the undersurface of the AV valves and prevent them from turning inside out when the ventricles contract and push blood against the cusps. In the event that the chordae rupture or snap, the AV valve would resemble the umbrella, and blood would flow backward, from the ventricles into the atria.

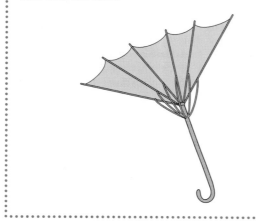

The **right atrioventricular (AV) valve** is located between the right atrium and the right ventricle. The right AV valve is called the **tricuspid valve** (trī-kŭs′pĭd vălv) because it has three cusps. When the tricuspid valve is open, blood flows freely from the right atrium into the right ventricle. When the right ventricle contracts, however, the tricuspid valve closes and prevents blood from flowing back into the right atrium. The valve ensures a forward flow of blood.

The **left atrioventricular (AV) valve** is located between the left atrium and the left ventricle. The left AV valve is called the **bicuspid valve** (bī-kŭs′pĭd vălv) because it has two cusps. It is also called the **mitral valve** (mī′trəl vălv) because it resembles a bishop's mitre, a hat with two flaps. When the mitral valve is open, blood flows from the left atrium into the left ventricle. When the left ventricle contracts, the mitral valve closes and prevents the flow of blood from the left ventricle back into the left atrium. The valve ensures a forward flow of blood.

Do You Know...

What happens when your heart valve becomes leaky?

A leaky, or incompetent, valve allows blood to leak back into the chamber from which it has just been pumped. In other words, the leaky valve allows the blood to flow in the wrong direction. This condition increases the workload of the heart because the heart must repeatedly pump the same blood. Over time, a leaky valve causes more serious heart problems. The defective valve must eventually be repaired or replaced.

Semilunar Valves

The two semilunar valves (exit valves) are the pulmonic valve and the aortic valve (see Fig. 14–5).

PULMONIC VALVE. The **pulmonic valve** is also called the **pulmonary valve** or the **right semilunar valve.** It is located between the right ventricle and the pulmonary artery. When the right ventricle relaxes, the valve is in a closed position. When the right ventricle contracts, blood from the ventricle forces the pulmonic valve open. Blood then flows through the open valve into the pulmonary artery, the large vessel that carries the blood from the right ventricle to the lungs. When the right ventricle relaxes, the pulmonic valve snaps closed and prevents any blood from returning to the right ventricle from the pulmonary artery.

AORTIC VALVE. The **aortic valve** or the **left semilunar valve** is located between the left ventricle and the aorta. When the left ventricle relaxes, the valve is in a closed position. When the left ventricle contracts, blood from the ventricle forces the aortic valve open. The blood flows through the open aortic valve into the aorta. When the left ventricle relaxes, the aortic valve snaps closed and prevents any backflow of blood from the aorta into the ventricle.

How do the semilunar valves close? The semilunar valves close when the pressure in the pulmonary artery and the aorta becomes greater than the pressure in the ventricles. The blood in these large blood vessels gets behind the flaps of the valves, snapping them closed. The closed semilunar valves prevent the backward flow of blood from the pulmonary artery and aorta into the ventricles.

Heart Sounds

The heart sounds (sounds like "lubb-dupp") are made by the vibrations caused by the closure of the valves. The first heart sound, lubb, is due to the closure of the AV valves at the beginning of ventricular contraction. The second heart sound, dupp, is due to the closure of the semilunar valves at the beginning of ventricular relaxation. When valves become faulty, the heart sounds change. Abnormal heart sounds are called **murmurs.** The positions of the valves can be located according to rib number (Fig. 14–6).

Pathway: Blood Flow Through the Heart

The arrows in Figure 14–4 indicate the pathway of blood as it flows through the heart. Unoxygenated (blue) blood enters the right atrium from the superior and inferior venae cavae. The blood flows through the tricuspid valve into the right ventricle. From the right ventricle, the blood flows through the pulmonic valve into the pulmonary artery. The right and left pulmonary arteries carry unoxygenated blood to the lungs for gas exchange. The blood releases carbon dioxide as waste and picks up a fresh supply of oxygen.

The oxygenated (red) blood flows through four pulmonary veins from the lungs into the left atrium. From the left atrium, the blood flows through the bicuspid, or mitral, valve into the left ventricle. Left ventricular contraction forces blood through the aortic valve into the aorta for distribution to the systemic circulation. The pathway of blood flow through the heart and pulmonary circulation is summarized in Figure 14–7.

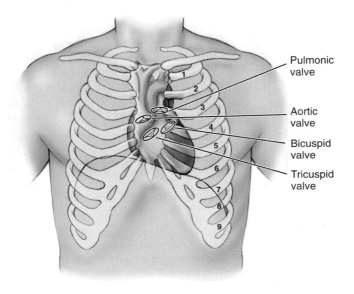

FIGURE 14–6 ● Location of heart valves. By counting ribs, you can locate each valve.

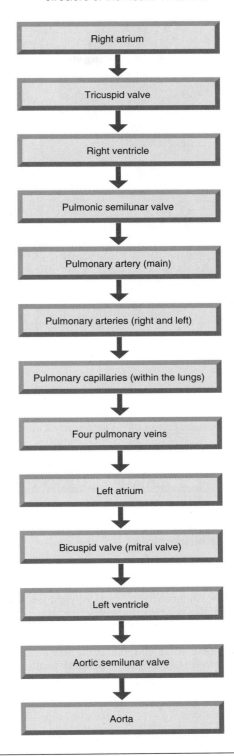

FIGURE 14–7 ● Blood flow through the heart and pulmonary circulation.

Blood Supply to the Myocardium

Although blood constantly flows through the heart, this blood does not nourish the myocardium. The blood supply that nourishes and oxy-

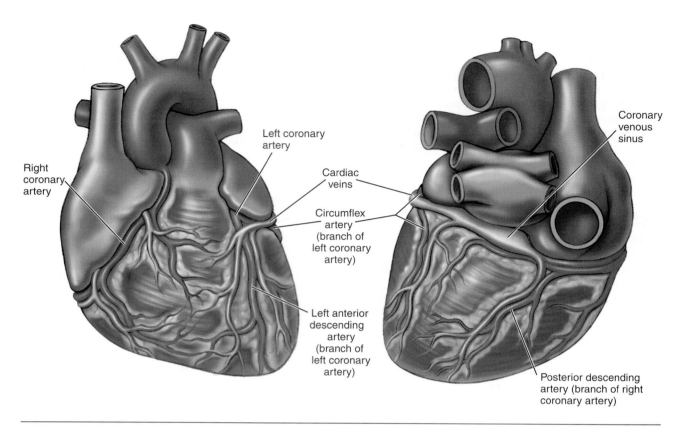

FIGURE 14–8 ● Blood supply to the myocardium: coronary blood vessels. The myocardium is supplied by the right and left coronary arteries. The left coronary artery branches into the left anterior descending artery and the circumflex artery. The coronary veins collect blood and empty it into the coronary venous sinus, which eventually empties into the right atrium.

Do You Know...

What happens if coronary blood flow becomes inadequate?

If coronary blood flow decreases, the myocardial cells are deprived of oxygen and cannot perform their work. This condition is called ischemia and is accompanied by a type of pain known as angina. If the oxygen deprivation is too severe, myocardial cell death (necrosis) may occur. This condition is a myocardial infarction, or a heart attack. Both ischemia and infarction may be caused by the development of fatty plaques in the coronary arteries. When atherosclerotic plaques narrow the coronary artery, the myocardium becomes ischemic. When the plaques completely block the coronary arteries, an infarct develops.

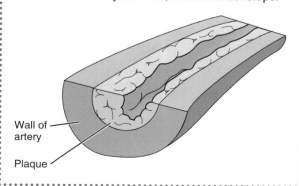

Wall of artery

Plaque

genates the myocardium is provided by the **coronary arteries** (Fig. 14–8). The arteries supplying the myocardium are called coronary arteries because they resemble a crown encircling the heart (the Latin word for crown is *corona*). The coronary arteries arise from the base of the aorta just above the aortic semilunar valve.

The two main coronary arteries are the **left** and the **right coronary arteries.** The right coronary artery nourishes the right side of the heart, especially the right ventricle. The left coronary artery branches into the **left anterior descending artery** and the **circumflex artery.** These arteries carry blood to the left side of the heart, especially the left

Do You Know...

Why are heart attacks treated with clot busters?

A blood clot may block the flow of blood through a coronary artery, causing myocardial damage. (This development is a heart attack.) The prompt administration of a new class of drugs called clot busters, or thrombolytics, dissolves the clot and restores coronary blood flow, thereby preventing further myocardial damage.

ventricular wall. The **coronary veins** collect the blood that nourishes the myocardium. The coronary veins carry the blood to the **coronary sinus,** which in turn empties the blood into the right atrium.

The myocardium depends on a constant supply of oxygenated blood. If coronary blood flow is interrupted even for a short period, the myocardium can be damaged. For instance, if a blood clot (thrombosis) occludes, or blocks, a coronary artery, myocardial cell death occurs. This event is a myocardial infarction (MI), or heart attack.

✳ **SUM IT UP!** The heart is a hollow muscular organ that pumps blood. The heart is a double pump. The right heart pumps unoxygenated blood to the lungs (pulmonic circulation). The left heart pumps oxygenated blood to the systemic circulation. The heart has four chambers, two atria and two ventricles. The two types of valves that direct blood flow in a forward direction are the atrioventricular valves (tricuspid and bicuspid) and the semilunar valves (pulmonic and aortic). The myocardium is nourished by the coronary blood vessels.

FUNCTION OF THE HEART: WHAT IT DOES

The heart is an efficient and adaptable pump. Together with the circulatory system, it maintains an adequate flow of blood to every cell in the body. How does the heart know when to pump and when to relax?

Cardiac Conduction System

The heart's conduction system initiates an electrical signal and then moves that signal along a pathway through the heart. Why is this electrical signal so important? The electrical signal stimulates the heart muscle to contract. No electrical signal means no myocardial contraction. The **cardiac conduction system** (kär′dē-ăk kən-dŭk′shən sĭs′təm) not only provides the stimulus for muscle contraction but also coordinates the pumping activity of the atria and ventricles. Both atria must contract at the same time. Simultaneous contraction of both ventricles then follows.

The conduction system is located within the walls of the heart and in the septum, which separates the right and left hearts. The conduction system consists of the following structures: the sinoatrial node, the atrial conducting fibers, the atrioventricular node, and the His-Purkinje system (Fig. 14–9).

Sinoatrial Node (SA Node)

The **sinoatrial (SA) node** is located in the upper posterior wall of the right atrium. An electrical

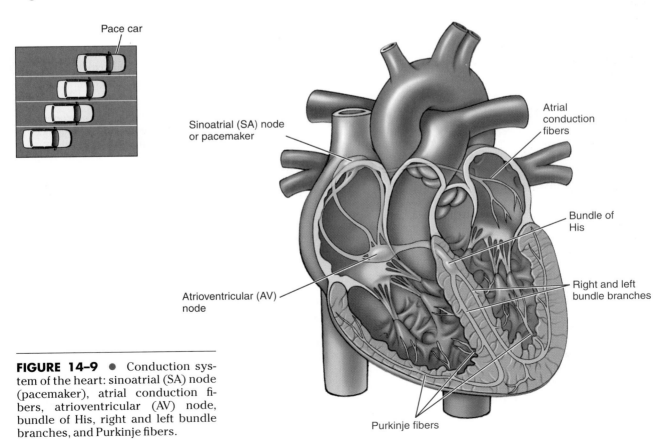

Pace car

Sinoatrial (SA) node or pacemaker

Atrioventricular (AV) node

Atrial conduction fibers

Bundle of His

Right and left bundle branches

Purkinje fibers

FIGURE 14–9 • Conduction system of the heart: sinoatrial (SA) node (pacemaker), atrial conduction fibers, atrioventricular (AV) node, bundle of His, right and left bundle branches, and Purkinje fibers.

signal originates within the SA node. The electrical signal is called the **action potential** or the **cardiac impulse.** In this text, we use the term *cardiac impulse.*

The SA node discharges, or fires, a cardiac impulse 60 to 100 times per minute (average 72 times). Because the firing of the SA node sets the rate at which the heart beats, or contracts, the SA node is called the **pacemaker** of the heart. Heart rate is set by this pacemaker just as the speed of a race is set by the pace car.

Atrial Conducting Fibers

The cardiac impulse spreads from the SA node through both atria along the atrial conducting fibers.

Atrioventricular Node (AV Node)

The **atrioventricular (AV) node** is located in the floor of the right atrium, near the interatrial septum. (Note: Do not confuse the AV *node* with the AV *valve.*) The cardiac impulse spreads from the SA node across the atrial fibers to the AV node. The cardiac impulse slows as it moves through the AV node into the **bundle of His,** the specialized conduction tissue located in the interventricular septum. The slowing of the cardiac impulse as it moves through the AV node is important. Its slow movement through the AV node delays ventricular activation, thereby allowing the relaxed ventricle time to fill with blood following atrial contraction.

His-Purkinje System

The bundle of His divides into two branches, the right and left bundle branches. The right and left bundle branches send out numerous long fibers called **Purkinje fibers** (pûr-kǐn'jē fī'bûrz). Purkinje fibers are distributed throughout the ventricular myocardium. The fibers making up the His-Purkinje system are fast-conducting fibers. Purkinje fibers conduct the cardiac impulse very rapidly throughout the ventricles, thereby ensuring a coordinated contraction of both ventricles. The pathway followed by the cardiac impulse is summarized in Figure 14–10.

The ability of cardiac tissue to create a cardiac impulse accounts for two characteristics of cardiac tissue: automaticity and rhythmicity. Because the cardiac impulse arises within cardiac tissue itself, cardiac tissue is said to have **automaticity.** Remember: a skeletal muscle cannot contract unless it is stimulated by a motor nerve. This is not true for cardiac muscle; no extrinsic nerve is necessary for the cardiac impulse to be fired; the impulse arises from within cardiac tissue.

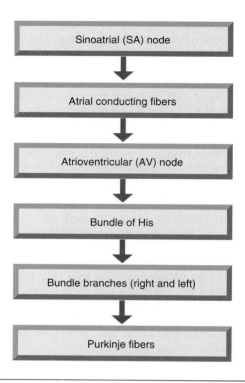

FIGURE 14–10 • Pathway followed by a cardiac impulse.

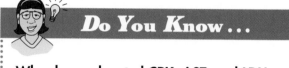

Do You Know...

Why do an elevated CPK, AST, and LDH indicate a heart attack (myocardial infarction)?

Creatine phosphokinase (CPK), aspartate aminotransferase (AST), and lactic dehydrogenase (LDH) are enzymes normally found in cardiac muscle cells. When the cardiac muscle cells are damaged, as in a heart attack, the enzymes leak out of the damaged cells into the blood. If a person complains of chest pain, a sample of blood is analyzed for the presence of these enzymes. If the enzymes are elevated, a heart attack is suspected.

Because cardiac tissue fires a cardiac impulse regularly, the heart is said to have **rhythmicity.** The SA node, for instance, fires at a rate of 60 to 100 times per minute. Your heart has rhythm. At times, the rhythm of the heart is disturbed; the heart is then said to be dysrhythmic (difficulty with rhythm). Some dysrhythmias are relatively harmless. Others are life-threatening and demand immediate attention. **Ventricular fibrillation** is one life-threatening dysrhythmia. A fibrillating muscle merely quivers rather than contracting. A fibrillating muscle cannot pump blood effectively.

The Case of the Wandering Pacemaker

The SA node is normally the site where the cardiac impulse arises. At times, however, other areas of the heart take over the role of the pacemaker. For example, the area outside the SA node can produce a cardiac impulse. This impulse is called an **ectopic focus** because it causes an ectopic beat to occur. (Ectopic means that the beat originates in an area other than the normal site, the SA node.) The AV node can also assume the role of pacemaker, as can other cells within the ventricular conduction system. Serious dysrhythmias occur when these other sites act as pacemakers.

Electrocardiogram

The cardiac impulse that stimulates muscle contraction is an electrical signal. This electrical activity of the heart can be measured by placing electrodes on the surface of the chest and attaching the electrodes to a recording device. The record of these electrical signals is called an **electrocardiogram** (ĕ-lĕk″trō-kär′dē-ə-grăm″) (ECG) (Fig. 14–11).

The components of the ECG include a P wave, a QRS complex, and a T wave. The **P wave** reflects the electrical activity associated with atrial depolarization. Depolarization occurs when the inflow of sodium ions (Na^+) makes the inside of the cell positive. Depolarization precedes and triggers contraction of the heart muscle. (See Chapter 9 for a review of polarization, depolarization, and repolarization.) The **QRS complex** reflects the electrical activity associated with ventricular depolarization. The **T wave** reflects the electrical activity associated with ventricular repolarization. (Repolarization refers to the return of the cell to its resting state where the inside of the cell is negative.)

In addition to identifying areas of depolarization and repolarization, the P, QRS, and T deflections of the ECG provide other useful information. For instance, the P-R interval represents the time it takes for the cardiac impulse to travel from the atria (P wave) to the ventricles (QRS complex). Other measurements include the width of the QRS complex, the length of the P-R interval, and the length of the S-T interval. The ECG provides valu-

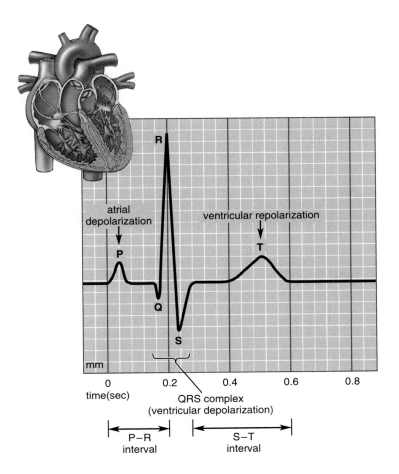

FIGURE 14–11 • Normal electrocardiogram (ECG) showing one cardiac cycle. The events are indicated by letters: P wave (atrial depolarization), QRS complex (ventricular depolarization), and T wave (ventricular repolarization).

able information about the electrical activity of the heart.

Note that the ECG is recorded on special graph paper that allows electrical events to be timed. The cardiologist can determine whether the electrical signals are moving too fast or are delayed for abnormally long periods. Abnormal patterns may indicate specific cardiac conditions.

✳ **SUM IT UP!** Together with the circulatory system, the heart maintains an adequate flow of blood to every cell in the body. Heart muscle contracts in response to an electrical signal called the cardiac impulse, which spreads throughout the heart, coordinating atrial and ventricular muscle contraction. The cardiac impulse normally arises within the SA node (the pacemaker) and spreads through both atria over specialized conduction tissue. The cardiac impulse then enters the AV node, where it is momentarily delayed before entering the conduction system in the ventricles (the His-Purkinje system). Because the cardiac impulse arises within cardiac tissue, the tissue is said to display automaticity (ie, it fires automatically). Because the cardiac impulse fires at a regular interval (60–100 times per minute), cardiac tissue displays rhythmicity.

Cardiac Cycle

The **cardiac cycle** (kär′dē-ăk sī′kəl) is the sequence of events that occurs during one heartbeat. A cardiac cycle is a coordinated contraction and relaxation of the chambers of the heart. Contraction of the heart muscle (myocardium) is called **systole** (sĭs′tə-lē). Systole squeezes blood out of a chamber. Relaxation of the myocardium is called **diastole** (dī-ăs′tə-lē). Blood fills a chamber during diastole.

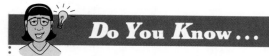

Do You Know...

Why can a rapid heart rate cause chest pain?

Coronary blood flow is greatest during myocardial relaxation (diastole). When the heart beats at a very rapid rate, the myocardium spends more of its time in the contracted state (systole). Because coronary blood flow is minimal during systole, the myocardium receives too little oxygen, causing chest pain and possibly myocardial damage.

Atrial muscle activity and ventricular muscle activity are closely coordinated. For instance, during atrial systole, the ventricles are in diastole. In this way, when the atria contract, they squeeze blood into the relaxed ventricles. With a heart rate of 70 beats per minute, the length of the cardiac cycle is 0.8 seconds. All chambers rest for 0.4 second. The cardiac cycle has three stages (Fig. 14–12):

- *Atrial systole:* The atria contract (systole) and pump blood into the ventricles (AV valves are open).
- *Ventricular systole:* At the end of atrial systole, the ventricles contract; this is called ventricular systole. As ventricular contractions begin, blood is forced against the AV valves, causing them to snap shut. The blood pushes the semilunar valves open, allowing blood to flow into the pulmonary artery and aorta.
- *Diastole:* For a brief period during the cardiac cycle, both the atria and the ventricles are in diastole. As the chambers relax, blood flows into the atria. Because the AV valves are open at this time, much of this blood also flows passively into the ventricles. The period of diastole therefore is a period of filling (of blood); atrial systole follows. The cycle then repeats itself.

Cardiac Output

Cardiac output (kär′dē-ăk out′po͞ot) is the amount of blood pumped by each ventricle in 1 minute. The normal cardiac output is about 5 liters per minute. Because the total blood volume is about 5 liters (5000 mL), the entire blood volume passes through the heart every minute.

Two factors determine cardiac output: heart rate and stroke volume, the amount of blood pumped by the ventricle per beat. The exact relationship is expressed as follows:

Cardiac output = heart rate × stroke volume

Heart Rate

The **heart rate** is the number of times the heart beats each minute. The heart rate reflects the rhythmic discharge, or firing, of the SA node. The normal adult resting heart rate is between 60 and 100 beats per minute, with an average of 72 beats per minute. The heart rate is commonly measured as the **pulse** (see Chapter 15). People's heart rates differ for many reasons: size, gender, age, level of exercise, stimulation of the autonomic nerves, hormonal influence, pathology, and various medications.

- *Size:* Size affects heart rate: generally, the larger the size, the slower the rate. Our feathered and furry friends dramatically reflect the difference size makes. The heart rate of a hummingbird, for instance, is greater than 200 beats per minute, whereas that of a grizzly is only about 30 beats per minute. Why do heart rates differ? The small hummingbird has a very high metabolism and

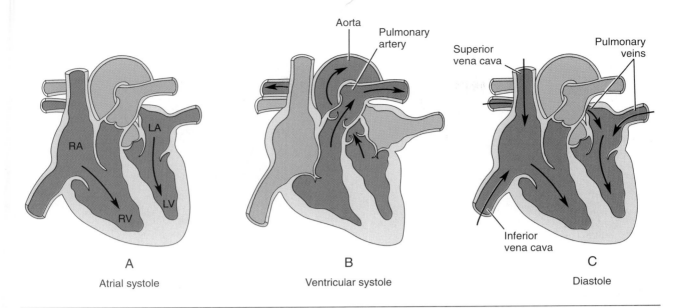

FIGURE 14-12 ● Stages of the cardiac cycle. A, Atrial systole: the atria contract and force blood into the relaxed ventricles (AV valves are open). B, Ventricular systole: the ventricles contract, forcing blood into the pulmonary artery and into the aorta (AV valves are closed, semilunar valves are open). C, Diastole: both atria and ventricles are relaxed and fill with blood (AV valves are open).

therefore requires a large amount of oxygen. The metabolism of a grizzly is much slower, requiring less oxygen.

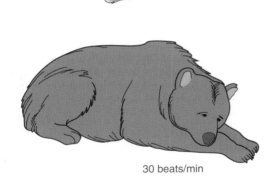

≥ 200 beats/min

30 beats/min

- *Gender:* Women have faster heart rates than men.
- *Age:* Generally, the younger the person, the faster the rate. The normal adult heart rate, for instance, is 70 to 80 beats per minute, whereas a normal child's heart rate is around 100 beats per minute. An infant's heart rate is about 120 beats per minute, and fetal heart rates are about 140 beats per minute.
- *Exercise:* Exercise increases heart rate. Check your pulse as you exercise and note the increase. Note also the decrease in pulse when you rest. At rest, the heart rate may be 65 but may increase over 100 beats per minute with exercise.
- *Stimulation of the autonomic nerves:* The heart is innervated by the autonomic nervous system. Firing of the sympathetic nerve stimulates the SA node, causing an increase in heart rate. Stim-ulation of parasympathetic fibers (vagus nerve) innervating the SA node causes a slowing of heart rate. (Note: The nerve impulse arises within the SA node and does not require outside nerves; cardiac tissue has automaticity. The autonomic nerves do not *cause* the nerve impulse; they can, however, *affect the rate* at which the cardiac impulse forms. See Chapters 10 and 15 about the role of autonomic innervation in cardiac function.)
- *Hormonal influence:* Several hormones affect heart rate. Epinephrine and norepinephrine, secreted by the adrenal gland, can increase heart rate. Thyroid hormone also increases heart rate.
- *Pathology:* Certain disease states can affect heart rate. For instance, a dysfunctional SA node may fire too slowly, thereby slowing the heart too much. Other pathologic conditions may increase heart rate, setting the stage for more serious life-threatening dysrhythmias.
- *Medications:* Certain drugs can affect heart rate. Digitalis slows the heart rate, while epinephrine (Adrenalin) increases the heart rate. Heavy coffee drinkers often experience palpitations (the heart feels as if it has extra beats) because of the stimulatory effect of caffeine on the heart. Because some drugs can profoundly alter heart rate, heart rate must be monitored when these drugs are used. For instance, if digitalis is administered when the pulse is less than 60 beats per minute, bradycardia and other serious cardiac dysrhythmias may develop.

Stroke Volume

Stroke volume (strōk vŏl'yo͞om), the amount of blood pumped by the ventricle per beat, is the

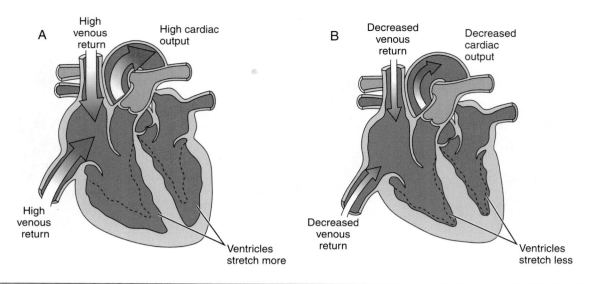

FIGURE 14–13 ● Starling's law of the heart: matching venous return with cardiac output. A, A large volume of blood is returned to the heart (venous return); this same large volume is pumped out of the heart (cardiac output). B, A smaller venous return (small arrow) is matched with a smaller cardiac output.

second factor affecting cardiac output. An average resting stroke volume is 60 to 80 mL per beat (about 2 ounces). The ventricles normally pump out only about 65% of the blood in the ventricles. Therefore, if the ventricles can be made to contract more forcefully, a greater percentage of the blood can be pumped per beat. In other words, a greater force of contraction can increase stroke volume.

The stroke volume can be altered in two ways: through Starling's law of the heart and through an inotropic effect.

STARLING'S LAW OF THE HEART

Starling's law of the heart (stär′lĭngz lō) depends on the degree of stretch of the myocardial fibers. The greater the stretch, the stronger is the force of contraction. For instance, an increase in the amount of blood entering the ventricle causes the ventricle to stretch (Fig. 14–13). This stretch increases the force of contraction, which, in turn, increases stroke volume. Conversely, a decrease in the amount of blood entering the ventricles causes less stretch. As a result, the force of contraction decreases, thereby decreasing stroke volume.

What is the purpose of Starling's law of the heart? It allows the heart to match cardiac output with the amount of blood returned to the heart from the veins (venous return). In other words, it allows the heart to pump out (cardiac output) the same amount of blood it receives (venous return).

INOTROPIC EFFECT. A second way to increase stroke volume is by strengthening the force of myocardial contraction without stretching the myocardial fibers. This is called a **positive (+) inotropic effect** (ĭn″ə-trŏp′ĭk ĕ-fĕkt′). Stimulation of the heart by sympathetic nerves can cause a positive (+) inotropic effect. Certain hormones

and medications can also cause this effect. Some medications, however, cause a negative (−) inotropic effect. A **negative (−) inotropic effect** is a decrease in the force of contraction, so that the strength of myocardial contraction is diminished. A diminished force of contraction can ultimately cause the heart to fail. Therefore, when administering a medication known to cause a negative (−) inotropic effect, cardiac function must be monitored and signs of cardiac failure noted.

COMPARING CAUSES OF ALTERED STROKE VOLUME. Both Starling's law of the heart and an inotropic effect can change the stroke volume. What is the difference between the two? Starling's law of the heart is caused by muscle stretching. The inotropic effect does not require stretching. It is due to other factors, primarily an increase in the amount of calcium entering the myocardium while it is contracting. (See Chapter 8 for a review of the role of calcium in muscle contraction.)

✳ **SUM IT UP!** Heart muscle contracts in response to an electrical signal called the cardiac impulse. The cardiac impulse originates in the SA node and spreads, through the atria, to the AV node, bundle of His, and Purkinje fibers. These structures are called the conduction system. A recording of the electrical events of the heart is called an electrocardiogram, or ECG. Cardiac tissue displays automaticity and rhythmicity. Cardiac muscle contraction is called systole; cardiac muscle relaxation is called diastole. The cardiac cycle is the sequence of events that occurs during one heartbeat. The cardiac cycle has three stages: atrial systole, ventricular systole, and diastole. Cardiac output is determined by heart rate and stroke volume. Stroke volume can be altered through Starling's law of the heart or through an inotropic effect.

As You Age

1. Contrary to popular opinion, no significant age-related decline occurs in resting cardiac output. When cardiac output declines, it is secondary to age-related disease processes such as arteriosclerosis.

2. An age-related decline occurs in exercise cardiac output. The heart cannot respond as quickly or as forcefully to the increased workload of the exercised heart. Exertion, sudden movements, and changes in position may cause a decrease in cardiac output, resulting in dizziness and loss of balance (falls).

3. Several structural changes in the heart contribute to the impaired response to exercise: heart muscle loses elasticity and becomes more rigid; heart valves become thicker and more rigid; the number of pacemaker cells decreases; and the aging heart cells have a decreased ability to use oxygen.

4. An age-related increase occurs in blood pressure, which increases the work the heart must do to pump blood into the systemic circulation.

Disorders of the Heart

Angina pectoris

From the Latin, meaning chest pain. The chest pain is due to inadequate oxygenation of the myocardium. The decreased oxygenation is generally caused by a decrease in coronary artery blood flow and is therefore called myocardial ischemia. Anginal pain is often triggered by exercise and emotional stress.

Cardiac dysrhythmias

Abnormal electrical conduction in the heart or abnormal changes in heart rate and rhythm. Fibrillation refers to an irregular, quivering, and ineffective type of myocardial contraction. Both the atria and the ventricles can fibrillate. Ventricular fibrillation causes a severe decrease in cardiac output and blood pressure with loss of consciousness; it is life-threatening and demands immediate treatment. Flutter refers to a regular but rapid pace (200–300 beats per minute). An atrioventricular block occurs when the electrical signal cannot pass from the atria to the ventricles. Blocks are classified as first-, second,- and third-degree.

Congenital heart defects

A heart defect present at birth but not necessarily hereditary. Heart defects often involve the atrial and ventricular septa. An interatrial septal defect is an opening between the two atria. Blood flows through the hole and does not follow the correct path through the heart. A ventricular septal defect is a hole in the ventricular septum; it allows blood to flow back and forth between the ventricles. Other congenital heart defects include tetralogy of Fallot and a patent ductus arteriosus.

Coronary heart disease

A commonly used term for any disease affecting the heart.

Inflammation of the heart

Inflammation of the layers of the heart. Pericarditis is inflammation of the pericardium. Myocarditis is inflammation of the heart muscle, the myocardium. Endocarditis is inflammation of the endocardium, the heart valves, and the inner lining of the blood vessels attached to the heart. Bacterial endocarditis is the most common infectious disease of the heart.

Myocardial infarction (MI)

Also called a heart attack. An infarct is an area of tissue that has died. A myocardial infarction is an area of dead myocardium caused by a lack of oxygenated blood. Coronary artery blood supply may be decreased because of fatty plaque buildup inside the arteries (atherosclerosis), a blood clot (coronary thrombosis), spasm of the blood vessel wall, or low blood pressure.

continued

Disorders of the Lung *continued*

Rheumatic fever	An infectious disease generally caused by a *Streptococcus* bacterium. The body develops antibodies to the streptococcal microorganism; then the antibodies attack the heart (particularly the valves) and joints, causing rheumatic heart disease.
Valvular heart disease	Dysfunction of any of the four valves. When blood flows through a diseased valve, it produces a characteristic sound called a murmur. Dysfunctional valves may produce regurgitation, or backflow of blood (eg, mitral insufficiency). Valves may also be narrowed or stenosed (mitral stenosis).

Summary Outline

The heart pumps blood through the blood vessels, supplying the cells of the body with oxygen and nutrients and carrying away the waste products of metabolism.

I. Structure of the Heart: What It Is

A. Location and Size
1. The heart is the size of a fist. It is located in the mediastinum and lies toward the left side of the body.
2. The heart is supported by a sling-like structure called the pericardium.

B. The Heart's Layers and Coverings
1. The heart is composed of three layers of tissue.
2. The endocardium is the innermost lining of the heart. It creates a shiny and smooth surface.
3. The myocardium is the thick middle layer composed of muscle tissue. It enables the heart to pump blood.
4. The epicardium is the outermost layer of the heart. The epicardium (at the apex of the heart) is continuous with the inner lining of the pericardium (sling). This arrangement forms the pericardial space.

C. A Double Pump and Two Circulations
1. The right heart pumps blood to the lungs for oxygenation. This process is the pulmonary circulation.
2. The left heart pumps blood throughout the rest of the body. This process is the systemic circulation.

D. The Heart's Chambers and Large Blood Vessels
1. The heart has four chambers, two atria and two ventricles. The atria receive the blood, and the ventricles pump the blood.
2. The right atrium receives blood from the venae cavae.
3. The right ventricle pumps unoxygenated blood to the lungs.
4. The left atrium receives blood from the lungs (pulmonary veins).
5. The left ventricle pumps blood into the aorta.

E. Heart Valves
1. The purpose of heart valves is to keep blood flowing in a forward direction.
2. Two atrioventricular (AV) valves are the tricuspid valve (right heart) and the bicuspid (mitral) valve (left heart). The cusps, or flaps, of the AV valves are held in place by tough fibrous bands called chordae tendineae.
3. The two semilunar valves are the pulmonic valve (right heart) and the aortic valve (left heart).

F. Heart Sounds
1. The heart sounds ("lubb-dupp") are made by the vibrations caused by closure of the valves.
2. The lubb is due to the closure of the AV valves at the beginning of ventricular systole. The dupp is due to the closure of the semilunar valves at the beginning of ventricular diastole.

G. Pathway: Blood Flow Through the Heart
1. The right heart receives blood from the venae cavae and pumps it to the lungs for oxygenation. The left heart receives oxygenated blood from the lungs and pumps it to the systemic circulation.
2. Blood flows in this sequence through the following structures: right atrium to tricuspid valve to right ventricle to pulmonic valve to pulmonary artery to pulmonary capillaries (lung) to pulmonary veins to left atrium to bicuspid (mitral) valve to left ventricle to aortic valve to aorta.

H. Blood Supply to the Myocardium
1. The left and right coronary arteries supply the myocardium with oxygen and nutrients. The left coronary artery branches into the left anterior descending artery and the circumflex artery.
2. The coronary veins drain the unoxygenated blood and empty it into the coronary sinus (which empties into the right atrium).

II. Functions of the Heart: What It Does

A. Conduction System
1. The heart generates an electrical signal (cardiac impulse) that moves throughout the heart in a coordinated way. The electrical signal causes the myocardium to contract.

Summary Outline, continued

II. Functions of the Heart: What It Does, *continued*

A. Conduction System, *continued*

2. The cardiac impulse originates in the sino-atrial node (SA node). The pathway followed by the cardiac impulse is SA node to AV node to bundle of His to right and left bundle branches (of His) to Purkinje fibers.
3. Cardiac muscle displays automaticity and rhythmicity.
4. The electrical activity of cardiac muscle is recorded as an electrocardiogram (ECG). The recordings include a P wave (atrial depolarization), a QRS complex (ventricular depolarization), and a T wave (ventricular repolarization).

B. Cardiac Cycle

1. The cardiac cycle is the sequence of events that occur during one heartbeat.
2. The cardiac cycle has three stages: atrial systole (contraction), ventricular systole, and diastole (relaxation).
3. The heart chambers fill with blood during diastole and empty during systole.

C. Cardiac Output

1. Cardiac output is the amount of blood pumped by each ventricle in 1 minute (5 liters per minute).
2. Cardiac output is determined by two factors: heart rate and stroke volume.

3. Heart rate refers to the number of times the heart beats per minute. The normal heart rate is between 60 and 100 beats per minute. Heart rate varies with body size, gender, age, level of exercise, autonomic activity, hormonal effects, pathology, and medications.
4. Stroke volume refers to the amount of blood ejected during one beat (mL per beat). The average resting stroke volume is 60 to 80 mL per beat, about 65% of the ventricular volume.
5. Stroke volume can be changed in two ways: by Starling's law of the heart and by an inotropic effect.
6. Starling's law of the heart changes the force of myocardial contraction (and stroke volume) by stretch. An increase in stretch causes an increase in the force of myocardial contraction and an increase in stroke volume. A decrease in stretch decreases stroke volume.
7. An inotropic effect refers to a change in the force of myocardial contraction that does not depend on stretch. A positive inotropic effect causes a greater force of contraction and an increase in stroke volume. A negative inotropic effect causes a decrease in stroke volume.

Review Your Knowledge

1. Give the terms that describe the following characteristics of the heart:
   a. Size
   b. Body cavity
   c. Location with respect to midline of body
   d. Location with respect to ribs
   e. Space between the lungs in which the heart is located
   f. Average number of times the heart pumps each minute

2. What is the sling-like structure that supports the heart?

3. Trace a drop of blood from the right atrium of the heart as it flows into the left atrium. What is this circulation called?

4. Explain why cardiac tamponade results in the heart being unable to pump a sufficient amount of blood to the body.

5. How is the pulmonary circulation different from the systemic circulation?

6. What is the difference between the following terms?
   a. Atria and ventricles
   b. Atrioventricular valves and semilunar valves
   c. Automaticity and rhythmicity
   d. Starling's law of the heart and positive inotropic effect

7. Why are the heart valves important? Can the heart function with leaky valves?

8. Why might a thrombus in a coronary artery cause sudden death?

9. What is the function of fluid in the pericardial sac?

10. Define systole, diastole, stroke volume, and cardiac cycle.

11. What is the function of the conduction system of the heart? Name the parts of the conduction system.

12. What are the noises that describe heart sounds? What causes the first and second heart sounds?

13. State how the following factors affect heart rate:
   a. Size
   b. Gender
   c. Age
   d. Exercise
   e. Autonomic nerve stimulation
   f. Hormones
   g. Pathology
   h. Medications

14. What two factors determine cardiac output?

15. Where does edema occur with left-sided heart failure? Where does edema occur with right-sided heart failure?

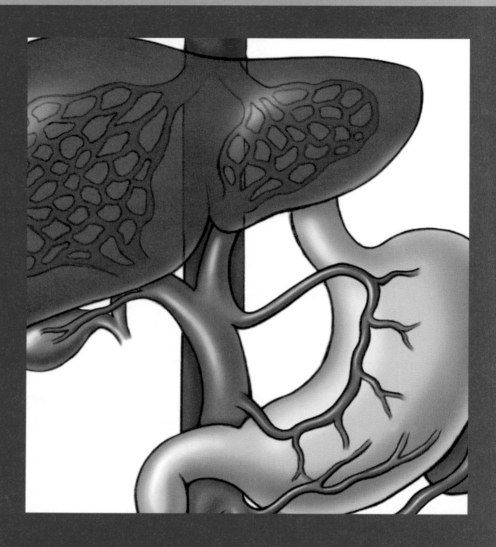

••• Selected terms in bold type in this chapter are defined in the Glossary.

15 BLOOD VESSELS AND CIRCULATION

Objectives

1. Describe the pulmonary and systemic circulations.

2. Describe the structure and function of arteries, capillaries, and veins.

3. List the three layers of tissue found in arteries and veins.

4. Explain the functions of conductance, resistance, exchange, and capacitance vessels.

5. List those major arteries of the systemic circulation that are branches of the ascending aorta, the aortic arch, and the descending aorta.

6. List the major veins of the systemic circulation.

7. Describe the following special circulations: blood supply to the head and brain, hepatic circulation, and fetal circulation.

8. Explain the factors that determine blood pressure.

9. List three factors that cause venous blood to flow back to the heart.

10. Explain rapidly acting mechanisms and slowly acting mechanisms that keep blood pressure within normal limits.

11. Describe capillary exchange.

STRUCTURE OF THE CIRCULATORY SYSTEM: WHAT IT IS

The circulatory system consists of the heart (described in Chapter 14) and blood vessels. The historical description of the heart and blood vessels is intriguing. The ancients knew that the heart played an important role in pumping blood through the body, but no one described the role of the blood vessels. The ancient Greeks thought that blood moved throughout the body like an ocean tide. Blood was seen as washing out from the heart through a series of blood vessels and then ebbing back to the heart through the same blood vessels, with impurities removed from the blood as it washed through the lungs. Not until the 17th century did the English physician William Harvey identify the system of blood vessels and thus provide the first accurate description of the circulation.

Circles, Circuits, and Circulations

The blood vessels are a series of connected hollow tubes that begin and end in the heart. The blood vessels form a path through the body, much like the system of highways and roads that enables us to travel from place to place. Note the path of the delivery truck in Figure 15–1. Leaving the bakery, the truck travels a major highway and exits onto a smaller road. The truck then arrives at a grocery store, where it makes a delivery. The empty truck then returns to the bakery through a number of connecting roads. Note the circle, or circuit, from bakery to grocery store to bakery, a path formed by various roads.

The heart and blood vessels also form a circuit. The heart pumps blood into the large artery. The blood flows through a series of blood vessels back to the heart. Moving from heart to blood vessels to heart, the blood forms a circuit, or circulation. This arrangement ensures a continuous one-way movement of blood. As Chapter 14 explained, the two main circulations are the pulmonary circulation and the systemic circulation.

The **pulmonary circulation** (pŭl′mə-nĕr″ē sûr″kyə-lā′shən) carries blood from the right ventricle of the heart to the lungs and back to the left atrium of the heart (see Fig. 14–3). The pulmonary circulation transports unoxygenated blood to the lungs, where oxygen is taken up, or loaded, and carbon dioxide is unloaded. Oxygenated blood then returns to the left side of the heart to be pumped into the systemic circulation.

The **systemic circulation** (sĭs-stĕm′ĭk sûr″kyə-lā′shən) is the larger circulation; it provides the blood supply to the rest of the body. The systemic circulation carries oxygen and other vital nutrients to the cells and picks up carbon dioxide and other waste from the cells.

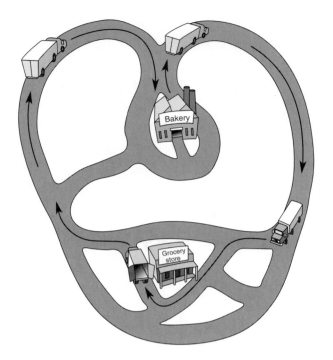

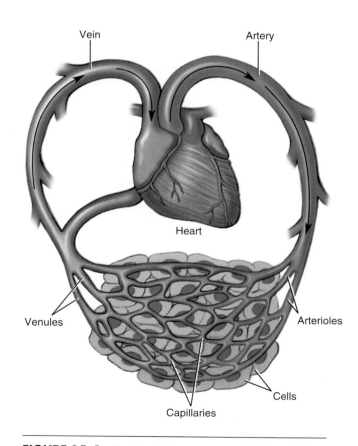

FIGURE 15–1 • Circulatory system. A delivery truck travels certain roads to a grocery store, where bread is delivered. The empty truck then travels back to the bakery over different roads, thereby completing a route, or circuit. The circulatory system also contains routes. The blood vessels are analogous to the roads and path followed by the truck. Note the route, or circuit, from the heart to the blood vessels and back to the heart.

Highways and Byways: Naming the Blood Vessels

Note the different types of blood vessels (Fig. 15–2), their relationship to the heart, and the color-coding. The blood vessels are the body's highways and byways; they are classified as arteries, capillaries, and veins (Table 15–1).

Arteries

Arteries (är′tə-rēz) are blood vessels that carry blood away from the heart. The large arteries repeatedly branch into smaller and smaller arteries as they are distributed throughout the en-tire body. As they branch, the arteries become much more numerous but smaller in diameter. The smallest of the arteries are called **arterioles** (är-tīr′ē-ōlz). The arteries are red in Figure 15–2 because they carry oxygenated blood.

Capillaries

Blood flows from the arterioles into the capillaries. The **capillaries** (kăp′ə-lěr″ēz) are, by far, the most numerous of all the blood vessels. Because the body has so many of them, a capillary is close to every cell in the body. This arrangement provides every cell with a continuous supply of oxygen and other vital nutrients. The capillaries are colored from red to purple to blue. Why the

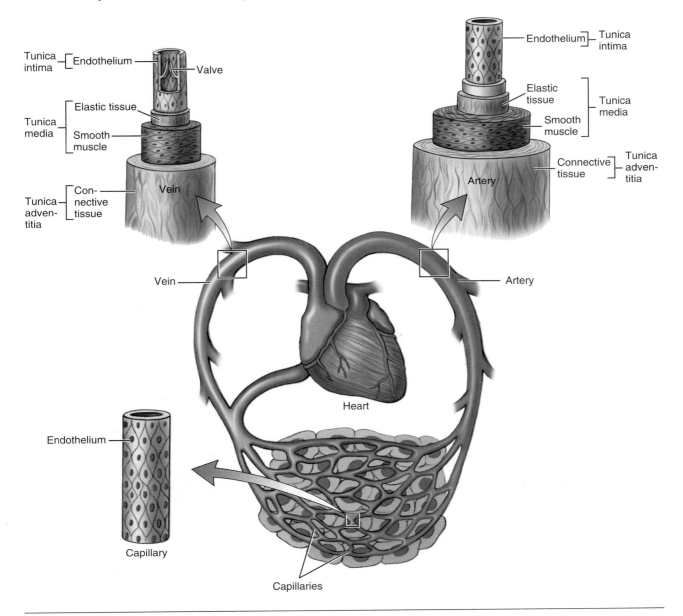

FIGURE 15–2 • Blood vessel wall layers. With the exception of the capillaries, the blood vessels contain three layers: tunica intima (inner layer), tunica media (middle layer), and tunica adventitia (outer layer). Compare the walls of the arteries and veins. Note that the veins also contain valves that help direct the flow of blood back to the heart. The capillary wall is composed of a single layer of cells (endothelium).

Table 15 ● 1	STRUCTURE AND FUNCTION OF BLOOD VESSELS	
VESSEL	**STRUCTURE**	**FUNCTION**
Artery	Thick wall with three layers: tunica intima (endothelial lining), tunica media (elastic tissue and smooth muscle), and tunica adventitia (connective tissue).	Called conductance vessels because they carry blood from the heart to the arterioles.
Arteriole	Thinner than the wall of an artery but with three layers, mostly smooth muscle.	Called resistance vessels because the contraction and relaxation of the muscle changes vessel diameter, which alters resistance to blood flow.
Capillary	Layer of endothelium.	Called "exchange" vessels because nutrients, gases, and wastes exchange between the blood and interstitial fluid.
Venule	Thin wall with less smooth muscle and elastic tissue than an arteriole.	Venules and veins collect and return blood from the tissues to the heart. They are called capacitance vessels because they hold or store blood (most of the blood is located in the venous side of the circulation).
Vein	Three layers (intima, media, and adventitia), but thinner and less elastic than an artery; contain valves.	

progression from red to blue? Because, at the capillary level, the blood gives up its oxygen to the tissues; the unoxygenated blood leaving the tissues is therefore bluish.

Veins

Blood flows from the capillaries into the veins. **Veins** (vānz) are blood vessels that carry blood back to the heart. The smallest of the veins are called **venules** (věn′yo͞olz). Venules receive blood from the capillaries. The small venules come together, or converge, to form fewer but larger veins. The large veins empty the blood into the right atrium of the heart. The veins are blue in Figure 15–2 because they transport unoxygenated blood.

Blood Vessel Walls: What They Are

With the exception of the capillaries, the blood vessels are composed of three layers of tissue, identified in Figure 15–2. The three layers are the tunica intima, the tunica media, and the tunica adventitia (*tunica* is Latin for sheath).

- Tunica intima. The **tunica intima** is the innermost coat, an endothelium. The endothelial lining forms a slick, shiny surface continuous with the endocardium, the inner lining of the heart. Blood flows easily and smoothly along this surface.
- Tunica media. The **tunica media** is the middle coat. It is the thickest coat and is composed primarily of elastic tissue and smooth muscle,

which varies according to the function of the blood vessel. The large arteries, for instance, contain considerable elastic tissue so that they can stretch in response to the pumping action of the heart. The smallest of the arteries, the arterioles, are composed primarily of smooth muscle. The muscle allows the arterioles to contract and relax, thereby changing the diameter of the arteriole.
- Tunica adventitia. The outer coat is called the **tunica adventitia.** It is made of tough connective tissue. Its main function is to support and protect blood vessels.

Blood Vessels: What They Do

Note how the structure of the blood vessels changes from artery to capillary to vein (see Fig. 15–2). As always, the structure is related to its function.

Arteries (Conductance Vessels)

The walls of the large arteries are thick, tough, and elastic because they must withstand the high pressure of the blood pumped from the ventricles. Because the primary function of the large arteries is to *conduct* blood from the heart to the arterioles, the large arteries are called **conductance vessels** (kən-dŭk′təns ves′əlz).

Arterioles (Resistance Vessels)

The arterioles are the smallest of the arteries. They are composed primarily of smooth muscle and spend most of their time contracting and relaxing. By changing their diameter, the arterioles affect resistance to the flow of blood. A narrow vessel offers an increased resistance to blood flow; a wider vessel offers less resistance to flow. Because of their effect on resistance, the arterioles are called **resistance vessels** (rĭ-zĭs′təns vĕs′əlz).

Capillaries (Exchange Vessels)

The capillaries have the thinnest walls of any of the blood vessels. The capillary wall is made up of a single layer of endothelium (simple squamous epithelium) lying on a delicate basement membrane. The thin capillary wall enables water and dissolved substances, including oxygen, to diffuse from the blood into the tissue spaces, where it becomes available for use by the cells. The capillary also allows waste from the metabolizing cell to diffuse from the tissue spaces into the capillaries for transport to the organs of excretion. Because the capillaries allow for an exchange of nutrients and waste, these vessels are called **exchange vessels** (ĕks-chānj′ vĕs′əlz).

Veins and Venules (Capacitance Vessels)

As the capillaries begin to converge, or join together, to form venules, the structure of the wall also changes. The venule wall is slightly thicker than the capillary wall. As the venules converge to form larger veins, the walls become even thicker. The tunica media of the vein, however, is much thinner than is the tunica media of the artery. This difference is appropriate because pressure within the veins is considerably less than the pressure in the arterial blood vessels.

In addition to thinner walls, the veins differ in another way: most veins contain one-way valves. These valves are located within the veins and direct the flow of blood toward the heart. The valves are most numerous in the veins of the lower extremities, where they prevent backflow, helping move blood away from the ankles toward the heart.

In addition to carrying blood back to the heart, the veins play another role. The veins store blood. In fact, about 70% of the total blood volume is found on the venous side of the circulation. Because the veins store blood, they are called **capacitance vessels** (kə-păs′ĭ-təns vĕs′əlz) (*capacitance* refers to storage).

Major Arteries of the Systemic Circulation

The major arteries of the systemic circulation include the aorta and the arteries arising from the aorta.

Aorta

The **aorta** (ā-ôr′tə) originates in the heart's left ventricle (Fig. 15–3). The aorta extends upward from the left ventricle, curves in an arch-like fashion, and then descends through the thorax (chest) and abdomen. The aorta descends just behind the heart, in front of the vertebral column. It penetrates the diaphragm as it descends into the abdomen. The aorta ends in the pelvic cavity as it splits, or bifurcates, into the iliac arteries.

The aorta is divided into segments, each named according to two systems. One system is the path that the aorta follows as it courses through the body. In this system, the aorta is divided into the **ascending aorta,** the **arch of the aorta,** and the **descending aorta.** In the second naming system, the aorta is named according to its location within the body cavities. Thus, we have the **thoracic aorta** and the **abdominal aorta.** In this text, we use both naming systems.

Branches of the Aorta

All systemic arteries are either direct or indirect branches of the aorta. In other words, the arteries arise directly from the aorta, or they arise from vessels that are themselves branches of the aorta. For instance, the coronary arteries arise directly from the ascending aorta. The brachial artery in the right arm, however, arises from the axillary artery. The axillary artery has its origin in the brachiocephalic artery, which arises from the arch of the aorta. The brachial artery therefore arises indirectly from the aorta.

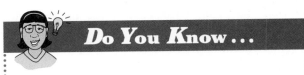

Do You Know . . .

Why is an aneurysm so dangerous?

An aneurysm is a weakening in the wall of an artery. The blood vessel is enlarged and appears as an outpouching in the wall. This condition may cause a rupture, resulting in a massive hemorrhage. If the ruptured aneurysm involves a cerebral artery, a hemorrhage into the brain may cause severe neurologic damage and death.

The systemic arteries are described in the order in which they arise from the aorta. Refer to Figure 15–4 as you read the text. You should be able to identify the arteries and the structures they supply.

BRANCHES OF THE ASCENDING AORTA. The ascending aorta arises from the left ventricle. It begins at the aortic semilunar valve and extends to the aortic arch. The **right** and **left coronary arteries** branch from the ascending aorta. The coronary ar-

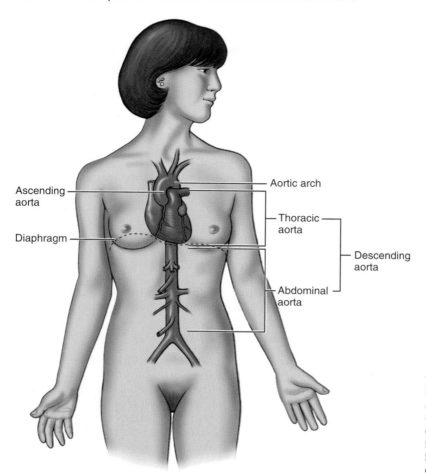

Ascending aorta

Aortic arch

Diaphragm

Thoracic aorta

Descending aorta

Abdominal aorta

FIGURE 15–3 ● Segments of the aorta. The two ways to name the aorta are (1) according to the path it follows (ascending aorta, aortic arch, and descending aorta) and (2) according to the cavity in which it is located (thoracic and abdominal aorta).

teries are distributed throughout the heart and supply oxygenated blood to the myocardium.

BRANCHES OF THE AORTIC ARCH. The aortic arch extends from the ascending aorta to the beginning of the descending aorta. Three large arteries arise from the aortic arch:

- The **brachiocephalic artery** is a large artery on the right side of the body. It supplies blood to the right side of the head and neck, right shoulder, and right upper extremity. Refer to Figure 15–4 for the names of the arteries that extend from, or branch off, the brachiocephalic artery. These arteries supply the right side of the head and neck and the arm and hand regions.
- The **left common carotid artery** extends upward from the highest part of the aortic arch and supplies the left side of the head and neck. Note that the left common carotid artery arises directly from the aorta, while the right common carotid arises from the brachiocephalic artery. (There is no left brachiocephalic artery.)
- The **left subclavian artery** supplies blood to the left shoulder and upper arm.

BRANCHES OF THE DESCENDING AORTA (THORACIC AORTA). The thoracic aorta is the upper portion of the descending aorta. It extends from the aortic arch to the diaphragm. **Intercostal arteries** arise from the aorta and supply the intercostal muscles

of the ribs. Other small arteries supply the organs in the thorax, including the esophagus and some of the respiratory passages.

Do You Know...

Why is coronary artery bypass surgery done?

A person may develop atherosclerosis, a condition involving the coronary arteries. In atherosclerosis, fatty plaques build up on the inner lining of the coronary arteries. The plaque buildup may be so severe that the lumen of the coronary artery becomes occluded. Consequently, blood flow to the myocardium is severely reduced, producing anginal pain, ischemia, and possibly a myocardial infarction. Sometimes it is possible to bypass the blocked arteries with a graft. A vein from the leg (the saphenous vein is usually the donor vein) is grafted onto the clogged artery, creating a detour around the block. This procedure restores blood supply to the myocardium and generally relieves anginal pain and ischemic episodes.

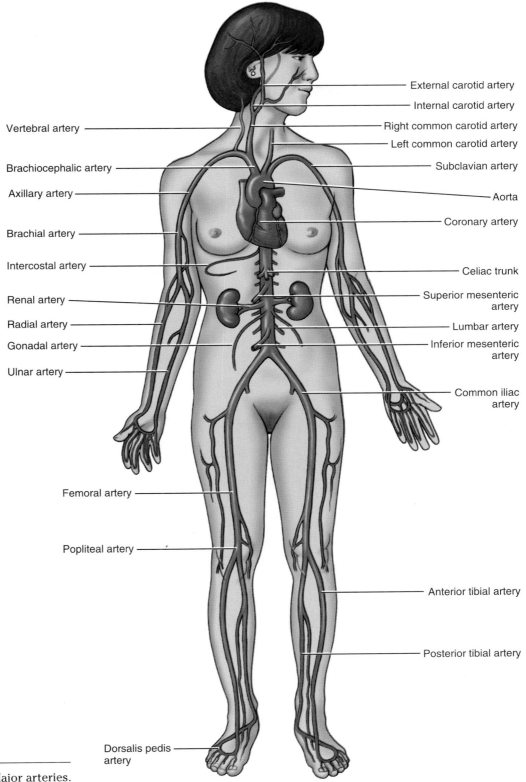

Vertebral artery

Brachiocephalic artery

Axillary artery

Brachial artery

Intercostal artery

Renal artery

Radial artery

Gonadal artery

Ulnar artery

External carotid artery

Internal carotid artery

Right common carotid artery

Left common carotid artery

Subclavian artery

Aorta

Coronary artery

Celiac trunk

Superior mesenteric artery

Lumbar artery

Inferior mesenteric artery

Common iliac artery

Femoral artery

Popliteal artery

Anterior tibial artery

Posterior tibial artery

Dorsalis pedis artery

FIGURE 15–4 ● Major arteries.

BRANCHES OF THE DESCENDING AORTA (ABDOMINAL AORTA). The abdominal aorta extends from the thoracic aorta to the lower abdomen. Branches of the abdominal aorta include

• The **celiac trunk,** a short artery that further divides into three smaller arteries: the **gastric** artery, which supplies the stomach; the **splenic artery,** which supplies the spleen; and the **hepatic artery,** which supplies the liver.

• The two mesenteric arteries, the superior and inferior segments. The **superior mesenteric artery** supplies blood to most of the small intestine and part of the large intestine. The other part of the large intestine receives its blood supply from the **inferior mesenteric artery.**

- The two **renal arteries,** which supply blood to the right and left kidneys.

Other branches of the abdominal aorta include the **gonadal arteries** and the **lumbar arteries.**

The distal abdominal aorta bifurcates, or splits, into the **right** and **left common iliac arteries,** which supply the thigh and lower extremities. Identify the major arteries of the thigh and leg—the femoral, popliteal, anterior, and posterior tibial arteries—on Figure 15–4. The **anterior** and **posterior tibial arteries** give rise to arteries that supply the foot. The **anterior tibial artery** becomes the **dorsalis pedis artery** at the ankle.

Major Veins of the Systemic Circulation

If you look at the back of your hand, you can see several veins but no arteries. Why is this? The arteries are usually located in deep and well-protected areas. Many of the veins, however, are located more superficially and can be seen. These are called **superficial veins.** Other veins are located more deeply and usually run parallel to the arteries. These are called **deep veins.** With few exceptions, the names of the deep veins are identical to the names of the companion arteries. For instance, the femoral artery in the thigh is accompanied by the femoral vein. In Figure 15–5, note the similarity in the names of many of the arteries and veins. So, the good news is this: if you learned the names of the arteries, you also know most of the names of the veins.

Venae Cavae

The veins carry blood from all parts of the body to the venae cavae for delivery to the heart. While the arteries arise from and diverge (spread out) from the aorta, the veins converge and empty into the venae cavae.

The **vena cava** (vē'nə kǎ'və) is the largest vein in the body. It is divided into the **superior vena cava (SVC)** and the **inferior vena cava (IVC).** Veins draining blood from the head, shoulders, and upper extremities empty into the superior vena cava. Veins draining the lower part of the body empty into the inferior vena cava. The superior and inferior venae cavae empty into the right atrium. Locate the individual veins on Figure 15–5.

Veins That Empty Into the Superior Vena Cava

The superior vena cava (SVC) receives blood from the head, shoulder, and upper extremities.

Veins may drain directly or indirectly into the SVC. For instance, the brachiocephalic veins empty directly into the SVC. The axillary vein, however, drains into the subclavian vein, which drains into the brachiocephalic vein, which in turn drains into the SVC. Refer to Figure 15–5 so that you can trace the flow of venous blood from a distal site to the vena cava:

- The **cephalic vein** is a superficial vein that drains the lateral arm region and carries blood to the axillary vein towards the SVC.
- The **basilic vein** is a superficial vein that drains the medial arm region. The cephalic and the basilic veins are joined by the **median cubital vein** (anterior aspect of the elbow). When a sample of blood is needed for testing, a needle is often inserted into the median cubital vein.
- The **subclavian veins** receive blood from the axillary veins and from the external jugular veins. Blood is carried by these veins to the brachiocephalic veins, which empty into the superior vena cava.
- The **internal jugular veins** drain blood from the brain.
- The **brachiocephalic veins** are large veins. They receive blood from the subclavian and internal jugular veins. The right and left brachiocephalic veins drain into the SVC.
- The **azygos vein** is a single vein that drains the thorax and empties directly into the SVC.

Veins That Empty Into the Inferior Vena Cava

The inferior vena cava (IVC) returns blood to the heart from all regions of the body below the diaphragm. Follow the venous drainage in the lower leg in Figure 15–5.

- The **tibial veins** and the **peroneal veins** drain the calf and foot regions. The **posterior tibial vein** drains into the **popliteal vein** (in the knee) and then the **femoral vein** (in the thigh). The femoral vein enters the pelvis as the **external iliac vein** and empties into the **common iliac vein.** The common iliac vein continues as the IVC.
- The **great saphenous veins** are the longest veins in the body. They begin in the foot, ascend along the medial side, and merge with the femoral vein (in the thigh) to become the external iliac vein. These veins receive drainage from the superficial veins of the leg and thigh region. These are the veins sometimes "borrowed" for use in cardiac bypass surgery. Portions of saphenous vein are surgically removed and transplanted into the heart. They are used to bypass clogged coronary arteries.

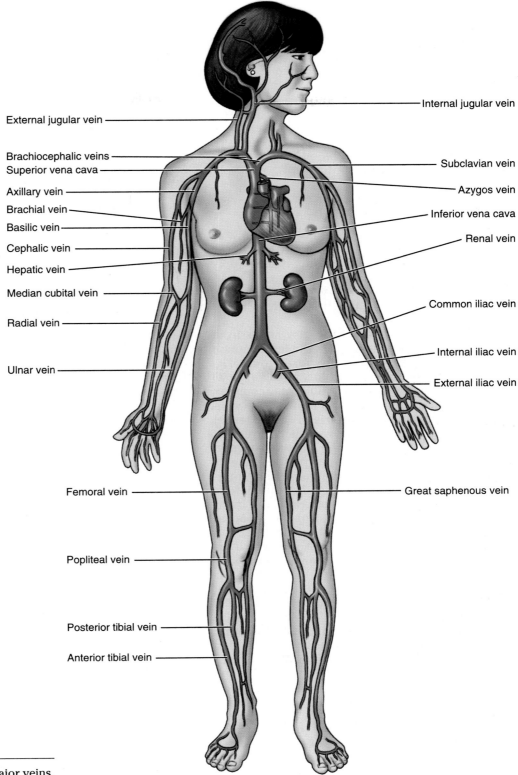

External jugular vein

Brachiocephalic veins
Superior vena cava

Axillary vein
Brachial vein
Basilic vein
Cephalic vein
Hepatic vein
Median cubital vein

Radial vein

Ulnar vein

Femoral vein

Popliteal vein

Posterior tibial vein

Anterior tibial vein

Internal jugular vein

Subclavian vein

Azygos vein

Inferior vena cava

Renal vein

Common iliac vein

Internal iliac vein

External iliac vein

Great saphenous vein

FIGURE 15–5 ● Major veins.

- The internal and external iliac veins unite to form the common iliac veins. The common iliac veins converge to form the inferior vena cava. The inferior vena cava ascends through the abdominal and thoracic regions to the right atrium of the heart.

- The **renal veins** drain the right and left kidneys, emptying blood directly into the IVC.
- The **hepatic veins** drain the liver. The hepatic veins are a part of the larger **hepatic portal circulation,** a unique venous system associated with the liver.

Special Circulations

Although the pulmonic and systemic circulations are the principal divisions of the circulatory system, several organs in the systemic circulation have unique characteristics. These are called *special circulations*. They include the blood supply to the head and brain, the blood supply to the liver, and the arrangement of the blood vessels in the unborn child (fetal circulation).

Blood Supply to the Head and Brain

The brain requires a continuous supply of blood; even a few minutes without oxygen causes irreversible brain damage. To ensure a rich supply of blood, the head is supplied by two pairs of arteries, carotid arteries and vertebral arteries. Thus, blood arrives at the brain through two routes (Fig. 15–6A).

The right common carotid artery arises from the brachiocephalic artery while the left common carotid arises directly from the aortic arch (Fig. 15–6B). (There is no left brachiocephalic artery.) At about the level of the mandible, the common carotid arteries bifurcate, or split, into the external and internal carotid arteries. The **external carotid arteries** supply the superficial areas of the neck, face, and scalp. The **internal carotid arteries** extend to the front part of the base of the brain. Once inside the cranium, each internal carotid artery divides, sending numerous branches to various parts of the brain. The internal carotid arteries supply most of the blood to the brain.

ARTERIES OF THE HEAD AND NECK. **Vertebral arteries** pass upward toward the brain from the subclavian arteries toward the back of the neck. As the vertebral arteries extend up into the cranium, they join to form a single **basilar artery** (see Fig. 15–6B). Numerous branches from the basilar artery supply areas of the brain around the brain stem and cerebellum. The basilar artery also sends branches that connect, or anastomose, with branches of the internal carotids.

The branches from the internal carotid arteries and the basilar artery form a circle of arteries at the base of the brain. This circular arrangement of arteries is an **anastomosis** (ə-năs″tə-mō′sĭs), or connection, called the **circle of Willis** (see Fig. 15–6B). Arising from the circle of Willis are many branches that penetrate the brain tissue and maintain a rich supply of blood to the brain.

Most of the blood supply to the brain runs through the internal carotid arteries. If the carotid arteries become blocked, the vertebral arteries cannot supply enough blood to the brain to maintain life. Remember: Without an adequate supply of oxygenated blood, the organ dies. Thus, a clogged internal carotid artery can lead to irreversible brain death. A clogged carotid artery is a serious but, unfortunately, common occurrence.

VENOUS DRAINAGE OF THE HEAD AND BRAIN. The **external** and **internal jugular veins** are the two major veins that drain blood from the head and neck (Fig. 15–6C). The external jugular veins are more superficial and drain blood from the posterior head and neck region. They empty into the subclavian veins. The internal jugular veins drain the anterior head, face, and neck. The deep internal jugular veins drain most of the blood from the venous sinuses of the brain. The internal jugular veins on each side of the neck join with the subclavian veins to form the brachiocephalic veins. The brachiocephalic veins empty into the superior vena cava.

Blood Supply to the Liver and the Hepatic Portal Circulation

The blood vessels of the liver have a unique arrangement. Three groups of blood vessels are associated with the portal circulation; they are the portal vein, the hepatic veins, and the hepatic artery.

The purpose of the hepatic portal circulation is to carry blood rich in digestive end-products from the organs of digestion to the liver (Fig. 15–7). Because it plays such a critical role in metabolism, the liver needs easy access to the the digestive end-products. As the blood flows through the liver, many of the nutrients are extracted from the blood or modified in some way.

The **portal vein** is a large vein that carries blood from the organs of digestion to the liver. It is formed by the union of two large veins: the superior mesenteric vein and the splenic vein. The **superior mesenteric vein** receives blood from the small intestine, where most digestion and absorption occur, and the first part of the large intestine. The **splenic vein** receives blood from the stomach, spleen, and pancreas. In addition, the splenic vein receives blood from the **inferior mesenteric vein,** which drains the last part of the large intestine.

In addition to the portal vein, the liver has two other blood vessels: the hepatic artery and the hepatic veins. The hepatic artery is a branch of the celiac trunk, a large artery that branches off the abdominal aorta (see Fig. 15–4). The hepatic artery carries oxygen-rich blood to the liver. The hepatic veins drain blood from the liver. Venous blood travels through the hepatic veins from the liver to the inferior vena cava (see Fig. 15–5).

Note that both the hepatic artery and the portal vein carry blood *toward* the liver. The hepatic artery carries oxygen, while the portal vein carries blood rich in the products of digestion to the liver. The hepatic veins carry blood *away from* the liver, toward the heart.

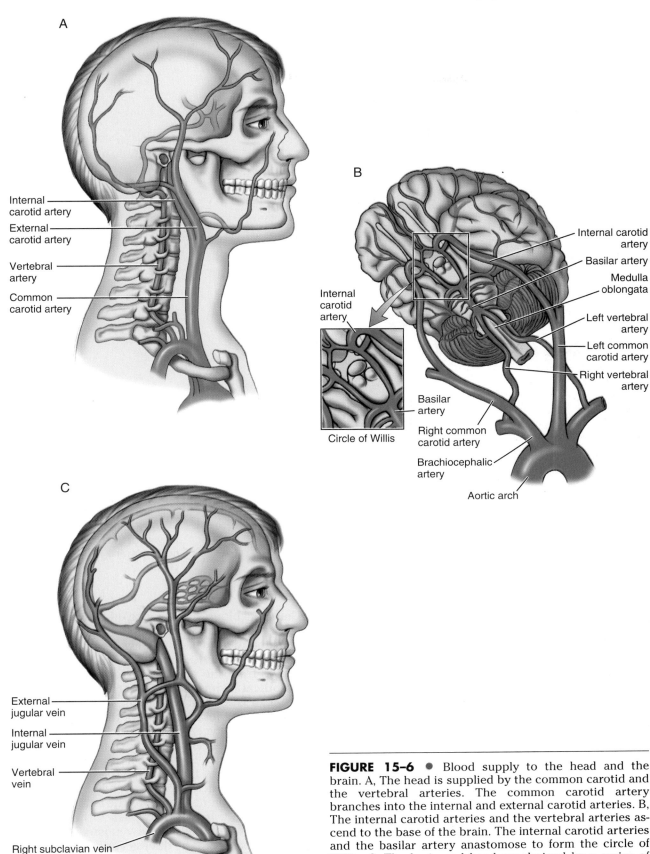

A

Internal carotid artery
External carotid artery
Vertebral artery
Common carotid artery

B

Internal carotid artery
Basilar artery
Medulla oblongata
Left vertebral artery
Left common carotid artery
Right vertebral artery

Internal carotid artery

Basilar artery
Right common carotid artery
Brachiocephalic artery
Aortic arch

Circle of Willis

C

External jugular vein
Internal jugular vein
Vertebral vein
Right subclavian vein
Right brachiocephalic vein

FIGURE 15–6 ● Blood supply to the head and the brain. A, The head is supplied by the common carotid and the vertebral arteries. The common carotid artery branches into the internal and external carotid arteries. B, The internal carotid arteries and the vertebral arteries ascend to the base of the brain. The internal carotid arteries and the basilar artery anastomose to form the circle of Willis. C, The brain and head are drained by a series of veins, the largest being the jugular veins.

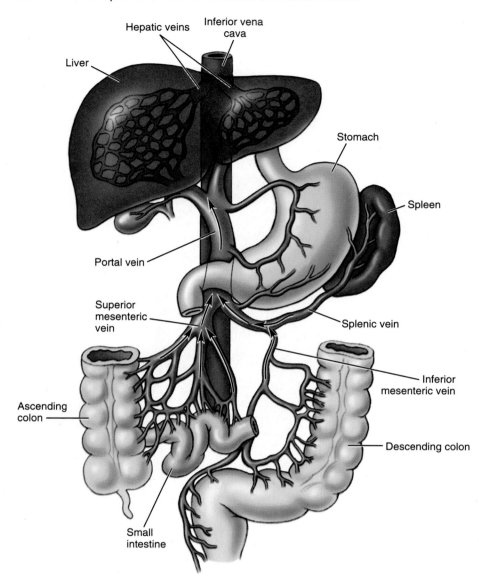

Liver

Hepatic veins

Inferior vena cava

Stomach

Spleen

Portal vein

Superior mesenteric vein

Splenic vein

Inferior mesenteric vein

Ascending colon

Descending colon

Small intestine

FIGURE 15–7 ● Hepatic portal system. The portal vein carries venous blood from the organs of digestion and spleen to the liver. The portal vein is formed as the splenic and the superior mesenteric veins merge. Venous blood leaves the liver by way of the hepatic veins and flows toward the inferior vena cava.

Fetal Circulation

Look at your "belly button," or **umbilicus.** At one time you had a long **umbilical cord,** a lifeline that attached you to a **placenta** embedded in the walls of your mother's uterus. Why was this attachment necessary? As a fetus, you were submerged in amniotic fluid and were unable to eat or breathe. All your nutrients and oxygen had to be supplied by your mother. Your mother also absorbed much of the waste produced by your tiny body and eliminated it through her excretory organs. The exchange of all your nutrients, gases, and waste occurred at a structure called the placenta.

Because of these special needs, the fetal heart and circulation have several modifications that make them different from the child's and adult's (Fig. 15–8). These modifications are summarized in Table 15–2.

- Umbilical blood vessels. The umbilical cord contains three blood vessels: one large umbilical vein and two smaller umbilical arteries. The **umbilical vein** carries blood rich in oxygen and nutrients from the placenta to the fetus. The two **umbilical arteries** carry carbon dioxide and other waste from the fetus to the placenta. (Note: In the fetal circulation the umbilical *vein* is carrying oxygen-rich blood, while the umbilical *arteries* are carrying oxygen-poor blood.)
- Ductus venosus. Blood flows through the umbilical vein into the fetus. Within the body of the fetus, the umbilical vein branches. Some blood flows through one branch to the fetal liver. Most of the blood, however, bypasses the liver and passes through the ductus venosus into the inferior vena cava. The **ductus venosus** is a vessel that connects the umbilical vein with the inferior vena cava. After birth, the ductus venosus closes and serves no further purpose.

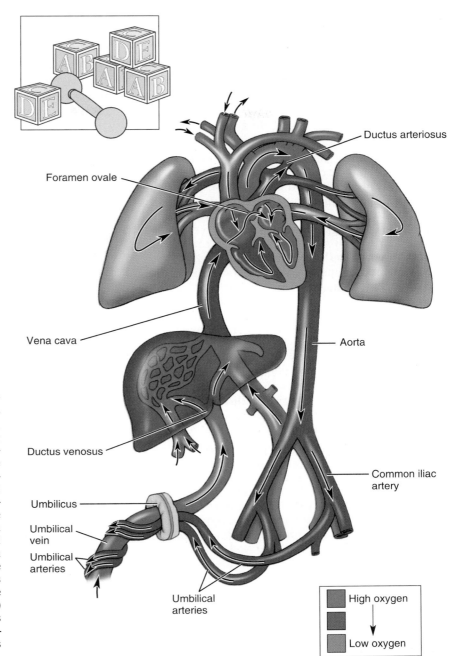

FIGURE 15–8 • Fetal circulation. Exchange between the fetal and maternal circulation occurs at the placenta. An umbilical vein carries oxygenated blood from the placenta into the fetus. Two umbilical arteries carry unoxygenated blood from the fetus to the placenta. Three structures are unique to the fetal circulation: the foramen ovale, the ductus arteriosus, and the ductus venosus. The foramen ovale (the opening between the right and left atria) and the ductus arteriosus (opening between the pulmonary artery and the aorta) allow most of the blood to bypass the lungs. The ductus venosus allows most of the blood to bypass the liver.

Table 15 • 2 SPECIAL FEATURES IN THE FETAL CIRCULATION

STRUCTURE	LOCATION	FUNCTION
Umbilical arteries (2)	Umbilical cord	Transport blood from fetus to the placenta
Umbilical vein (1)	Umbilical cord	Transports blood from the placenta to the fetus
Ductus venosus	Between the umbilical vein and the inferior vena cava	Carries blood from umbilical vein to inferior vena cava; allows the blood to bypass the liver
Foramen ovale	Septum between the right and left atria	Allows blood to go directly from the right atrium into the left atrium to bypass the pulmonary circulation
Ductus arteriosus	Between the pulmonary artery and the aorta	Allows blood in the pulmonary artery to go directly into the descending aorta and to bypass the pulmonary circulation

Because the deflated fetal lungs are not used for gas exchange, they have no need for blood pumped through the pulmonary circulation. Two modifications in the fetal heart and large vessels reroute most of the blood around the lungs. The two modifications are the foramen ovale and the ductus arteriosus:

- Foramen ovale. The **foramen ovale** is an opening in the interatrial septum. This opening allows most of the blood to flow from the right atrium directly into the left atrium. Remember: In the adult heart, blood flows from the right atrium to the right ventricle to the pulmonary artery to the pulmonary capillaries to the pulmonary veins to the left atrium.
- Ductus arteriosus. While most blood flows through the foramen ovale into the left atrium, some blood enters the right ventricle and is pumped into the pulmonary artery. How does this blood bypass the lungs? The fetus has a short tube, or opening, called the **ductus arteriosus,** which connects the pulmonary artery with the aorta. Blood pumped into the pulmonary artery bypasses the lungs by flowing through the ductus arteriosus directly into the aorta. After birth, these fetal structures close down, becoming nonfunctional.

Occasionally, the fetal structures do not close and appear as congenital heart defects. For instance, the ductus arteriosus may fail to close, thereby allowing blood continuously to shunt from the pulmonary artery into the aorta. In other words, a portion of the infant's blood bypasses the lungs and does not become oxygenated. This unoxygenated blood is then pumped through the systemic circulation, causing cyanosis. A child with this defect is sometimes called a "blue baby." The patent (open) ductus arteriosus can easily be repaired surgically.

A word about color coding in Figure 15–8. Blood vessels carrying oxygenated blood are colored red; these are usually the arteries. Vessels carrying unoxygenated blood are colored blue; these are usually veins. Color-coding in the fetal circulation differs. The umbilical vein is colored red, indicating oxygenated blood. The umbilical arteries are colored blue, indicating unoxygenated blood.

Note the color of the upper portion of the vena cava. The adult vena cava is colored blue because it contains unoxygenated blood. The fetal vena cava is colored violet, indicating that the blood is a mixture of unoxygenated blood (coming from the metabolizing fetal tissue) and oxygenated blood (coming from the umbilical vein). Note also the color of the blood in the fetal aorta; it is not the bright red color characteristic of the adult aorta. The adult aorta carries only oxygenated blood. The fetal aorta mixes oxygenated and unoxygenated blood. Remember: In the fetal circulation, the blood bypasses the lungs.

✳ **SUM IT UP!** The circulatory system is composed of the heart and the blood vessels. The heart pumps blood into the blood vessels and the blood vessels carry the blood through the body. The arteries distribute the blood to the millions of capillaries, where nutrients, gases, and waste material exchange, or move across, the capillary wall. The venous vessels drain the capillaries and bring the blood back to the heart. Blood flowing from the heart to the blood vessels and back to the heart completes a circuit, or circulation. The pulmonary and systemic circulations are the main circulatory systems. Several special circulations include the circulation to the brain (circle of Willis), the hepatic portal circulation, and the fetal circulation.

FUNCTION OF THE CIRCULATORY SYSTEM: WHAT IT DOES

The anatomy of the heart and the blood vessels is intimately related to its functioning. The circulatory system maintains an adequate flow of blood to every cell in the body. An important question is this: What causes the blood to move through the circulatory system?

Blood Pressure

Blood is pushed through the arterial blood vessels primarily because of the pressure produced by the contraction of the ventricles of the heart. As the heart contracts, blood is pushed into the arteries. **Blood pressure** is the force exerted by the blood against the walls of the blood vessels.

The maintenance of normal blood pressure is extremely important. If blood pressure becomes too low, blood flow to vital organs decreases, and the person is said to be in shock. Without immediate treatment, the person may die. If the blood pressure becomes elevated, the blood vessels may burst, or rupture. A ruptured blood vessel in the brain, for example, is a major cause of **stroke,** resulting in loss of speech, paralysis, and possible death. A long-term, or chronic, elevation of blood pressure, called **hypertension,** also causes serious problems. It puts added strain on the heart, damages the blood vessels in the kidneys, and damages the retina, causing loss of vision. Because of the importance of maintaining a normal blood pressure, you will frequently be asked to assess blood pressure in your patients.

Measurement of Blood Pressure

120/80 mmHg: WHAT IT MEANS. You just had a physical examination. The physician nodded approvingly that your blood pressure is normal at

120/80 mmHg. While you are thrilled to be normal, you ask what exactly 120/80 mmHg means.

The blood pressure in the large arteries is caused by the heart's pumping activity. When the ventricles contract, a volume of blood is ejected, or pushed, out of the ventricle into the artery, thereby increasing pressure. The pressure in the arteries at the peak of ventricular contraction **(systole)** is called the **systolic pressure;** it is the top number, 120 mmHg. The **diastolic pressure** is the pressure in the large arteries when the ventricles of the heart are relaxing **(diastole).** The diastolic reading is the bottom number, 80 mmHg.

By measuring blood pressure, you can also calculate pulse pressure. The **pulse pressure** is the difference between the systolic and the diastolic pressure. For instance, your blood pressure is 120/80 mmHg. Your pulse pressure is 40 mmHg (120 minus 80). Note that a blood pressure range of 100 to 140 mmHg (systolic) to 60 to 90 mmHg (diastolic) is considered normal for adult males. Any reading greater than 140/90 mmHg is consid-

ered hypertensive. Blood pressure readings vary according to age, gender, and size. For instance, the normal blood pressure of a 2-year-old child is 95/65 mmHg.

TAKING A BLOOD PRESSURE. Measurement of blood pressure provides valuable information regarding a person's general health (Fig. 15–9). You will be taking blood pressure readings on most of your patients. Blood pressure is most commonly measured over the brachial artery, in the upper arm. The pressures are expressed in mmHg (millimeters of mercury). Unless otherwise stated, the term *blood pressure* refers to the blood pressure in the large arteries.

The instrument used to take a blood pressure recording is the sphygmomanometer. The **sphygmomanometer** is a device with two basic components, a dial indicating the pressure and an inflatable cuff. The cuff is wrapped around the patient's upper arm and inflated with air until the brachial artery is compressed and the flow of blood through the artery is stopped. Then, with a stetho-

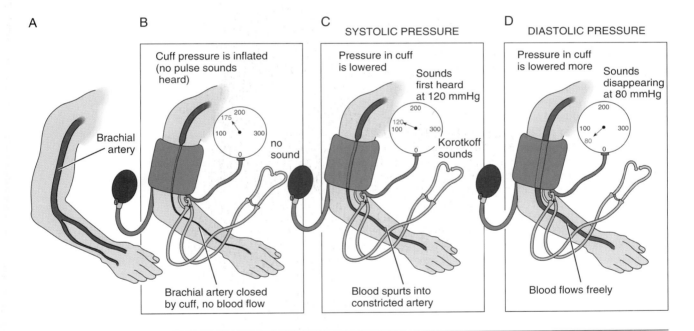

FIGURE 15–9 • Taking a blood pressure. The measurement of blood pressure requires a sphygmomanometer and a stethoscope. Follow the panels for an explanation of the systolic (120 mmHg) and diastolic (80 mmHg) pressures. A, Identify the location of the brachial artery. B, Inflate the cuff, thereby squeezing the upper arm. At this point, the cuff pressure has become greater than the blood pressure within the brachial artery. The cuff pressure collapses the brachial artery, thereby stopping the flow of blood. No sound can be heard through the stethoscope. C, As the pressure within the cuff gradually diminishes, the artery opens slightly, and blood spurts through the blood vessel in response to the pressure within the brachial artery. You can hear the spurting effect of the blood as soft tapping sounds. The number on the sphygmomanometer that corresponds to the tapping sounds is recorded as the systolic blood pressure (120 mmHg). With further reduction in cuff pressure, the brachial artery opens wider and allows blood flow through the artery to increase. The sound of the blood flowing through the partially opened artery sounds different from the tapping sounds of the spurting blood; it sounds louder and more distinct. D, As cuff pressure declines even further, the brachial artery opens completely, and normal blood flow through the artery resumes. At this point the sounds (stethoscope) disappear. The pressure at which the sounds disappear is read as the diastolic blood pressure (80 mmHg).

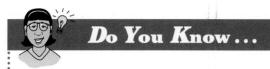

What is the meaning of "white coat" hypertension?

A routine physical examination generally includes an assessment of blood pressure. A person may have a normal blood pressure and yet be so anxious about the results of examination that blood pressure becomes elevated as soon as the physician begins the examination. The person is hypertensive only when the physician is taking the blood pressure. Because the physician is usually wearing a white coat, it is called "white coat" hypertension. At least three blood pressure elevations must be measured for the person to be classified as hypertensive.

scope placed over the brachial artery distal to, or below, the cuff, the examiner listens for various sounds. The sounds, called **Korotkoff sounds,** are caused by the flow of blood through the brachial artery. The measurement of blood pressure is illustrated and explained in Figure 15–9.

Blood Pressure in Different Blood Vessels

Blood pressures vary from one kind of blood vessel to the next (Fig. 15–10). Note that the blood pressure is highest in the aorta because it is closest to the left ventricle, which pumps blood with great force. The blood pressure gradually declines as the blood flows from the large arteries into the arterioles into the capillaries into the venules and finally into the veins. This difference in pressure causes blood to flow from the arterial side of the circulation to the venous side. Note that a blood pressure of 120/80 mmHg is normal only for large blood vessels. Capillary pressure is generally much lower. Pressure within the large veins is around 0 mmHg.

How Venous Blood Flows Back to the Heart

Although blood pressure is very high in the arterial circulation, it decreases to almost 0 mmHg in the veins. The blood pressure in the veins is so low, in fact, that it alone cannot return blood from the veins back to the heart. Other mechanisms accomplish the task of returning venous blood to the heart. Three mechanisms—skeletal muscle action, respiratory movements, and constriction of the veins—cause venous blood to return to the heart.

SKELETAL MUSCLE ACTION. As Figure 15–11 shows, the large veins in the leg are surrounded by skeletal muscles. As the skeletal muscles contract, they squeeze the large veins, thereby squirting

blood toward the heart. Note that, because of the closed valves, blood does not squirt backwards. Thus contraction of the skeletal muscles of the legs assists with the return of venous blood to the heart.

This mechanism is called the **skeletal muscle pump.** The pump helps explain the beneficial effects of exercise for your patients. Exercise improves venous blood flow, thereby preventing stagnation of blood and blood clot formation.

RESPIRATORY MOVEMENTS. The act of breathing is performed by the contraction and relaxation of the skeletal muscles of the chest. These respiratory movements cause the pressures in the chest to change. The changes in intrathoracic pressure assist the return of venous blood to the heart. The

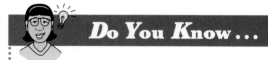

What do varicose veins look like?

Varicose veins are distended and twisted veins, usually involving the superficial veins in the legs. Varicosities can develop in other veins. Hemorrhoids, for instance, are varicose veins that affect the veins in the anal region. Persons who are alcoholic often develop varicose veins at the base of the esophagus. These are called esophageal varices. These varices are apt to rupture, causing a massive, life-threatening hemorrhage.

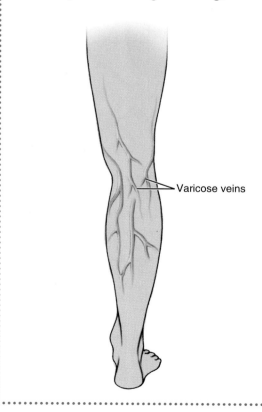

Varicose veins

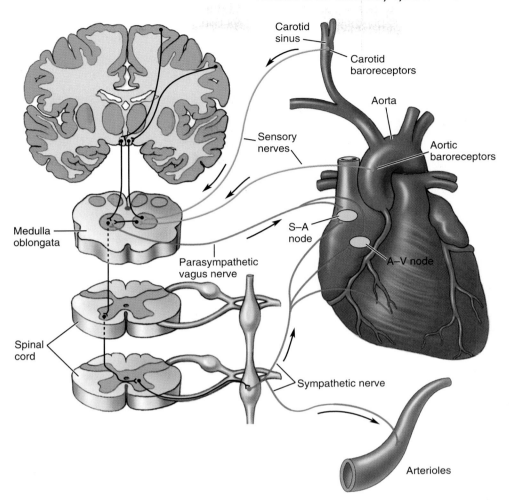

FIGURE 15–14 ● Baroreceptor reflex. The baroreceptor keeps the blood pressure within normal limits. The reflex consists of baroreceptors (aortic arch and carotid sinuses); nerves that carry sensory information to the brain; the medulla in the brain, which evaluates the information; and the nerves of the autonomic nervous system (sympathetic and parasympathetic), which carry the decision from the medulla to the heart and blood vessels.

cially the arterioles. Several mechanisms regulate blood pressure. The most important rapidly acting mechanism is the baroreceptor reflex. When blood pressure declines, the baroreceptor reflex causes a discharge of the sympathetic nervous system. Firing of the sympathetic nerves results in an increase in blood pressure, restoring blood pressure to normal. When blood pressure increases above normal, the baroreceptor reflex causes a discharge of the parasympathetic nerves. These, in turn, help to lower blood pressure. The renin-angiotensin–aldosterone mechanism is concerned with the long-term regulation of blood pressure.

Distribution of Blood Flow

While the blood vessels' ability to dilate (causing vasodilation) and constrict (causing vasoconstriction) plays an important role in the regulation of blood pressure, vasodilation and vasoconstriction also play an important role in the distribution of blood flow. As Figure 15–15 shows, blood flow to a particular area of the body can change. For instance, in the resting state, the skeletal muscle receives 20% of the total blood flow, and the kidney and the abdomen receive 19% and 24%, respectively. Note what happens during strenuous exercise. Blood flow is shunted, or redirected; the percentage of blood flow pumped to skeletal muscle greatly increases (to 71% of total flow). The percentage that flows through the kidney and abdomen considerably decreases (3.5% of total flow). In other words, the blood is directed to sites where it is most needed, to the skeletal muscle. Note also that the blood flow to the skin increases from 9% to 11% of total flow. This change is related to the dissipation of body heat by the skin (see Chapter 6).

How does blood flow adjust itself? When the person starts to exercise, the autonomic nerves

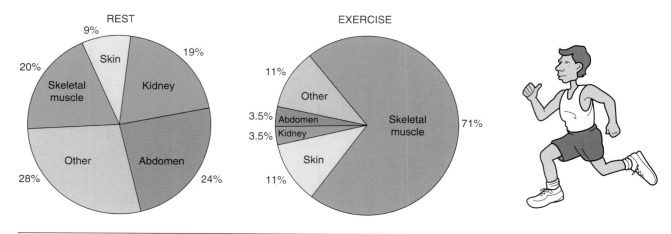

FIGURE 15–15 ● Distribution of blood flow at rest and during exercise. The circle on the left illustrates the distribution of blood flow in a person at rest. The skeletal muscle receives 20% of the total blood flow. The circle on the right illustrates the distribution of blood flow during strenuous exercise; strenuous exercise causes blood flow to the skeletal muscles to increase to 71% of the total flow. Note the blood flow adjustments for other organs.

and various chemical substances act on the blood vessels to cause either vasodilation or vasoconstriction. During exercise, blood vessels to the skeletal muscles dilate, thereby increasing blood flow. The blood vessels to the kidneys and abdominal area constrict, thereby decreasing blood flow and allowing more blood to be directed to the skeletal muscles. At the completion of the exercise, the blood vessels change again, thereby redirecting the flow of blood to resting status.

Pulse

What is the pulse? The ventricles pump blood into the arteries an average of 72 times per minute. The blood causes an alternating expansion and recoil of the arteries with each beat of the heart. This alternating expansion and recoil creates a pressure wave (similar to vibration), which travels through all the arteries. This wave is called the **pulse.**

Because it is due to the rhythmic contraction of the ventricles of the heart, the pulse is often described as a heartbeat that can be felt at an arterial site. Although a pulse can be felt in any artery lying close to the surface of the body, the site most often used to feel the pulse is the radial artery in the wrist area. Determine your own radial pulse and then try feeling a pulse at several pulse points identified in Figure 15–16.

The normal resting pulse rate is about 72 beats per minute (range 60–100 beats per minute). Many factors can affect pulse rate. Some of the more important factors include size, gender, age, level of exercise, strong emotions, various hor-

mones, pathologic states, and a wide variety of drugs. (These factors are described in Chapter 14.)

What can you learn about the patient by feeling the pulse? You can determine the heart rate. A normal heart rate is about 72 beats per minute. You can detect a **tachycardia** (a heart rate in excess of 100 beats per minute). You can detect a **bradycardia** (a slow rate, less than 60 beats per minute). You can also determine if the heart is beating regularly or rhythmically. By assessing the rhythm or regularity of the pulse, you may detect a cardiac dysrhythmia.

You can also assess the pulse for its strength. Does the pulse feel strong or weak? At times the heart contracts so weakly that the heartbeat cannot be felt over the radial artery, which happens in a person who has lost a lot of blood and is in shock. Lastly, you may not be able to detect a pulse in a particular artery. The pulse may be absent in a blocked or occluded artery. For instance, if a person has poor arterial circulation to the feet, as occurs with many diabetic persons, the dorsalis pedis pulse may be undetectable. Thus, a correct assessment of the pulse can provide much useful information about the patient's condition.

Capillary Exchange

Capillaries are the most numerous of the blood vessels. Estimates suggest that there are about 10 billion capillaries in the body. If all of the capillaries in the body were lined up end-to-end, they would encircle the earth 2½ times. The capillaries are also the smallest blood vessels. They

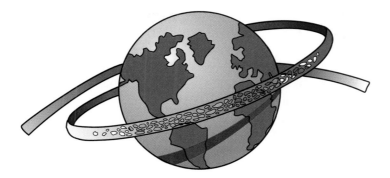

connect the arterioles with the venules, but they do much more than act as connecting vessels between the arteries and veins. The capillaries act as exchange vessels.

What is an exchange vessel? An exchange vessel makes deliveries and pick-ups, much like a

waiter (Fig. 15–17A). For instance, a waiter drops off trays of food to hungry guests. After a period has passed, the waiter picks up the waste—the empty trays, dirty dishes, and leftover food. Note the exchange part: trays of food dropped off and waste picked up.

How Capillaries Work

The capillaries are sites for the exchange of nutrients and waste (Fig. 15–17B). As blood flows through the capillaries, substances move out of the capillary into the surrounding tissue spaces (interstitium). These substances include oxygen, water, electrolytes, and various nutrients such as glucose; they are the substances the cell needs to live and grow.

These substances are taken up and used by the cells. As the cells carry on their work, they produce waste material such as carbon dioxide. The cellular waste diffuses out of the cell, into the interstitium. The waste and the water in which it is dissolved then move into the capillaries. The blood carries the waste away from the capillary to the organs of excretion, such as the kidneys and the lungs.

What has been accomplished at the capillary site? Like the waiter, the blood has delivered substances necessary for cell function. The cells are the hungry guests. After a while, the capillary, like the waiter, has picked up the waste so that it can be carried away and eliminated. An exchange has taken place. Therefore, the capillaries are called *exchange vessels*.

Why Capillaries Are Good Exchange Vessels

Three characteristics make the capillaries good exchange vessels: thin capillary walls, holes in the capillary walls, and large numbers of capillaries (Fig. 15–18).

THIN CAPILLARY WALLS. The capillary wall consists of a single layer of epithelium that sits on a delicate basement membrane. This single layer creates a very thin wall and allows many substances to move easily from the blood to the tissue space.

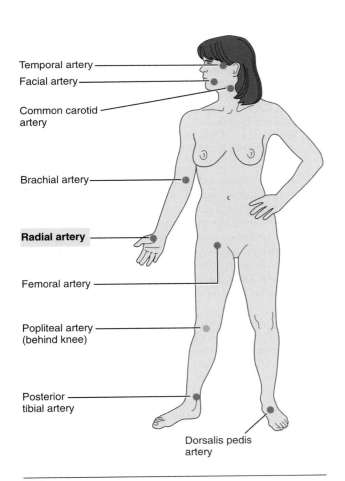

Temporal artery
Facial artery
Common carotid artery
Brachial artery
Radial artery
Femoral artery
Popliteal artery (behind knee)
Posterior tibial artery
Dorsalis pedis artery

FIGURE 15–16 • Pulses. These are the sites where the pulses can be easily felt, or palpated. Note the wrist where the radial pulse is located. The brachial artery pulse is the site over which you place the stethoscope when taking a blood pressure.

A

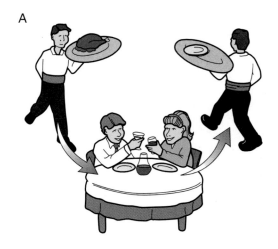

B

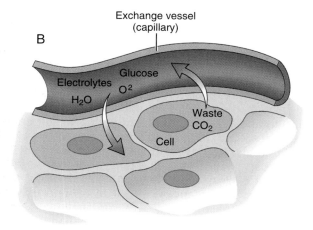

FIGURE 15-17 ● Capillary exchange: deliveries and pick-up. A, A waiter delivers food to hungry guests; later he picks up the dirty dishes and waste. He has exchanged the food for waste. B, The blood in the capillary delivers O_2, water, electrolytes, and glucose to the "hungry" cells. The capillary blood also picks up waste and carries it away for disposal. Oxygen and nutrients are exchanged for carbon dioxide and other waste.

HOLES IN THE CAPILLARY WALLS. The capillary walls contain tiny holes, or pores. The size of the pore determines which substances can cross the wall. Note that substance X is smaller than the pore and can therefore leave the capillary through the pore. Substance X might represent water, various electrolytes, and glucose. Substance Z, however, is larger than the pore and cannot fit through the hole. Substance Z is, therefore, confined to the

capillary. Plasma proteins, for instance, are normally too large to fit through the pores. The plasma proteins thus remain in the capillaries.

The size of the pores varies from tissue to tissue. For instance, capillary pores in skeletal muscle are much smaller than the pores of the capillaries in the liver, spleen, and bone marrow. The pore size in the liver, in fact, is so large that even the large plasma proteins and red blood cells can leave

1. Very thin capillary wall (only one cell thick)

2. Capillary walls have holes or pores

3. Millions of capillaries have slow velocity of flow of blood

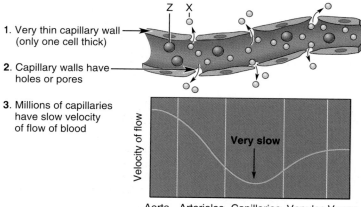

FIGURE 15-18 ● Why capillaries are good exchange vessels. (1) Capillary walls are very thin. Substances exchange very easily across the single layer wall. (2) Capillary walls have holes, or pores, through which substances move. (3) Blood flow in the capillaries is very slow. This slow movement of blood allows adequate time for substances to exchange.

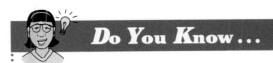

Do You Know...

What do a prune and a dehydrated person have in common?

A prune is a dehydrated plum. As water is removed from the plum, the skin assumes a shriveled appearance. The same process occurs in a person who is dehydrated. As fluid is lost from the body, water moves from the interstitium (tissue spaces), into the blood vessels in an attempt to maintain adequate blood volume and blood pressure. As water is lost from the interstitium, the overlying skin appears shriveled, much like a prune. The dehydrated patient is said to have poor skin turgor.

the capillary easily and mix freely with the tissue fluid; the blood literally bathes the hepatic cells. These capillaries are so different that they have a special name; they are called **hepatic sinusoids.**

LARGE NUMBERS OF CAPILLARIES. With so many capillaries, every cell in the body has a capillary near it. This arrangement ensures continuous nourishment of the cells. The large numbers of capillaries also affect the rate of blood flow. The more capillaries there are, the slower the blood flow. Blood flow within the capillaries is very slow. This slow rate of blood flow increases the time that the blood remains in the capillary. More time in the capillary means more exchange.

Running Downhill, Pushing and Pulling

What are the forces that cause cellular substances (glucose, oxygen, and waste) to move, or exchange, across the capillary wall? How do these substances move from the blood into the tissue spaces and then back into the blood? Two processes are exchange involving diffusion and exchange involving a filtration-osmosis balancing act.

EXCHANGE INVOLVING DIFFUSION: RUNNING DOWNHILL. Diffusion is the primary process causing substances to move across the capillary wall. **Diffusion** means that a substance moves from an area of high concentration to an area of low concentration. In other words, the diffusing substance runs down its diffusion gradient. For instance, the concentration of oxygen is higher in the capillary than in the tissue fluid. Thus, oxygen diffuses from the capillary into the interstitium (space between the cells). On the other hand, carbon dioxide concentration is higher in the interstitium than in the capillaries. Thus, carbon dioxide diffuses from the interstitium into the capillary.

EXCHANGE INVOLVING FILTRATION-OSMOSIS: THE PUSH AND PULL OF EXCHANGE. A secondary process of exchange involves filtration-osmosis. This process is very important for the movement of water and dissolved substances across the capillary. Filtration is illustrated in the syringe in Figure 15–19A. A syringe is loaded with water. If you were to punch holes in the side of the syringe and push on the plunger, what would happen? Not only would water flow out of the needle-end, but it would also squirt out of the side of the syringe in response to the pressure.

The plunger and syringe are similar to the heart and capillaries (Fig. 15–19B). The heart pushes, or pumps, blood through the capillaries. Because of the blood pressure, blood moves forward from the arterial to the venous circulation. Because of the holes, or pores, in the capillary wall, however, water and the smaller substances (eg, electrolytes, glucose) squirt into the interstitium.

The *pushing* of the water and dissolved substances through the pores is filtration. Note that the cause of filtration is blood pressure, or the pumping action of the heart. Note also the direction. In response to the pressure in the capillary, water and the dissolved substances are pushed out of the capillary into the interstitium. What happens to all the material pushed into the interstitium? It is used by the cell as needed.

The waste from the cell dissolves in the water in the interstitial space. What then? The water and dissolved waste must return to the capillaries. This effect involves osmosis. Figure 15–19C shows that the osmotic pressure in the capillary is higher than in the interstitium. The capillary osmotic pressure is higher because of the plasma proteins trapped within the capillaries. (Recall that the plasma proteins are too large to fit through the capillary pores.) The plasma proteins create a high osmotic pressure and pull the water from the interstitium into the capillary. Any excess water that the plasma proteins cannot pull back into the capillary is removed from the interstitium by the lymphatic vessels. (See Chapter 16.)

What is the balancing act? The exact amount of water pushed out of, or filtered, at one end of the capillary is pulled in, or reabsorbed, at the other end. The balancing act is important. If the amount of water filtered out of the capillary exceeds the amount reabsorbed from the tissue space, fluid collects in the tissue space. Excess fluid collection in the interstitium is called **edema.** If more water is reabsorbed from the tissue space than was filtered, the tissue space appears dehydrated.

✳ **SUM IT UP!** As blood flows through the capillaries, an exchange of nutrients and gases occurs between the capillary blood and the interstitium. Nourishing substances are continuously delivered to the cells, while waste products are removed from the interstitium for eventual elimination from the body. The processes of diffusion, filtration, and osmosis play key roles in the exchange and distribution of these substances.

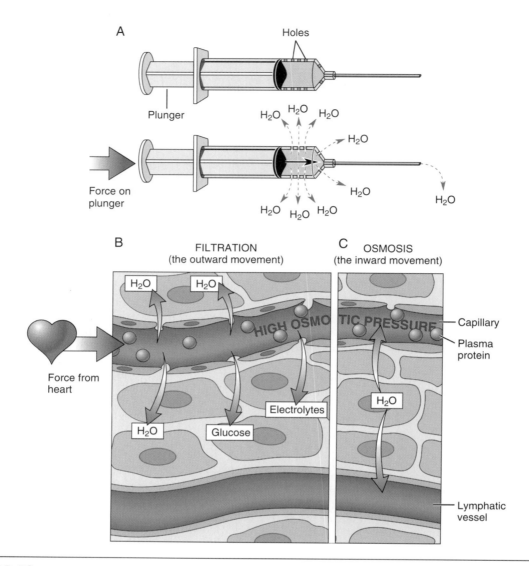

FIGURE 15–19 ● Filtration and osmosis. A, A syringe is filled with water. The barrel of the syringe is punctured, forming little holes. Note how water squirts through the holes on the side of the syringe when the plunger is pushed. B, When the heart contracts, it forces blood through the capillaries. Water and dissolved substances squirt through the capillary holes into the interstitium. C, The high osmotic pressure in the capillaries pulls the water and dissolved substances back into the capillary from the interstitium. Water also leaves the interstitium through the lymphatic vessels.

As You Age

1. The circulatory system is one of the body systems most affected by age. The walls of the arteries thicken and become less elastic and more stiff. There are two major consequences: blood flow to vital organs (eg, the brain) decreases and blood pressure increases.

2. Changes occur in both the walls and the valves of the veins. As a result, the elderly are more prone to the development of varicose veins.

3. The inner surface of the blood vessels becomes roughened because of age-related changes in the vessel wall and the development of fatty plaques. As a result, elderly persons are more prone to thrombus formation.

4. The baroreceptors become less sensitive. Cardiovascular adjustments to changes in position are slowed, and the person may become dizzy and tend to fall.

Disorders of Blood Vessels and Circulation

Aneurysm
A bulging of a weakened arterial wall most often affecting the aorta. The major concern is that the aneurysm will rupture, causing a massive hemorrhage. Rupture of a cerebral aneurysm causes a stroke.

Arterial occlusive disease
Narrowing of the arterial vessels, commonly affecting the lower extremities. The narrowing is due to changes in the arterial wall structure and the development of fatty plaques on the inner wall.

Arteriosclerosis
Hardening, or calcification, of arterial walls often causing the blood pressure to increase.

Atherosclerosis
From the Greek meaning porridge and hardening. The arterial walls fibrose, harden, and accumulate lipids. Atherosclerosis is a major cause of myocardial infarction, stroke, and occlusive arterial disease of the lower extremities. The narrowing of the arteries decreases blood flow, deprives the cells of nutrients and oxygen, and causes gangrene (death). Persons with diabetes mellitus are particularly prone to arterial occlusive disease; it is a major cause of toe, foot, and leg amputations in the diabetic patient.

Hypertension
A persistent, abnormally elevated blood pressure. By itself, hypertension causes no symptoms and is therefore called the silent killer. Hypertension is serious because it increases the risk of stroke, heart attack, and kidney failure.

Phlebitis
An inflammation of a vein, causing pain and swelling. Thrombophlebitis is caused by thrombotic (clot) occlusion of a vein. A serious consequence is the dislodging of the thrombus, which causes a fatal pulmonary embolus.

Shock
A condition characterized by inadequate blood flow to the tissues. Shock is often caused by hemorrhage and a severe decrease in blood pressure. The persistent low blood pressure impairs tissue oxygenation. Unless the hypotensive state is corrected, the patient develops irreversible shock and dies.

Summary Outline

The circulatory system is a series of blood vessels, or hollow tubes, that begin and end in the heart. The circulatory system delivers blood to all the body's cells and then returns the blood to the heart.

I. Structure of the Circulatory System

A. Two Circulations
1. The pulmonary circulation carries blood from the right ventricle to the lungs and to the left atrium. The pulmonary circulation oxygenates the blood.
2. The systemic circulation supplies blood to the rest of the body and then returns the blood to the heart.

B. Names of Blood Vessels
1. Arteries carry blood away from the heart. The smallest arteries are the arterioles.
2. Capillaries are the smallest and most numerous of the blood vessels. There is a capillary close to every cell in the body.

3. Veins carry blood from the capillaries back to the heart. Small veins are called venules.
4. The usual sequence of blood flow is this: heart (left side) to arteries to arterioles to capillaries to venules to veins to heart (right side).

C. Layers of Blood Vessels
1. The tunica intima is the innermost layer and forms a smooth and shiny endothelium.
2. The tunica media is the middle layer that contains elastic tissue and smooth muscle.
3. The tunica adventitia is the outermost layer of connective tissue.

D. Blood Vessels: What They Do
1. Arteries conduct blood from the heart to the organs and are called conductance vessels.
2. The arterioles constrict and dilate, thereby determining resistance to the flow of blood. The arterioles are called resistance vessels.

continued

Summary Outline *continued*

I. Structure of the Circulatory System, *continued*

D. Blood Vessels: What They Do, *continued*

3. Capillaries are concerned with the exchange of water and dissolved substances between the blood and tissue fluid. Capillaries are called exchange vessels.
4. Veins and venules return blood to the heart from the body. The veins also store blood and are therefore called capacitance vessels.

E. Major Arteries of the Systemic Circulation

1. The major arteries include the aorta and the arteries arising from the aorta.
2. See Figure 15–4 for the names and locations of the major arteries.

F. Major Veins of the Systemic Circulation

1. The major veins include the venae cavae and the veins that empty into them.
2. See Figure 15–5 for the names and locations of the major veins.

G. Special Circulations

1. The head and brain are supplied by two sets of arteries: the carotid arteries and the vertebral arteries. The internal carotid arteries and the basilar artery form the circle of Willis. Blood from the head and brain drains into the jugular veins.
2. The blood supply to the liver is composed of the portal vein, the hepatic artery, and the hepatic veins. The hepatic artery brings oxygen-rich blood to the liver. The portal vein carries blood from the digestive tract to the liver. The hepatic veins carry blood from the liver to the inferior vena cava.
3. The fetal circulation has several unique features. The fetus uses the placenta as lungs. The umbilical blood vessels carry blood between the placenta and the fetus. Three special structures are the ductus venosus, the foramen ovale, and the ductus arteriosus.

II. Functions of the Circulatory System

A. The Circulatory System and Blood Pressure

1. The circulatory system maintains a blood pressure to ensure an adequate flow of blood to the body.
2. The normal blood pressure is 120/80 mm Hg; 120 is the systolic reading, and 80 is the diastolic reading. The pulse pressure is the difference between the systolic and diastolic reading (120 − 80 = 40).
3. Blood pressure varies throughout the circulatory system. Blood pressure is highest in the aorta and lowest in the venae cavae. The normal blood pressure of 120/80 mmHg is the blood pressure in a large artery.
4. Blood pressure is determined by the action of the heart and the blood vessels. The heart affects blood pressure by increasing or decreasing heart rate or stroke volume, or both. The blood vessels affect blood pressure by constricting or dilating the arterioles.
5. Blood pressure is regulated on a day-to-day basis by the baroreceptor reflex. Other mechanisms can correct blood pressure more slowly. The most important is the renin-angiotensin-aldosterone mechanism.

B. The Circulatory System and the Distribution of Blood

1. Blood flow to a part of the body can be altered according to need (eg, blood flow to exercising muscles increases).
2. Alterations in blood flow occur when the autonomic nervous system and various chemicals tell the arterioles to constrict or dilate.

C. The Circulatory System and Capillary Exchange

1. The capillaries are the site of exchange of nutrients and waste between the blood and the tissue fluid.
2. Factors that make the capillaries ideal exchange vessels are the large surface area, thin walls with holes, and slow rate of blood flow through the capillaries.
3. Water and dissolved substances move out of the capillary into the tissue spaces by diffusion and filtration. The capillary pressure pushes water out of the capillaries. Water and dissolved waste move from the tissue fluid into the capillaries by osmosis.

D. The Circulatory System and the Pulse

1. The pulse is due to the alternating expansion and recoil of the artery creating a pressure wave (similar to vibration).
2. The pulse is caused by the pumping of the heart; pulse rate therefore reflects heart rate.
3. The normal pulse is an average of 72 beats per minute (range 60 to 100 beats per minute).

 Review Your Knowledge

1. Why are the walls of the arteries so much thicker than those of the corresponding veins?

2. Trace a drop of blood from the left ventricle of the heart to the wrist of the right hand and back to the heart. Trace a drop of blood from the heart to the dorsum of the right foot and back to the right side of the heart.

3. Describe the structure of the capillary walls. How is their structure related to their function?

Review Your Knowledge *continued*

4. What two paired vessels provide arterial blood to the brain? What name describes the communication between them?

5. What is the function of the hepatic portal circulation? Why is a portal circulation a "strange" circulation?

6. Define pulse.

7. Identify the artery palpated at the following pressure points: wrist, front of the ear, side of the neck, groin, back of the knee.

8. Define blood pressure, systolic pressure, and diastolic pressure.

9. What vital role does blood pressure play?

10. Two elements determine blood pressure: cardiac output and vascular resistance, or friction in the blood vessels. Name two factors that increase cardiac output. Name three factors that increase vascular resistance.

11. What is the effect of hemorrhage on blood pressure? Why?

12. What are varicose veins?

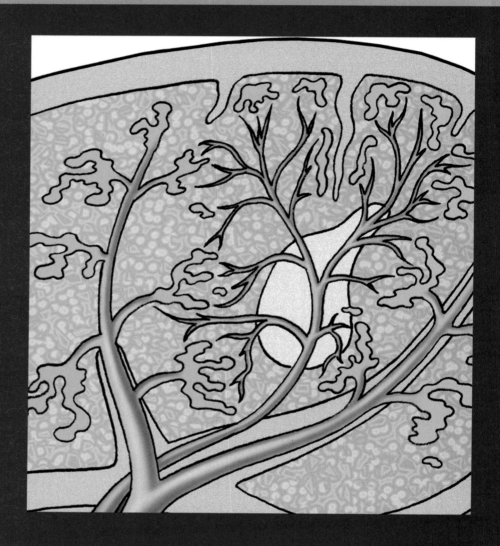

16 LYMPHATIC SYSTEM

*O*bjectives

1. List three functions of the lymphatic system.

2. Describe the composition of lymph.

3. Describe the flow path for lymph.

4. List three factors that help lymph move through the lymphatic vessels.

5. Describe the four lymphoid organs: lymph nodes, tonsils, thymus gland, and spleen.

6. List two functions of the lymphoid organs.

7. State the location of the following lymph nodes: cervical nodes, axillary nodes, and inguinal nodes.

8. Describe the function of the following lymph nodes: cervical nodes, axillary nodes, and inguinal nodes.

The woman in Figure 16–1 has a condition called elephantiasis. The name is an obvious reference to the size and shape of her leg. The condition is caused by the invasion and blockage of the lymphatic vessels by small worms called filariae. The tremendous swelling of the leg illustrates the importance of the lymphatic system, which drains fluid from our tissue spaces.

The lymphatic system contains lymph, lymphatic vessels, lymphoid organs, and lymphoid tissue widely scattered throughout the body. The three main functions of the lymphatic system are these:

• The lymphatic vessels return tissue fluid to the blood. The elephantiasis shown in Figure 16–1 provides ample evidence for the importance of adequate drainage.
• Specialized lymphatic vessels play an important role in the intestinal absorption of fats and fat-soluble vitamins.
• Lymphoid tissue helps the body defend itself against disease.

THE LYMPHATIC SYSTEM

Lymph: What It Is, Where It Comes From

Lymph (lĭmf) is a clear fluid that resembles plasma. Lymph is composed primarily of water, electrolytes, waste from metabolizing cells, and some protein that leaks out of the capillaries of the systemic circulation. Where does lymph come from? It is formed from the plasma during capillary exchange. Where does it go? It leaves the tissue space, or interstitium, through the lymphatic

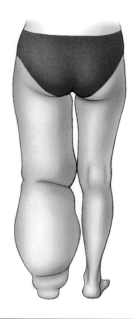

FIGURE 16–1 • Elephantiasis, a form of lymphedema, develops with inadequate drainage of lymph.

vessels. The lymphatic vessels carry the lymph toward the heart and eventually empty it into the blood.

Fluid and dissolved substances are continuously filtered out of the blood capillaries into the interstitium to form tissue fluid. Approximately 90% of this tissue fluid moves back into the blood capillaries and is carried away as part of the venous blood. What about the 10% of the tissue fluid that does not re-enter the blood capillaries? This fluid is drained by the lymphatic capillaries that surround the blood capillaries (Fig. 16–2). The tissue fluid entering the lymphatic vessels is the lymph.

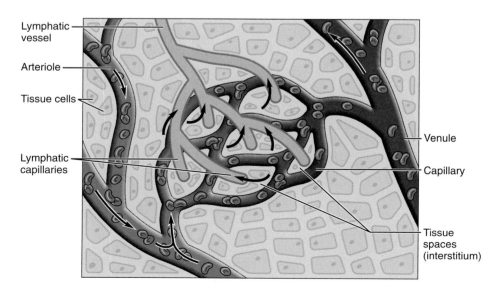

Lymphatic vessel

Arteriole

Tissue cells

Lymphatic capillaries

Venule

Capillary

Tissue spaces (interstitium)

FIGURE 16–2 • Lymph capillaries in the tissue space (interstitium). Tissue fluid is formed from the blood that flows through the blood capillaries. Most of the fluid is reabsorbed by the blood capillaries. Excess fluid is drained by the lymph capillaries.

Lymphatic Vessels

The **lymphatic vessels** (lĭm-făt'ĭk ves'əlz) include lymphatic capillaries and several larger lymphatic vessels. Like the blood vessels, the lymphatic vessels form an extensive network. The distribution of lymphatic vessels is similar to the distribution of veins. Every organ in the body has a rich supply of lymphatic vessels. They pick up tissue fluid and transport that fluid toward the heart. Figure 16–3 shows the relationship between the circulatory system and the lymphatic system.

The walls of the lymphatic capillaries are made up of a single layer of epithelium; the epithelium, or endothelium, has large holes, or pores. This large-pore structure allows the lymphatic capillaries to drain tissue fluid and proteins, thereby forming lymph. Once absorbed by the lymphatic capillaries, the lymph flows toward the heart through a series of larger and larger lymphatic vessels until it reaches the large lymphatic ducts.

For example, lymph from the right arm and the right side of the head and thorax drains into the **right lymphatic duct** (lĭm-făt'ĭk dŭkt). Lymph

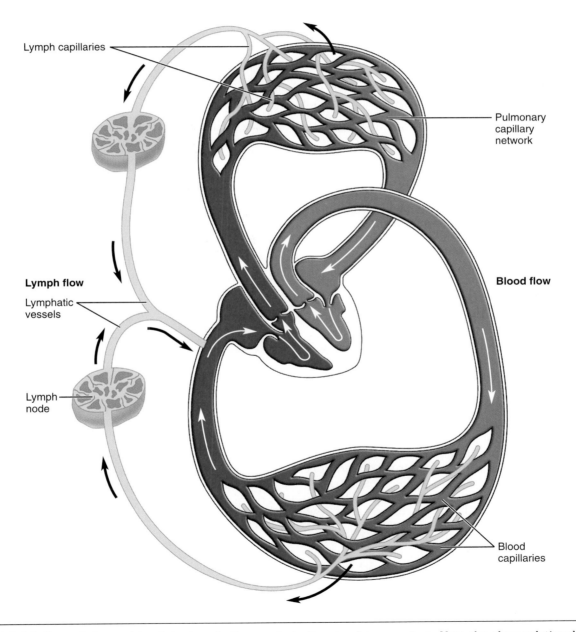

Lymph capillaries

Pulmonary capillary network

Lymph flow

Blood flow

Lymphatic vessels

Lymph node

Blood capillaries

FIGURE 16–3 ● Relationship of the lymphatic vessels to the circulatory system. Note the close relationship between the distribution of the lymphatic vessels (green) and the venous blood vessels (blue). Tissue fluid is drained by the lymphatic capillaries and transported by a series of larger lymphatic vessels toward the heart. The lymph eventually drains into the venous blood close to the heart.

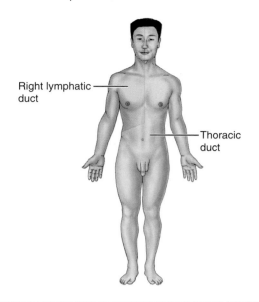

Right lymphatic duct

Thoracic duct

FIGURE 16–4 ● Areas of the body drained by the main lymphatic ducts. The shaded area represents the area drained by the right lymphatic duct. The unshaded area represents the area drained by the thoracic duct.

from the rest of the body drains into the **thoracic duct** (thə-răs′ĭk dŭkt) (Fig. 16–4). Both ducts empty the lymph into the subclavian veins. The right lymphatic duct drains lymph into the right subclavian vein; the thoracic duct drains lymph into the left subclavian vein.

Movement Through the Lymphatic Vessels

Whereas blood moves, or flows, because it is pumped by the heart, lymph depends on other means for movement. Lymph moves in response to

- The milking action of the skeletal muscles. As the skeletal muscles contract, they squeeze the surrounding lymphatic vessels. This milking action pushes lymph toward the heart.
- The movement of the chest during respiration. Contraction and relaxation of the chest muscles cause changes in the pressure within the thorax. The changes in intrathoracic pressure affect the flow of lymph.
- The rhythmic contraction of the smooth muscle in the lymphatic vessels. The alternating contraction and relaxation of the smooth muscle cause lymph to flow.

The lymphatic vessels form a one-way path. Lymph flows from the tissue spaces toward the heart. Why? Like the veins, the lymphatic vessels contain valves. Valves prevent any backflow of lymph; if lymph moves at all, it must move toward the heart.

✳ **SUM IT UP!** Lymphatic vessels accompany venous blood vessels throughout the body. They drain fluid and protein from tissue spaces as lymph; the lymph is eventually returned to venous blood by larger lymphatic vessels. Lymph is cleansed as it flows through the many lymph nodes associated with the lymphatic vessels.

LYMPHOID ORGANS

The **lymphoid organs** include the lymph nodes, the tonsils, the thymus gland, and the spleen (Fig. 16–5). Lymphoid tissue is also found scattered throughout the body in many other or-

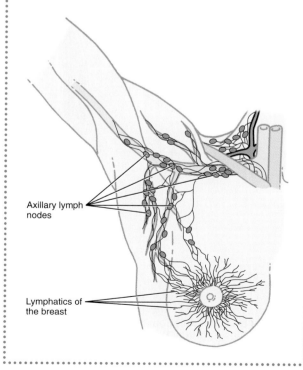

Do You Know...

Why are the axillary lymph nodes removed during a mastectomy (surgical breast removal)?

Cancer of the breast often spreads, or metastasizes, to the axillary lymph nodes. In an attempt to rid the body of all cancer cells, the surgeon removes the breast and the associated axillary lymph nodes. Each lymph node is then biopsied; further treatment often depends on how many of the lymph nodes are positive (ie, are cancerous, or malignant). Removal of the axillary lymph nodes frequently impairs lymphatic drainage. Consequently, the woman may develop edema of the affected arm and shoulder.

Axillary lymph nodes

Lymphatics of the breast

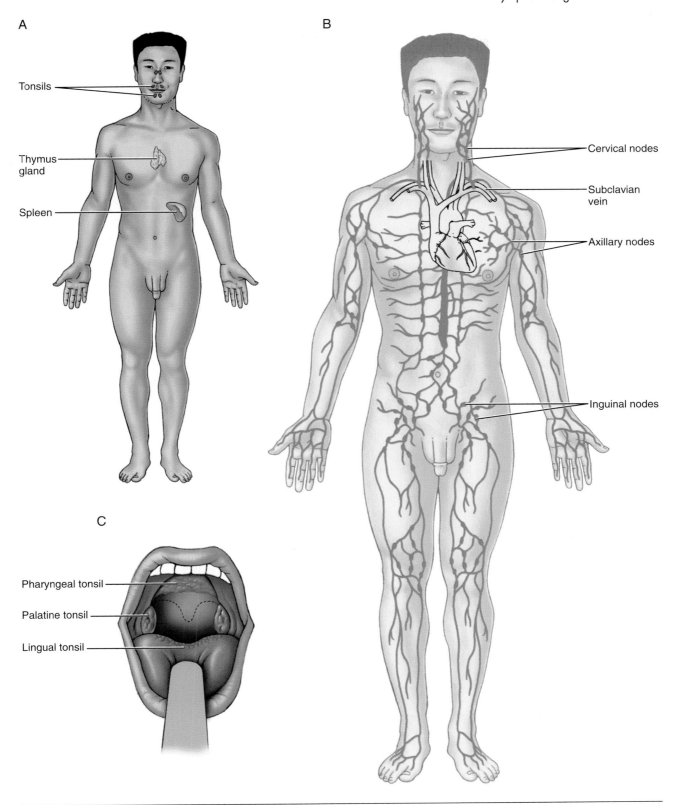

FIGURE 16–5 ● Location of lymphoid tissue. A, The lymphoid organs: tonsils, thymus gland, and spleen. B, Distribution of lymph nodes. Three major clusters of lymph nodes are the cervical lymph nodes, the axillary lymph nodes, and the inguinal lymph nodes. C, Tonsils: pharyngeal, palatine, and lingual. (The soft palate has been removed to show the pharyngeal tonsils.)

gans. In general, the lymphoid organs and lymphoid tissue help defend the body against disease by filtering particles such as pathogens and cancer cells from the lymph, tissue fluid, and blood and by supporting the activities of the lymphocytes, which provide immunity against disease.

Lymph Nodes

Lymph nodes (lĭmf nōdz) are small pea-shaped patches of lymphatic tissue strategically located so as to filter the lymph as it flows through the lymphatic vessels. Lymph nodes tend to appear in clusters (Fig. 16–5B). The larger clusters include the following:

- **Cervical lymph nodes,** which drain and cleanse lymph coming from the head and neck areas. Enlarged, tender cervical lymph nodes often accompany upper respiratory infections.
- **Axillary lymph nodes** located in the axillary area, or armpit. These nodes drain and cleanse lymph coming from the upper extremities, the shoulder, and the breast area. Cancer cells that escape from the breast are often trapped in the axillary lymph nodes.
- **Inguinal lymph nodes** located in the groin region. These nodes drain and cleanse lymph from the lower extremities and from the external genitalia.

What does a lymph node look like? A lymph node contains several compartments, called **lymph nodules,** separated by lymph sinuses (Fig. 16–6). The lymph nodules are masses of lymphocytes and macrophages. These cells are defensive cells; they are concerned with immunity and phagocytosis (the ingestion and removal of foreign substances). They protect the body against disease. The lymph nodules are separated by **lymph sinuses;** these are lymph-filled spaces. Afferent lymphatic vessels carry lymph into the node for cleansing. The lymph leaves the node through the efferent lymphatic vessels as it continues its journey toward the heart.

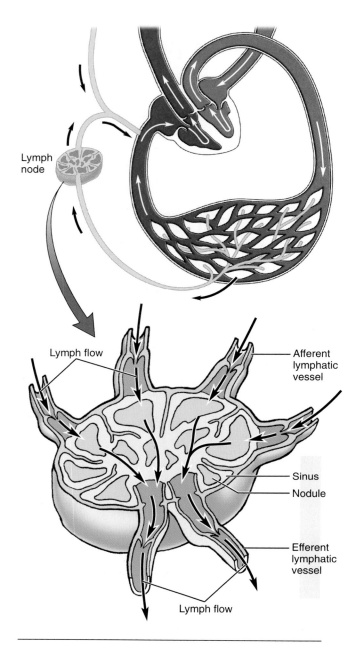

FIGURE 16–6 ● Cross section of a lymph node. Lymph flows into the node through the afferent lymphatic vessels (arrows). As the lymph flows through the sinuses, it is cleansed. The lymph then flows out of the node through the efferent lymphatic vessels.

Do You Know...

What is the "kissing disease"?

Infectious mononucleosis, or "mono," is an acute viral infection that involves the lymphatic tissue. Frequently, the cervical lymph nodes are enlarged. Mononucleosis frequently occurs in the young adult population. The causative organism is often spread by close contact, such as kissing; hence the name.

Tonsils

Tonsils (tŏn′səlz) are partially encapsulated lymph nodes in the throat area (see Fig. 16–5A). They filter tissue fluid contaminated by pathogens that enter the body through the nose or mouth or both. The three sets of tonsils are

- **Palatine tonsils,** small masses of lymphoid tissue located at the opening of the oral cavity into the pharynx. The palatine tonsils are what is

Do You Know...

Why do you sometimes get swollen glands when you have a sore throat?

As the lymph drains from the throat, it flows through the closest lymph nodes, where it is cleansed by the resident phagocytes. The lymph nodes may become tender and enlarged as they work to kill the pathogens. This condition is called **lymphadenitis.** Calling the condition swollen glands is somewhat misleading. The swelling and tenderness are associated with the enlarged lymph nodes and not with glands.

commonly referred to when we use the term *tonsils.* A tonsillectomy is most often performed on this particular set of tonsils.
- **Pharyngeal tonsils,** also called the **adenoids.** They are located near the opening of the nasal cavity in the upper pharynx. Enlargement of the adenoids may interfere with breathing and require surgical removal (called adenoidectomy).
- **Lingual tonsils** located at the back of the tongue.

Thymus Gland

The **thymus gland** (thī′məs glănd) is located in the upper thorax behind the sternum and below the thyroid gland (see Fig. 16–5A). Most active during early life, the thymus gland plays a crucial role in the development of the immune system before birth and in the first few months after birth. After puberty, the gland shrinks and is replaced by connective tissue and fat. It is concerned with the processing and maturation of special lymphocytes called T cells (see Chapter 17).

The thymus gland secretes hormones called **thymosins.** Thymosins promote the maturation of lymphocytes within the thymus gland. They also promote the growth and activity of lymphocytes in lymphoid functions throughout the body.

Spleen

The **spleen** (splēn) is the largest lymphoid organ in the body. It is located in the upper left quadrant of the abdominal cavity, just beneath the diaphragm and is normally protected by the lower rib cage (Fig. 16–7). Although the spleen is much larger, its shape and structure are similar to those of a lymph node.

The spleen filters blood rather than lymph. The spleen is composed of two types of tissue called white pulp and red pulp. The **white pulp** is

lymphoid tissue consisting primarily of lymphocytes surrounding arteries. The **red pulp** contains venous sinuses filled with blood and disease-preventing cells such as lymphocytes and macrophages. Blood enters the spleen through the splenic artery. The blood is cleansed as it slowly flows through the spleen. Microorganisms trapped by the spleen are destroyed by the leukocytes within the spleen. The cleansed blood leaves the spleen through the splenic vein.

Do You Know...

Why can an overactive spleen cause serious blood problems?

The spleen plays an important role in the removal of old, worn-out red blood cells and platelets from the circulation. If the spleen becomes too aggressive, however, blood cells are removed from the circulation prematurely. This process causes a low red blood cell count (anemia) and a low platelet count, resulting in thrombocytopenia and bleeding.

In addition to its cleansing role, the spleen has other functions. The spleen acts as a reservoir for blood. In other words, blood is stored within the spleen. When blood is needed by the body in an emergency, such as hemorrhage, the muscles in the spleen contract, forcing blood out of the spleen into the general circulation. The spleen also destroys and phagocytoses old, worn-out red blood cells. Finally, the spleen plays a role in erythropoiesis, as a site of red blood cell production before birth.

✳ **SUM IT UP!** Lymphocyte-containing organs, called lymphoid organs, include the lymph nodes, tonsils, thymus gland, and spleen. Lymphoid tissue, in general, plays a crucial role in the prevention of disease.

As You Age

1. Lymphoid tissue reaches its peak development at puberty and then progressively shrinks with age.
2. After puberty, the thymus gland involutes, or shrivels up, and is replaced by connective tissue. This process involves a decrease in the amount of thymosin produced. Because of these changes, the defensive mechanisms of the body diminish with age.

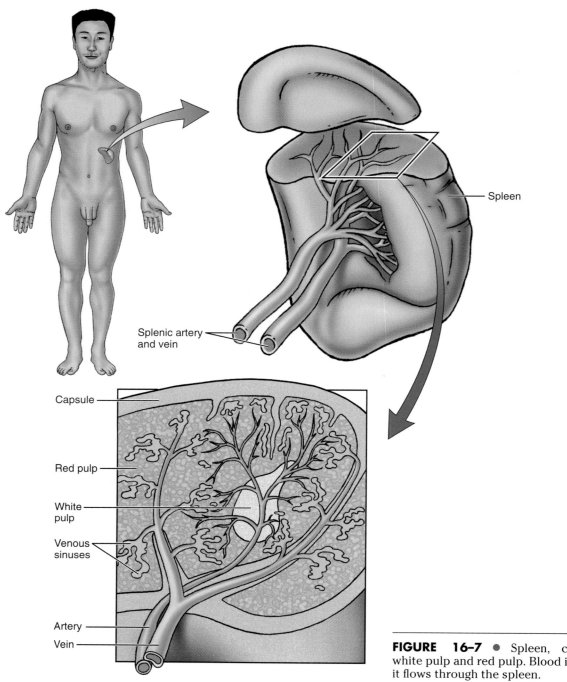

Capsule

Red pulp

White pulp

Venous sinuses

Artery

Vein

Splenic artery and vein

Spleen

FIGURE 16–7 ● Spleen, composed of white pulp and red pulp. Blood is cleansed as it flows through the spleen.

Disorders of the Lymphatic System

Cancer

Several types of malignant tumors affect lymphatic tissue. Lymphosarcoma is a malignant tumor of lymphoid tissue (involving the connective tissue). Most lymphomas (tumors that occur in lymphoid tissue) are malignant. Hodgkin's disease and non-Hodgkin's disease are malignant lymphomas. Both are characterized by painless and progressive enlargement of lymphoid tissue.

Lymphadenitis

Inflammation of the lymph nodes. The nodes become swollen and tender as they fight an infection. With a sore throat there is often a cervical lymphadenitis.

continued

Disorders of the Lymphatic System, *continued*

Lymphadenopathy   Disease of the lymph nodes. Lymphadenopathy often accompanies infection and cancer. HIV infection involves generalized lymphadenopathy.

Lymphangitis   Inflammation of the lymphatic vessels characterized by fine red streaks from the affected area to the groin or axilla. The condition is usually due to a staphylococcal or streptococcal infection.

Summary Outline

The main functions of the lymphatic system are defense of the body against infection, return of fluid from the tissue spaces to the blood, and absorption of fat and fat-soluble vitamins from the digestive tract.

I. The Lymphatic System
A. Lymph
1. Lymph is a clear fluid containing water, electrolytes, waste, and some protein.
2. Water and electrolytes are filtered from the plasma into the tissue spaces. Water leaves the tissue spaces by way of the lymphatic vessels (within the lymphatic vessels the fluid is known as lymph).

B. Lymphatic Vessels
1. Lymphatic vessels are similar in structure and distribution to the blood capillaries and the veins. The large holes in the lymphatic capillaries absorb fluid and protein from the tissue spaces.
2. Lymph from the right arm and right side of the head and thorax drains into the right lymphatic duct. The rest of the lymphatic vessels drain into the thoracic duct. Both large lymphatic vessels drain into the subclavian veins.

C. Movement of Lymph
1. Lymph is not pumped like blood (by the heart).
2. Lymph moves in response to skeletal muscle contraction (through milking action), chest movement, and contraction of smooth muscle in the lymphatic vessels.

II. Lymphoid Organs
The lymphoid organs are the lymph nodes, tonsils, thymus gland, and spleen.

A. Lymph Nodes
1. Lymph nodes are arranged in large clusters; major clusters of lymph nodes are the cervical, axillary, and inguinal nodes.
2. Lymph nodes help protect the body against infection.

B. Tonsils
1. Tonsils are encapsulated lymph nodes.
2. The tonsils are the palatine, pharyngeal, and lingual tonsils.

C. Thymus Gland
1. The thymus gland produces and helps to differentiate the lymphocytes.
2. The thymus gland secretes thymosins.

D. Spleen
1. The spleen is the largest lymphoid organ in the body and functions as a large lymph node.
2. The two types of splenic tissue are red pulp and white pulp.
3. The spleen helps filter blood; microorganisms are killed by the resident leukocytes in the spleen. The spleen also removes old worn-out red blood cells and platelets.

Review Your Knowledge

1. Name three functions of the lymph system.
2. Where does lymph come from?
3. How are lymphatic vessels different from blood vessels?
4. Through what ducts and veins does the lymph flow to arrive at the heart?
5. What three mechanisms assist in the movement of lymph? What prevents the backflow of lymph?
6. Name four lymphoid organs.
7. What are the locations and functions of the following lymph nodes: cervical, axillary, and inguinal?
8. What cells are found in lymph nodes?
9. What are the three types of tonsils? Which tonsils are the ones you can see most clearly when you open your mouth?
10. What is the largest lymphoid organ in the body?

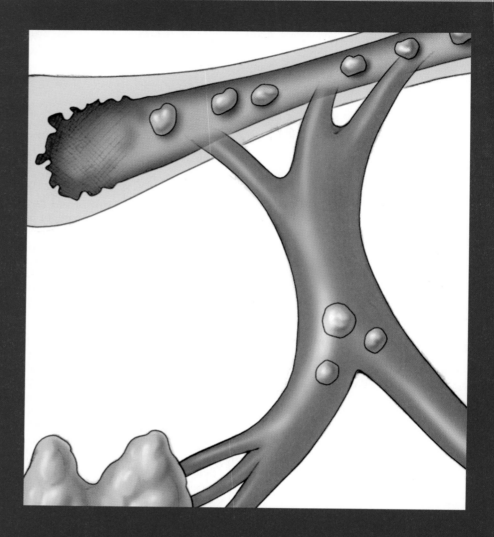

• • • Key Terms

Active immunity (ăk′tĭv ĭ-myōō′nĭ-tē)

Allergen (ăl′ər-jən)

Antibody (ăn′tĭ-bŏd″ē)

Antibody-mediated immunity
(ăn′tĭ-bŏd″ē mē′dē-āt″əd ĭ-myōō′nĭ-tē)

Antigen (ăn′tĭ-jən)

Artificially acquired immunity
(är″tə-fĭsh′əl-lē ə-kwīrd′ ĭ-myōō′nĭ-tē)

Autoimmunity (ô″tō-ĭ-myōō′nĭ-tē)

B cell (B lymphocyte) (bē sĕl *or* lĭm′fə-sīt)

Cell-mediated immunity
(sĕl′mē″dē-āt″əd ĭ-myōō′nĭ-tē)

Clone (klōn)

Complement proteins (kŏm′plə-mĕnt prō′tēn″)

Immunity (ĭ-myōō′nĭ-tē)

Immunoglobulin (ĭm′yōō-nō-glŏb′yə-lĭn)

Inflammation (ĭn″flə-mā′shən)

Interferon (ĭn″tər-fĭr′ŏn″)

Macrophage (măk′rə-fāj)

Naturally acquired immunity
(năch′ər-əl-lē ə-kwīrd′ ĭ-myōō′nĭ-tē)

Passive immunity (păs′ĭv ĭ-myōō′nĭ-tē)

Reticuloendothelial system (RES)
(rĭ-tĭk′yə-lō-ĕn″də-thē′lē-əl sĭs′təm)

T cell (T lymphocyte) (tē sĕl *or* lĭm′fə-sīt)

Tissue macrophage system
(tĭ′shōō măk′rə-fāj sĭs′təm)

Vaccine (văk-sēn′)

• • • Selected terms in bold type in this chapter are defined in the Glossary.

17 IMMUNE SYSTEM

Objectives

1. Differentiate between specific and nonspecific immunity.

2. Describe the process of phagocytosis.

3. Explain the causes of the signs of inflammation: redness, heat, swelling, and pain.

4. Explain the role of fever in fighting infection.

5. Describe two groups of protective proteins: interferons and complement proteins.

6. Describe the relationship of antigens to specific immunity.

7. Describe the development and function of T cells (T lymphocytes) and B cells (B lymphocytes).

8. Explain the role of T cells in cell-mediated immunity.

9. Explain the role of B cells in antibody-mediated immunity.

10. List the three most common immunoglobulins.

11. Describe the actions of antibodies.

12. Describe the two main categories of immunity: genetic immunity and acquired immunity.

13. Give examples of naturally and artificially acquired active and passive immunity.

14. Summarize the process of an allergic reaction.

oey was born with severe combined immunodeficiency disease (SCID); his immune system was not functioning well. This condition put Joey at high risk for life-threatening infections. As a result of this constant danger of infection, Joey spent most of his life in the sterile environment of a bubble. The bubble protected him from a world of microorganisms. For persons with healthy immune systems, microorganisms are harmless, but for Joey, the same microorganisms became dangerous pathogens. Understandably, the young child rebelled at life in a bubble and opted to live on the outside. Soon after leaving the bubble at the age of 12, however, Joey succumbed to an overwhelming infection.

Today, the use of bone marrow transplants has eliminated the life-long use of bubbles and has offered new hope for children with immune deficiency disease, who, unlike most of us, cannot share the world with millions of microorganisms. Without a functioning immune system, such children face a constant threat of infection and disease.

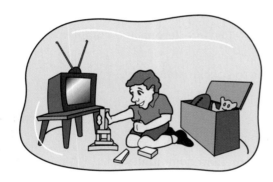

The human body is constantly bombarded by an army of microorganisms. Many of these microorganisms try to gain entrance to the body, but most are turned away. Some enter the body and live harmoniously within. Our intestines, for instance, harbor many microorganisms; some even perform helpful tasks, such as the bacterial synthesis of vitamin K. Other microorganisms, however, can cause serious problems if they gain entrance. Ask any tourist who has experienced "Montezuma's revenge," a gastrointestinal response to a microorganism common in southern North America.

Pathogens, or disease-producing organisms, are a major concern for the body's elaborate defense mechanisms. In addition to protecting the body from pathogens, these defense mechanisms protect the body from all other foreign agents, including pollens (like ragweed), toxins (like bee sting venom), and our own cells that have gone astray (cancer cells). This defense capacity is called **immunity** (ĭ-myoō′nĭ-tē). The **immune system** includes all of the structures and processes that mount a defense against foreign agents.

Do You Know...

How does stress affect the immune system?

"Stressed-out" persons secrete excessive amounts of steroids, one of which is cortisol. Cortisol suppresses the immune response. This response explains, in part, why persons who are stressed out experience a higher rate of upper respiratory infections. Some scientists have suggested that high levels of stress might encourage the development of cancer.

CLASSIFICATION OF THE IMMUNE SYSTEM

The defense mechanisms are classified as nonspecific and specific immunity. (Table 17–1 lists the many types of cells involved in the immune response.) **Nonspecific immunity** protects the body against many different types of foreign agents. With nonspecific immunity, the body need not recognize the specific foreign agent. **Specific immunity** homes in on a foreign substance and provides protection against one specific substance but no others.

Nonspecific Immunity

A number of defense mechanisms are included in the category of nonspecific immunity (Fig. 17–1). Nonspecific immunity can be divided into lines of defense. The first line of defense includes mechanical barriers, chemical barriers, and certain reflexes. The second line of defense includes phagocytosis, inflammation, fever, protective proteins (interferons and complement proteins), and natural killer (NK) cells. Remember: The nonspecific defense mechanisms work against all foreign agents; *no recognition of a specific agent is necessary.*

Mechanical and Chemical Barriers

Intact skin and mucous membranes serve as **mechanical barriers;** pathogens cannot cross these structures and enter the body. Mechanical barriers are the body's first line of defense, and destruction of mechanical barriers is an invitation to invasion and subsequent infection (see Fig. 17–1). Assisting the skin and mucous membranes with their defensive functions are their secretions; the secretions are the **chemical barriers.**

For example, tears, saliva, and perspiration provide chemical barriers that wash away mi-

Table 17•1   CELLS INVOLVED IN IMMUNITY

CELL TYPE	PRODUCTION SITE	FUNCTION
Leukocytes (WBCs)		
Neutrophils	Bone marrow	Phagocytosis
Basophils	Bone marrow	Secrete histamine and heparin
Eosinophils	Bone marrow	Destroy parasites
Monocytes	Bone marrow	Phagocytosis; enter tissues and are transformed into macrophages
Lymphocytes	Bone marrow, thymus gland, and other lymphoid organs	
B cells		Antibody-mediated immunity; produce plasma cells, which secrete antibodies
T cells		Cell-mediated immunity
Killer T cells		Kill cells
Helper T cells		Secrete substances (lymphokines), which activate B cells, and other cells
Suppressor T cells		Inhibit B cell and T cell activity (help control immune response)
Natural killer (NK) cells		Kill cells
Plasma cells	B lymphocytes	Secrete antibodies
Macrophages	Almost all organs and tissues	Phagocytosis; present antigens to helper T cells
Mast cells	Almost all organs and tissues, especially liver and lungs	Release histamine and other chemicals involved in inflammation
Memory cells	From activated B and T cells	Involved in "remembering" the antigen for a faster response when the antigen is introduced a second time

croorganisms. They also establish a hostile environment, thereby killing the potential pathogens. The acid and digestive enzymes secreted by the cells of the stomach kill most of the microorganisms swallowed. Tears secrete a substance called lysozyme, which discourages the growth of pathogens on the surface of the eye.

Other secretions make the environment sticky and so provide another kind of chemical barrier. The mucus secreted by the mucous membranes of the respiratory tract sticks to and traps inhaled foreign material. Then the cilia, which line most of the respiratory structures, sweep the entrapped material toward the throat so that inhaled material can eventually be coughed up and eliminated. In addition to the mechanical and chemical barriers, certain reflexes assist in the removal of pathogens. Sneezing and coughing help to remove pathogens from the respiratory tract, while vomiting and diarrhea help to remove pathogens from the digestive tract.

Mechanical and chemical barriers are not an adequate defense against all pathogens, however. If a pathogen penetrates this first line of defense, it encounters processes that make up the second line of defense.

Phagocytosis

Some of the white blood cells can ingest and destroy pathogens and other foreign substances by a process called **phagocytosis** (which means cellular eating). Phagocytosis involves special cells, called **phagocytes,** that accomplish this task. Some phagocytes, the neutrophils and monocytes, are motile; they wander around the body through the blood and tissue fluid, doing their job. Other phagocytes are confined within a particular tissue and are called fixed.

Traveling through the blood to the site of infection, the neutrophils and monocytes can squeeze through the tiny gaps between the endothelial cells of the capillary walls and enter the tissue spaces at the site of infection. The process of squeezing through the tiny gaps is called **diapedesis.** How do the neutrophils and monocytes know where to go? Chemicals released by injured cells attract them to the injured site. This signaling to attract phagocytes is called **chemotaxis.** This process is similar to a bloodhound tracking a scent. The hound picks up the signal (odor), which directs him to its source.

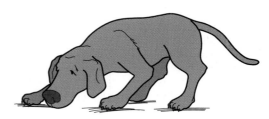

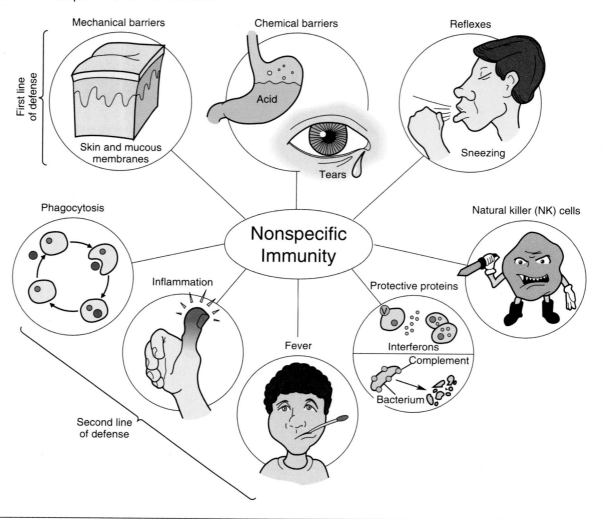

FIGURE 17-1 ● Nonspecific immunity. The first line of defense includes mechanical barriers, chemical barriers, and reflexes. Processes involved in the second line of defense are phagocytosis, inflammation, fever, protective proteins (complement proteins and interferons), and natural killer (NK) cells.

What does a phagocyte do? A phagocyte engulfs, or eats, particles or pathogens much like an ameba does (see Fig. 17–1). The phagocyte's plasma membrane sends out "false feet," called pseudopods, which surround the pathogen. The surfaces of the plasma membrane then fuse, thereby capturing the pathogen within the phagocyte. The entrapped pathogen soon encounters a lysosome. The lysosomal membrane fuses with the pathogen, releasing potent lysosomal enzymes around it. The lysosomal enzymes destroy the pathogen. The process of phagocytosis can be summarized as *eaten and digested.*

One group of the phagocytic cells, the monocytes, deposit themselves in various organs and give rise to **macrophages** (măk′rə-fāj″əz). As the name implies, the macrophages are big eaters. They become fixed within a particular organ and are thus nonmotile. They can, however, divide and

produce new macrophages at their fixed site. The Kupffer cells (in the liver), for instance, are fixed to the walls of the sinusoids (large capillaries). As blood flows through the hepatic sinusoids, pathogens and other foreign substances are removed from the blood and phagocytosed. The liver, spleen, lungs, and lymph nodes have a particularly rich supply of fixed phagocytes. This diffuse, or widely scattered, group of macrophages is called the **reticuloendothelial system (RES)** (rĭ-tĭk′yə-lō-ĕn″də-thē′lē-əl sĭs′təm), or **tissue macrophage system** (tĭ″shoo̅ măk′rə-fāj sĭs′təm).

Inflammation

Inflammation (ĭn″flə-mā′shən) refers to the responses the body makes when confronted by an irritant. The irritant can be almost anything; common irritants include pathogens, friction, excessive heat or cold, x-rays, injuries, and chemicals. If the irritant is caused by a pathogen, the inflammation is called an **infection.**

Inflammation is characterized by the following signs: redness, heat, swelling, and pain (see Fig. 17–1). What are the causes of these symptoms? When the tissues are injured or irritated, injured cells release histamine and other substances. These substances cause the blood vessels in the injured tissue to dilate. The dilated blood vessels bring more blood to the area. The increased blood flow causes redness and heat. The histamine and other substances also cause the blood vessel walls to leak; fluid and dissolved substances leak out of the blood vessels into the tissue spaces. This leaking causes the swelling. Fluid and irritating chemicals accumulating at the injured site also stimulate pain receptors; therefore the person experiences pain. Redness, heat, swelling, and pain are the classic signs of inflammation.

The increased blood flow also carries an increased number of phagocytic cells (neutrophils and monocytes) to the injured site. As the phagocytes do their job, many are killed in the process. In a severe infection, the area becomes filled with dead leukocytes, pathogens, injured cells, and tissue fluid. This thick, yellowish accumulation of dead material is called **pus.** The presence of pus indicates that the phagocytes are doing their job.

Because of the leaky blood vessels, fluid collects in the tissue spaces. This tissue fluid contains some of the blood-clotting factors, such as fibrinogen, a protein present in plasma. Fibrinogen creates fibrin threads within the tissue spaces. Later, fibroblasts, the cells that form connective tissue, may also invade the injured area. The connective tissue helps to contain, or restrict, the area of inflammation and thereby prevents the infection from spreading throughout the body. Fibroblastic activity is also involved in tissue repair.

Fever

As phagocytes perform their duty, they release fever-producing substances called **pyrogens** (from the Latin word for fire). The pyrogens stimulate the hypothalamus (in the brain) to reset the body's temperature, producing a fever. The elevation in temperature is thought to be beneficial in several ways: a fever stimulates phagocytosis and decreases the ability of certain pathogens to multiply. In fact, the elimination of mild fevers may do more harm than good.

Ample evidence suggests that the reduction of fever prolongs an infection. Note, however, that a very high fever must be reduced because high body temperature may cause severe and irreversible brain damage. High fever, especially in children, is frequently accompanied by seizures. Because these seizures are due to an elevated body temperature, they are called febrile seizures.

Protective Proteins

Two groups of protective proteins, the interferons and the complement proteins, act nonspecifically to protect the body (see Fig. 17–1). **Interferons** (ĭn″tər-fîr′ŏnz) are a group of proteins secreted by cells infected by a virus. The interferons prevent further viral replication, thereby protecting the surrounding cells from infection. Researchers first found interferon in cells infected by the influenza virus. They called it interferon because it interfered with viral replication. In general, interferons boost the immune system.

A second group of proteins that protect the body are the complement proteins. **Complement proteins** (kŏm′plə-měnt prō′tēnz) circulate in the blood in their inactive form. When the complement proteins are activated against a bacterium, they swarm over it. The complement attaches to the bacterium's outer membrane and punches holes in it. The holes in the membrane allow fluid and electrolytes to flow into the bacterium, causing it to burst and subsequently die. The activated complements perform other functions that enhance phagocytosis and the inflammatory response.

Natural Killer (NK) Cells

Natural killer (NK) cells are a special type of lymphocyte that act nonspecifically to kill certain cells. NK cells are particularly effective against virus-infected and cancer cells. The NK cells, like many nonspecific mechanisms, cooperate with the specific defense mechanisms to mount the most effective defense possible.

✳ **SUM IT UP!** Figure 17–2 summarizes the functions of the nonspecific defense mechanisms. The wall of the fortress is the first line of defense. It protects the body from invaders such as bacteria, fungi, and viruses. Parts of this first line of defense are mechanical barriers (intact skin and mucous membrane), chemical barriers (saliva, tears, gastric juice, mucus), and reflexes (coughing, sneezing, vomiting). Behind the wall of the fortress is the second line of defense, processes that cause inflammation and fever, protective proteins, and the NK cells. The body's arsenal is truly impressive, but there is more.

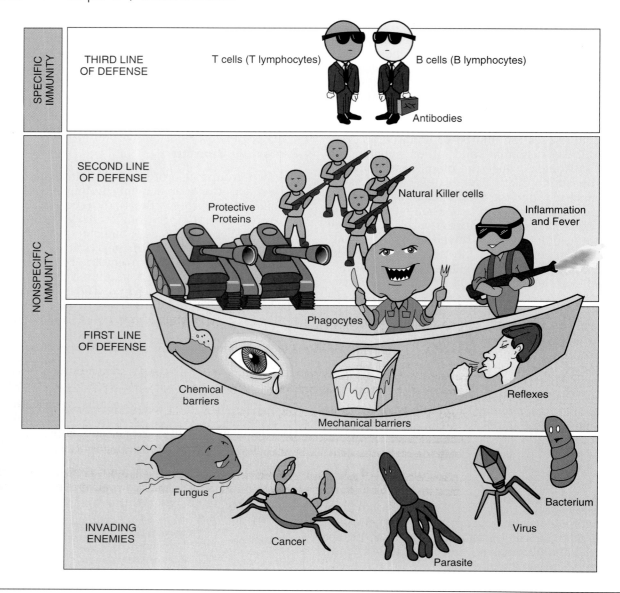

FIGURE 17–2 • The immune system wages its battle with lines of defense. Fungus, bacterium, virus, and cancer cell represent the invading enemy. The enemy must first penetrate the wall of the fortress: the mechanical/chemical barriers and the reflexes. Behind the wall is the second line of defense represented by the various warriors: phagocytosis, inflammation, fever, protective proteins, and natural killer (NK) cells. The B and T lymphocytes (B and T cells), assisted by the macrophages, form the third line of defense.

Specific Immunity

Specific immunity refers to defense mechanisms with very specific actions (Table 17–2). They protect against a specific foreign agent, such as the measles virus (a specific pathogen) or the pollen that comes from ragweed. The two cells that play key roles in these specific mechanisms are the lymphocytes and the macrophages (see Table 17–1). Understanding the function of lymphocytes requires an understanding of antigens.

Antigens

Foreign substances to which lymphocytes respond are called **antigens** (ăn'tĭ-jənz). Antigens are generally large and complex molecules; most are proteins, but a few are polysaccharides and lipids. Antigens are found on the surface of many substances, such as pathogens, red blood cells, pollens, foods, toxins, and cancer cells. Foreign substances that display antigens are described as antigenic. Antigenic substances are attacked by lymphocytes.

Table 17•2	CHARACTERISTICS OF T AND B CELLS (LYMPHOCYTES)	
CHARACTERISTICS	**T CELLS**	**B CELLS**
Site of production	Bone marrow	Bone marrow
Site of maturation and differentiation	Thymus gland	Bone marrow (probably the fetal liver)
Primary function	Cell-mediated immunity: T cells interact with antigen *directly*	Antibody-mediated immunity; B cells interact with antigen *indirectly* by secreting antibodies; also called humoral immunity
Subgroups	Killer T cells Helper T cells Suppressor T cells Memory T cells	Plasma cells Memory B cells
% of blood lymphocytes	70–80%	20–30%
Secretions	Lymphokines	Antibodies

Self and Nonself: Is That Me?

Before birth, your lymphocytes somehow get to know who belongs and who does not. In effect, your lymphocytes learn to recognize you (self) and take steps to eliminate not you (nonself, or foreign agent). Your body perceives your own cells and secretions as nonantigenic and other cells as antigenic. The antigenic cells are subsequently eliminated. Recognition of self is called **immunotolerance.**

Sometimes a person's immune system fails to identify self and mounts an immune attack against its own cells. This attack is the basis of the autoimmune diseases such as rheumatoid arthritis, myasthenia gravis, multiple sclerosis, and systemic lupus erythematosis.

Lymphocytes

The two types of lymphocytes are **T lymphocytes** (tē lĭm′fə-sītz) and **B lymphocytes** (bē lĭm′fə-sītz), or **T cells** (tē sĕlz) and **B cells** (bē sĕlz). Although they both come from the stem cells in the bone marrow, they differ in their development and functions. Table 17–2 compares T and B cells.

WHY THE NAMES T AND B CELLS? During fetal development, stem cells in the bone marrow produce lymphocytes (Fig. 17–3). The blood carries lymphocytes throughout the body. About one half of the lymphocytes travel to the thymus gland, where they mature and differentiate. These cells are transformed and become T lymphocytes (thymus-derived lymphocytes), or T cells. Eventually, the blood carries T cells away from the thymus gland to various lymphoid tissues, particularly the lymph nodes, thoracic duct, and spleen. T cells

live, work, and reproduce in the lymphoid tissue. Some T cells also circulate in the blood and make up 70% to 80% of the blood's lymphocytes.

What about the B lymphocytes? Lymphocytes that do not reach the thymus gland are processed in another part of the body, probably the fetal liver and bone marrow (the B is for bone marrow). These cells mature and differentiate into B lymphocytes, or B cells. Like the T cells, the B cells take up residence in lymphoid tissue. B cells make up 20% to 30% of the circulating lymphocytes.

Both T cells and B cells attack antigens, but they do so in different ways. T cells attack antigens directly, through cell-to-cell contact. This immune response is called **cell-mediated immunity** (sĕl′mē″dē-āt″əd ĭ-myōo′nĭ-tē). B cells, on the other hand, interact with the antigen indirectly, through the secretion of **antibodies** (ăn′tĭ-bŏd″ēz). This response is called **antibody-mediated immunity** (ăn′tĭ-bŏd″ē me′dē-āt″əd ĭ-myōo′nĭ-tē). Because the antibodies are carried by the blood and other tissue fluid (the body humors), this type of immunity is also called **humoral immunity.**

CELL-MEDIATED IMMUNITY: T CELL FUNCTION. Cell-mediated immunity is especially effective against pathogens, fungi, cancer cells, protozoan parasites, and foreign tissue such as organ transplants. Refer to Figure 17–4 as you read about the steps in cell-mediated immunity.

- Step 1: The antigen, on the surface of the pathogen, is engulfed, or phagocytosed, by a macrophage. The macrophage digests the antigen and pushes the antigen to its surface. The macrophage's ability to push the antigen to its surface is called **antigen presentation.**
- Step 2: T cells that have receptor sites bind to the antigen and become activated. This process

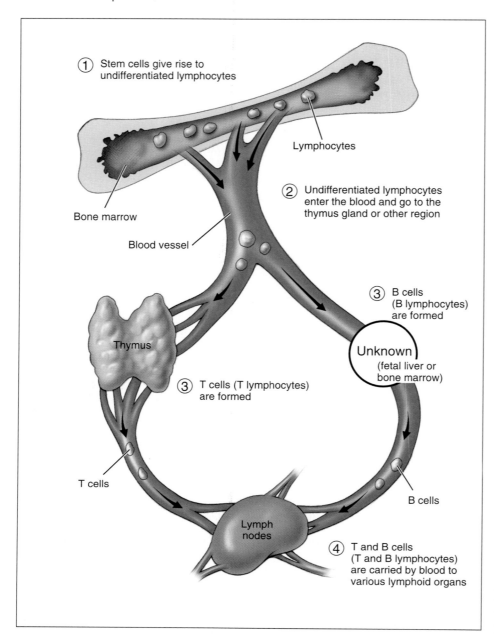

① Stem cells give rise to undifferentiated lymphocytes

Lymphocytes

Bone marrow

Blood vessel

② Undifferentiated lymphocytes enter the blood and go to the thymus gland or other region

③ B cells (B lymphocytes) are formed

Unknown (fetal liver or bone marrow)

Thymus

③ T cells (T lymphocytes) are formed

T cells

Lymph nodes

B cells

④ T and B cells (T and B lymphocytes) are carried by blood to various lymphoid organs

FIGURE 17–3 ● Formation of lymphocytes (T and B cells). (1) Stem cells give rise to undifferentiated lymphocytes in the bone marrow. (2) Undifferentiated lymphocytes leave the bone marrow by way of the blood. (3) Some lymphocytes travel to the thymus gland, where they mature and are transformed into T lymphocytes, or T cells. Some lymphocytes go to another part of the body, probably the fetal liver or bone marrow. Here they mature and become B lymphocytes, or B cells. (4) T and B cells travel to other lymphoid tissue, such as lymph nodes, where they live, work, and reproduce.

is called **T-cell activation.** Activation of the T cell always requires an antigen-presenting cell, such as a macrophage.

- Step 3: The activated T cell divides repeatedly, resulting in large numbers of T cells. This group of T cells is called a **clone** (klōn), a group of identical cells formed from the same parent cell. There are four subgroups within the clone: killer T cells, helper T cells, suppressor T cells, and memory T cells.

The **killer T cells** destroy the antigen (pathogen) by two mechanisms: by punching holes in the antigen's cell membrane and by secreting substances called **lymphokines,** which enhance phagocytic activity. The killer T cells engage in cell-to-cell

combat. The **helper T cells** also secrete a lymphokine that stimulates both T cells and B cells and, in general, enhances the immune response. The **suppressor T cells** inhibit, or stop, the immune response when the antigen has been destroyed. The suppressor T cells control B and T cell activity.

The **memory T cells** do not participate in the destruction of the antigen. These cells "remember" the initial encounter with the antigen. If the antigen is presented at some future time, the memory cells can proliferate, or quickly reproduce, and thus allow a faster immune response to occur.

ANTIBODY-MEDIATED IMMUNITY: B CELL FUNCTION. B cells engage in antibody-mediated immunity. Ac-

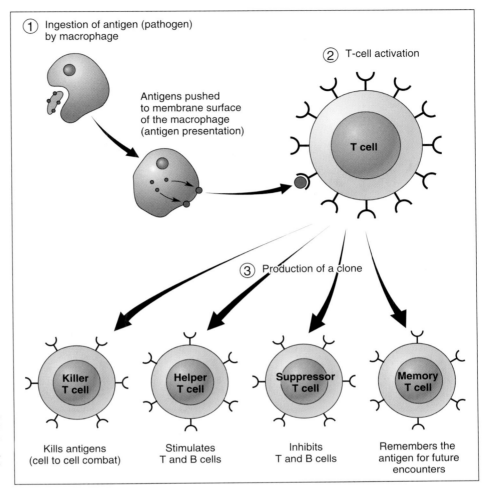

FIGURE 17–4 ● Cell-mediated immunity: T cell function. (1) The macrophage ingests the antigen (pathogen). The macrophage processes the antigen and pushes the antigen to its surface (antigen presentation). (2) The T cell is activated. (3) A clone is produced. The clone includes the four subgroups of the activated T cell: killer T cells, helper T cells, suppressor T cells, and memory T cells.

tivated B cells produce a clone of cells that secrete antibodies. (A clone is a group of identical cells formed from the same parent cell.) The antibodies, in turn, are carried by the blood and body fluids to the antigen-bearing cells (pathogens). Individual B cells can produce over 10 million different antibodies, each of which reacts against a specific antigen. The large numbers of antibodies allow the body to develop immunity against many different diseases. Follow Figure 17–5 as you read about the steps in antibody-mediated immunity.

- Step 1: A macrophage engulfs and processes antigen. The antigen is pushed to the surface of the macrophage and presented to both the B cell and the helper T cell.
- Step 2: The presented antigens bind to both the B cell and the helper T cell, activating both cells. Only those B cells and helper T cells with the proper receptors are activated.
- Step 3: The activated helper T cells secrete a lymphokine that stimulates the B cells to reproduce, producing a clone. The two subgroups of the clone include plasma cells and memory B cells. Plasma cells produce large quantities of

antibodies that travel through the blood to the antigens (pathogens). The memory B cells do not participate in the attack; they remember the specific antigen during future encounters and allow a quicker response to the invading antigen.

Note that B and T cell activation both depends on helper T cell activity. Human immunodeficiency virus (HIV) attacks the helper T cells, thereby producing severe impairment of the immune system. This syndrome is called acquired immunodeficiency syndrome (AIDS). Because of the impairment of their immune system, persons with HIV infection and AIDS experience numerous bouts of infection.

What Antibodies Are. The antibodies secreted by the B cells are proteins called **immunoglobulins** (ĭm′yōō-nō-glŏb″yə-lĭnz). The immunoglobulins are found primarily in the plasma in the gamma globulin part of the plasma proteins. There are five major types of immunoglobulins. The three most abundant immunoglobulins are immunoglobulin G, immunoglobulin A, and immunoglobulin M. A fourth immunoglobulin, immunoglobulin E, is involved in hypersensitivity reactions and is described later.

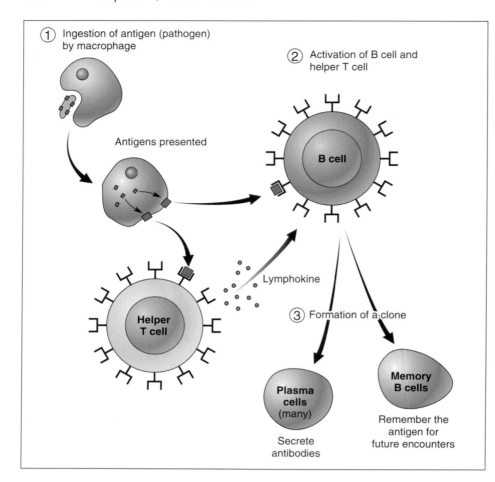

① Ingestion of antigen (pathogen) by macrophage

Antigens presented

② Activation of B cell and helper T cell

B cell

Helper T cell

 Lymphokine

③ Formation of a clone

Plasma cells (many)

Secrete antibodies

Memory B cells

Remember the antigen for future encounters

FIGURE 17–5 ● Antibody-mediated immunity: B cell function. (1) The macrophage ingests the antigen (pathogen). The macrophage processes the antigen and pushes it to the macrophage surface (antigen presentation). (2) Both B and helper T cells are activated. The helper T cell secretes a lymphokine, which further stimulates the B cell. (3) A clone is produced. The clone includes the two subgroups of the B cell: plasma cells and memory B cells. The function of each cell is identified.

- **Immunoglobulin G (IgG)** is an antibody found in plasma and body fluids. It is particularly effective against certain bacteria, viruses, and various toxins. It also activates complement proteins.
- **Immunoglobulin A (IgA)** is an antibody found primarily in the secretions of exocrine glands. IgA in milk, tears, and gastric juice helps protect against infection. Breast milk contains IgA antibodies; these antibodies help the infant to ward off infection.
- **Immunoglobulin M (IgM)** is an antibody found in blood plasma. The anti-A and anti-B antibodies associated with red blood cells are a type of IgM antibody. IgM is capable of activating complement.

What Antibodies Do. Antibodies destroy antigens. They accomplish this task directly by attacking the membrane and indirectly by activating complement proteins that, in turn, facilitate the attack on the antigens.

When antibodies react with antigens directly, the antibodies bind to, or interact with, antigens. This process is called an **antigen-antibody reaction.** By engaging in an antigen-antibody reaction,

Do You Know...

What is an abscess?

When an area becomes infected, the cells involved in the inflammatory response do two things. First, they kill the pathogens. As the war continues, dead cells (including phagocytes, injured cells, and pathogens) and secretions accumulate in the area as pus. Second, the cells build a wall of tissue around the infected debris. This walled-off area is an abscess. An abscess performs a beneficial role in that it restricts the spread of the infection throughout the body. A large abscess may require a surgical procedure in which the abscess is lanced and drained.

the antigen-antibody components clump together, or **agglutinate.** Agglutination makes it easier for the phagocytic cells to destroy the antigen. Under normal conditions, *direct* attack by the antibodies

Table 17 ● 3	SOME CHEMICAL MEDIATORS INVOLVED IN IMMUNITY

CHEMICAL MEDIATOR	DESCRIPTION AND FUNCTION
Complement	A group of plasma proteins. When activated they kill pathogens directly, and enhance phagocytosis.
Cytokines	General term for protein chemicals that regulate the immune response. Cytokines that are secreted by lymphocytes are called lymphokines.
Histamine	Secreted primarily by mast cells; acts on the blood vessels to cause vasodilation and "leaky" capillaries; responsible for some of the signs of inflammation. Also released in response to allergic reactions
Immunoglobulins	Antibodies secreted by plasma cells (B cells): IgA, IgD, IgE, IgG, and IgM
Interferons	Proteins that nonspecifically inhibit viral reproduction

is not very helpful in protecting the body against invasion by pathogens.

A more effective way for antibodies to attack an antigen is through activation of the complement proteins. These activated complement proteins cause a variety of effects: they stimulate chemotaxis (attract more phagocytes), promote agglutination, make pathogens more susceptible to phagocytosis, and encourage lysis, or rupture of the pathogen's cell membrane. Direct and indirect attacks by antibodies provide an effective defense against foreign agents. Complement proteins are among the chemical mediators that control the immune response. (Table 17–3 lists other chemical mediators.)

Remember Me? Primary and Secondary Responses. Activated when exposed to an antigen, B cells produce many plasma cells and memory cells. The plasma cells secrete antibodies. This initial response to antigen is called the **primary response.** It is graphed in Figure 17–6. Note that the primary response is associated with a slow development and a relatively low plasma level of antibodies. Note what happens when the immune system is challenged for a second time by the same antigen. The immune system responds quickly and produces a large number of antibodies. This second challenge is called the **secondary response.** Compare the plasma levels of antibodies in the primary and secondary responses.

Why is the secondary response so much greater? The initial exposure to the antigen has stimulated the formation of both antibody-secreting plasma cells and memory cells. The memory cells, which live for a long time in the plasma, are activated very quickly on the second exposure. The activated memory cells, in turn, induce the formation of many antibody-secreting plasma cells. This fast reaction accounts for the larger number of antibodies associated with the secondary response.

What does the secondary response mean for you? It means that you won't get the disease a second time because you are immune to that disease. For example, if you had measles as a child, you developed measles antibodies and many memory cells. If you are then exposed to the measles virus later in life, the memory cells "remember" the first exposure and produce antibody-secreting plasma cells very quickly. The measles antibodies, in turn, attack the measles virus and prevent you from becoming ill.

The level of antibodies in your blood is called an antibody **titer.** If you have had measles, for instance, your measles antibody titer is higher than the titer of someone who has never had measles.

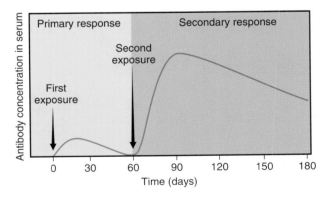

FIGURE 17–6 ● Primary and secondary responses. The primary response occurs when an antigen initially activates a B cell. The B cell forms antibody-secreting plasma cells and memory B cells. The secondary response occurs when the memory B cells (formed during the primary response) are exposed to the same antigen for a second time. The secondary response is faster and produces more antibodies than does the primary response.

TYPES OF IMMUNITY

The two main categories of immunity are genetic immunity and acquired immunity (Fig. 17–7).

Genetic Immunity

Do you ever wonder why you have never had hoof and mouth disease or why your dog did not pick up chickenpox from you? As a human, you have inherited immunity to certain diseases, such as hoof and mouth disease; you are immunologically protected from your pet cow. Likewise, your dog will never contract chickenpox; she is immunologically protected from you. Another comforting thought: Neither you nor your dog is in danger of contracting Dutch elm disease from your tree. Each of you was born with genetic information that conveys immunity to certain diseases. **Genetic immunity** is also called inborn, innate, or species immunity. As you can see, your species protects you from diseases that afflict other species.

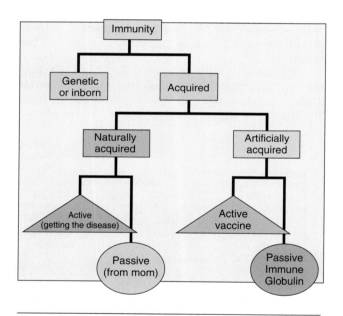

FIGURE 17–7 ● Types of immunity. Immunity is either genetic or acquired. Immunity is acquired either naturally or artificially. Naturally acquired immunity can be either active (triangles) or passive (circles). Artificially acquired immunity can also be either active or passive. The means by which you achieve a particular type of immunity is indicated in the triangles and circles. You can acquire active immunity (triangle) by getting the disease (so the immunity is naturally acquired) or by the use of a vaccine (so the immunity is artificially acquired). You can acquire passive immunity (circle) through a gift of antibodies from your mother (through placental transfer or breast milk) or from another donor who gives you immune globulin.

Acquired Immunity

Unlike genetic immunity, **acquired immunity** is received during a person's lifetime. Acquired immunity comes either naturally or artificially.

Naturally Acquired Immunity

You can acquire immunity naturally in two ways. The first is by getting the disease. As a child you probably had one of the childhood diseases, such as chickenpox. Your body responded to the specific pathogen by developing antibodies. After that first exposure, you never became ill with chickenpox again because your immune system had a ready supply of antibodies and memory cells with which to respond quickly to the second invasion of the chickenpox virus. Because your own body produced the antibodies, this type of **naturally acquired immunity** (năch′ər-əl-lē ə-kwīrd ĭ-myoo′nĭ-tē) is called **active immunity** (ăk′tĭv ĭ-myoo′nĭ-tē). Active immunity is generally long-lasting.

The second way to acquire immunity naturally is by receiving antibodies from your mother. Some antibodies (IgG) crossed the placenta from your mother into you as a fetus. Your mother developed these antibodies in response to the pathogens she encountered throughout her lifetime. Because your immune system did not produce these antibodies (you received them as a gift from your mother), this type of immunity is called **passive immunity** (păs′ĭv ĭ-myoo′nĭ-tē). Antibodies can also be transferred passively from mother to infant through breast milk. Breast milk contains IgA antibodies.

Unlike active immunity, which often lasts a lifetime, passive immunity is short-lived. The antibodies are broken down and eliminated from the baby's body. The mother's antibodies afford protection to the infant for about the first 6 months after birth. Breastfeeding may extend the length of immunoprotection.

Artificially Acquired Immunity

You can acquire immunity artificially in two ways. The first is by way of a vaccine. The second is by injection of immune globulin. Both provide **artificially acquired immunity** (är″tə-físh′əl-lē ə-kwīrd ĭ-myoo′nĭ-tē).

A **vaccine** (văk-sēn′) is an antigen-bearing substance (eg, a pathogen) injected into a person in an attempt to stimulate antibody production. The antigen is usually an altered form of the pathogen. For instance, the measles virus is first killed or weakened (attenuated). The attenuated virus cannot cause the disease (eg, measles) when injected into the person, but it can still act as an antigen and stimulate the person's immune system to produce antibodies. The use of dead or at-

Table 17 • 4

TYPES OF ACQUIRED IMMUNITY

TYPE	STIMULUS	RESULT
Naturally acquired		
Active immunity	Exposed to live pathogens (eg, get the disease)	Long-term immunity; makes antibodies; symptoms of disease appear
Passive immunity	Antibodies are passed from mother to infant (across placenta and/or by breastfeeding)	Short-term immunity (lasts approximately first 6 months and for duration of breast-feeding); does not stimulate the production of antibodies
Artificially acquired		
Active immunity	Vaccination	Long-term immunity; makes antibodies
Passive immunity	Injection with gamma globulin (antibodies)	Short-term immunity; does not stimulate the production of antibodies

tenuated pathogen to stimulate antibody production is **vaccination,** or **immunization.** The solution of dead or attenuated pathogens is the vaccine. Because the use of a vaccine stimulates the body to produce its own antibodies, vaccines induce active immunity.

A vaccine can also be made from the toxin secreted by the pathogen. The toxin is altered to reduce its harmfulness, but it can still act as an antigen to induce immunity. The altered toxin is called a **toxoid.** Because a toxoid stimulates the production of antibodies, it causes active immunity.

Review Figure 17–6. The purpose of vaccination is to provide an initial exposure and stimulate the formation of memory cells (the primary response). The purpose of a booster shot is to stimulate the secondary response by administering another dose of the vaccine.

Many vaccines have almost eradicated certain diseases. For instance, infants routinely receive a series of DTP injections. DTP injections stimulate active immunity for diphtheria (*d*iphtheria toxoid), and tetanus (*t*etanus toxoid), pertussis, or whooping cough (*p*ertussis vaccine). MMR vaccine (*m*easles-rubeola, *m*umps, and *r*ubella) is also used preventively during early childhood.

Immune globulin differs from a vaccine. Immune globulin is obtained from a donor (human or animal) and contains antibodies (immune globulins). The antibodies are formed in the donor in response to a specific antigen. These preformed antibodies are taken from the donor and injected into a recipient, thereby conveying passive immunity.

Why might this procedure be done? Let us assume that you are not immune to hepatitis B and so do not have antibodies against the hepatitis B virus. You are then exposed to the virus. Because you have no immunity to the virus, you may receive immune globulin (antibodies) in an attempt to provide immediate protection against the virus. Because this is a form of passive immunity, the immunity is short-lived. Immune globulins are available for rubella (German measles), hepatitis A and B, rabies, and tetanus. A comparison of the different types of acquired immunity appears in Table 17–4.

Other forms of passive immunity are commonly used to prevent the disease or to prevent the development of severe symptoms of the disease. **Antitoxins** contain antibodies that neutralize the toxins secreted by the pathogens but have no effect on the pathogens themselves. Examples of antitoxins include tetanus antitoxin (TAT) and the antitoxins for diphtheria and botulism. Antivenoms contain antibodies that combat the effects of the poisonous venom of snakes.

Do You Know...

What's so serious about stepping on a rusty nail?

By stepping on a rusty nail, you accomplish two things. First, you may allow a potentially lethal pathogen, *Clostridium tetani (Cl. tetani),* to enter your body. Second, you have a wound that encourages the growth of the pathogen. The deep puncture wound introduces the pathogen into the deep tissue of the foot. Because little bleeding is associated with a puncture wound, the pathogen is not washed out of the wound. More importantly, however, a deep puncture wound prevents air (oxygen) from entering the wound. Because the *Cl. tetani* pathogen grows anaerobically (without oxygen), the conditions associated with a puncture wound are ideal. These conditions are the reason you are immunized against tetanus.

OTHER IMMUNOLOGIC RESPONSES

Normally, the immune system protects the body from nonself; foreign agents are recognized and eliminated. Sometimes, however, the immune system goes awry: it attacks self, causing autoimmune disease, or it overreacts, causing **allergies.**

Allergic Reactions

The immune system sometimes forms antibodies to substances not usually recognized as foreign. This response forms the basis of **allergic reactions.** The two common allergic reactions are the delayed-reaction allergy and the immediate-reaction allergy.

The **delayed-reaction allergy** is so named because it usually takes about 48 hours to occur; its onset is delayed. This type of allergic response can occur in anyone. It usually results from the repeated exposure of the skin to chemicals, such as household detergents. Repeated exposure to the chemical activates T cells, which eventually accumulate in the skin. Local tissue response to T cell activity causes skin eruptions and other signs of inflammation. This skin response is called **contact dermatitis.** Other forms of contact dermatitis are associated with poison ivy, poison oak, certain cosmetics, and soaps.

The **immediate-reaction allergy,** as its name implies, occurs rapidly in response to its stimulus. It is more commonly called an immediate **hypersensitivity reaction** and involves immunoglobulin E, the IgE antibodies. **Allergens** (ăl′ər-jənz), substances capable of inducing allergy, that are apt to be involved in this type of allergic response include pollens, such as ragweed, venom from insects, drugs such as penicillin, and the antigens on red blood cells. An **allergen** is an antigen capable of causing an allergic reaction. Figure 17–8 illustrates the steps involved in the development of an immediate hypersensitivity reaction.

- Step 1: An allergen activates a B cell.
- Step 2: The activated B cell forms a clone of antibody-secreting plasma cells.
- Step 3: The plasma cells secrete large amounts of IgE antibodies against the specific allergen.
- Step 4: The IgE antibodies bind to the mast cells in body tissues.
- Step 5: More of the allergen invades the body. The allergen binds with the IgE antibodies on the mast cells. The mast cells release large amounts of histamine and other chemicals that cause systemic effects. The systemic effects can be severe; they include a massive vasodilation, which causes a sharp drop in blood pressure and severe constriction of the respiratory passages (bronchoconstriction), making breathing extremely difficult and, in some cases, impossible. This severe form of the immediate hypersensitivity reaction is called **anaphylaxis** or **anaphylactic shock.** Persons allergic to penicillin are at risk for anaphylaxis. As a result, always ask a person about allergies to medications before administering any type of drug, particularly antibiotics.

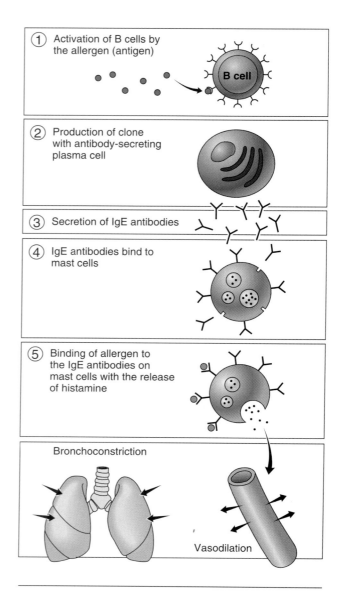

① Activation of B cells by the allergen (antigen)

B cell

② Production of clone with antibody-secreting plasma cell

③ Secretion of IgE antibodies

④ IgE antibodies bind to mast cells

⑤ Binding of allergen to the IgE antibodies on mast cells with the release of histamine

Bronchoconstriction

Vasodilation

FIGURE 17–8 • Immediate-reaction allergy (immediate hypersensitivity reaction.) (1) An allergen (antigen) binds to the receptor on a B cell; this event activates the B cell. (2) The activated B cell produces a clone, including plasma cells. (3) The plasma cells secrete IgE antibodies. (4) The IgE antibodies bind to mast cells. (5) When additional allergen is introduced, the allergen binds to the antibody on the mast cells. This process releases a dangerous amount of histamine into the blood. The lowest panel illustrates the effects of histamine. Histamine causes a narrowing of the respiratory passages. This narrowing, in turn, decreases the amount of air that can be inhaled and causes severe wheezing. Histamine also causes widespread dilation of the blood vessels and a severe drop in blood pressure.

Autoimmune Disease

Sometimes a person's T cell attacks self, causing extensive tissue damage and organ dysfunction. This process is **autoimmunity** (ô″tō-ĭ-myoo′nĭ-tē). Diseases that develop in response to

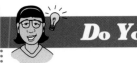

Do You Know...

Why can a person die of a bee sting?

This person has become sensitized to bee venom, which is an allergen. IgE antibodies to the bee venom are attached to the surface of the person's mast cells. When the person is stung, the bee venom allergen binds to the IgE antibodies on the mast cells, causing a massive release of histamine and other histamine-like chemicals. These chemicals cause an anaphylactic reaction. Unless treated immediately, the person is apt to die in anaphylactic shock. Treatment is usually an injection of epinephrine (Adrenalin), which opens breathing passages and elevates blood pressure. Steroids (cortisol) are also given to suppress the immune response.

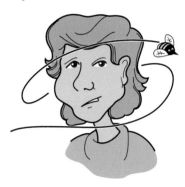

system recognizes the donated kidney as foreign and mounts an immune attack against it. When the immune attack is successful, the organ is destroyed and is said to be rejected.

There are several ways to prevent organ rejection. The physician first selects a donor organ that is immunologically similar to the recipient's tissues. The physician then administers drugs that suppress the recipient's immune system. Cyclosporine is a commonly used immunosuppressant that inhibits the secretion of certain lymphokines, which, in turn, diminishes the immune attack against the donated organ. Unfortunately, these measures are not always successful, and the recipient may ultimately reject the organ.

✳ **SUM IT UP!** Specific immunity forms the third line of defense of the immune response. It allows the immune system to recognize and destroy specific foreign, or nonself, agents called antigens. The lymphocytes (B and T cells) and the macrophages are the most important cells associated with specific immunity. T cells engage in cell-to-cell combat (cell-mediated immunity) while B cells fight at a distance through the mediation of antibodies. Macrophages not only engage in phagocytosis but also present the antigen to the lymphocytes. Immunity is classified as either genetic or acquired. Immunity may be acquired naturally or artificially. If a person makes antibodies within his or her own body, the immunity is active. If the person merely receives antibodies that were made by another person or animal, the immunity is passive. While the immune system normally works to protect the body, it can go awry, causing allergic reactions and autoimmune disease.

self attack are called **autoimmune diseases.** A surprisingly large number of diseases are considered autoimmune. A partial list includes thyroiditis, myasthenia gravis, systemic lupus erythematosis, rheumatic fever, rheumatoid arthritis, and some forms of diabetes mellitus.

Consider this. The immune system is affected by both your endocrine system and your nervous systems. Your endocrine and nervous systems are both affected by your emotional state (eg, happy, sad, angry). What are the chances that your emotional state can affect your immune system and hence your physical well-being? In other words, does happiness promote health, while anger and depression cause disease? A new branch of science called **psychoneuroimmunology** seeks to explore this relationship. In the meantime, be happy!

Organ Rejection

Organ transplants have become common means of dealing with organ failure. A patient in kidney failure, for instance, may receive a kidney transplant. One of the greatest problems associated with this new surgical technology is the problem of organ rejection. The recipient's immune

As You Age

1. T cell and B cell function are somewhat deficient in the elderly. Depressed lymphocyte function is accompanied by a decrease in macrophage activity. Consequently, the elderly are more prone to develop infections, and they recover more slowly. Depressed lymphocyte function might also explain the higher incidence of cancer in the elderly population.

2. The elderly have increased levels of circulating autoantibodies (antibodies directed against self). This increase explains, in part, why the elderly are more prone to the development of autoimmune disease.

3. The elderly frequently take drugs or have therapies that depress the immune system. For instance, the use of steroids in the treatment of arthritis and the use of drugs and radiation in the treatment of cancer all cause immunosuppression.

Disorders of the Immune System

Allergic responses	Delayed hypersensitivities and immediate hypersensitivities. These include contact dermatitis and anaphylaxis.
Autoimmune disorders	An immune system disorder in which the person's immune system produces antibodies against its own cells. There are many autoimmune diseases, including rheumatoid arthritis, Hashimoto thyroiditis, diabetes mellitus (Type 1), and rheumatic fever. Rheumatic fever is an immune disorder in which the antibodies produced in response to a streptococcal infection attack the heart muscle and its valves.
Immunodeficiencies	An incompetent or deficient immune system. Immunodeficiencies can be congenital or acquired. Severe combined immunodeficiency disease (SCID) is a congenital type of immunodeficiency. Children are defenseless against most pathogens and readily succumb to minor infections unless isolated from the environment of microorganisms. Immunodeficiency disease can also be acquired. The acquired immunodeficiency syndrome (AIDS) is an example of a virally induced immunodeficiency.
Infection	A condition in which the body or part of the body is invaded by a pathogen (bacterium, virus, parasite, fungus) that multiplies and causes harm. There may be a localized response (inflammation) and/or a systemic response (fever, malaise, leukocytosis).

Summary Outline

The immune system is a defense system that protects the body from foreign agents such as pathogens, pollens, toxins, and cancer cells.

I. Nonspecific Immunity
Nonspecific immune mechanisms protect the body against many different types of foreign agents and do not require recognition of the specific agent.

A. Lines of Defense
1. The first line of defense includes mechanical barriers (intact skin and mucous membrane), chemical barriers (tears, saliva, perspiration, mucus, stomach acid), and certain reflexes (coughing, sneezing, diarrhea, blinking).
2. The second line of defense includes phagocytosis (the motile neutrophils and monocytes and the fixed macrophages), inflammation (redness, heat, swelling, pain), fever, protective proteins (interferons and complement proteins), and natural killer (NK) cells.

II. Specific Immunity
Specific immunity protects the body against specific foreign agents and requires recognition of the specific agent involved.

A. Structures Involved With Specific Immunity
1. Specific immunity is considered the third line of defense.

2. Specific immunity is accomplished through the coordinated activity of macrophages and T and B cells.

B. T Cells, or T Lymphocytes
1. The T cells make up 70% to 80% of the blood's lymphocytes and live, work, and reproduce in lymphoid tissue (the T is for thymus gland).
2. T cells engage in cell-mediated immunity (T cells attack antigens directly through cell-to-cell contact).
3. The macrophage presents the antigen, thereby activating the T cell. The activated T cell produces a clone of T cells (killer T cells, helper T cells, suppressor T cells, and memory T cells).

C. B Cells, or B Lymphocytes
1. B cells make up 20% to 30% of the blood's lymphocytes and live in lymphoid tissue (the B is for bone marrow).
2. B cells engage in antibody-mediated immunity (B cells attack antigens indirectly, through the secretion of antibodies).
3. The macrophage presents the antigen to the B and T cells, thereby activating the B cells and the helper T cells. This process, in turn, produces a clone (memory cells and plasma cells). The plasma cells secrete antibodies that travel through the blood to the antigens.

Summary Outline, continued

II. Specific Immunity, *continued*

   C. B Cells, or B Lymphocytes, *continued*

   4. The antibodies are called immunoglobulins (IgG, IgA, IgM and IgE).

III. Types of Immunity

   A. Genetic or Acquired Immunity

   1. With genetic immunity, a person is genetically immune to an antigen.
   2. A person can acquire immunity naturally or artificially.
   3. A person can acquire immunity naturally in two ways: by getting the disease or by receiving antibodies from the mother across the placenta and/or through breast milk.
   4. Immunity can be acquired artificially in two ways: by the use of a vaccine or by injection of immune globulin made by another person or animal.

   B. Active or Passive Immunity

   1. Active immunity means that a person's body makes the antibodies. Active immunity is long-lasting.
   2. Passive immunity means that the antibodies are made by another animal and then injected into a patient's body. Passive immunity is short-lived.

IV. Other Immunologic Responses

   A. Allergic Reactions

   1. Allergic reactions are due to the formation of antibodies to substances usually not recognized as foreign.
   2. There are two types of allergic reactions: delayed-onset allergy and immediate-reaction allergy.
   3. A delayed-onset allergy takes about 48 hours to develop. Contact dermatitis to a household chemical is a common example.
   4. An immediate-reaction allergy (also called an immediate hypersensitivity reaction) is often due to exposure to pollens and drugs such as penicillin. The most severe form is anaphylaxis.

   B. Autoimmunity and Tissue or Organ Rejection

   1. Autoimmune disease develops when the immune system mounts an attack against self.
   2. Tissue or organ rejection occurs when the immune system of an organ transplant recipient recognizes the organ as foreign and immunologically attacks it.

Review Your Knowledge

1. What is the difference between specific immunity and nonspecific immunity?

2. Explain the difference between first and second lines of defense. Which type of defense includes mechanical barriers, chemical barriers, and reflexes? Which type includes phagocytosis, inflammation, fever, and interferons?

3. List two examples of mechanical barriers and two examples of chemical barriers.

4. How do reflexes assist in the removal of pathogens?

5. Explain how chemotaxis is similar to a bloodhound tracking a scent.

6. Which four organs have an especially rich supply of fixed phagocytes?

7. Explain the causes of redness, heat, swelling, and pain in the process of inflammation.

8. How is a mild or moderate fever helpful to the body in fighting infection?

9. Explain how interferons and complement proteins act nonspecifically to protect the body.

10. Which cells mature and differentiate in the thymus gland? Which lymphocytes are processed in the bone marrow?

11. Explain the difference between cell-mediated immunity and antibody-mediated immunity.

12. What is the difference between helper T cells and suppressor T cells?

13. How do IgG, IgA, and IgM assist the body's immune system?

14. List four ways that activated complement proteins help protect the body against invasion by pathogens.

15. What is the importance of an antibody titer for measles?

16. What is the difference between genetic and acquired immunity? What is the difference between active and passive immunity?

17. What type of immunity is conferred when you receive a vaccination? What type of immunity is conferred when you receive an injection of gamma globulin?

18. List the five steps involved in the development of an immediate hypersensitivity reaction.

19. What is an autoimmune disease?

20. Name two ways to prevent organ rejection in a transplant.

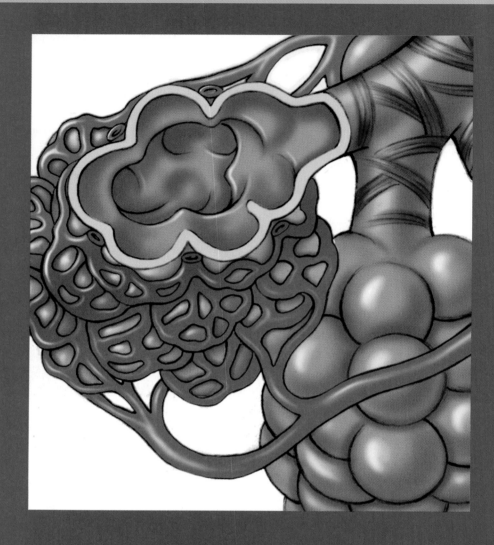

••• Key Terms

Alveolus (pl. alveoli) (ăl-vē′ə-ləs)

Bronchus (pl. bronchi) (brŏng′kəs)

Carbaminohemoglobin
  (kär-băm″ĭ-nō-hē′mə-glō″bĭn)

Epiglottis (ĕp″ĭ-glŏt′ĭs)

Exhalation (ĕks″hə-lā′shən)

Glottis (glŏt′ĭs)

Hyperventilation (hī′pər-vĕn-tĭl-ā′shən)

Hypoventilation (hī″pō-vĕn-tĭl-ā′shən)

Inhalation (ĭn″hə-lā′shən)

Intrapleural pressure
  (ĭn″trə-plŏŏr′əl prĕsh′ər)

Larynx (lăr′ĭngks)

Mediastinum (mē″dē-ə-stī′nəm)

Oxyhemoglobin (ŏk″sē-hē′mə-glō″bĭn)

Partial pressure (pär′shəl prĕsh′ər)

Pharynx (făr′ĭngks)

Pleura (plŏŏr′ə)

Surfactant (sər-făk′tənt)

Tidal volume (tĭd′l vŏl′yŏŏm)

Trachea (trā′kē-ə)

Vital capacity (vīt′l kə-păs′ĭ-tē)

••• Selected terms in bold type in this chapter are defined in the Glossary.

18 RESPIRATORY SYSTEM

Objectives

1. Describe the structure and functions of the organs of the respiratory system.

2. Trace the movement of air from the nostrils to the alveoli.

3. List the three steps of respiration.

4. Explain how breathing functions through neural and chemical controls.

5. Explain conditions that determine whether lungs collapse or expand.

6. Describe the role of pulmonary surfactants in reducing surface tension.

7. Explain the role of pressure in maintaining expanded lungs.

8. Describe the relationship of Boyle's law to ventilation.

9. Explain how respiratory muscles affect thoracic volume.

10. List three conditions that make the alveoli well suited for the exchange of oxygen and carbon dioxide.

11. Explain how respiratory gases diffuse.

12. Describe how oxygen and carbon dioxide move to and from the lungs.

13. List lung volumes and capacities.

14. Describe common variations and abnormalities of breathing.

15. Describe the respiratory regulation of acid-base balance.

Is he breathing? This is the first question asked about a person who has been seriously injured. The question indicates the importance of each breath. To breathe is to live; not to breathe is to die. Each breath is a breath of life.

Throughout history, people have acknowledged the importance of breathing. Because of its close connection with life, ancient peoples attributed the act of breathing to the divine. Even the phases of breathing are called inspiration and expiration, references to a divine spirit moving into and out of our lungs. The creation story in Genesis, in which God breathed life into the little clay figure Adam, vividly expresses an image of divine breath. Poetry also describes breathing as the life force. For example, the great Persian poet Sa'di echoed the sacredness of breath in a prayer: "Each respiration holds two blessings. Life is inhaled, and stale, foul air is exhaled. Therefore, thank God twice every breath you take."

Most of us equate breathing with respiration. Respiration includes breathing, but it is more than breathing; it involves the entire process of gas exchange between the atmosphere and the body cells. Respiration includes three steps:

- Movement of air into and out of the lungs, called **ventilation,** or breathing. Two phases of ventilation are **inhalation** (ĭn″hə-lā′shən) and **exhalation** (ĕks″hə-lā′shən). Inhalation, also called inspiration, is the breathing-in phase. During inhalation, oxygen-rich air moves into tiny air sacs in the lungs. Exhalation, also called expiration, is the breathing-out phase. During exhalation, air rich in carbon dioxide is moved out of the lungs. One inhalation and one exhalation makes up one **respiratory cycle.**
- The exchange of respiratory gases oxygen and carbon dioxide. The two sites of exchange are in the lungs and in the cells of the body.
- The transport of oxygen and carbon dioxide between the lungs and body cells. Blood accomplishes this transport of gases.

STRUCTURE: ORGANS OF THE RESPIRATORY SYSTEM

The respiratory system contains the upper respiratory and the lower respiratory tracts (Fig. 18–1). The upper respiratory tract contains the respiratory organs located outside the chest cavity: the nose and nasal cavities, pharynx, larynx, and upper trachea. The lower respiratory tract consists of organs located in the chest cavity: the lower trachea, bronchi, bronchioles, alveoli, and lungs. The lower parts of the bronchi, bronchioles, and alveoli are all located in the lungs. The pleural membranes and the muscles that form the chest cavity are also part of the lower respiratory tract.

Most of the respiratory organs are concerned with conduction, or movement, of air through the respiratory passages. This process constitutes ventilation. The alveoli are the tiny air sacs located at the end of the respiratory passages. They are concerned with the exchange of the oxygen and carbon dioxide between the air and the blood.

Nose and Nasal Cavities

The **nose** includes an external portion that forms part of the face and an internal portion called the **nasal cavities.** The nasal cavities are separated into right and left halves by a partition called the **nasal septum.** The septum is made of bone and cartilage. Air enters the nasal cavities through two openings called the **nostrils,** or **nares.** Nasal hairs in the nostrils filter large particles of dust that might otherwise be inhaled. In addition to its respiratory function, the nasal cavity contains the receptor cells for the sense of smell. The olfactory organs cover the upper parts of the nasal cavity and a part of the nasal septum.

Three bony projections called **nasal conchae** appear on the lateral walls of the nasal cavities. The conchae increase the surface area of the nasal cavities and support the ciliated mucous membrane, which lines the nasal cavities. The mucous membrane contains many blood vessels and mucus-secreting cells. The rich supply of blood warms and moistens the air, while the sticky mucus traps dust and pollen and other small particles, thereby cleansing the air as it is inhaled. Because the nose helps to warm, moisten, and cleanse the air, breathing through the nose is better than mouth breathing.

The nasal cavities contain several drainage openings. Mucus from the **paranasal sinuses** drains into the nasal cavity. The paranasal sinuses include the maxillary, frontal, ethmoidal, and sphenoidal sinuses (see Chapter 7). Tears from the nasolacrimal ducts also drain into the nasal cavities. As you know, crying means a runny nose.

In some persons, the nasal septum may bend toward one side or the other, thereby obstructing the flow of air and making breathing difficult. The abnormal positioning of the septum is called a **deviated septum.** Surgical repair of the deviated septum (septoplasty) corrects the problem.

Pharynx

The **pharynx** (făr′ĭngks), or throat, is behind the oral cavity and between the nasal cavities and the larynx (Fig. 18–2). The pharynx includes three parts: an upper section called the **nasopharynx,** a middle section called the **oropharynx,** and a lower section called the **laryngopharynx.** The oropharynx and the laryngopharynx are part of both the digestive system and the respiratory system and function as a passageway for both food

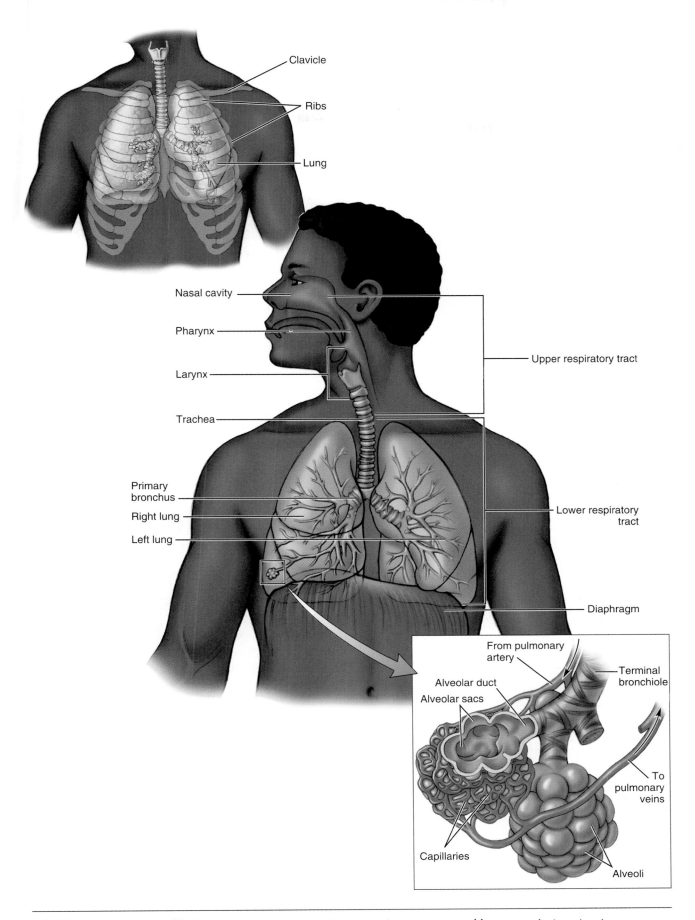

FIGURE 18-1 ● Organs of the respiratory system: upper respiratory tract and lower respiratory tract.

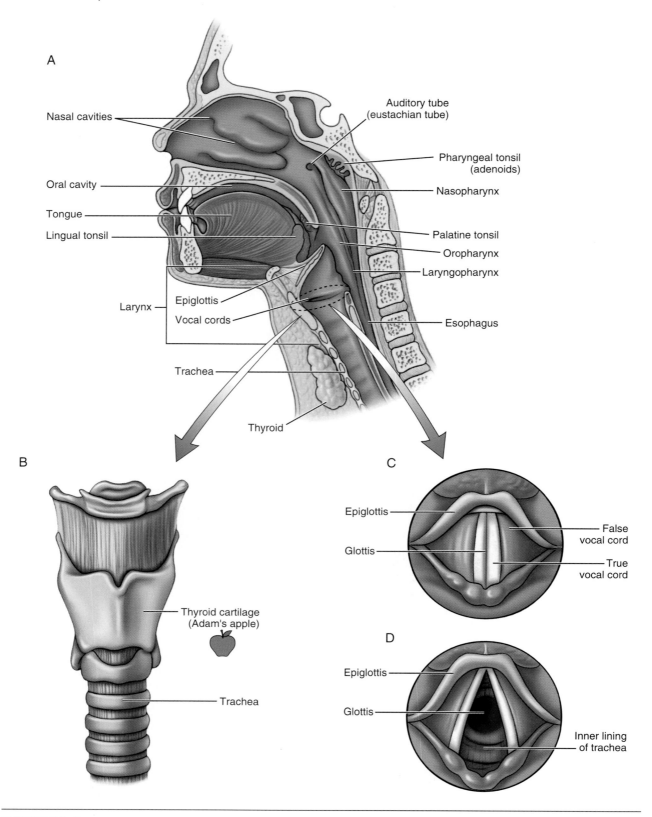

FIGURE 18–2 ● A, Organs of the upper respiratory tract. B, Larynx showing the thyroid cartilage (Adam's apple). C, Vocal cords and glottis (closed). D, Vocal cords and glottis (open). Note that the epiglottis prevents food from entering the respiratory structures.

Do You Know...

Why are tiny toys not good for tiny tots?

Young children generally put toys in their mouths. The tiny toy may become lodged in the larynx or bronchus, causing an acute respiratory obstruction. The Heimlich maneuver, or abdominal thrust, is a simple technique to help dislodge a tiny toy. The Heimlich maneuver is performed differently in adults and infants.

Here are the steps for the adult:

1. Stand behind the choking person and wrap your arms around the person's waist.
2. Position your hands (fist position) between the person's navel and the bottom of the rib cage.
3. Press your fist into the abdomen with a quick upward movement.
4. Repeat several times as necessary.

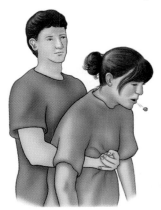

Heimlich maneuver (adult)

Here are the steps for the infant:

1. Hold the infant downward, "sandwiched" in your arms.
2. Deliver five back blows between the shoulder blades.
3. Turn the baby over, give five chest thrusts (compressions) with first two fingers.
4. Repeat sequel several times as necessary, until the foreign object is removed.

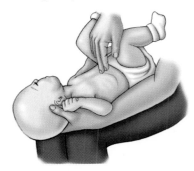

Heimlich maneuver (infant)

and air. The pharynx conducts food toward the esophagus (the food tube, or passageway for food to enter the stomach). The pharynx also conducts air to the larynx as it moves toward the lungs.

The pharynx contains two other structures: the openings from the eustachian tubes (auditory tubes) and the tonsils. The eustachian tube connects the nasopharynx with the middle ear. The eustachian tube helps keep the air pressure equal on both sides of the tympanic membrane. The tonsils are clusters of lymphoid tissue that help protect us from disease (see Chapter 16). The pharyngeal tonsils, or adenoids, are close to the eustachian tubes. The palatine tonsils are on the lateral walls of the oropharynx; they are on either side of the uvula. The lingual tonsils are on the posterior surface of the tongue.

Larynx

The **larynx** (lăr′ĭngks), also called the **voicebox,** is located between the pharynx and the trachea (see Fig. 18–2A). The larynx has three functions: it acts as a passageway for air during breathing; it produces sound, your voice (hence the name *voicebox*); and it prevents food and other foreign objects from entering the breathing structures (eg, trachea). The larynx is a triangular structure made primarily of cartilage, muscles, and ligaments (see Fig. 18–2B).

The largest of the cartilaginous structures in the larynx is the **thyroid cartilage.** It is a tough hyaline cartilage and protrudes in the front of the neck. Thyroid means shield, the shape of the thyroid cartilage. The thyroid cartilage is larger in men and is called the **Adam's apple.**

The **epiglottis** (ĕp″ĭ-glŏt′ĭs) is another cartilagenous structure, located at the top of the larynx (see Fig. 18–2A). The epiglottis is an elastic cartilage and extends from the larynx toward the tongue. The epiglottis acts as a flap, a very important flap.

Down the Wrong Way

As Figure 18–2A shows, the pharynx acts as a passageway for food, water, and air. Food and water in the pharynx, however, should not enter the larynx. How is food and water normally kept out of the larynx? At the top of the larynx is a hole called the **glottis** (glŏt′ĭs). When you breathe in air, the glottis opens, and air moves through the glottis into tubes that carry it to the lungs.

When you swallow food, however, a flap called the epiglottis covers the glottis, thereby preventing food from entering the lower respiratory passages. Instead, the food enters the esophagus, the tube that empties into the stomach. How does this happen? During swallowing, the larynx moves upward and forward while the epiglottis moves downward. If you place your fingers on your larynx as you swallow, you can feel the larynx move upward and forward. In addition to movement of the epiglottis, the glottis closes. Compare the size of the glottis in Figure 18–2C and D.

The larynx is called the voicebox because it contains the **vocal cords** (see Figs. 18–2A and C). The vocal cords are folds of tissue composed of muscle and elastic ligaments and covered by mucous membrane. The cords stretch across the upper part of the larynx. The glottis is the space between the vocal cords.

The two types of vocal cords are the false and the true vocal cords. The **false vocal cords** are called false because they do not produce sounds. Instead, the muscle fibers in this structure help to close the airway during swallowing. The **true vocal cords** produce sound. Air flowing from the lungs through the glottis during exhalation causes the true vocal cords to vibrate, thereby producing sound.

The loudness of your voice depends on the force with which the air moves past the true vocal cords. The pitch of your voice depends on the tension exerted on the muscles of the true vocal cords. You form sound into words with your pharynx, oral cavity, tongue and lip movement. The nasal cavities, sinuses, and the pharynx act as resonating chambers, thereby altering the quality of your voice. Listen to the different voices of your friends. One voice may sound high and squeaky while another may sound low and booming.

How was "dumb plant" used to control gossip (without, of course, killing the gossiper)?

A tea made from *Dieffenbachia* (dumb plant) was given to Roman slaves before they were sent to the market to shop. The tea caused the slave's tongue and mouth to swell and paralyzed the throat. The slave was therefore unable to speak and gossip about household affairs. It is still used by some African tribes as a punishment for gossip. An overdose of the poison causes excessive swelling, obstruction of the respiratory passageways, and death by suffocation.

From Boy to Young Man

Why is Jack's voice lower than Jill's? At puberty, under the influence of testosterone, the male larynx enlarges, and the vocal cords become longer and thicker. The larger and thicker the vocal cords are, the deeper the voice is. Changes in the larynx and vocal cords cause the boy's voice to "break" as he matures into a young man. In an earlier period in history, young choir boys with beautiful high voices were castrated. Castration,

the surgical excision of the testes, removes the source of testosterone and prevents thickening of the vocal cords. These unfortunate castrated boys would not experience any break in their voices and would continue to sing beautifully as members of the castrati choir. For obvious reasons, this practice eventually disappeared.

Trachea

The **trachea** (trā′kē-ə), or **windpipe,** is a tube 4 to 5 inches (10–12.5 cm) long and 1 inch (2.5 cm) in diameter (Fig. 18–3). The trachea extends from

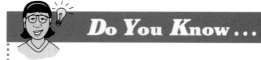

What is a tracheostomy?

Sometimes a part of the upper respiratory tract becomes blocked, thereby obstructing the flow of air into the lungs. To restore airflow, an emergency tracheostomy may be performed. This procedure is the insertion of a tube through a surgical incision into the trachea, below the level of the obstruction. The tracheostomy bypasses the obstruction and allows air to flow through the tube into the lungs.

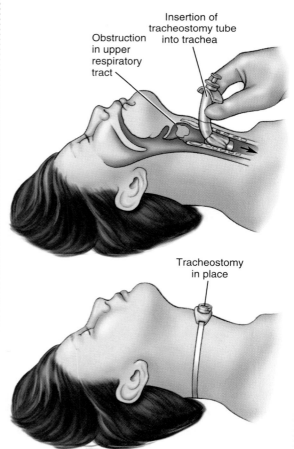

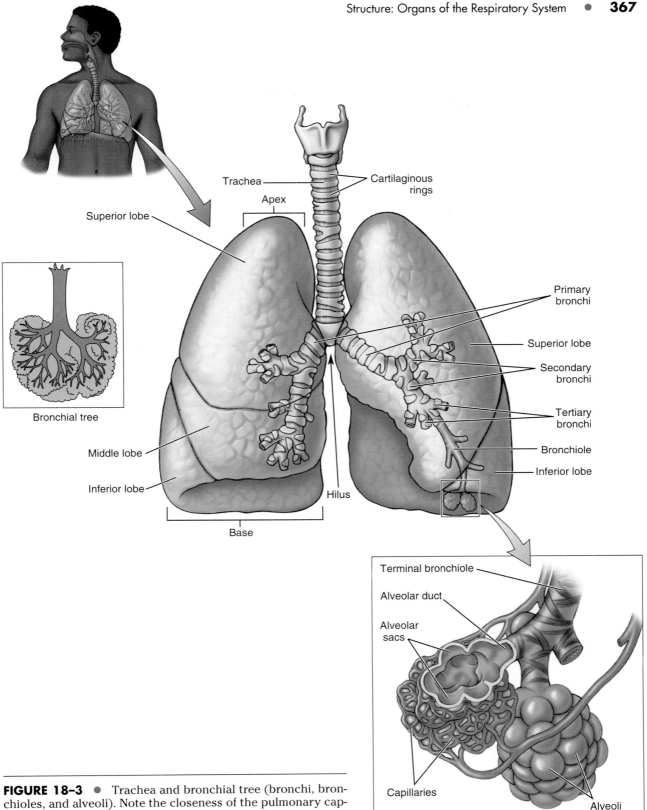

FIGURE 18-3 ● Trachea and bronchial tree (bronchi, bronchioles, and alveoli). Note the closeness of the pulmonary capillaries to the alveolus.

the lower edge of the larynx downward into the thoracic cavity, where it splits into the right and left bronchi (singular, **bronchus** [brŏng′kəs]). The trachea is in front of the esophagus, the food tube. The trachea conducts air to and from the lungs.

C-shaped rings of cartilage partially surround the trachea for its entire length and serve to keep it open. The rings are open on the back side of the trachea, so that the esophagus can bulge forward as food moves along the esophagus to the stomach. You can feel the cartilaginous rings if you run your fingers along the front of your neck. Without this strong cartilaginous support, the trachea would collapse and shut off the flow of air through the respiratory passages. Because of the cartilaginous rings, a tight collar or necktie does not collapse the trachea. A severe blow to the anterior neck, however, can crush the trachea and cause an acute respiratory obstruction.

Bronchial Tree: Bronchi, Bronchioles, and Alveoli

The bronchial tree consists of the bronchi, the bronchioles, and the alveoli. It is called a tree because the bronchi and their many branches resemble an upside-down tree (see Fig. 18–3). Most of the bronchial tree is in the lungs.

Bronchi

The right and left primary bronchi are formed as the lower part of the trachea divides into two tubes. The primary bronchi enter the lungs at a region called the **hilus.** The primary bronchi branch into secondary bronchi, which branch into smaller tertiary bronchi. Because the heart lies toward the left side of the chest, the **left bronchus** is narrower and positioned more horizontally than the right bronchus. The **right bronchus** is shorter and wider than the left bronchus and extends downward in a more vertical direction. Because of the differences in the size and positioning of the bronchi, food particles and small objects are more easily inhaled, or aspirated, into the right bronchus.

The upper segments of the bronchi have C-shaped cartilaginous rings, which help to keep the bronchi open. As the bronchi extend into the lungs, however, the amount of cartilage decreases and finally disappears. The finer and more distal branches of the bronchi contain no cartilage.

Bronchioles

The bronchi divide repeatedly into smaller tubes called **bronchioles.** The walls of the bronchioles contain smooth muscle and no cartilage. The bronchioles regulate the flow of air to the alveoli. Contraction of the bronchiolar smooth muscle causes the bronchioles to constrict, thereby decreasing the bronchiolar lumen and so decreasing airflow. Relaxation of the bronchioles causes the lumen to increase, thereby increasing air flow.

An asthma attack illustrates the effect of bronchiolar smooth muscle constriction. In a person with asthma, the bronchioles hyperrespond to a particular allergen. The bronchiolar smooth muscle then constricts, decreasing the flow of air into the lungs. The person complains of a tight chest and expends much energy trying to force air

through the constricted bronchioles into the lungs. Forced air causes a wheezing sound often heard on inhalation. Bronchiolar smooth muscle relaxants are medications that cause bronchodilation, thereby improving airflow and relieving the wheezing.

Alveoli

The bronchioles continue to divide and give rise to many tiny tubes called **alveolar ducts** (see Fig. 18–3). These ducts end in microscopic grapelike structures called alveoli (singular, **alveolus** [ăl-vē′ə-ləs]). The alveoli are tiny air (alveolar) sacs that form at the ends of the respiratory passages. A pulmonary capillary surrounds each alveolus. The alveoli function to exchange oxygen and carbon dioxide across the alveolar-pulmonary capillary membrane.

Certain respiratory diseases may destroy alveoli or cause a thickening of the alveolar wall. As a result, the exchange of gases is slowed. Oxygenation of the blood may decrease, causing hypoxemia, and the blood may retain carbon dioxide, causing a disturbance in acid-base balance.

✳ **SUM IT UP!** Breathing, or ventilation, consists of inhalation and exhalation. Breathing involves the movement of air through the following structures: from the nasal cavities to the pharynx to the larynx to the trachea to the bronchi to the bronchioles to the alveoli. When the air reaches the alveoli, the tiny air sacs at the end of the bronchial tree, the respiratory gases, oxygen and carbon dioxide, diffuse across the alveolar-pulmonary capillary membrane. Most of the respiratory structures conduct air to and from the lungs. Only the alveoli function in the exchange of the respiratory gases between the outside air and the blood.

Lungs

The two lungs, located in the thoracic cavity, extend from an area just above the clavicles to the diaphragm. The lungs are soft cone-shaped organs so large that they occupy most of the space in the thoracic cavity (see Fig. 18–3). The lungs are subdivided into lobes. The right lung has three lobes: the superior, middle, and inferior lobes. Because of the location of the heart in the left side of the chest, the left lung has only two lobes: the superior lobe and the inferior lobe.

The upper rounded part of the lung is called the **apex,** while the lower portion is called the **base.** The base of the lung rests on the diaphragm. As organs in which the exchange of respiratory gases takes place, the lungs contain the bronchial tree. The area between the two lungs is called the **mediastinum** (mē″dē-ə-stī′nəm). It contains the heart, large blood vessels (aorta, pulmonary artery, and venae cavae), esophagus, trachea, and lymph nodes.

The amount of air the lungs can hold varies with a person's body build, age, and physical conditioning. For instance, a tall person has larger lungs than a short person. A swimmer generally has larger lungs than a "couch potato." And the trained singer has larger lungs than the singer whose talents are heard only in the shower.

Pleural Membranes

Pleural Cavity: A Potential Space

The outside of each lung and the inner chest wall are lined with a continuous serous membrane called the **pleura** (ploor′ə) (Fig. 18–4). The pleura is named according to its location. The membrane on the outer surface of each lung is called the **visceral pleura.** The membrane lining the chest wall is called the **parietal pleura.** The visceral pleura and the parietal pleura are attracted to each other like two flat plates of glass whose surfaces are wet. The plates of glass can slide past one another but offer some resistance when you try to pull them apart.

Between the visceral pleura and the parietal pleura is a potential space called the **intrapleural space,** or **pleural cavity.** The pleural membranes secrete a thin layer of serous fluid that creates the intrapleural space. The serous fluid lubricates the pleural membranes and allows the two pleural membranes to slide past one another with little friction and discomfort. The intrapleural space is

called a potential space. Under abnormal conditions, this space has the *potential* to accumulate excess fluid, blood, and air.

Expanded Lungs/Collapsed Lungs

Figure 18–4 shows that the lungs occupy most of the thoracic cage, but this statement must be qualified: the *expanded* lungs occupy most of the thoracic cage. Under normal conditions, the lungs expand like inflated balloons. Under certain abnormal conditions, however, the lung may collapse. What determines whether or not the lungs collapse or expand?

WHY LUNGS COLLAPSE. If the thoracic cavity is entered surgically, the lungs collapse. Why does this happen? Consider a balloon and a lung (Fig. 18–5A). If you blow up a balloon but fail to tie off the open end, the air rushes out, and the balloon collapses. The balloon collapses because of the arrangement of its elastic fibers. When the elastic fibers stretch, they remain stretched only when tension is applied (eg, the air blown into the balloon stretches the balloon). If the end of the balloon is not tied off, the elastic fibers recoil, forcing air out and collapsing the balloon. The same can be said of the lung. The arrangement of the lung's elastic tissue is similar to the arrangement of the elastic fibers in the balloon. The elastic tissue of the lung can stretch, but it recoils and returns to its unstretched position if tension is released (Fig. 18–5B).

The lung (in the open thoracic cavity) can also collapse for a second reason, a force called **surface tension.** The single alveolus in Figure 18–5C illustrates surface tension. A thin layer of water lines the inside of the alveolus. Water is a polar molecule; one end of the water molecule has a positive (+) charge, while the other end of the molecule has a negative (−) charge. Note how the water molecules line up. The positive (+) end of one water molecule is attracted to the negative (−) charge on the second water molecule. Each water molecule pulls on the other. The electrical attraction of the water molecules is the surface tension. As the water molecules pull on one another, they tend to make the alveolus smaller; in other words, they collapse the alveoli. Thus, the lungs collapse for the two reasons: the arrangement of the elastic fibers in the lung and the surface tension in the alveoli.

Note: the surface tension of pure water is normally very high. In the mature, normal lung, certain cells secrete pulmonary surfactants. **Surfactants** (sər-fǎk′tənts) are lipoproteins secreted by special alveolar cells. Pulmonary surfactants act like detergents. They decrease surface tension by interfering with the electrical attraction between the water molecules on the inner surface of the alveolus (see Fig. 18–5C). While surfactants lower surface tension, they do not eliminate it. Surface tension remains a force that acts to collapse the alveoli.

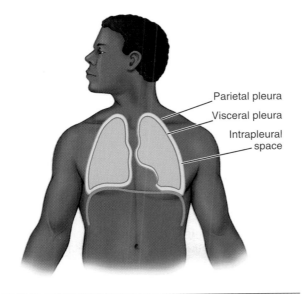

Parietal pleura

Visceral pleura

Intrapleural space

FIGURE 18–4 ● Lungs and the pleural membranes: parietal pleura, visceral pleura, and the intrapleural space.

A

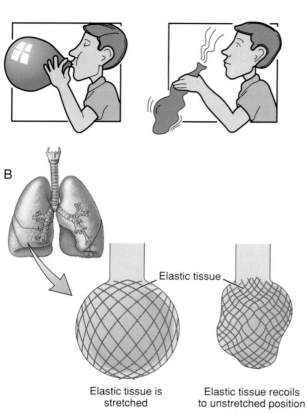

B

Elastic tissue

Elastic tissue is
stretched

Elastic tissue recoils
to unstretched position

C

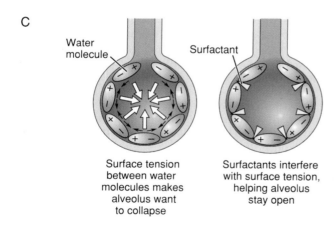

Water
molecule

Surfactant

Surface tension
between water
molecules makes
alveolus want
to collapse

Surfactants interfere
with surface tension,
helping alveolus
stay open

FIGURE 18-5 ● A and B, Like the alveolus, a balloon
is made of elastic fibers that remain expanded as long as
air pressure maintains tension. C, Surface tension tends
to collapse the alveolus, but pulmonary surfactants decrease surface tension, preventing alveolar collapse.

WHY LUNGS EXPAND. If the elastic fibers and the
surface tension act to collapse the lungs, why do
they remain expanded (in the normal closed thorax)? Lung expansion depends on pressure within
the chest cavity. A series of diagrams in Figure
18–6 illustrates this point. There are three pres-

Do You Know...

Why is a premature infant more apt than a full-term infant to develop respiratory distress syndrome?

Surfactant-secreting cells appear only during
the later stages of fetal development. An infant
born 2 to 3 months prematurely generally has insufficient surfactant-secreting cells. As a result,
surface tension within the alveoli is excessively
high, the alveoli collapse, and the infant experiences respiratory distress. The infant may die in
respiratory failure. This condition is commonly
called **respiratory distress syndrome.** Premature
infants are given surfactants through inhalation in
an attempt to prevent this life-threatening condition.

sures (see Fig. 18–6A) labeled P1, P2, and P3. P1 is
the pressure outside the chest (eg, the pressure
in the room), also called the **atmospheric pressure.** P2 is the pressure in the lung; it is called the
intrapulmonic pressure. P3 is the pressure in the
intrapleural space, also called the **intrapleural
pressure** (ĭn″trə-plo͞or′əl prĕsh′ər). Note in Figure 18–6A that the lungs are normally expanded.

Figures 18–6B and C explain why the lungs expand. To illustrate this point, a hole is created in
the right chest wall, so that the right lung collapses. Note the pressures. Because of the hole in
the chest wall, all the pressures are equal. In other
words, P1=P2=P3. In Figure 18–6C, a tube is inserted through the hole of the right chest wall,
into the intrapleural space. The tube is attached to
a pump, which removes air from the intrapleural
space. As air moves from the intrapleural space,
the intrapleural pressure (P3) decreases and becomes negative. This negative intrapleural pressure (P3) merely means that it is less than either
the atmospheric pressure (P1) or the intrapulmonic pressure (P2).

What is the effect of a negative intrapleural
pressure? Because P2 (intrapulmonic pressure) is
greater than P3 (intrapleural pressure), the lung is
pushed toward the chest wall causing the lung to
expand. Also, because P1 (atmospheric pressure)
is greater than P3, the chest wall is pushed inward
toward the lung. When the chest wall and the
lungs meet, the lung is expanded (see Figs. 18–6C
and D). The important point is this: the lung expands and remains expanded because the intrapleural pressure is negative.

What happens if the pump is removed,
thereby recreating the hole in the chest wall? Because P1 is greater than P3, air rushes into the intrapleural space through the hole and eliminates

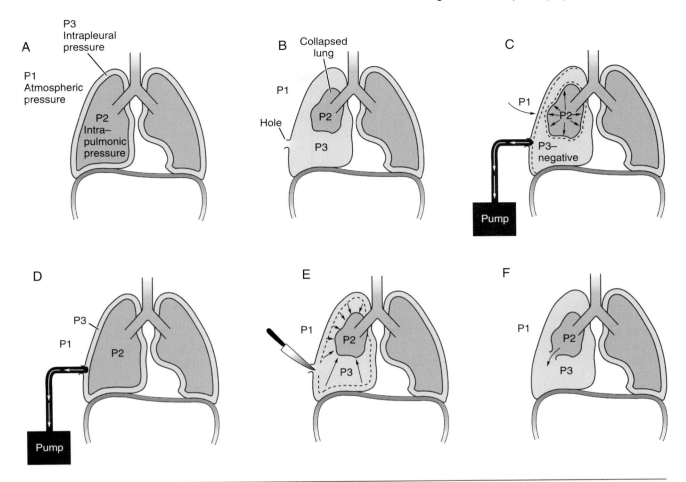

FIGURE 18–6 ● Lung expansion and collapse. A, The lungs expanded. B, The right lung collapses because of the hole in the chest wall. C, Air is pumped out of the intrapleural space, creating a negative intrapleural pressure. D, The lung expands because of the negative intrapleural pressure. E, The lung collapses because of the hole (knife wound) in the chest wall. F, The lung collapses because of a hole in the lung.

the negative intrapleural pressure. As a result, the lung collapses. Remember: the lung expands only when the intrapleural pressure is negative.

Figure 18–6E illustrates the effects of a stab wound to the chest. The hole created by the knife allows the air to rush into the intrapleural space and eliminate the negative intrapleural pressure. The introduction of air into the intrapleural space and subsequent collapse of the lung is called a **pneumothorax** (*pneumo* means air; *thorax* means chest). Air in the intrapleural space is also the reason that the lungs collapse when a surgical incision is made into the chest wall.

Figure 18–6F shows the effect of a hole in the lung. Because the intrapulmonic pressure (P2) is greater than the intrapleural pressure (P3), air rushes into the intrapleural space through the hole in the lung, thereby eliminating the negative intrapleural pressure and collapsing the lung. Sometimes persons with emphysema develop blebs, or blisters, on the outer surface of their lungs. The blebs rupture and create a hole be-

tween the intrapulmonic and the intrapleural spaces, causing air to rush into the intrapleural space and collapsing the lung.

What can be done for a collapsed lung? The physician inserts a tube through the chest wall into the intrapleural space and pulls air out of the intrapleural space. As the air leaves the intrapleural space, negative pressure is reestablished, and the lung expands. Sometimes the physician inserts a large needle into the intrapleural space to aspirate, or withdraw, air, blood, and pus. This procedure is called a **thoracentesis.** It facilitates lung expansion. Note: the intrapleural pressure remains negative only when no hole exists in either the chest wall or the lungs.

✳ **SUM IT UP!** The expanded lungs normally fill the thoracic cavity. Unless pressure conditions in the pleural cavity are correct, the lungs collapse. The tendency of the lungs to collapse is due to two factors: the arrangement of the elastic fibers of the lungs and the alveolar surface tension. If the lungs tend to collapse, why do the lungs stay expanded? The expansion of the lungs is due to a negative intrapleural pressure within the chest cavity. If the negative intrapleural pressure is eliminated, the lungs collapse.

RESPIRATORY FUNCTION

Three Steps in Respiration

The organs of the respiratory system and the pressure in the chest cavity maintain the lungs in an expanded condition. Now let us see how the whole system works, its physiology. Respiration involves three steps:

- Ventilation, or breathing
- Exchange of oxygen and carbon dioxide between the air sacs and the blood and the exchange of oxygen and carbon dioxide between the blood and the cells of the body
- Transport of oxygen and carbon dioxide by the blood

Ventilation, or Breathing

PRESSURE/VOLUME: BOYLE'S LAW. To understand ventilation, you need some background information. You need to know the relationship between pressure and volume, a relationship called **Boyle's law.** Note the two tubes in Figure 18–7. Tube A is a small tube that fits into a bicycle tire. When filled, the tube can hold 1 liter of air. Tube B is larger and fits into a truck tire. When filled, it can hold 10 liters of air. Thus, the volume of the truck tube (B) is 10 times greater than the volume of the bicycle tube (A).

In the upper panel of Figure 18–7, both tubes are empty. Let us add 1 liter of air to each tube and measure the pressure in each tube. By touching the surfaces of the tubes, you can get a rough estimate of the pressures. Tube A feels firm, while tube B feels soft. In other words, the pressure in tube A is greater than the pressure in tube B. Both tubes received the same amount of air, so why are the pressures different? The different volumes of the tubes cause the different pressures. The pressure is higher in tube A because the volume of tube A is small; the 1 liter of air completely fills the tube. The pressure in tube B is lower because its

A

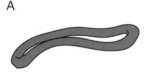

Deflated bicycle tube

B

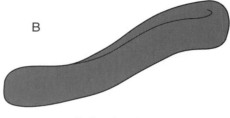

Deflated truck tube
(10X volume of bicycle tube)

FIGURE 18–7 • Boyle's law: relationship between pressure and volume. A, A bicycle tube deflated (upper panel) and inflated with 1 liter of air (lower panel). The tube is firm, indicating a high pressure. B, A truck tube deflated (upper panel) and partially inflated with 1 liter of air. The tube is not firm, indicating less pressure in tube B than in tube A.

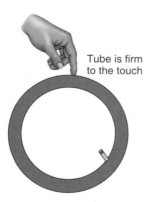

Tube is firm to the touch

Bicycle tube inflated with 1 liter of air

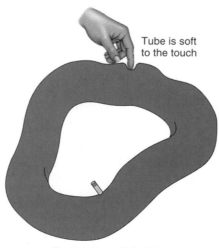

Tube is soft to the touch

Truck tube partially inflated with 1 liter of air

volume is large (10 liters). The 1 liter of air only partially fills the truck tube. The important point is this: the smaller the volume, the higher the pressure, or the greater the volume, the lower the pressure. If volume changes, the pressure changes. This is Boyle's law, the principle upon which ventilation is based.

Do You Know...

Why does this person's chest look like a barrel?

This person has **emphysema,** a condition characterized by damaged tissue in the lower respiratory structures and overinflated alveoli. As a result, the lungs cannot exhale the proper amount of air, and the air remains trapped in the alveoli. Consequently, the alveoli and lungs become overinflated and cause the chest to be shaped like a barrel. A person with severe emphysema is described as barrel-chested.

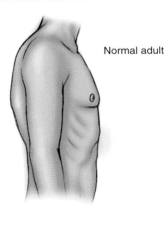

Normal adult

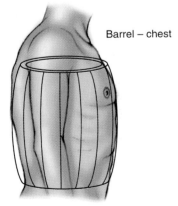

Barrel – chest

BOYLE'S LAW AND BREATHING. What does Boyle's law have to do with ventilation? On inhalation (breathing in), air flows into the lungs. What is the force that causes the air to flow in? Place your hands on your rib cage. Inhale. Notice that the thoracic cage moves up and out on inhalation (Fig. 18–8A and B). This movement increases the volume of the thoracic cavity and lungs. As the volume in the lung increases, the pressure in the lung (P2) decreases (satisfying Boyle's law). As a result, P2 becomes less than P1 (atmospheric pressure, the air you breathe). Air flows from high pressure to low pressure, through the nose into the lungs.

What happens on exhalation? Another change in lung volume. Place your hands on your rib cage and exhale. The thoracic and lung volumes decrease as the rib cage returns to its resting position (Fig. 18–8C and D). The decreased lung volume causes the pressure within the lungs (P2) to increase. Now P2 is greater than P1, and air flows out of the lungs through the nose. Let us clarify the relationship between Boyle's law and ventilation.

- Air flows in response to changes in pressure. As the lung volume increases on inhalation, the intrapulmonic pressure (P2) decreases, and air flows into the lungs.
- On exhalation, lung volume decreases, intrapulmonic pressure (P2) increases, and air flows out of the lungs.
- Air flows in response to pressure changes. Pressure changes occur in response to changes in volume. Inhalation is associated with an increase in thoracic volume; exhalation is associated with a decrease in thoracic volume.

MUSCLES OF RESPIRATION. What causes the thoracic volume to change? The change in thoracic volume is due to the contraction and relaxation of the respiratory muscles (see Fig. 18–8A and B). On inhalation, the respiratory muscles, the diaphragm, and the intercostal muscles contract. The **diaphragm** is a dome-shaped muscle that forms the floor of the thoracic cavity and separates the thoracic cavity from the abdominal cavity. The diaphragm is the chief muscle of inspiration. Contraction of the diaphragm flattens the muscle and pulls it downward, toward the abdomen. This movement increases the length of the thoracic cavity. During quiet breathing, the diaphragm accounts for most of the increase in the thoracic volume.

The two intercostal muscles, the external and internal intercostals, are between the ribs. When the external intercostal muscles contract, the rib cage moves up and out, thereby increasing the width of the thoracic cavity. Note that the size of the thoracic cavity increases in three directions: from front to back, from side to side, and lengthwise. Why is this increase in thoracic volume so important? As the thoracic volume increases, so does the volume of the lungs. According to Boyle's law, the increase in volume decreases the pressure in the lungs, and as a result, air flows into the lungs. During exertion, some of the accessory

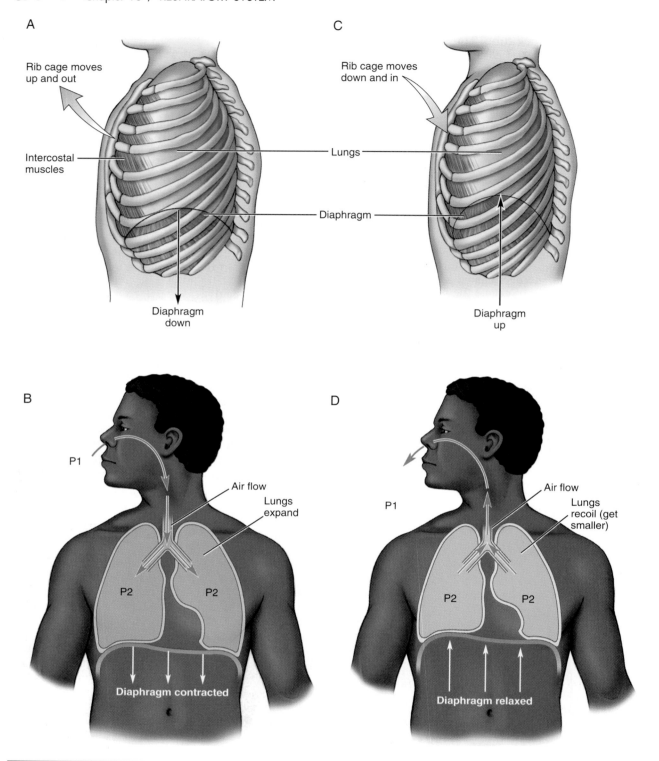

A

Rib cage moves
up and out

Intercostal
muscles

Lungs

Diaphragm

Diaphragm
down

C

Rib cage moves
down and in

Lungs

Diaphragm

Diaphragm
up

B

P1

Air flow

Lungs
expand

P2   P2

Diaphragm contracted

D

P1

Air flow

Lungs
recoil (get
smaller)

P2   P2

Diaphragm relaxed

FIGURE 18–8 ● Inhalation and exhalation. A and B, The thoracic volume increases, and air rushes into the lungs. C and D, The thoracic volume decreases, and air rushes out of the lungs.

muscles of respiration, located in the neck and chest, can move the rib cage further.

On exhalation, the muscles of respiration relax and allow the ribs and the diaphragm to return to their original positions (Fig. 18–8C and D). This movement decreases thoracic and lung volume and increases pressure in the lungs. Consequently, air flows out of the lungs. Elastic recoil of lung tissue and surface tension within the alveoli aid with exhalation. Forced exhalation uses the accessory muscles of respiration. These include the muscles of the abdominal wall and the internal intercostal muscles. Contraction of the accessory muscles of respiration pulls the bottom of the rib cage down and in, and it forces the abdominal viscera upward toward the relaxed diaphragm. These actions force additional air out of the lungs.

How much energy does it take to breathe? Inhalation is due to the contraction of the respiratory muscles. It is an active process. The muscles use up energy (ATP) as they contract. Exhalation associated with normal quiet breathing is passive. Exhalation is due to muscle relaxation. No energy is required for muscle relaxation. Thus, in normal quiet breathing, we use up energy on only half the respiratory cycle, inhalation. We rest on exhalation. During forced exhalation (as in exercise), however, the accessory muscles of respiration must contract, and exhalation becomes energy-using, or active.

With certain lung diseases, such as emphysema, exhalation can be achieved only when the accessory muscles of respiration are used. The patient with emphysema, therefore, uses energy during both inhalation and exhalation. This process is physically exhausting, and these patients usually complain of being very tired.

NERVES THAT SUPPLY THE RESPIRATORY MUSCLES. Ventilation occurs in response to changes in the thoracic volume, and the changes in thoracic volume are due to muscle contraction and relaxation. To contract, the respiratory muscles, being skeletal muscles, must be stimulated by motor nerves. The motor nerves supplying the respiratory muscles are the phrenic nerve and the intercostal nerves. The phrenic nerve exits from the spinal cord at the level of C4, travels within the cervical plexus, and is distributed to the diaphragm. Firing of the phrenic nerve stimulates the diaphragm to contract. The intercostal nerves supply the intercostal muscles. Thus, inhalation is initiated by the firing of the phrenic and intercostal nerves.

You will be caring for patients whose nerve-muscle function is impaired. For instance, if the spinal cord is severed above C4, the phrenic nerve cannot fire. As a result, the skeletal muscles cannot contract. The person not only is quadriplegic but also can breathe only with the assistance of a ventilator. Other patients experience difficulty in breathing because of the effects of certain drugs. Curare, for instance, is a drug commonly used during surgery to cause muscle relaxation. It is a neuromuscular blocking agent that interferes with the transmission of the signal from nerve to muscle. The block occurs within the neuromuscular junction. The patient is not only unable to move the body voluntarily but also is unable to breathe.

✳ **SUM IT UP!** The three steps in respiration are ventilation, exchange of oxygen and carbon dioxide in the lungs and the cells, and transport of oxygen and carbon dioxide by the blood. Ventilation occurs in response to changes in thoracic volumes, which, in turn, cause changes in intrapulmonic pressures. Inhalation (breathing in) occurs when the respiratory muscles contract and enlarge the thoracic cage. Exhalation (breathing out) occurs when the respiratory muscles relax, allowing the thorax to return to its smaller, resting thoracic volume. The muscles of respiration contract in response to stimulation of the phrenic and intercostal nerves.

Gas Exchange

During ventilation, inhalation delivers fresh oxygen-rich air to the alveoli, and exhalation removes carbon dioxide–laden air from the alveoli. The second step of respiration is the exchange of the respiratory gases. Exchange occurs at two sites: in the lungs and at the cells (Fig. 18–9).

GAS EXCHANGE WITHIN THE LUNGS. Gas exchange occurs in the lungs and specifically across the membranes of the alveolus and the pulmonary capillary. What makes the alveoli so well suited for the exchange of oxygen and carbon dioxide? Three conditions promote gas exchange at the alveoli: a large surface area, thin alveolar walls, and a close relationship between the alveoli and the pulmonary capillaries.

 Do You Know...

Why can a failing heart cause the alveoli to fill with water?

After blood becomes oxygenated in the lungs, it flows toward the left side of the heart through the pulmonary veins. If the left side of the heart becomes weakened and fails, the blood cannot be pumped out of the left ventricle. Instead, the blood backs up into the pulmonary veins and capillaries. The pulmonary capillaries then become congested, and water is pushed from the pulmonary capillaries across the alveolar wall into the alveoli. This condition is called **pulmonary edema.** The water in the alveoli impairs gas exchange. The person is dyspneic and hypoxic, has a wet cough, and generally has to sit upright to breathe, a condition called **orthopnea.** Drugs that improve cardiac performance (eg, digitalis) and increase the excretion of water (eg, diuretics) help to relieve pulmonary edema.

• Large surface area. Millions of alveoli, approximately 350 million per lung, create a total surface area about one half the size of a tennis court. The large surface increases the amount of oxygen and carbon dioxide exchanged across the alveolar membranes.

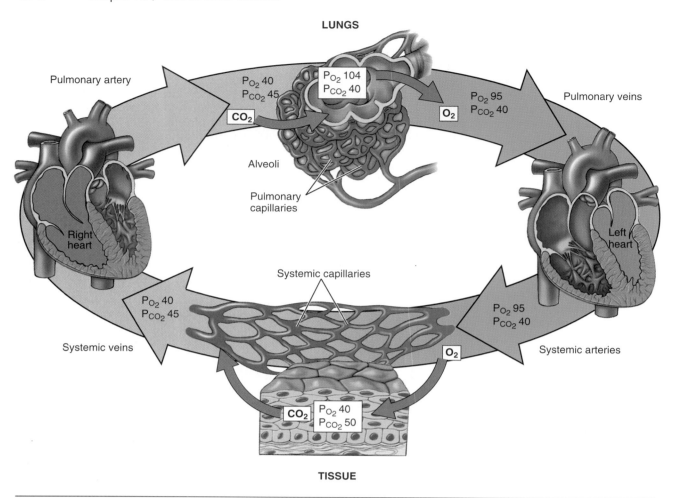

LUNGS

Pulmonary artery

P_{O_2} 40
P_{CO_2} 45

P_{O_2} 104
P_{CO_2} 40

CO_2

O_2

P_{O_2} 95
P_{CO_2} 40

Pulmonary veins

Alveoli

Pulmonary
capillaries

Right
heart

Left
heart

Systemic capillaries

P_{O_2} 40
P_{CO_2} 45

P_{O_2} 95
P_{CO_2} 40

Systemic veins

O_2

Systemic arteries

CO_2

P_{O_2} 40
P_{CO_2} 50

TISSUE

FIGURE 18–9 • Partial pressures of oxygen and carbon dioxide. Within the lungs: P_{O_2} is higher in the alveoli than in the blood. O_2 diffuses into the blood. The P_{CO_2} is highest in the pulmonary capillary and therefore diffuses into the alveoli for excretion. Within the tissues, P_{O_2} is highest in the blood and diffuses into the tissues for use by the metabolizing cells. P_{CO_2} is highest in the tissues and therefore diffuses from the tissues into the blood.

- Thin alveolar walls. The alveoli are composed of simple squamous epithelial cells, making the alveolar wall very thin. The wall of the pulmonary capillary is also very thin. The thin walls favor diffusion because they do not offer much resistance to the movement of oxygen and carbon dioxide across the membranes.
- Closeness of the alveoli to the pulmonary capillaries. Each alveolus is very close to a pulmonary capillary. This closeness promotes diffusion. The diffusion of oxygen and carbon dioxide occurs fastest when the diffusion distances are short. For diffusion, closeness ensures quickness.

What causes the respiratory gases to diffuse? Chapter 3 describes how molecules diffuse from an area of greater concentration to an area of lesser concentration. For gases such as oxygen and carbon dioxide, however, concentration is related to pressure. When the molecules of a gas are

highly concentrated, the gas creates a high pressure in a contained space. Consequently, we can talk about diffusion from areas of high pressure to areas of low pressure.

PRESSURES AND PARTIAL PRESSURES. Ordinary room air is a gas composed of 78% nitrogen, 21% oxygen, and 0.04% carbon dioxide. Each part of the gas contributes to the total pressure. The amount of pressure each gas contributes is called the **partial pressure** (pär′shəl prĕsh′ər). The partial pressure of oxygen is symbolized as the P_{O_2}; the partial pressure of carbon dioxide is symbolized as the P_{CO_2}. (Because the body does not use nitrogen, we can ignore it.)

Partial Pressures Within the Lungs. Let us analyze the partial pressures of the respiratory gases in the alveoli and the pulmonary capillary (see Fig. 18–9). The P_{O_2} of air in the alveoli is 104 mmHg, while the P_{O_2} of venous blood (the blue end of the pulmonary capillary) is 40 mmHg. Oxygen diffuses from the area of high pressure (the alveolus) to the area of low pressure (the pulmonary capillary). Note that the P_{O_2} in the blood goes from 40 mmHg (blue) to 95 mmHg (red). The partial pressure of oxygen increases because the blood has been oxygenated.

As for the waste, the carbon dioxide (CO_2), the P_{CO_2} in the blood (blue capillary) is 45 mmHg, while the P_{CO_2} in the alveolus is only 40 mmHg. CO_2 diffuses from the capillary, the area of high pressure, to the alveolus, the area of low pressure. Because of the diffusion of CO_2 out of the blood, the P_{CO_2} of the blood goes from 45 mmHg (the blue end of the capillary) to 40 mmHg (the red end of the capillary). What has been accomplished? The blood coming from the right side of the heart (blue) has been oxygenated and the oxygenated blood (red) eventually returns to the left side of the heart so that it can be pumped throughout the body. As oxygenation occurs, CO_2 has been removed; it leaves the lungs during exhalation.

PARTIAL PRESSURES AT THE CELLS. What happens to the gases at the tissues, or body cells? Two events occur. First, oxygen leaves the blood and diffuses into the cells, where it can be used during cell metabolism. Second, carbon dioxide diffuses into the blood as metabolism occurs in the cell.

What partial pressures cause these events to happen? The P_{O_2} of the arterial blood is 95 mmHg while the cellular P_{O_2} is only 40 mmHg. During gas exchange, oxygen diffuses from the blood into the space surrounding the cells. The P_{CO_2} of the cells is 50 mmHg while the arterial P_{CO_2} is only 40 mmHg. CO_2 therefore diffuses from the cells into the blood. The blood then carries the CO_2 to the lungs for excretion. Thus, oxygenated blood from the lungs carries the oxygen to the cells; the oxygen then diffuses from the blood into the cells. The CO_2, the waste produced by the metabolizing cells, diffuses into the blood, which carries the CO_2 to the lungs for excretion. Note the venous blood leaving the cells. The P_{O_2} is 40 mmHg because the O_2 has been used up by the cells. The P_{CO_2} is 45 mmHg because the waste (CO_2) was removed from the cells.

Transport of Oxygen and Carbon Dioxide

The third step in respiration is the blood's mechanism for transporting oxygen and carbon dioxide between the lungs and body cells. Although the blood transports both oxygen and carbon dioxide, the way in which blood transports each gas differs.

OXYGEN TRANSPORT. Almost all of the oxygen (98%) is transported by the hemoglobin in the red blood cells. (You can review hemoglobin in Chapter 13.) The remaining 2% of the oxygen is dissolved in the plasma. As soon as oxygen enters the blood in the pulmonary capillaries, it immediately

forms a loose bond with the iron portion of the hemoglobin molecule. This new molecule is **oxyhemoglobin** (ŏk″sē-hē′mə-glō″bĭn). As the oxygenated blood travels to the cells throughout the body, the oxygen splits, or unloads from the hemoglobin molecule and diffuses across the capillary walls to the cells. The oxygen is eventually used up by the metabolizing cells.

CARBON DIOXIDE TRANSPORT. Blood carries carbon dioxide from the metabolizing cells to the lungs, where it is exhaled. Blood carries carbon dioxide in three forms:

- Ten percent of the carbon dioxide is dissolved in plasma.
- Twenty percent of the carbon dioxide combines with hemoglobin to form **carbaminohemoglobin** (kär-băm″ĭ-nō-hē′mə-glō″bĭn). Note that the hemoglobin carries both oxygen and carbon dioxide, but by different parts of the hemoglobin molecule. The oxygen forms a loose bond with the iron portion of the hemoglobin, while the carbon dioxide bonds with the globin, or protein portion, of the hemoglobin.
- Seventy percent of the carbon dioxide is converted to the **bicarbonate ion** (HCO_3^-). Note that the blood carries most of the carbon dioxide in the form of bicarbonate.

✳ **SUM IT UP!** The exchange of the respiratory gases occurs at two sites: in the lungs and in the cells. Oxygen diffuses from the alveoli into the pulmonary capillaries. Carbon dioxide diffuses from the pulmonary capillaries into the alveoli. At the cellular sites, oxygen diffuses from the capillaries into the cells; carbon dioxide diffuses from the cells into the capillaries. Blood transports oxygen and carbon dioxide. Hemoglobin carries most of the oxygen as oxyhemoglobin. The blood carries most of the carbon dioxide in the form of bicarbonate ion (HCO_3^-).

Lung Volumes and Capacities

Lung Volumes

Think about all the ways you can vary the amount of air you breathe. For instance, you can inhale a small amount of air, or you can take a deep breath. How are you breathing now? Probably slowly and effortlessly. With strenuous exercise, you would breathe more rapidly and deeply. If you become anxious, your breathing pattern becomes more rapid and shallow. With certain diseases, your respirations might increase or decrease. In other words, the amount, or volume, of air you breathe can vary significantly.

The different volumes of air you breathe have names. The four pulmonary volumes are tidal volume, inspiratory reserve volume, expiratory reserve volume, and residual volume. A spirometer

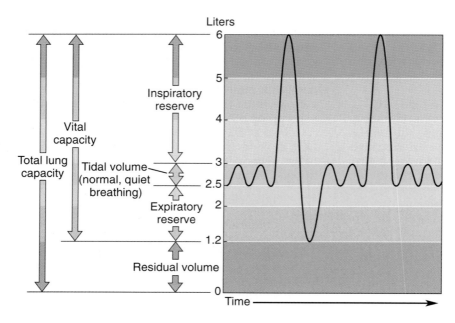

FIGURE 18-10 • Pulmonary volumes.

measures pulmonary volumes. The patient blows into the spirometer, and it measures the amount of air and prints the results on graph paper. A recording of the volumes appears in Figure 18–10 and is summarized in Table 18–1.

- Tidal volume. Breathe in and out. The amount of air moved into or out of the lungs with each breath is called the **tidal volume** (tĭd′l vŏl′yo̅o̅m). The average tidal volume during normal quiet breathing is about 500 mL.
- Inspiratory reserve volume. Inhale a normal volume of air. Now, in addition to this normal amount of air, inhale as much as you possibly can. The additional volume of air is called the **inspiratory reserve volume.** This extra volume is approximately 3000 mL.
- Expiratory reserve volume. Exhale a normal amount of air. Now in addition to this normal amount of air, exhale as much as you possibly can. The extra volume of exhaled air is called the **expiratory reserve volume.** It is about 1100 mL.
- Residual volume. Even after a forced exhalation, about 1100 mL of air remains in the lungs. This remaining air is the **residual volume.** Residual air remains in the lungs at all times, even between breaths. Note in Figure 18–10 that the

Table 18 • 1	LUNG VOLUMES AND CAPACITIES	
NAME	**DESCRIPTION**	**AMOUNT (mL)**
Volumes		
Tidal volume	The volume of air moved into or out of the lungs during one respiratory cycle.	500
Residual volume	The volume of air that remains in the lungs after a forceful exhalation.	1200
Inspiratory reserve volume	The volume of air that can be forcefully inhaled after normal inhalation.	3000
Expiratory reserve volume	The volume of air that can be forcefully exhaled after normal exhalation.	1100
Capacities		
Vital capacity	The maximum volume of air that can be exhaled following maximal inhalation.	4600
Functional residual capacity	The amount of air remaining in the lungs following exhalation during quiet breathing.	2300
Total lung capacity	The total amount of air in the lung following a maximal inhalation.	5800

four pulmonary volumes add up to the **total lung capacity.**

Lung Capacities

In addition to four pulmonary volumes are four pulmonary capacities. A **pulmonary capacity** is a combination of pulmonary volumes. For instance, **vital capacity** (vīt′l kə-păs′ĭ-tē) (4600 mL) refers to the combination of tidal volume (500 mL), inspiratory reserve volume (3000 mL), and expiratory reserve volume (1100 mL). The measurement of vital capacity is a commonly used pulmonary function test.

You can measure vital capacity as follows. Take the deepest breath possible. Exhale all the air you possibly can into a spirometer. The spirometer measures the amount of air you exhale. The amount exhaled should be approximately 4600 mL. In other words, vital capacity is the maximal amount of air exhaled after a maximal inhalation. Vital capacity measures pulmonary function in patients with lung diseases such as emphysema and asthma. Other pulmonary capacities are listed in Table 18–1.

Dead Space

Some of the air you inhale never reaches the alveoli. It stays in the conducting passageways of the trachea, bronchi, and bronchioles. Because this air does not reach the alveoli, it is not available for gas exchange and is said to occupy **anatomical dead space.** The dead space holds about 150 mL of air. Breathing slowly and deeply increases the amount of well-oxygenated air that reaches the alveoli. Conversely, rapid panting delivers a poorer quality of air to the alveoli because a greater percentage of the inhaled volume of air remains in the anatomical dead space. Therefore, when you encourage your patients to take deep breaths, you are also helping to supply the alveoli with well-oxygenated air.

Control of Breathing

Normal breathing is rhythmic and involuntary. For instance, as you read, you are breathing effortlessly, about 16 times per minute. (The normal respiratory rate ranges from 12 to 20 breaths per minute in an adult and from 20 to 40 breaths per minute in the child, depending on the age and size of the child.) You do not have to remember to breathe in and out. Nor do you have to calculate how deeply to breathe. Fortunately, breathing occurs automatically. You do not have to think about it.

For instance, if you were to get up and exercise, your breathing would automatically increase. Why? Breathing automatically adjusts to deliver more oxygen to the working cells and to remove carbon dioxide, the waste product of metabolism. In other words, the body regulates breathing

moment-to-moment to respond to changes in cellular activity.

You can voluntarily control breathing, up to a point. Hold your breath for 5 seconds. Now hold your breath for 3 minutes. You can't do it; you must breathe. The need to breathe means that Sammy should not hold you hostage with his temper tantrums. No matter how good his performance and how long he holds his breath, he will eventually take a really deep breath and live.

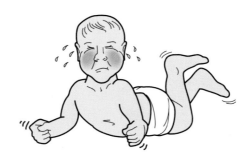

Neural Control of Respiration

How does the body control breathing? The two mechanisms that control breathing are nervous and chemical mechanisms. The nervous mechanism involves several areas of the brain, the most important being the brain stem. Special groups of neurons are widely scattered throughout the brain stem, particularly in the medulla oblongata and the pons (Fig. 18–11). The main control center for breathing, in the medulla, is called the **medullary respiratory control** center. It sets the basic breathing rhythm.

Inhalation occurs when the inspiratory neurons in the medulla fire, giving rise to nerve impulses. The nerve impulses travel from the medulla along the phrenic and intercostal nerves to the muscles of respiration. Contraction of the respiratory muscles causes inhalation. Exhalation occurs when the expiratory neurons in the medulla oblongata fire and shut down the inspiratory neurons. This process inhibits the formation of nerve impulses and causes the respiratory muscles to relax. Thus breathing is due to the alternate firing of the inspiratory and expiratory neurons: the inspiratory neurons fire and cause inhalation, the expiratory neurons fire and cause exhalation, the inspiratory neurons fire and cause inhalation, and so on.

Although the medulla is the main control center for breathing, the pons also plays an important role. The pons contains the **pneumotaxic center** and the **apneustic center.** These areas in the pons modify and help to control breathing patterns.

The medullary respiratory center is very sensitive to the effects of narcotics. Narcotics, such as morphine, depress the medulla and slow respirations. If the narcotic overdose is large enough, respirations may even cease, causing respiratory arrest and death. Because of the profound effect of narcotics on respirations, you must check the pa-

tient's respiratory rate before administering narcotics.

Although the brain stem normally determines
the basic rate and depth of breathing, other areas
of the brain can also affect breathing patterns.
These areas include the hypothalamus and the
cerebral cortex. For instance, the hypothalamus
processes our emotional responses, such as anxiety and fear. The hypothalamus, in turn, stimulates the brain stem and changes the breathing
pattern. Rapid breathing, a response to anxiety or
fear, is part of the fight or flight response. The

cerebral cortex can also affect respirations; cortical activity allows us voluntarily to control the
depth and rate of breathing.

Several other nervous pathways affect the respiratory system. For instance, the vagus nerve
carries nerve impulses from the lungs to the brain
stem. When the lungs become inflated, nerve impulses travel to the brain stem, inhibiting the inspiratory neurons. This response is called the
Hering-Breuer reflex. It prevents overinflation of
the lungs. The nervous structures not only control
breathing patterns but also affect several reflexes

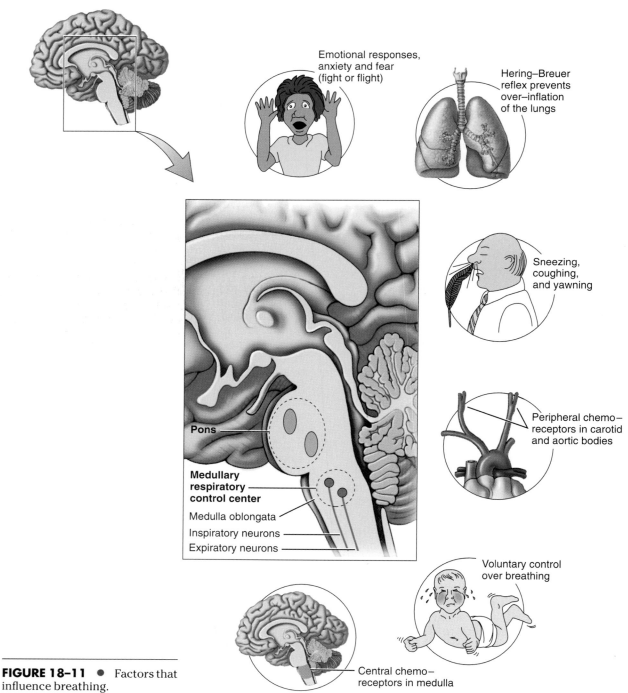

FIGURE 18–11 ● Factors that
influence breathing.

Disorders of the Respiratory System

Asthma	A condition due to a hyperresponsiveness of the bronchiolar smooth muscle. Asthma causes difficulty with breathing (especially affecting the inhalation phase of respiration). Generally, the bronchiolar constriction is triggered by an allergen in the air but may be related to exercise or various pathogens.
Atelectasis	Incomplete expansion of the lung or a portion of the lung. The patient experiences varying degrees of dyspnea and hypoxia, depending on the extent of the atelectasis. Many respiratory diseases, such as cancer of the lung, mucous plugs (asthma), and pneumonia cause atelectasis.
Cancer of the lung	Bronchogenic carcinoma is a common form. As the tumor grows, it obstructs the air passages, causing them to collapse and eventually become infected. As the tumor grows and replaces normal lung tissue, less oxygen can be exchanged, and the person becomes dyspneic and hypoxic. Metastasis is common.
Chronic obstructive pulmonary disease (COPD)	Various combinations of asthma, chronic bronchitis, and emphysema. The most serious complications of COPD are heart and respiratory failure.
Common cold	Also called acute coryza. The common cold is the most common respiratory disease.
Emphysema	Means "puffed up" alveoli. As the lungs lose their elastic tissue, the airways collapse during exhalation, thereby obstructing the outflow of air. Overinflation of the lungs causes a permanently expanded "barrel chest."
Inflammation of the respiratory tract	An inflamed part of the respiratory system. Most inflammations are caused by pathogens. Common inflammations include sinusitis (inflammation of the mucous membranes lining the paranasal sinuses), rhinitis (inflammation of the mucous membrane lining the nasal cavity), pharyngitis (sore throat), and laryngitis (hoarseness or lack of voice due to inflammation of the lining of the larynx).
Influenza	Also called flu. The flu is a contagious upper respiratory infection of viral origin. The flu may spread to the lungs, causing a severe form of pneumonia that is especially serious in the elderly population.
Pleurisy	Pleuritis. Occasionally, the pleural membranes become inflamed and dry out. As the inflamed pleural membranes slide past one another, friction arises between the two membranes, and the person experiences pain on breathing.
Pneumonia	Inflammation of the lungs in which the alveoli become filled with exudate. The exudate consists of serum and pus (products of infection). As the alveoli become filled with exudate, oxygenation decreases and the patient becomes hypoxemic.

Summary Outline

I. Structures: Organs of the Respiratory System

The respiratory system consists of the upper respiratory tract and the lower respiratory tract.

A. Nose and Nasal Cavities
1. The nose is supported by bone and cartilage. The nares, or nostrils, are the openings in the nose.
2. The nasal septum divides the nasal cavity into two passages. Mucous membranes line the nasal cavities. The membranes filter, warm, and moisten the incoming air.
3. Olfactory receptors in the nasal cavities respond to chemicals in the inhaled air.
4. The paranasal sinuses drain into the nasal cavities.

B. Pharynx, the Throat
1. The nasopharynx forms a passage for air only.
2. The oropharynx and laryngopharynx form passageways for both air and food.

continued

I. Structures: Organs of the Respiratory System, *continued*

C. Larynx, the Voicebox

1. The larynx conducts air between the pharynx and the trachea, prevents foreign objects from entering the trachea, and produces sound.
2. Composed of muscle and cartilage, the larynx is lined with mucous membrane. The thyroid cartilage (Adam's apple) is the largest and most anterior cartilage of the larynx.
3. The epiglottis is the uppermost cartilage. It covers the larynx during swallowing.
4. Air passes through the glottis and causes vocal cords to vibrate, thereby producing sound.

D. Trachea, the Windpipe

1. Extending into the chest cavity, the trachea branches into the right and left bronchi.
2. A series of tough C-shaped rings of cartilage keeps the trachea open.

E. Bronchial Tree

1. The bronchial tree contains the bronchi, bronchioles, and alveoli.
2. The large primary bronchi branch into smaller, secondary and tertiary bronchi. The tertiary bronchi continue to branch into smaller tubes, called bronchioles.
3. The bronchioles conduct air between the bronchi and the alveoli. The bronchioles are composed primarily of bronchiolar smooth muscle. Contraction and relaxation of the bronchioles determine the size of the respiratory air passages and therefore affect the amount of air that can enter the alveoli.
4. The alveoli are tiny grape-like air sacs surrounded by pulmonary capillaries. Gas exchange occurs across the thin walls of the alveoli.

F. Lungs

1. The right lung has three lobes. Because of the location of the heart on the left side of the chest, the left lung has only two lobes. A space called the mediastinum separates the lungs.
2. The lungs contain the structures of the lower respiratory tract, blood vessels, and connective tissue.

G. Pleural Membranes

1. The serous membranes in the chest cavity, called the pleural membranes, are the parietal pleura, which lines the inside of the chest wall, and the visceral pleura, which lines the outside of the lungs.
2. Serous fluid between the pleural membranes prevents friction and keeps the membranes together during breathing.
3. The potential space between the pleural membranes is the intrapleural space. For the lungs to remain expanded, pressure in the intrapleural space must be negative (less than atmospheric pressure). When the negative pressure in the intrapleural space is eliminated (eg, by a stab wound to the chest), the lung collapses.

II. Respiratory Function

The three steps of respiration are ventilation, exchange of respiratory gases, and transport of respiratory gases in the blood.

A. Ventilation (Breathing)

1. The two phases of ventilation are inhalation and exhalation. One respiratory cycle refers to one inhalation and one exhalation.
2. Ventilation occurs in response to changes in the thoracic volume (Boyle's law).
3. On inhalation, thoracic volume increases. As a result, intrapulmonic pressure decreases, and the greater atmospheric pressure forces air to move into the lungs. Inhalation is due to the contraction of the respiratory muscles, the diaphragm, and the intercostal muscles.
4. On exhalation, thoracic volume decreases. As a result, the intrapulmonic pressure increases and forces air out of the lungs. Elastic lung recoil and surface tension in the alveoli aid with exhalation. Exhalation is due to the relaxation of the respiratory muscles.
5. The phrenic and intercostal nerves are motor nerves that supply the diaphragm and the intercostal muscles. Stimulation of the nerves causes the muscles to contract, thereby increasing thoracic volume causing inhalation. When the nerves stop firing, the respiratory muscles relax, and thoracic volume decreases, thereby causing exhalation.
6. Inhalation is an active process, meaning that energy is used during muscle contraction. Unforced exhalation is passive, meaning that no muscle contraction and energy consumption is necessary. Forced exhalation is due to the contraction of the internal intercostal and abdominal muscles. Because of the contraction of the muscles, forced exhalation is considered active.

B. Exchange of Gases

1. Exchange of respiratory gases occurs in the alveoli and pulmonary capillaries.
2. Gases diffuse from an area of high pressure to an area of low pressure.
3. Oxygen diffuses from the air in the alveoli (PO_2 = 104 mm Hg) into the blood of the pulmonary capillaries (PO_2 = 40 mm Hg). Carbon dioxide diffuses from the pulmonary capillaries (PCO_2 = 45 mm Hg) into the alveoli (PCO_2 = 40 mm Hg).
4. Exchange of gases also occurs at the cells. Oxygen diffuses from the capillaries (PO_2 = 95 mm Hg) to the cells (PO_2 = 40 mm Hg). Carbon dioxide diffuses from the cells (PCO_2 = 45 mm Hg) into the capillaries. Carbon dioxide diffuses into the blood, where it is transported to the lungs for excretion.

C. Transport of Gases in the Blood

1. Blood transports oxygen and carbon dioxide.
2. Most of the oxygen is transported by the hemoglobin in the red blood cell, where oxygen forms a loose bond with the iron portion of the hemoglobin molecule and is called oxyhemoglobin.
3. The blood transports most carbon dioxide in the form of bicarbonate ion (HCO_3^-). Smaller amounts of carbon dioxide are dissolved in plasma and bound to hemoglobin as carbaminohemoglobin.

Summary Outline, continued

III. Lung Volumes and Capacities

A. Pulmonary Volumes (Amounts of Air)

1. Tidal volume is the volume of air that moves in or out during one respiratory cycle.
2. Inspiratory reserve volume is the additional air that can be inhaled after a normal inhalation.
3. Expiratory reserve volume is the additional air that can be exhaled after a normal exhalation.
4. Residual volume is the volume of air remaining in the lungs at all times.

B. Vital Capacity and Dead Space

1. Vital capacity is the amount of air that can be exhaled after a maximal inhalation. It combines tidal volume, inspiratory reserve volume, and expiratory reserve volume.
2. Air remaining in the large conducting passageways is unavailable for gas exchange. This area is called dead space; it holds about 150 mL of air.

IV. Control of Breathing

A. Normal Breathing: Rhythmic and Involuntary

1. The respiratory center is located in the brain stem, primarily the medulla oblongata (the medullary respiratory center) and the pons.
2. The medullary respiratory center contains inspiratory and expiratory neurons. Nerve impulses travel along the phrenic and intercostal nerves to the muscles of respiration. This process causes muscle contraction and inhalation. Firing of the expiratory neurons inhibits the firing of the inspiratory neurons and leads to muscle relaxation and exhalation. The rhythmic breathing pattern is established by the alternating firing of the inspiratory and expiratory neurons.
3. The pneumotaxic center and the apneustic center are in the pons. These centers help to control the medullary respiratory center to produce a normal breathing pattern.
4. Two other areas of the brain can affect respirations: the hypothalamus (the seat of the emotions) and the cerebral cortex (which allows for the voluntary control of emotions).

B. Factors Affecting Respirations

1. Chemicals, stretching of the lung tissue, emotional states, and voluntary input can all affect respirations.
2. Central chemoreceptors, associated with the respiratory center, are stimulated by blood levels of hydrogen ion and carbon dioxide. Stimulation increases the rate of breathing.
3. Peripheral chemoreceptors are sensitive to low concentrations of oxygen and hydrogen ion in the blood. Stimulation of the peripheral chemoreceptors stimulates breathing.

Review Your Knowledge

1. Trace the movement of air from the nares to the alveoli.

2. What are the three steps of respiration?

3. Why is it better to be a nose breather than a mouth breather?

4. What is the function of the epiglottis?

5. How do the right and left bronchus differ in structure?

6. What happens to the bronchioles during an asthma attack?

7. What is the area between the two lungs called?

8. Why do lungs collapse?

9. Why do lungs expand?

10. What happens if there is a hole in the lung?

11. How does Boyle's law relate to ventilation?

12. What causes the thoracic volume to change?

13. Which two nerves initiate inhalation?

14. What are three conditions that make the alveoli well suited for the exchange of oxygen and carbon dioxide?

15. What is the difference between tidal volume and vital capacity?

16. Is the control of breathing voluntary or involuntary?

17. How do narcotics affect respirations?

18. How do central and peripheral chemoreceptors control respiration?

19. What are six common variations in respirations?

20. Why is orthopnea described in "pillow" terms?

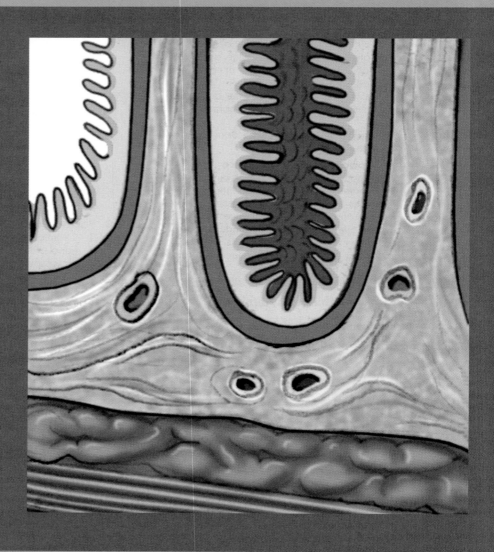

19 DIGESTIVE SYSTEM

Objectives

1. List four functions of the digestive system.

2. Describe the four layers of the digestive tract.

3. List three functions of the peritoneal membranes.

4. List, in sequence, the parts of the alimentary canal from the mouth to the anus.

5. Describe the structure and functions of the organs of the digestive tract.

6. Describe the structure and functions of the accessory organs of the digestive tract.

7. List nine functions of the liver.

8. Explain the physiology of digestion and absorption.

9. List the major enzymes involved in digestion.

10. Describe the role of bile in the digestion of fats.

11. Discuss basic concepts of nutrition.

12. Describe five categories of nutrients.

13. List six factors that affect metabolic rate.

Most of us have no difficulty in eating our way through the Thanksgiving holiday turkey dinner, although the hours after the feeding frenzy can be a digestive challenge. Our digestive systems work very efficiently to digest and absorb as much of the food as possible. Before the holiday is over, the turkey dinner will be a part of every cell in your body.

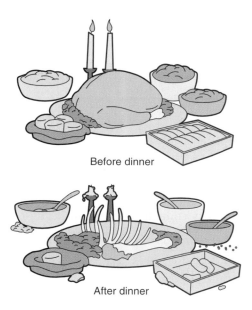

Before dinner

After dinner

Every cell requires a constant supply of nutrients and energy. Food is their source. The purpose of the digestive system is to break down (digest) the food into particles small and simple enough to be absorbed. **Digestion** (dī-jĕs′chən) is the process by which food is broken down into smaller particles suitable for absorption. Digestion takes place within the digestive tract. **Absorption** (əb-sôrp′shən) is the process by which the end-products of digestion move across the walls of the digestive tract into the blood for distribution throughout the body.

OVERVIEW OF THE DIGESTIVE SYSTEM

The digestive tract and the accessory organs of digestion make up the digestive system. The digestive tract is a hollow tube extending from the mouth to the anus. It is also called the **alimentary canal** or the **gastrointestinal tract** (Fig. 19–1). The structures of the digestive tract include the mouth, pharynx, esophagus, stomach, small intestine, large intestine, rectum, and anus.

The accessory organs include the salivary glands, teeth, liver, gallbladder, and pancreas. The salivary glands empty their secretions into the mouth while the liver, gallbladder, and pancreas empty their secretions into the small intestine. The four functions of the digestive system are ingestion, digestion, absorption, and elimination.

The two forms of digestion are mechanical and chemical. **Mechanical digestion** is the breakdown of large food particles into smaller pieces, or particles, by physical means. This process is usually achieved by chewing and by the mashing, or squishing, actions of the muscles in the digestive tract. **Chemical digestion** is the chemical alteration of food. For instance, a protein changes chemically into amino acids. Chemical substances such as digestive enzymes, acid, and bile accomplish chemical digestion.

The end-products of digestion are absorbed by moving across the lining of the digestive tract into the blood. Digested nutrients eventually reach every cell in the body. The food that cannot be digested and absorbed is eliminated from the body as feces. Elimination of waste products is the last stage of the digestive process. Some water is also eliminated in the feces.

Layers of the Digestive Tract

Although modified for specific functions in different organs, the wall of the digestive tract has a similar structure throughout its length (Fig. 19–2). The wall of the digestive tract has four layers: the mucosa, the submucosa, the muscle layer, and the serosa.

Mucosa

The innermost layer of the digestive tract, the **mucosa,** is composed of mucous membrane. Specialized cells (glands) secrete mucus, digestive enzymes, and hormones. Ducts from the exocrine glands empty into the lumen of the digestive tract.

Submucosa

A thick layer of loose connective tissue, the **submucosa,** lies next to the mucosa. The submucosa contains blood vessels, nerves, glands, and lymphatic vessels.

Muscle Layer

The third layer of the digestive tract is the muscle layer. Two layers of smooth muscles are an inner circular layer and an outer longitudinal layer. Autonomic nerve fibers also lie between the two layers of muscles. The muscle layer is responsible for several types of movements in the digestive tract. Mixing movements occur in the stomach. Repeated contraction and relaxation of the stomach muscles mechanically digest the food and mix the particles with digestive juices.

A second type of muscle movement is **peristalsis** (pĕr″ĭ-stäl′sĭs), a rhythmic alternating contraction and relaxation of the muscles. Peristalsis pushes the food through the digestive tract from one segment to the next. Peristalsis moves

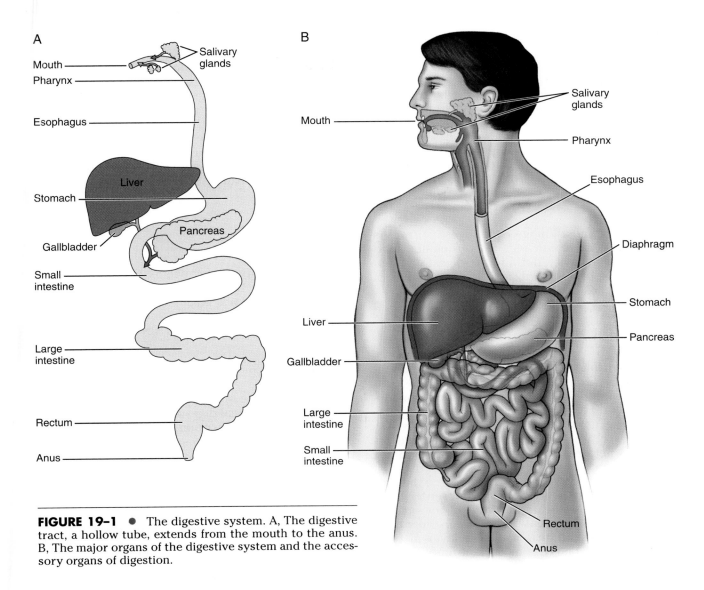

FIGURE 19–1 ● The digestive system. A, The digestive tract, a hollow tube, extends from the mouth to the anus. B, The major organs of the digestive system and the accessory organs of digestion.

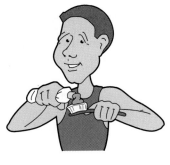

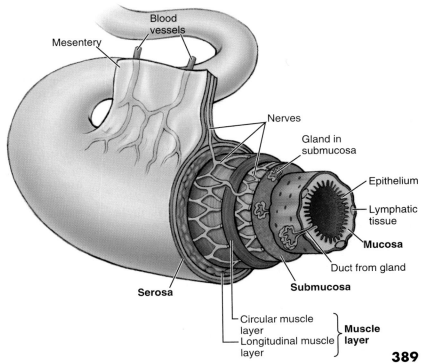

FIGURE 19–2 ● Wall of the digestive tract. The four layers are the mucosa, submucosa, muscle layer, and serosa. Note that the glands empty their secretions into the lumen of the digestive tract by way of ducts. Note also that the serosa extends as the mesentery. Peristalsis resembles the movement of toothpaste as it is squeezed through the tube.

389

food in the same way that toothpaste squirts from a tube. The toothpaste squirts in a forward direction because the bottom of the tube is squeezed. Peristaltic waves squeeze the food from behind and push it forward. Peristaltic waves are stimulated by the presence of food. Muscle activity is also responsible for other types of movement, such as swallowing **(deglutition)** and **defecation,** the elimination of waste from the digestive tract.

Serosa

The outermost lining of the digestive tract is the **serosa.** The serosa secretes serous fluid into the abdominal cavity, not into the digestive tract. This process provides lubrication, so that the abdominal organs do not rub against each other.

Peritoneal Membranes

The peritoneal membranes within the abdominal cavity are extensions of the serosa. These form large flat and folded structures that perform several important functions. They help anchor the digestive organs in place; carry blood vessels, lymph vessels, and nerves to the abdominal organs; and help restrict the spread of infection in the abdominal cavity.

The peritoneal membranes, located behind the digestive organs, are called the **mesentery** and **mesocolon.** When located in front of the organs, they are called the **greater** and **lesser omentum.** The greater omentum is a double layer of peritoneum that contains a considerable amount of fat and resembles an apron draped over the abdominal organs.

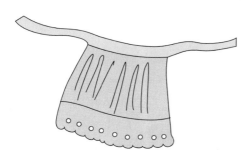

✳ **SUM IT UP!** The digestive system is made up of the digestive tract (a hollow tube from the mouth to the anus) and the accessory organs of digestion (teeth, glands, liver, gallbladder, and pancreas). The digestive system has four functions: ingestion, digestion, absorption, and elimination. Although modified for specific functions in different organs, the wall of the digestive tract has a similar structure throughout its length. The wall of the digestive tract has four layers: mucosa, sub-

mucosa, muscle layer, and serosa. The muscle layer enables the digestive tract to mix, mash, and move food through the tract; the forward movement of food is due to peristalsis. Large, flat peritoneal membranes in the abdominal cavity serve three functions: they help anchor digestive organs in place; they carry blood vessels, lymph vessels, and nerves to the digestive organs; and they help prevent the spread of infection in the abdominal cavity.

Mouth

The digestive tract begins with the mouth, also known as the **oral cavity** or **buccal cavity.** The mouth contains structures that assist in the digestive process. These include the teeth, tongue, salivary glands, and several other structures.

Teeth

The purpose of the teeth is to chew food and to begin mechanical digestion. During the process of chewing, or **mastication,** the teeth break down large pieces of food into smaller fragments. Once moistened by the secretions in the mouth, these smaller fragments are easily swallowed.

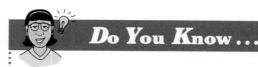

What are wisdom teeth?

Several back molars appear later in life (at 17–25 years of age when you have become wiser) and are therefore called **wisdom teeth.** In many individuals, the wisdom teeth remain imbedded in the jawbone and are said to be impacted. Because impacted teeth serve no function and are often a source of infection, they are frequently removed.

During a lifetime, a person will have two sets of teeth, deciduous and permanent. The **deciduous teeth** are also called baby teeth or milk teeth. There are 20 deciduous teeth. They begin to appear at the age of 6 months and are generally in place by the age of 2½ years. Between the ages of 6 and 12 years, these teeth are pushed out and replaced by the permanent teeth. There are 32 permanent teeth (Fig. 19–3A).

Note the positions and names of the teeth: the incisors, cuspids (canines), premolars (bicuspids), and molars (including wisdom teeth). The shape and location of each tooth determines its function. For instance, the sharp chisel-shaped in-

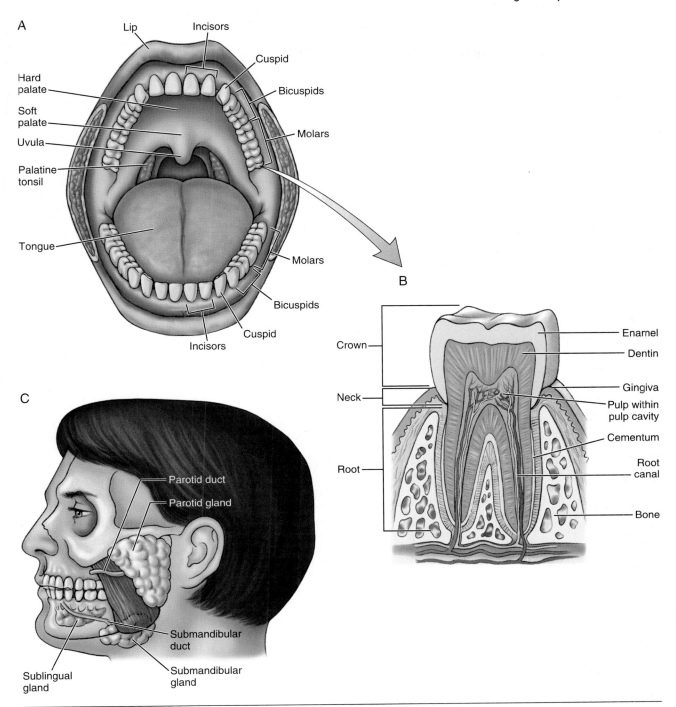

A

Lip
Incisors
Cuspid
Bicuspids
Molars
Hard palate
Soft palate
Uvula
Palatine tonsil
Tongue
Molars
Bicuspids
Cuspid
Incisors

B

Crown
Neck
Root
Enamel
Dentin
Gingiva
Pulp within pulp cavity
Cementum
Root canal
Bone

C

Parotid duct
Parotid gland
Submandibular duct
Sublingual gland
Submandibular gland

FIGURE 19–3 ● Oral cavity. A, Structures in the mouth. B, Longitudinal section of a tooth. C, Location of the salivary glands.

cisors and cone-shaped cuspids are front teeth used to tear or grasp food. The larger, flatter molar, a back tooth, is more suited for grinding food.

A tooth has three parts: the crown, the neck, and the root (Fig. 19–3B). The **crown** of the tooth is above the level of the gum, or **gingiva,** and is covered with a hard brittle **enamel.** The **neck** connects the crown with the root of the tooth. The **root** is that part of the tooth embedded in the jaw-

bone. The outer surface of the root is anchored to the periodontal membrane by **cementum.** This holds the tooth in place. The bulk of the tooth consists of a bone-like material called **dentin.** Nerves, blood vessels, and connective tissue, called **pulp,** penetrate the dentin through the pulp cavity and supply the tooth with sensation and nutrients. As the pulp cavity extends into the root, it is called the **root canal.**

Tongue

The **tongue** is a muscular organ that occupies the floor of the mouth and serves two major roles in the digestive process. First, it facilitates chewing and swallowing by continuously moving and repositioning the food in the mouth. As swallowing begins, the tongue pushes the food, which it has molded into a ball-like mass called a **bolus,** toward the pharynx. Second, the tongue allows us to taste food (taste is described in Chapter 11).

If you look under your tongue in the mirror, you will notice two structures. One is a small piece of mucous membrane, called the **frenulum,** which anchors the tongue to the floor of the mouth and is the reason people cannot swallow their tongues. The second structure is an extensive capillary network that provides the sublingual (under the tongue) area with a rich supply of blood. Because the blood supply is so good, medications are absorbed rapidly when administered sublingually.

Salivary Glands

Three pairs of salivary glands secrete their contents into the mouth: the parotid glands, the submandibular glands, and the sublingual glands (Fig. 19–3C). The **parotid glands** are the largest of the three glands and lie below and anterior to the ears. These are the glands infected by the mumps virus; the result is a chipmunk appearance. The **submandibular glands** are located on the floor of the mouth. The **sublingual glands** are located under the tongue and are the smallest of the salivary glands. Secretions from the salivary glands reach the mouth by way of tiny ducts. The salivary glands secrete **saliva,** a watery fluid that contains mucus and one digestive enzyme called salivary amylase, or ptyalin. Approximately 1 liter of saliva is secreted per day. The most important function of saliva is to soften and moisten food and thereby facilitate swallowing.

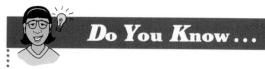

What is mumps?

Mumps is a viral infection of the parotid glands and is characterized by pain and swelling. If mumps occurs in postadolescent males, the infection may spread to the testes and cause sterility.

Occasionally, one of the salivary ducts becomes obstructed by a stone. The condition is called sialolithiasis (*lithos* means stone) and is characterized by intense pain on eating when the salivary juices start to flow.

Other Structures Within the Mouth

The **hard** and **soft palates** form the roof of the mouth (see Fig. 19–3A). The anterior hard palate separates the oral cavity from the nasal passages, while the posterior soft palate separates the oral cavity from the nasopharynx. The soft palate extends toward the back of the oral cavity as the **uvula,** the V-shaped piece of soft tissue that hangs down from the upper back region of the mouth. The uvula plays a role in swallowing. The **palatine tonsils** are masses of lymphoid tissue located along the sides of the posterior oral cavity. These play a role in the body's defense against infection (see Chapter 16).

Pharynx

The tongue pushes the food from the mouth into the **pharynx,** commonly called the throat. The pharynx is involved in swallowing, a reflex action called deglutition. The three parts of the pharynx are the nasopharynx, the oropharynx, and the laryngopharynx (Fig. 19–4). Only the oropharynx and laryngopharynx are part of the digestive system.

The pharynx communicates with nasal, respiratory, and digestive passages. The act of swallowing normally directs food from the throat into the **esophagus,** a long tube that empties into the stomach. Food does not normally enter the nasal or respiratory passages because swallowing temporarily closes off the openings to both. For instance, during swallowing, the soft palate moves toward the opening to the nasopharynx. Similarly, the laryngeal opening is closed when the trachea moves upward and allows a flap of tissue, called the **epiglottis,** to cover the entrance to the respiratory passages. You can see this process as the up and down movement of the Adam's apple, part of the larynx.

Failure of the epiglottis to cover the opening allows food to enter the respiratory passages, causing aspiration, which makes a person choke. An episode of coughing usually follows to clear the airway and reestablish the flow of air.

Esophagus

The esophagus is a tube that carries food from the pharynx to the stomach (see Fig. 19–1). The esophagus, approximately 10 inches (25 cm) in length, descends through the chest cavity and penetrates the diaphragm. The act of swallowing pushes the bolus of food into the esophagus. The presence of food within the esophagus stimulates peristaltic activity and causes the food to move into the stomach. Glands within the mucosa of the

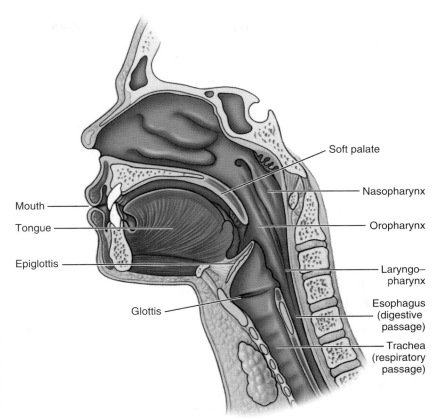

FIGURE 19-4 ● Eating and swallowing: from mouth to pharynx to esophagus. Food follows a path as it is ingested and swallowed. Note the epiglottis, the structure that prevents the entrance of food into the respiratory passages.

esophagus secrete mucus, which lubricates the bolus of food and facilitates its passage along the esophagus.

Do You Know...

What is a tracheoesophageal fistula (TE fistula)?

Occasionally, an infant is born with an opening between the trachea (respiratory passage) and the esophagus (digestive passage). This condition is a **tracheoesophageal fistula (TE fistula).** When the infant eats, food enters the trachea and lungs through this fistula. When this condition occurs, the infant experiences severe respiratory distress with violent coughing and deep cyanosis. Surgical correction is necessary for survival.

The two esophageal sphincters are the **pharyngoesophageal sphincter** located at the top of the esophagus, and the **gastroesophageal,** or **lower esophageal, sphincter (LES),** a thickening at the base of the esophagus (Fig. 19–5). Swallowing pushes food past the pharyngoesophageal sphincter into the esophagus. Relaxation of the LES keeps the base of the esophagus open, thereby allowing the passage of food into the stomach. When contracted, however, the LES closes the base of the esophagus, thereby preventing reflux, or regurgitation, of stomach contents back into the esophagus.

Occasionally, reflux of stomach contents into the esophagus causes heartburn, or pyrosis. The burning sensation is a result of the high acidity of stomach contents. (Note that the word *pyrosis* is related to the word *pyromaniac,* a person who loves to set fires, and to the word *pyretic,* referring to fever.)

Stomach

The stomach is a pouch-like organ that lies in the upper left part of the abdominal cavity, just under the diaphragm (see Fig. 19–1).

The stomach performs five important digestive functions:

- Digestion of food.
- Secretion of gastric (stomach) juice, which includes digestive enzymes and hydrochloric acid as its most important substances.
- Secretion of gastric hormones and intrinsic factor.
- Regulation of the rate at which the partially digested food is delivered to the small intestine.
- Absorption of small quantities of water and dissolved substances. The stomach is not well

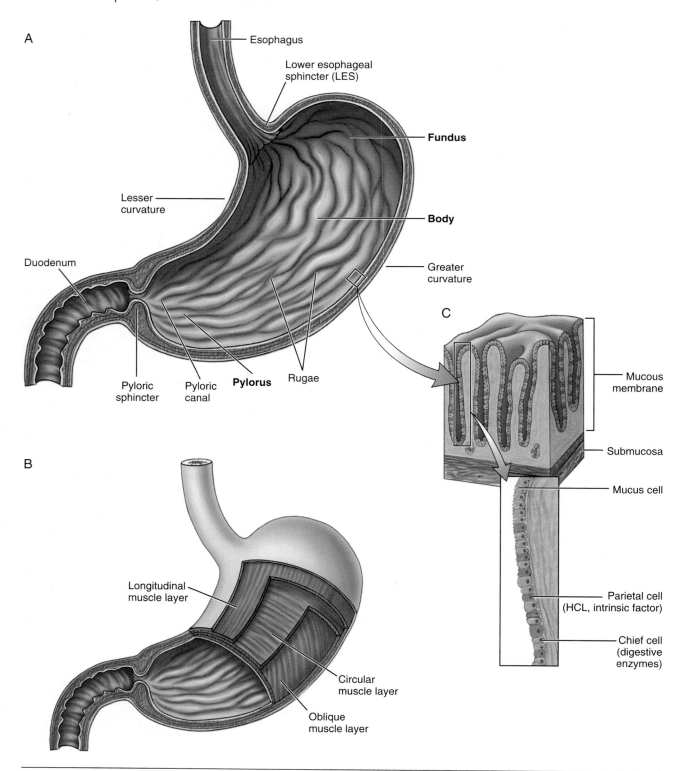

FIGURE 19–5 ● Stomach. A, Regions of the stomach: fundus, body, and pylorus. B, Three muscle layers of the stomach. C, Mucosa of the stomach showing the mucus, parietal, and chief cells.

suited for an absorptive role. It can, however, absorb alcohol efficiently. Therefore, the consumption of alcoholic beverages on an empty stomach can quickly increase blood levels of alcohol.

Regions of the Stomach

The major regions of the stomach include the **fundus,** the **body,** and the **pylorus** (see Fig. 19–5A). The pylorus continues as the **pyloric canal.** A **pyloric sphincter** is located at the end of the pyloric canal and helps regulate the rate at which gastric contents are delivered to the small intestine. Other landmarks of the stomach include the **greater curvature** and the **lesser curvature.**

How big can your stomach get? The empty stomach lies in thick accordion-like folds called **rugae.** The rugae allow the stomach to expand. For instance, when the stomach is empty, it is shaped like a sausage. Following a large meal, however, the stomach may be expanded to approximately 1 liter. Think of your turkey dinner sitting in your very expanded stomach. Sadly, the stomach can stretch in response to continued overeating.

Muscles of the Stomach

The stomach has three layers of muscles that lie in three directions: longitudinal, oblique, and circular (see Fig. 19–5B). (Note that the stomach has a thicker muscle layer than the rest of the digestive tract.) This arrangement allows the stomach to churn and mix the food with gastric juice to create a thick paste-like mixture called **chyme** (kīm). The muscles of the stomach also generate peristaltic waves that push the food toward the pylorus.

Nerves of the Stomach

The stomach is innervated (receives nerve impulses) primarily by the vagus nerve, part of the parasympathetic nervous system. Stimulation of the vagus nerve increases the motility of the stomach and the secretory rate of the gastric glands. Several drugs and surgical procedures interfere with vagal activity and therefore alter gastric secretion and motility.

Glands of the Stomach

The mucous membrane of the stomach contains gastric glands (see Fig. 19–5C). These glands contain three types of secretory cells: the **mucus cells,** which secrete mucus, the **chief cells,** which secrete digestive enzymes, and the **parietal cells,** which secrete hydrochloric acid (HCl) and intrinsic factor. The secretions of the gastric glands are called **gastric juice.** In addition to the gastric juice,

other cells secrete a thicker mucus that adheres closely to the stomach lining. This secretion forms a protective coating for the stomach lining and prevents the acidic gastric juices from digesting the stomach itself.

When the Stomach Is Not Working Right

The stomach gets a lot of attention clinically. Let us look at some conditions involving the stomach (Fig. 19–6):

- Ulcer (A). A healthy digestive tract has an intact inner mucous membrane. The stomach lining may erode, or break down, thereby creating a lesion called an **ulcer.** Some ulcers are thought to be caused by the *Helicobacter pylori (H. pylori)* microorganism and are painful and prone to bleeding. An antiulcer drug plan for this type of ulcer includes an antibiotic in addition to antacids.
- Hiatal hernia (B). The stomach is located in the abdominal cavity. The esophagus enters the abdominal cavity through an opening in the diaphragm. If that opening is weakened or enlarged, the stomach may protrude, or herniate, from the abdominal cavity into the thoracic cavity. This condition is called a **hiatal hernia.**
- Nasogastric tube (C). Food particles normally move from the stomach into the duodenum. Many conditions require that a **nasogastric tube** be inserted through the nasal passages into the stomach. Most often the nasogastric tube is used to empty the stomach to prevent vomiting. When a person cannot eat normally, a tube may be surgically inserted through the abdominal wall into the stomach. Food is introduced directly into the stomach through this tube. This procedure is called a **gastrostomy.**
- Gastric resection (D). An important function of the stomach is to regulate the rate at which chyme is delivered to the duodenum. A person with cancer of the stomach may require a surgical procedure that removes the stomach or part of it. The procedure is called a **gastric resection,** or **gastrectomy.** A serious consequence of gastric resection is the inability to regulate the rate at which chyme is delivered to the duodenum. Because food (chyme) is literally dumped into the duodenum (because there is no stomach), a condition called dumping syndrome develops. Dumping syndrome is characterized by severe nausea, perspiration, dizziness, and tachycardia.
- Pyloric stenosis (E). The digestive tract is a hollow tube that must remain open. Occasionally during infancy, the pylorus is too narrow and impedes the movement of food out of the stomach. This condition is **pyloric stenosis** (*stenosis* means narrowing). Pyloric stenosis is characterized by projectile vomiting immediately after

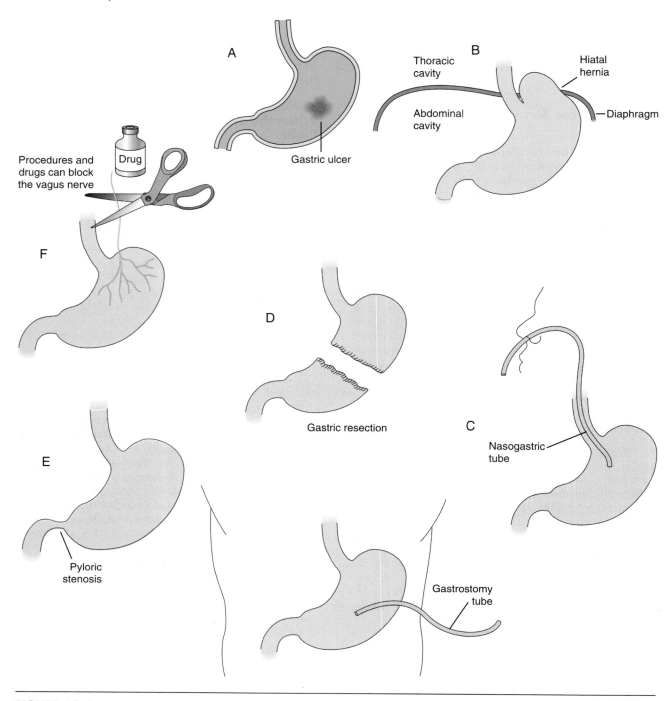

FIGURE 19–6 ● Stomach. Some clinical conditions that involve the stomach.

feeding. Fortunately, a simple surgical procedure corrects the defect.
- Gastric hyperactivity (F). Stimulation of the vagus nerve increases gastric secretion and motility. Certain drugs block the effects of the vagus nerve, thereby decreasing gastric secretion and motility. For instance, **gastric hyperactivity,** which occurs with some ulcers and a nervous stomach, may be treated with a drug that slows gastric motility and secretions. Atropine-like drugs are drugs that have a vagolytic effect and are used widely in the treatment of gastric hypermotility disorders. In addition, the vagus nerve may be severed by a surgical procedure called a **vagotomy.**

✳ **SUM IT UP!** The mouth begins the process of mechanical and chemical digestion.

The chewing action of the teeth physically breaks large pieces of food into smaller particles (mechanical digestion). The salivary juice (water, ions, mucus, and amylase) begins chemical digestion. The bolus of food is swallowed and moves from the mouth, through the pharynx and esophagus, and into the stomach. The stomach continues the digestive process. The muscle activity of the stomach mashes the food and mixes it with gastric juice into a paste-like consistency called chyme. Gastric juice (including enzymes, hydrochloric acid, and mucus) helps to chemically break down food. Although the stomach plays an important role in mechanical digestion, it plays a relatively minor role in chemical digestion. Most chemical digestion occurs in the small intestine, the structure into which the stomach pushes the chyme.

Small Intestine

An acidic chyme is expelled from the stomach into the small intestine (see Fig. 19–1). The small intestine is called small because its diameter is smaller than the diameter of the large intestine. The word *small* does not refer to its length; the small intestine is considerably longer than the large intestine. The small intestine is about 20 feet (6 m) long and the large intestine is about 5 feet (1.5 m) long. The small intestine is located in the central and lower abdominal cavity and is held in place by the **mesentery,** an extension of the peritoneum. The small intestine is concerned primarily with chemical digestion and the absorption of food. The small intestine consists of three parts: the duodenum, the jejunum, and the ileum.

Structures of the Small Intestine: What It Is

The **duodenum** (dōō″ə-dē′nəm) is the first segment of the small intestine. The word duodenum literally means twelve (*duo* means two, *denum* means ten). In this instance, the reference is to the width of 12 fingers. Thus, the length of the duodenum is 12 fingerbreadths or approximately 10 inches (25 cm).

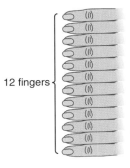

12 fingers

Why is the duodenum considered the meeting point for digestion? In addition to receiving chyme from the stomach, the duodenum also receives secretions from several accessory organs of digestion such as the liver, gallbladder, and pancreas (see Fig. 19–1). These secretions, in addition to those from the mouth, stomach, and duodenum are responsible for the digestion of all food. *Most digestion and absorption occur in the duodenum.*

The **jejunum** (jə-jōō′nəm) is the second segment of the small intestine. It is approximately 8 feet (2.4 m) in length. Some digestion and absorption of food occurs in the first part of the jejunum.

The **ileum** (ĭl′ē-əm) is the third segment of the small intestine and is approximately 12 feet (3.6 m) in length. It extends from the jejunum to the ileocecal valve. The **ileocecal valve** prevents the reflux of contents from the cecum (part of the large intestine) back into the ileum. The lining of the ileum contains numerous patches of lymphoid tissue called **Peyer's patches.** Peyer's patches diminish the bacterial content in the digestive system.

Functions of the Small Intestine: What It Does

What is so special about the wall of the small intestine? The wall of the small intestine forms circular folds with finger-like projections called **villi** (vĭl′ī) (singular, villus) (Fig. 19–7). The epithelial cells of each villus form extensions called **microvilli.** The large number of villi and microvilli increases the surface area of the small intestine. Why is a large surface area so important? The increased surface area increases the number of digested food particles that the small intestine can absorb. The villi and microvilli also give the inside of the small intestine a velvety appearance. Because of their appearance, these cells are called the **brush border.**

What is a villus? Each villus consists of a layer of epithelial tissue that surrounds a network of blood capillaries and a lymphatic capillary called a **lacteal** (see Fig. 19–7B). The villus absorbs the end-products of digestion into either the blood capillaries or the lacteal. The capillary blood within the villus drains into the hepatic portal vein and then into the liver. Thus, the end-products of carbohydrate and protein digestion first go to the liver for processing before being distributed throughout the body. The end-products of fat digestion enter the lacteal, forming a milky white lymph called **chyle.** The chyle empties directly into the lymphatic system. (Do not confuse the words chyle and chyme.) (The hepatic portal system is described in Chapter 15.)

In addition to forming a site for absorption, the brush border cells also secrete several digestive enzymes and two important hormones, secretin and cholecystokinin (CCK). Table 19–1 lists the major intestinal enzymes and hormones.

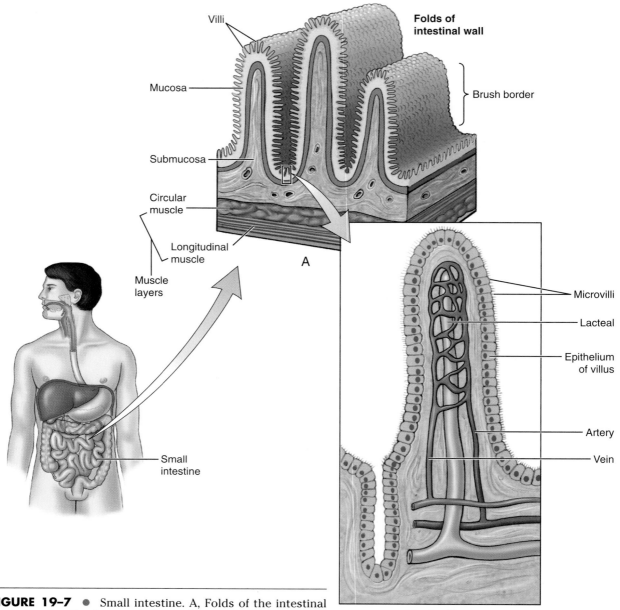

FIGURE 19-7 ● Small intestine. A, Folds of the intestinal wall showing the layers of the wall and the brush border (villi). B, Single villus showing the blood capillaries, the lacteal (lymph capillary), and the microvilli.

Large Intestine

The large intestine is approximately 5 feet (1.5 m) long and extends from the ileocecal valve to the anus (Fig. 19–8). The cecum, colon, rectum, and anal canal are parts of the large intestine.

Structure of the Large Intestine: What It Is

The first part of the large intestine is the **cecum** (sē′kəm). The cecum is located in the lower right quadrant and ascends on the right side as the **ascending colon** (kō′lən). Attached to the cecum is the **appendix** (ə-pĕn′dĭks), a worm-like structure that plays no known physiologic role.

Occasionally, the appendix becomes inflamed, causing appendicitis, and must be surgically removed through an appendectomy. Failure to remove an inflamed appendix causes it to rupture. The discharge of fecal material into the peritoneal cavity causes peritonitis, a life-threatening condition.

The ascending colon ascends on the right side and curves acutely near the liver (at the hepatic flexure). As it traverses, or crosses, the upper ab-

Table 19•1

MAJOR SECRETIONS OF THE DIGESTIVE SYSTEM

NAME	SOURCE	DIGESTIVE FUNCTION
Enzymes		
Salivary enzyme		
Amylase (ptyalin)	Salivary glands	Begins carbohydrate digestion to disaccharides
Gastric enzyme		
Pepsin	Gastric glands	Begins digestion of protein
Pancreatic enzymes		
Amylase	Pancreas	Digests polysaccharides to disaccharides
Lipase	Pancreas	Digests fats to fatty acids and glycerol
Proteases	Pancreas	Digest proteins to peptides
Trypsin		
Chymotrypsin		
Intestinal enzymes		
Peptidases	Intestine	Digest peptides to amino acids
Disaccharidases	Intestine	Digest disaccharides to monosaccharides
Sucrase		
Lactase		
Maltase		
Lipase	Intestine	Digests fats to fatty acids and glycerol
Enterokinase	Intestine	Activates trypsinogen to trypsin
Digestive Aids		
Hydrochloric acid	Stomach	Helps to unravel proteins; kills microorganisms that are ingested in food
Intrinsic factor	Stomach	Assists in the absorption of vitamin B_{12}
Bile	Liver	Emulsifies fats; aids in the absorption of fatty acids and the fat-soluble vitamins (A, D, E, K)
Mucus	Entire digestive tract	Softens food; lubricates food and eases its passage through the digestive tract
Hormones		
Gastrin	Stomach	Stimulates gastric glands to secrete gastric juice
Cholecystokinin (CCK)	Duodenum	Stimulates the gallbladder to contract and release bile; stimulates release of pancreatic digestive enzymes
Secretin	Duodenum	Stimulates the pancreas to secrete sodium bicarbonate

domen, it is known as the **transverse colon.** The colon then bends near the spleen (at the splenic flexure) to become the descending colon. The **descending colon** descends on the left side of the abdomen into an S-shaped segment called the **sigmoid colon.** Structures distal to the sigmoid colon include the rectum, anal canal, and anus. The anal canal ends at the anus, a structure composed primarily of two sphincter muscles (an involuntary internal sphincter and a voluntary external sphincter). The sphincters are closed except during the expulsion of the feces. Feces is waste composed primarily of nondigestible food residue; it forms the stool, or bowel movement (BM). Expulsion of feces is called defecation.

Functions of the Large Intestine: What It Does

The four functions of the large intestine are

• Absorption of water and certain electrolytes

• Synthesis of certain vitamins by the intestinal bacteria (especially vitamin K and certain B vitamins)
• Temporary storage site of waste (feces)
• Elimination of waste from the body (defecation)

PERISTALSIS

Intermittent and well-spaced peristaltic waves move the fecal material from the cecum into the ascending, transverse, and descending colon. As the fecal material moves through the colon, water is continuously reabsorbed from the feces, across the intestinal wall, into the capillaries. Consequently, as the feces enters the rectum, it has changed from a watery consistency to a semi-solid mass. Feces that remain in the large intestine for an extended period lose excess water, and the person experiences **constipation.** Rapid movement through the intestine allows insufficient time for water reabsorption, causing **diarrhea.**

Drugs may be administered to increase or decrease the motility of the large intestine. For in-

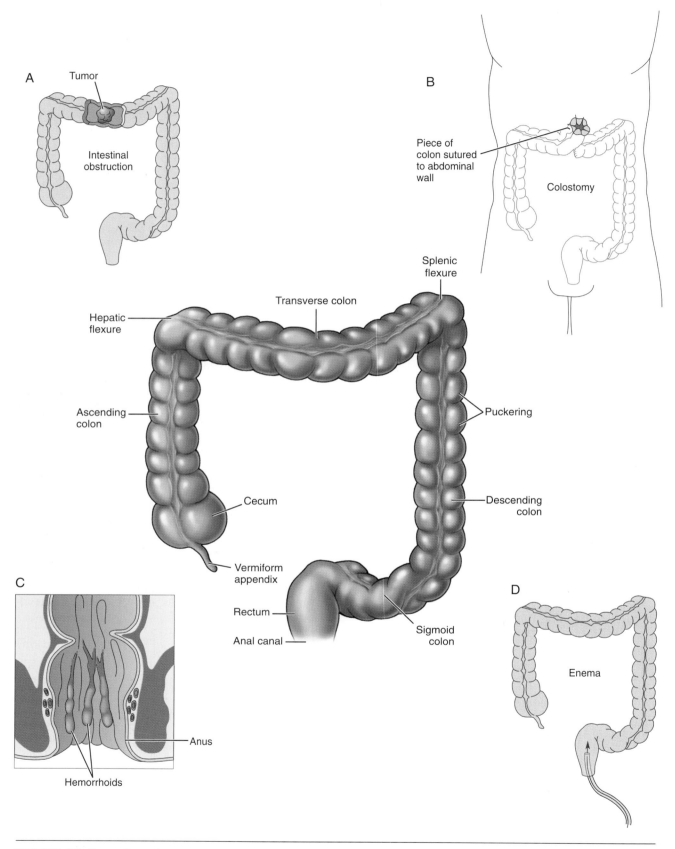

A, Tumor
Intestinal
obstruction

B, Piece of
colon sutured
to abdominal
wall
Colostomy

Splenic
flexure
Transverse colon
Hepatic
flexure
Ascending
colon
Puckering
Cecum
Descending
colon
Vermiform
appendix
Rectum
Anal canal
Sigmoid
colon

C
Anus
Hemorrhoids

D
Enema

FIGURE 19–8 ● Large intestine (center), with structures of the large intestine (periphery) and some clinical conditions that affect the large intestine. A, Intestinal obstruction by a tumor. B, Colostomy. C, Hemorrhoids. D, Placement of tube for an enema.

stance, a person with diarrhea may take a drug that slows motility. Slower motility allows for more water reabsorption and the formation of a drier stool. In contrast, a person with constipation requires an increase in motility, so as to prevent additional water reabsorption. Thus, a laxative, which increases motility, is frequently prescribed to relieve constipation.

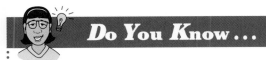

Do You Know...

What is paralytic ileus?

After surgery, intestinal peristalsis is often sluggish and may actually cease. This condition is called **paralytic ileus.** When this happens, food, gas, and liquid accumulate within the digestive tract, creating a life-threatening situation that demands immediate intervention.

BACTERIAL ACTION. What do bacteria do in the large intestine? The bacterial content within the feces is normally high. (The presence of bacteria in the intestinal tract is normal and is called the **normal flora.**) Some of these bacteria, *Escherichia coli (E. coli)* for instance, synthesize vitamins (vitamin K and certain of the B complex vitamins). Although *E. coli* is normal (and beneficial) in the intestinal tract, it can cause serious medical conditions in urine and blood. Bacteria are also responsible for the formation of malodorous molecules that provide stools with their characteristic aroma. Finally, digestion of food residue in the intestine by the bacteria generates gas, which when eliminated is called **flatus.**

When the Large Intestine Is Not Working Right

The large intestine is a common site of clinical disorders and discomfort. Let us examine some clinical conditions and procedures involving the large intestine (see Fig. 19–8).

Because the digestive tract is a hollow tube that extends from the mouth to the anus, it occasionally becomes blocked, or occluded (see Fig. 19–8A). For instance, a tumor may grow large enough to block a segment of the large intestine completely. Or the bowel may become twisted upon itself (causing a volvulus) and occlude the lumen of the bowel. Both conditions result in intestinal obstruction, whereby the movement of feces is impaired.

In the event of an intestinal obstruction, a surgical procedure may be performed to relieve the obstruction (see Fig. 19–8B). An incision into the colon and the rerouting of the colon onto the surface of the abdomen **(colostomy)** allows the feces to bypass the obstruction. Because of insufficient

water reabsorption, a colostomy performed on the ascending colon is characterized by drainage of a liquid feces. Because of adequate water reabsorption along the length of the large intestine, however, a colostomy performed on the sigmoid colon is characterized by a well-formed stool.

All organs receive a supply of oxygen-rich blood from the arteries and are drained by veins. The walls of the veins are thin and may become damaged by excessive pressure. Sometimes the veins that drain the anal region become stretched and distorted (causing varicosities). These varicosities are called **hemorrhoids** (see Fig. 19–8C).

For several reasons (eg, constipation, preparation for x-ray examination) cleansing of the rectum or colon may be necessary. This procedure is accomplished by infusing water through a tube inserted into the rectum **(enema)** (see Fig. 19–8D). The water stimulates the contraction of the muscle of the bowel, causing evacuation of its contents. Once the bowel is cleansed of fecal material, barium may be infused into the lower bowel (a procedure called a **barium enema**). The white translucent barium appears on x-ray and outlines any tumor or other abnormality.

✳ **SUM IT UP!** Chyme is discharged from the stomach into the duodenum, the first segment of the small intestine, where most digestion and absorption occur. The end-products of digestion are absorbed across the duodenal wall into the intestinal villi. The monosaccharides, primarily glucose, and the amino acids are absorbed into the capillaries of the villi. The fats and the fat-soluble vitamins are absorbed into the lacteals (lymphatic vessels). Unabsorbed material moves from the duodenum through the jejunum and the ilium, the second and third segments of the small intestine. Contents are discharged through the ileocecal valve into the large intestine. The large intestine consists (in order) of the cecum, ascending colon, transverse colon, descending colon, sigmoid colon, rectum, and anal canal. The large intestine is concerned with absorption of water and electrolytes and with defecation.

ACCESSORY DIGESTIVE ORGANS

Three important organs—the liver, the gallbladder, and the pancreas—empty their secretions into the duodenum (Fig. 19–9). These secretions are vital for the digestion of food.

Liver

The liver is a large, reddish-brown organ located in the right upper abdominal cavity (see Fig. 19–9A). The liver is the largest gland in the body and lies immediately below the diaphragm, tucked

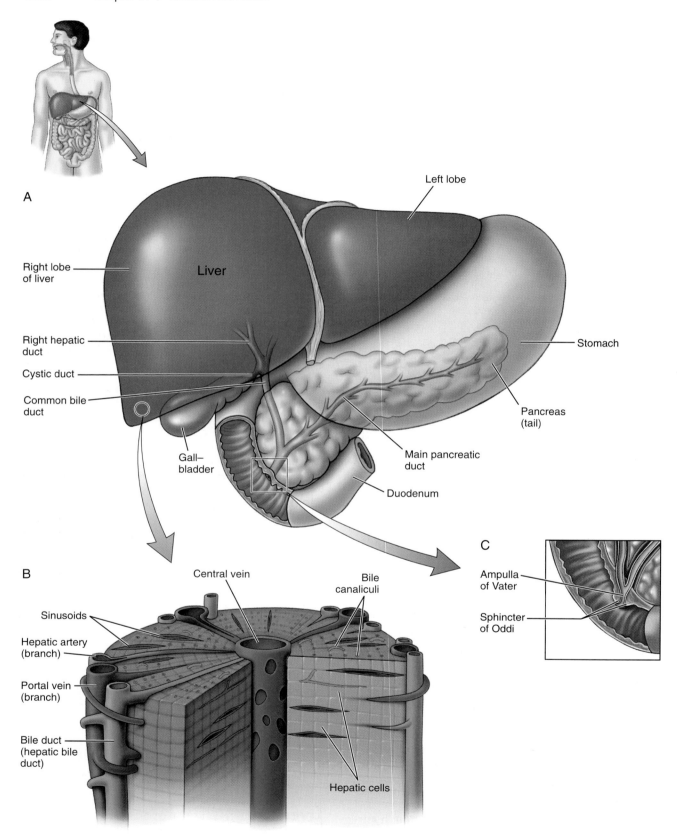

A

Left lobe

Right lobe
of liver

Liver

Right hepatic
duct

Cystic duct

Common bile
duct

Gall—
bladder

Stomach

Pancreas
(tail)

Main pancreatic
duct

Duodenum

B

Central vein

Bile
canaliculi

Sinusoids

Hepatic artery
(branch)

Portal vein
(branch)

Bile duct
(hepatic bile
duct)

Hepatic cells

C

Ampulla
of Vater

Sphincter
of Oddi

FIGURE 19–9 ● Liver, gallbladder, and pancreas. A, The relationship of the liver, gallbladder, and pancreas to the duodenum. Note the ducts that make up the biliary tree. B, Liver lobule, the functional unit of the liver. Note the blood flow into the liver (portal vein and hepatic artery), the formation of bile from the blood, and the secretion of bile into the bile ducts.

up under the right rib cage. The liver has two main lobes, a larger right lobe and a smaller left lobe separated by a ligament. This ligament secures the liver to the anterior abdominal wall and to the undersurface of the diaphragm. The liver is encapsulated by a tough fibrous membrane. The word *hepatic* refers to liver.

Functions of the Liver: What It Does

The liver is essential for life and performs many vital functions:

- Synthesis of bile salts and secretion of bile. Bile salts play an important role in fat digestion and in the absorption of fat-soluble vitamins. Bile secretion is the main digestive function of the liver.
- Synthesis of plasma proteins. The plasma proteins play an important role in maintaining blood volume and controlling blood coagulation (hemostasis).
- Storage. The liver stores many substances: glucose in the form of glycogen, the fat-soluble vitamins (A, D, E, and K), and vitamin B_{12}.
- Detoxification. The liver plays an important role in the detoxification of drugs and other harmful substances. The liver changes these toxic substances into substances that can be more easily eliminated from the body, generally through the kidneys.
- Excretion. The liver excretes many substances, including bilirubin, cholesterol, and drugs.
- Metabolism of carbohydrates. The liver plays an important role in the regulation of blood glucose levels. If blood glucose levels rise above normal, the liver can take the glucose out of the blood, convert it to glycogen, and then store it for future use. If the blood glucose levels decline below normal, the liver can make glucose from glycogen and from nonglucose substances and release it into the blood.
- Metabolism of protein. The liver can make a variety of different amino acids. Also, because only the liver contains the urea cycle enzymes, nitrogen (from ammonia) is converted to urea in the liver for eventual excretion by the kidneys. Free ammonia is extremely toxic to humans.
- Metabolism of fats. The liver can break down fatty acids, synthesize cholesterol and phospholipids, and convert excess dietary protein and carbohydrates to fat.
- Phagocytosis. The Kupffer cells can phagocytose bacteria and other substances.

Blood Supply to the Liver

THE HEPATIC PORTAL SYSTEM. The liver has a unique arrangement of blood vessels called the **hepatic portal system** (see Fig. 15–7). The liver receives a lot of blood, approximately 1.5 liters per minute, from two sources: the portal vein (which provides most of the blood) and the hepatic artery. The portal vein drains blood from all of the organs of digestion while the hepatic artery delivers oxygen-rich blood from the aorta to the liver. Thus, the portal vein brings blood rich in digestive end-products to the liver. Blood leaves the liver through the hepatic veins and empties into the vena cava, where it is returned to the heart for recirculation. (The hepatic portal system is described in detail in Chapter 15. Review the hepatic portal system so that you can understand absorption.)

LIVER LOBULES. The liver contains thousands of liver lobules, the functional unit of the liver (see Fig. 19–9B). The liver lobules consist of a special arrangement of blood vessels and hepatic cells. Note the central vein and the rows of hepatic cells that radiate away from the central vein. These cells are bathed by blood that enters the lobule from both the hepatic artery and the portal vein.

Blood from these two blood vessels mixes in the liver in spaces called **sinusoids.** The hepatic cells extract water and dissolved substances from the sinusoidal blood. Hepatic cells then secrete a green-yellow substance called bile into tiny canals called **canaliculi.** These tiny bile canals merge with canals from other lobules to form larger hepatic bile ducts. Bile exits from the liver through the **hepatic bile ducts.**

Bile

Bile (bīl) is a green-yellow secretion produced by the liver and stored in the gallbladder. Bile is composed primarily of water, electrolytes, cholesterol, bile pigments, and bile salts. The bile pigments **bilirubin** and **biliverdin** are formed from the hemoglobin of worn-out red blood cells. The **bile salts** are the most abundant constituents of the bile. Only the bile salts have a digestive function; they play an important role in fat digestion and in the absorption of fat-soluble vitamins. Bile salts also give the stool a brownish color. Between 800 and 1000 mL of bile is secreted in a 24-hour period.

Biliary Tree

The ducts that connect the liver, gallbladder, and duodenum are called the **biliary tree** (bĭl′ē-ĕr′ē trē) (see Fig. 19–9A). This network of ducts include the **hepatic bile ducts,** the **cystic duct,** and the **common bile duct.** The hepatic ducts receive bile from the canaliculi within the liver lobules. The hepatic ducts merge with the cystic duct to form the common bile duct, which carries bile from both the hepatic ducts (liver) and the cystic duct (gallbladder) to the duodenum.

The base of the common bile duct swells to form the **hepatopancreatic ampulla (ampulla of Vater)** (see Fig. 19–9C). The main pancreatic duct joins the common bile duct at this point. The **hepatopancreatic sphincter (sphincter of Oddi)** encircles the base of the ampulla, where it enters the duodenum. This sphincter is sensitive to nervous, hormonal, and pharmacologic control. The sphincter helps regulate the delivery of bile to the duodenum.

Gallbladder

The **gallbladder** is a pear-shaped sac attached to the underside of the liver (see Fig. 19–9A). The cystic duct connects the gallbladder with the common bile duct. Bile, produced in the liver, flows through the hepatic ducts and into the cystic duct and gallbladder. The gallbladder concentrates and stores approximately 2.5 pints (1.2 liters) of bile per day.

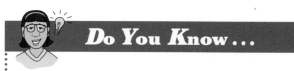

Do You Know...

Why do persons with gallbladder disease develop gray or clay-colored stools?

With gallbladder disease, a gallstone sometimes becomes lodged in the common bile duct and blocks the flow of bile into the duodenum. Because bile salts normally color the stool brown, the absence of bile salts gives rise to colorless, gray, or clay-colored stools.

The fat in the duodenum stimulates the release of a hormone, **cholecystokinin (CCK).** This hormone enters the bloodstream and circulates back to the gallbladder, where it causes the smooth muscle of the gallbladder to contract. When the gallbladder contracts, the bile is ejected into the cystic duct and then into the common bile duct and duodenum.

Pancreas

The **pancreas** is an accessory organ of digestion located just below the stomach (see Fig. 19–9A). Most of the pancreas lies posterior to the parietal peritoneum; its location is thus described as retroperitoneal. The head of the pancreas rests in the curve of the duodenum while the tail lies near the spleen in the upper left quadrant of the abdominal cavity. The main pancreatic duct, which travels the length of the pancreas, joins with the common bile duct at the ampulla of Vater. The large pancreatic duct carries digestive enzymes from the pancreas to the duodenum, the meeting point for digestion.

The pancreas secretes both endocrine and exocrine substances. The exocrine secretions include the digestive enzymes and an alkaline secretion. The pancreatic enzymes are the most important of all the digestive enzymes. They are secreted by the pancreatic **acinar cells** in their inactive forms and travel through the large main pancreatic duct to the duodenum.

In addition to the digestive enzymes, the pancreas also secretes an alkaline juice rich in **bicarbonate.** The bicarbonate neutralizes the highly acidic chyme coming from the stomach into the duodenum. This neutralization is important because the digestive enzymes in the duodenum work best in an alkaline environment.

The secretion of the digestive enzymes and bicarbonate is under nervous and hormonal control. The presence of food in the stomach and duodenum is the stimulus for the nervous and hormonal responses. For instance, the presence of chyme in the duodenum stimulates the release of the hormone CCK from the duodenal walls. CCK travels by way of the blood to the pancreas, stimulating the release of pancreatic digestive enzymes. Note that CCK affects both the gallbladder and the pancreas (see Table 19–1). The acid in the duodenum stimulates the release of a second hormone, **secretin,** from the duodenal walls. Secretin travels by way of the blood to the pancreas, stimulating release of the bicarbonate-rich juice.

When Accessory Digestive Organs Are Not Working Right

Disorders involving the liver, gallbladder, biliary tree, and pancreas are common. Let us examine several clinical conditions (Fig. 19–10):

- **Jaundice** (jŏn′dĭs). The liver secretes bile, which is stored in the gallbladder for future use in the duodenum. When needed, bile travels through bile ducts (hepatic ducts, cystic duct, and common bile duct) to the duodenum. If the bile ducts become blocked, as with stones in the common bile duct, the flow of bile stops. The bile backs up into the liver. The bile pigments, especially bilirubin, accumulate in the blood and are eventually carried throughout the body, where they are deposited in the skin. The skin turns yellow, and the person is described as being jaundiced. Because the jaundice is due to an obstruction, it is called **obstructive jaundice** (in contrast to hemolytic jaundice, which is caused by the rapid breakdown of red blood cells; see Chapter 13). Jaundice can also occur in response to liver disease (hepatitis). A person with hepatitis may become jaundiced because the swollen, or inflamed, hepatic tissue causes the tiny bile canaliculi to swell and close. This closure diminishes the excretion of bile from the liver and causes backup of bilirubin in the blood.

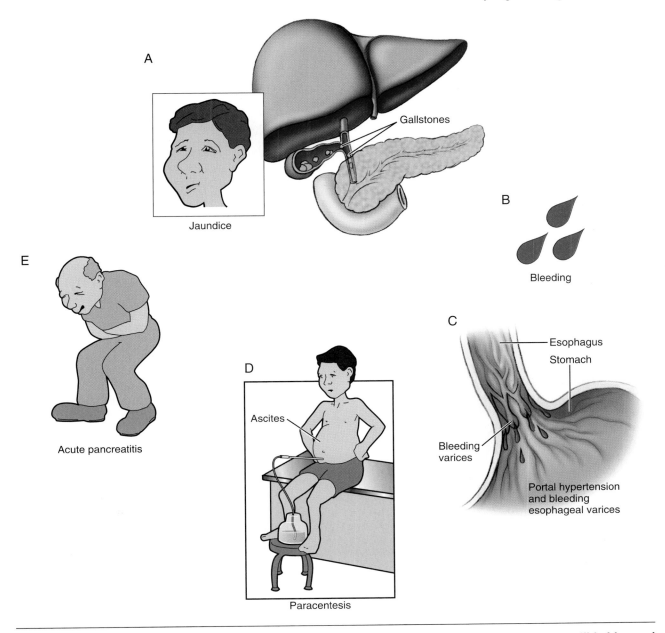

FIGURE 19-10 • Liver, gallbladder, and pancreas. Some clinical conditions that affect the liver, gallbladder, and pancreas.

• Bleeding. The liver synthesizes clotting factors such as prothrombin (Fig. 19–10B). What can make a person hypoprothrombinemic (a diminished amount of prothrombin in the blood)? A gallstone lodged in the common bile duct is a common cause of hypoprothrombinemia. Because bile is necessary for the absorption of fat-soluble vitamins, bile duct obstruction causes diminished absorption of vitamin K. Vitamin K is necessary for the hepatic synthesis of a number of clotting factors, including prothrombin. Thus, common bile duct obstruction diminishes the hepatic synthesis of prothrombin, causing hypoprothrombinemia and bleeding.

• Portal hypertension and hemorrhage. The liver receives a large flow of blood from the portal vein. Normally, the blood passes through the liver quickly and easily with very little resistance to the flow of blood. In alcoholic cirrhosis, however, the liver is so damaged that the flow of portal blood through the liver is greatly impeded. The blood backs up in the portal vein, elevating the pressure in the vein and causing portal hypertension. The increased portal pressure is felt not only by the portal vein but also by all the veins that drain into the portal vein, including the small veins at the base of the esophagus (Fig. 19–10C). If the portal pressure becomes too great, the thin, weaker varicosed veins (esophageal varices) at the base of the esophagus may rupture, causing a massive hemorrhage.

- Portal hypertension and ascites. In alcoholic cirrhosis, the increased portal vein pressure may also cause fluid to seep across the blood vessel into the peritoneal cavity. This process, called **portal hypertension,** causes accumulation of a large amount of clear yellow plasma-like fluid. The collection of fluid in the peritoneal cavity is **ascites** (Fig. 19–10D). The ascites may be so severe that the accumulated fluid pushes up on the diaphragm and interferes with breathing. The fluid may be siphoned off by the insertion of a tube into the peritoneal cavity. This procedure is called **paracentesis.**

- Pancreatitis. The pancreas secretes potent digestive enzymes in their inactive forms. These inactive enzymes normally flow through the main pancreatic duct into the duodenum, where the enzymes are activated. Sometimes, the enzymes become activated within the pancreas and digest the pancreatic tissue, causing severe inflammation in the form of acute pancreatitis. This condition is very painful and dangerous. It demands immediate intervention (Fig. 19–10E).

✳ **SUM IT UP!** The accessory digestive organs include the liver, gallbladder, and pancreas. These organs secrete substances that are eventually emptied into the duodenum, the meeting place for digestion. The liver performs many functions. It initially receives all of the blood that has passed through the digestive organs. The special arrangement of blood vessels that carries the digestive end-products to the liver is called the hepatic portal system. The liver's primary digestive role is the secretion of bile, which it synthesizes. Bile is then carried to the gallbladder, where it is concentrated and stored. The hormone cholecystokinin (CCK) is secreted by the walls of the duodenum when fat is present. Blood then carries the CCK to the gallbladder, which contracts and forces bile into the cystic duct, common bile duct, and finally the duodenum. The pancreas secretes the most potent digestive enzymes. The pancreatic enzymes empty into the base of the common bile duct and then into the duodenum. In addition to the digestive enzymes, bicarbonate-rich pancreatic secretions assist the digestive process.

DIGESTION AND ABSORPTION

The primary purpose of the digestive system is to break down large pieces of food into small particles suitable for absorption. Food is digested mechanically and chemically. Mechanical digestion is the physical breakdown of food into small fragments. It is achieved by the chewing activity of the mouth and by the mixing and churning activities of the muscles of the digestive organs.

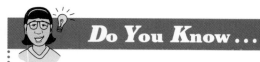
Do You Know . . .

Why should an infant not be given honey to eat?

Botulism spores are sometimes found in honey. The digestive tract of an infant allows the spores to grow. As the spores grow, they release a deadly toxin that is absorbed from the infant's stomach into the blood, causing botulism. The infant becomes lethargic, has no muscle control, and experiences breathing difficulty. With increasing age, the digestive tract destroys the botulism spores from honey. Therefore older children and adults can eat honey without developing botulism.

Chemical digestion is the chemical change occurring primarily in response to the digestive enzymes. Whereas mechanical digestion refers to a breakdown in the size of the piece of food, chemical digestion refers to a change in the chemical composition of the food molecule.

Food is made of carbohydrates, proteins, and fats. Digestive enzymes and several digestive aids (mucus, hydrochloric acid, and bile) play key roles in chemical digestion. Specific enzymes digest each type of food (see Table 19–1). (Before studying this section, review the structures of carbohydrates, protein, and fat in Chapter 4.)

Carbohydrates and Carbohydrate-Splitting Enzymes

Carbohydrates are organic compounds composed of carbon, hydrogen, and oxygen; they are classified according to size (see Fig. 4–2). **Monosaccharides** are single (mono) sugars (saccharide). The three monosaccharides are glucose, fructose, and galactose. Glucose is the most important of the three monosaccharides. **Disaccharides** are double (di) sugars. The three disaccharides are sucrose (table sugar), lactose, and maltose. **Polysaccharides** are many (poly) glucose molecules linked together. The shorter monosaccharides and disaccharides are called **sugars.** The longer-chain polysaccharides are **starches.**

A polysaccharide is digested in two stages (Fig. 19–11A). First, enzymes, called **amylases** (ăm′ə-lās″əz), break the polysaccharide into disaccharides. The two amylases are **salivary amylase (ptyalin)** and **pancreatic amylase.** Second, disaccharidases break disaccharides into monosaccharides. The three disaccharidases are sucrase, lactase, and maltase. (The ending *ase* indicates an enzyme.) The cells of the intestinal villi (brush border cells) secrete disaccharidases. Disaccharides therefore split into monosaccharides in the

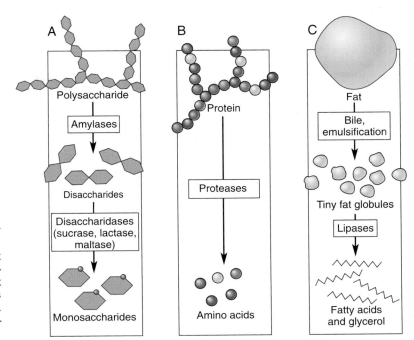

FIGURE 19–11 ● Chemical digestion. A, Amylases and disaccharidases break carbohydrates down into monosaccharides. B, Proteases and peptidases break proteins down into amino acids. C, Lipases break fats down to fatty acids and glycerol. The large fat globule must first be emulsified by bile.

duodenum at the surface of the villus. They are immediately absorbed across the villus into the blood capillaries.

Certain carbohydrates (eg, cellulose) cannot be digested and therefore remain within the lumen of the digestive system. While providing no direct nourishment, dietary cellulose is beneficial in that it provides fiber and bulk to the stool.

Many persons suffer from a deficiency of the enzyme lactase. They are unable to digest the sugar found in milk (lactose) and are said to be lactose intolerant. This enzyme deficiency prevents lactose-intolerant people from ingesting milk and many milk products.

Protein and Protein-Splitting Enzymes

The building blocks of proteins are **amino acids.** Several amino acids linked together form a **peptide.** Many amino acids linked together form a polypeptide. **Proteins** are very long polypeptide chains; some proteins contain more than one polypeptide chain (Fig. 19–11B). To be absorbed across the wall of the digestive tract, these chains must be uncoiled and broken down into small peptides and amino acids.

Enzymes called **proteases** (prō′tē-ās-əz), or **proteolytic enzymes,** digest proteins. Proteases are secreted by three organs: the stomach secretes pepsin; the intestinal brush border cells secrete enterokinase; and the pancreas secretes trypsin and chymotrypsin. The pancreatic proteases are the most potent proteases. Proteins are broken down into amino acids and are absorbed across the intestinal villi into the blood capillaries.

Gastric hydrochloric acid (HCl) also aids protein digestion. First, the HCl unravels the strands of protein, making the protein fragments more sensitive to the proteases. Second, the HCl activates a gastric proteolytic enzyme, pepsinogen (pepsinogen then creates pepsin). Pepsin then facilitates breaking protein into small chain peptides.

Fats and Fat-Splitting Enzymes

Fats are long-chain molecules composed of carbon, hydrogen, and oxygen. Enzymes called **lipases** (lī′pās-əz) digest fats. The most important is pancreatic lipase (Fig. 19–11C). The end-products of fat digestion are fatty acids and glycerol; fat is absorbed into the lacteals of the villus.

Bile aids fat digestion. Why is bile necessary (see Fig. 19–11C)? Fats, unlike carbohydrates or proteins, are not soluble in water; they tend to clump together into large fat globules when added to water. If, for instance, oil and water are placed in a test tube, the oil and water separate; the oil rises to the surface while the water settles at the bottom. Oil and water simply do not mix. The same separation occurs in the digestive tract. Dietary fat tends to form large fat globules. The lipase cannot readily digest the fat. It can attack only the outside surface of the fat globule.

Bile solves the large fat globule problem. Bile can split the large fat globule into thousands of tiny fat globules. This process is **emulsification.** Because of emulsification, the lipases can work on the surfaces of all the tiny fat globules, thereby digesting more fat. Bile performs two other important roles. Bile salts prevent the fatty acids (end-products of fat digestion) from reforming large fat globules in the intestine before they can be absorbed across the intestinal villi. Bile salts also help the absorption of the fat-soluble vitamins A, D, E, and K.

PUTTING THE DIGESTIVE SYSTEM TOGETHER

How is a turkey dinner digested and absorbed (Fig. 19–12)? ① In the mouth, food is chewed into tiny pieces and salivary amylase (ptyalin) begins the digestion of the carbohydrate into disaccharides. ② The smaller pieces of food are transported through the esophagus to the stomach, where they are mixed, mashed, and churned into chyme. In the stomach, pepsin begins the digestion of protein. The amount of digestion and absorption occurring in the mouth and stomach is minimal.

③ The partially digested food (chyme) squirts into the duodenum, where it mixes with bile and the pancreatic and intestinal enzymes. Pancreatic amylase and the disaccharidases digest the polysaccharides (carbohydrates) to monosaccha-

rides. The pancreatic proteases (trypsin and chymotrypsin) and the intestinal proteases digest the proteins to amino acids. A pendulum-like (swaying back and forth) peristaltic motion washes the digested food across each villus, thereby enhancing absorption. ④ The simple sugars and the amino acids are absorbed into the blood capillaries of the villi. These capillaries eventually empty into the portal vein, a vessel that carries blood to the liver.

Bile emulsifies the fats, and the pancreatic and intestinal lipases digest them. The end-products of fat digestion are fatty acids and glycerol. The fat products are absorbed into the lacteals of the villus. Most of the digestion and absorption occurs in the duodenum, the meeting point for digestion. ⑤ The unabsorbed food material moves along the jejunum and ileum, and into the large intestine. ⑥ A large volume of water and certain electrolytes are absorbed along this route, and a semisolid stool is formed. Several times per day, the solid material in the large intestine moves toward the rectum. ⑦ The presence of the fecal material in the rectum gives rise to an urge to defecate, or expel the contents. The major enzymes and digestive aids and their locations and functions are listed in Table 19–1.

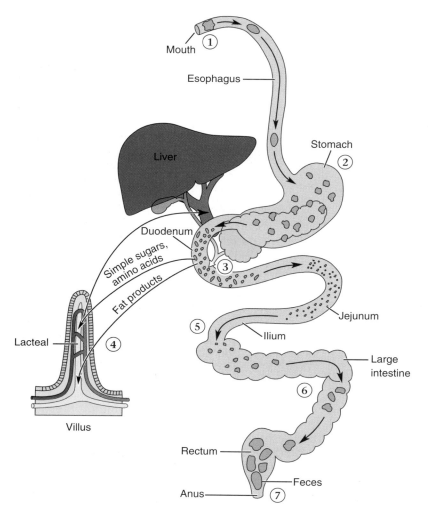

FIGURE 19–12 ● The digestion and absorption of the turkey meal. The food is mechanically and chemically digested and pushed through the various parts of the digestive tract. The nutrients are absorbed from the upper small intestine, primarily the duodenum, into the blood capillaries and lacteals. Blood that is rich in digestive end-products flows to the liver. Water is absorbed along the entire intestinal tract. The undigestible or nonabsorbable food particles accumulate in the rectum as waste.

✳ **SUM IT UP!** The primary purpose of the digestive system is to break down food (physically and chemically) into substances that can be absorbed. Most of the digestion takes place in the duodenum. The most important digestive enzymes are secreted by the pancreas. Carbohydrates are broken down into monosaccharides (primarily glucose) by the enzymatic actions of amylases and disaccharidases. The proteins are broken down to amino acids by proteases, especially trypsin and chymotrypsin. Fats are broken down to fatty acids and glycerol. Fats must first be emulsified by bile and then chemically split by lipase. Digestive end-products are absorbed across the intestinal villi into the blood (which absorbs glucose and amino acids) and lymph (which absorbs fats).

NUTRITION: CONCEPTS TO KNOW

Nutrition is the science that studies the relationship of food to the functioning of the body. Food consists of **nutrients,** substances the body uses to promote normal growth, maintenance, and repair. The five categories of nutrients are carbohydrates, proteins, lipids, vitamins, and minerals.

Carbohydrates

Dietary carbohydrates are classified as **simple sugars** and **complex carbohydrates.** A simple sugar is composed of monosaccharides and disaccharides. Glucose, the simplest carbohydrate, is the major fuel used to make adenosine triphosphate (ATP) in most body cells. Most of the carbohydrates come from plants. The sugars are derived primarily from fruit, sugar cane, and milk.

The complex carbohydrates are larger sugar molecules (polysaccharides) and consist primarily of starch and fiber. The starch is found in cereal grains (wheat, oats, corn, barley), legumes (peas, beans), and root vegetables (potatoes, rice, pasta). Fiber, or cellulose, is found primarily in vegetables. Cellulose cannot be digested by humans but is beneficial nutritionally because it provides bulk in the stool and aids in defecation.

Proteins

Dietary proteins supply the body with amino acids. Because the body cannot store amino acids, a daily supply is necessary. Amino acids are classified as essential and nonessential. An **essential amino acid** cannot be synthesized by the body and must therefore be consumed in the diet. A **nonessential amino acid** can be synthesized by the body. It is not essential that these amino acids be consumed in the diet. Of the 20 amino acids, nine are essential.

Proteins are classified as complete or incomplete. A **complete protein** contains all essential amino acids. Complete proteins are found in animal sources. Meat, eggs, and dairy products are complete proteins. **Incomplete proteins** do not contain all of the essential amino acids. Vegetable proteins are incomplete proteins. These include nuts, grains, and legumes. Vegetable proteins, if eaten in combinations, can supply a complete complement of amino acids. For instance, a favorite Mexican dish containing rice and beans is complete in that it supplies all the essential amino acids, even though both the rice and the beans are incomplete proteins.

Fats (Lipids)

Most dietary lipids are **triglycerides,** molecules that contain glycerol and fatty acids. Fatty acids are classified as saturated or unsaturated. A **saturated fatty acid** (eg, butter, lard) is solid at room temperature. Also included in this group are artificially hardened, or hydrogenated, fats such as vegetable shortening and margarine. Saturated fats come primarily from animal sources. An **unsaturated fat** is liquid at room temperature. Unsaturated fats are generally called oils.

The body can synthesize all fatty acids, with one exception, linoleic acid. Linoleic acid is a necessary component of cell membranes. Because the body cannot synthesize it, linoleic acid is an **essential fatty acid** and so must be included in the diet.

The American Heart Association recommends that no more than 30% of the daily caloric intake be fat and further that no more than 10% of the fat be saturated. The average American diet is currently 40% fat, 20% of which is unsaturated. Because the ingestion of fat, particularly saturated fat, has been linked to a number of health problems, health care providers now encourage Americans to cut fat intake.

Foods high in fat come from both animal and plant sources. Animal sources, however, tend to contain more saturated fat. They include meat (beef, lamb, pork), eggs, butter, and whole-milk products such as cheese. Plant sources include coconut oil and palm oil. Hydrogenated vegetable oils in shortening and margarine are also high in saturated fat. In addition to the fat content, these foods also tend to be high in cholesterol.

Vitamins

Vitamins (vī′tə-mĭnz) are small organic molecules that help regulate cell metabolism (Table 19–2). Vitamins are parts of enzymes or other organic substances essential for normal cell func-

Table 19•2 — SELECTED VITAMINS

VITAMIN	FUNCTION	DEFICIENCY
Fat-Soluble		
Vitamin A	Necessary for skin, mucous membranes, and night vision	Night blindness; dry scaly skin, disorders of mucous membranes
Vitamin D (calciferol)	Necessary for the absorption of calcium and phosphorus	Rickets in children; osteomalacia in adults
Vitamin E	Necessary for health of cell membrane	None defined
Vitamin K	Needed for the synthesis of prothrombin and other clotting factors	Bleeding
Water-Soluble		
Thiamine (Vitamin B_1)	Helps release energy from carbohydrates and amino acids; needed for growth	Beriberi; alcohol-induced Wernicke's syndrome
Riboflavin (Vitamin B_2)	Essential for growth	Skin and tongue disorders; dermatitis
Niacin (Vitamin B_3)	Helps release energy from nutrients	Pellagra with dermatitis, diarrhea, mental disorders
Pyridoxine (Vitamin B_6)	Participates in the metabolism of amino acids and proteins	Nervous system and skin disorders
Vitamin B_{12}	Helps form red blood cells and DNA	Anemias, particularly pernicious anemia
Folic acid	Participates in the formation of hemoglobin and DNA	Anemia; neural tube defects in embryo
Ascorbic acid (Vitamin C)	Necessary for synthesis of collagen; helps maintain capillaries; aids in the absorption of iron	Scurvy; poor bone and wound healing

tion. Vitamins are classified as fat soluble or water soluble. The **fat-soluble vitamins** include vitamins A, D, E, and K. Bile is necessary for the absorption of the fat-soluble vitamins. Because the body stores fat-soluble vitamins, excess intake **(hypervitaminosis)** may result in symptoms of toxicity.

The **water-soluble vitamins** include vitamins B and C. These vitamins do not depend on bile for absorption and, for the most part, are not stored by the body. Excess water-soluble vitamins are generally excreted in the urine. Excretion, however, does not rule out the possibility of toxicity in response to megadosing with water-soluble vitamins.

You can best appreciate the roles vitamins play by observing the effects of specific vitamin deficiencies. For instance, vitamin A is necessary for healthy skin. It also plays a vital role in night vision. Vitamin A deficiency is characterized by various skin lesions and by **night blindness,** the inability to see in a darkened room. Vitamin D is necessary for the absorption of calcium and the development and formation of strong bones. Vitamin D deficiency causes **rickets** in children, a condition in which the bones are soft and often bow in response to weight bearing. Because the skin can synthesize vitamin D in response to exposure to ultraviolet radiation, the incidence of rickets is higher in places with little sunlight.

Vitamin K plays a crucial role in hemostasis. It is necessary for the synthesis of prothrombin and

several other clotting factors. A deficiency of vitamin K causes a **hypoprothrombinemia** (diminished amount of prothrombin in the blood) and a tendency to bleed excessively.

Finally, vitamin C is necessary for the integrity of the skin and mucous membranes. A deficiency of vitamin C causes **scurvy,** a condition involving skin lesions and inability of the tissues to heal. Historically, scurvy was common on ships that were at sea for months at a time. Having determined that limes prevented scurvy, the British sailors traveled around the world sipping lime juice. In response to this habit, they were dubbed limeys. Other vitamin deficiencies are included on Table 19–2.

Minerals

Minerals (mĭn′ər-əlz) are inorganic substances necessary for normal body function (Table 19–3). Minerals have numerous functions, ranging from regulation of plasma volume (eg, sodium, chloride) to bone growth (eg, calcium) to oxygen transport (eg, iron) to the regulation of metabolic rate (eg, iodine).

Mineral deficiencies can cause serious health problems. For instance, because iodine is necessary for the synthesis of the thyroid hormone thyroxine, iodine deficiency can cause an enlarged thyroid gland (goiter) and hypothyroidism. Because iron is necessary for the synthesis of hemo-

Table 19•3	**SELECTED MINERALS**	
MINERAL	**FUNCTION**	**DEFICIENCIES**
Potassium (K)	Nerve and muscle activity	Nerve and muscle disorders
Sodium (Na)	Water balance; nerve impulse conduction	Weakness, cramps, diarrhea, dehydration, confusion
Calcium (Ca)	Component of bones and teeth, nerve conduction, muscle contraction, blood clotting	Rickets, tetany, bone softening
Phosphorus (P)	Component of bones and teeth, component of adenosine triphosphate, nucleic acids, and cell membranes	Bone demineralization
Iron (Fe)	Component of hemoglobin (red blood cells)	Anemia, dry skin
Iodine (I)	Necessary for synthesis of thyroid hormones	Hypothyroidism; iodine-deficient goiter
Magnesium (Mg)	Component of some enzymes; important in carbohydrate metabolism	Muscle spasm, dysrhythmias, vasodilation
Fluorine (F)	Component of bones and teeth	Dental caries
Trace minerals Zinc (Zn) Copper (Cu) Manganese (Mn) Selenium (Se)	Small amounts required for certain specific functions	

globin, iron deficiency can cause anemia. This anemic state is characterized by fatigue and, depending on its severity, a diminished ability to transport oxygen around the body.

Health and a Balanced Diet

A balanced diet contains all the essential nutrients and includes a variety of foods. The proportion of each type of food is illustrated in the food pyramid (Fig. 19–13). Note especially the liberal use of breads and cereals and the limited use of fats and sweets.

Many health problems are thought to originate in poor dietary choices. For instance, a diet high in cholesterol or fats, or both, has been implicated in coronary artery disease. Fatty plaques develop along the inside walls of the blood vessels and eventually occlude the flow of blood to the heart, causing a heart attack. Fatty plaques can also form within the blood vessels that supply the brain, causing a stroke and paralysis. A diet high in saturated fat has also been implicated in diabetes and cancer.

While overeating, especially eating fats, has been linked with health problems, a number of health problems are related to a deficiency of certain foods. For instance, infants who are fed fat-poor diets (eg, skim milk) may become deficient in fats essential for the development of nervous tissue. Fat deficiency may cause nerve damage and developmental delay. In poverty-stricken areas of the world, protein-deficiency diseases are common. Kwashiorkor, for example, is a protein-deficient state in which protein intake is inadequate to synthesize plasma proteins, muscle protein, and the protein necessary for healthy skin. The condition is characterized by edema formation, particularly ascites, muscle wasting, and dermatitis. The ascites appears as the distended abdomen of a starving child.

For the most part, malnutrition means starvation or a profound weight loss due to a caloric deficiency. Although malnutrition certainly takes this form in countries with limited food supplies, in the United States malnutrition appears most often in the overfed. The American diet and sedentary lifestyle have contributed to obesity, a national health problem. The magnitude of the problem is evident in the numbers of weight-reduction diets. The problem is so common that we now have a routine phrase, *couch potato,* to describe a sedentary person, one who may well be obese.

Body Energy

Need for Energy

Energy is essential for two reasons: it provides the body the power to do its work, and it maintains body temperature. For instance, the contraction of skeletal muscle for movement requires energy, as does the secretion of enzymes for digestion. During metabolism, a portion of the energy is transferred to ATP, but most is discharged as heat. Energy is therefore the source of heat for body temperature.

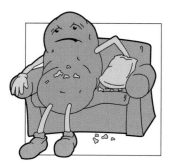

FIGURE 19–13 ● Food pyramid with the proportion and types of food that constitute a healthy diet.

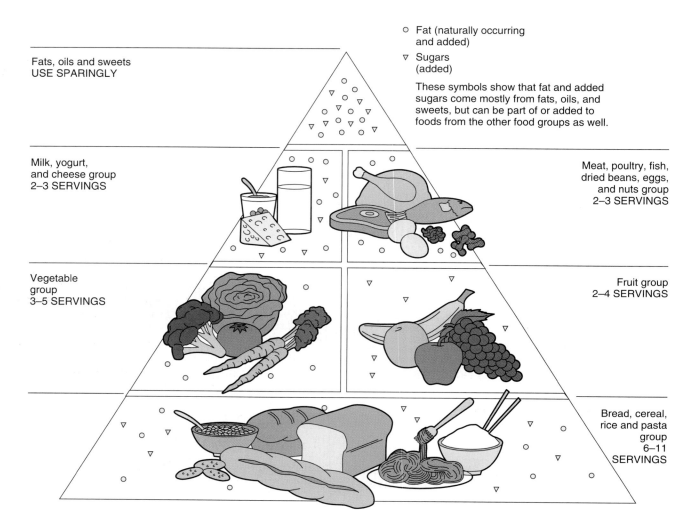

○ Fat (naturally occurring and added)

▽ Sugars (added)

These symbols show that fat and added sugars come mostly from fats, oils, and sweets, but can be part of or added to foods from the other food groups as well.

Fats, oils and sweets
USE SPARINGLY

Milk, yogurt, and cheese group
2–3 SERVINGS

Meat, poultry, fish, dried beans, eggs, and nuts group
2–3 SERVINGS

Vegetable group
3–5 SERVINGS

Fruit group
2–4 SERVINGS

Bread, cereal, rice and pasta group
6–11 SERVINGS

Measurement of Energy

Energy is measured in units called kilocalories (kcal), meaning the "large calorie." (A capital C means a "large calorie.") One **Calorie** is the amount of energy required to raise the temperature of 1 kg of water 1 degree Celsius. The energy yield of the three food groups, carbohydrates, proteins, and fats is expressed in calories:

carbohydrate yields 4 Cal/gram
protein yields 4 Cal/gram
fat yields 9 Cal/gram

Note that the metabolism of 1 gram of fat yields twice as many Calories as the metabolism of 1 gram of carbohydrate or protein.

Energy Balance

Energy balance occurs when the input of energy equals the output of energy, or in other words, when food intake equals energy expenditure. Energy balance is not always achieved. If, for instance, food intake exceeds energy expenditure, the excess energy is converted to and stored as fat, causing weight gain. Conversely, if food intake is less than the energy expended, weight loss occurs. Weight management programs, therefore, encourage both dietary restriction and exercise regimens.

Energy Expenditure

Energy expenditure differs depending on whether the body is in a resting or a nonresting state. The amount of energy the body requires per unit time to perform essential activities at rest is the **basal metabolic rate** (bā′səl mĕt″ə-bŏl′ĭk rāt) **(BMR).** These activities include breathing, kidney function, cardiac muscle contraction—whatever minimal functions the body must perform to remain alive.

Several factors affect BMR (Fig. 19–14). These include gender, age, body surface area, emotional state, overall health status, and several hormones, the most important being thyroxine (T$_4$). Men have a higher BMR than do women. An adolescent has a higher BMR than an elderly person. A tiny bird has a higher BMR than an elephant. A person livid with rage has a higher metabolism than a peaceful person. A patient with an infection has a higher BMR than the infection-free person. The thyroid hormone thyroxine exerts the most profound effect on BMR. The hyperthyroid patient has a higher BMR than a euthyroid (normal thyroid) person. The metabolism of a hyperthyroid patient can be so high that the patient can consume in excess of 6000 Cal/day and still lose weight. In contrast, the hypothyroid patient has a lower-than-normal BMR and frequently consults a physician because of loss of energy and weight gain.

The body needs a certain amount of energy to maintain minimal function but requires additional energy when the person engages in activity above and beyond the resting state. For instance, after ingestion of a meal, the body needs additional energy to digest and absorb the food. More importantly, the exercising skeletal muscles greatly increase metabolic rate. In general, the more active the person is, the higher the metabolic rate and the greater the expenditure of energy.

✳ **SUM IT UP!** The body uses food for energy, repair, and maintenance. A balanced diet contains specific amounts and types of nutrients: carbohydrates, proteins, fats, vitamins, and minerals. A food pyramid illustrates the proportion of food types. Failure to ingest certain nutrients causes malnutrition, deficiency states, and illness.

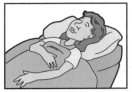
Basal metabolic rate (BMR)

Factors Affecting Metabolic Rate

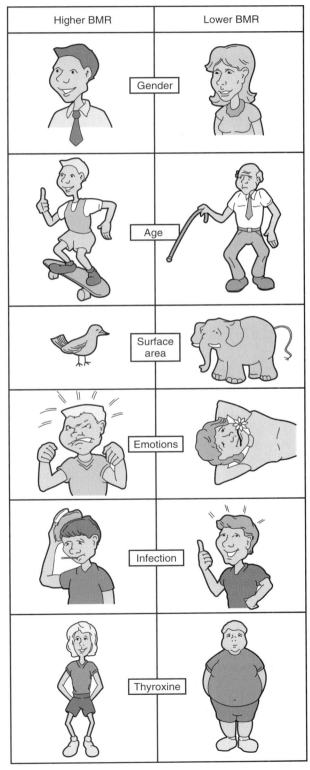

FIGURE 19–14 ● Metabolic rate. Basal metabolic rate (BMR) is the resting rate. Factors that affect BMR are gender, age, body surface area, emotional state, effects of disease (infection), and influence of thyroid hormone.

As You Age

1. The muscular wall of the digestive tract loses tone, causing constipation due to a slowing of peristalsis.

2. Secretion of saliva and digestive enzymes decreases, thereby decreasing digestion. The decrease in secretions also impairs the absorption of vitamins (vitamin B_{12}) and minerals (iron and calcium).

3. The sensations of taste and smell diminish with age. Consequently, food tastes different, and appetite may be affected.

4. The loss of teeth and an inability to chew food effectively makes eating difficult. The loss of teeth may also affect the choice of food, causing the elderly person to select a less nutritious diet, such as tea and toast.

5. Peristalsis in the esophagus is no longer triggered with each swallow, and the lower esophageal sphincter relaxes more slowly. These changes hamper swallowing and cause an early feeling of fullness.

6. A weakened gag reflex increases the risk of aspiration.

7. The liver shrinks and receives a smaller supply of blood. The rate of drug detoxification by the liver declines, thereby prolonging the effects of drugs and predisposing the person to a drug overdose. (Remember: The liver is the chief organ of drug inactivation.)

Disorders of the Digestive System

Anorexia	Loss of appetite due to many causes, ranging from simple emotional upset to serious diseases and adverse drug reactions. Anorexia nervosa is a severe psychologic disorder characterized by a fear of becoming obese. A significant loss of weight is achieved through starvation and a binge-purge routine called bulimia, another eating disorder.
Cirrhosis	A chronic disease of the liver in which the liver cells are replaced by scar tissue. Cirrhosis is often caused by chronic alcoholism or hepatitis. Cirrhosis leads to progressive loss of liver function, a life-threatening increase in portal pressure, ascites, esophageal varices, and massive hemorrhage.
Diverticulitis	An inflammation of the pouches (diverticula) in the lining of the intestinal wall.
Hepatitis	An inflammation of the liver commonly caused by a virus. There are many types of hepatitis, designated types A, B, C, D, and E. All cause hepatic cell damage; some increase the risk of cirrhosis and cancer of the liver. All forms of hepatitis are serious.
Inflammation of the Lining of the Gastrointestinal (GI) Tract	Inflamed lining of the GI tract has many causes. Gastritis, an inflammation of the stomach lining, is commonly caused by an infection (food poisoning), ingestion of ulcer-causing drugs (such as steroids, aspirin, nonsteroidal anti-inflammatory drugs [NSAIDs]), and smoking of tobacco. Enteritis is an inflammation of the intestinal lining commonly caused by infection. Gastroenteritis refers to an inflammation of the stomach and intestinal lining.
Inflammatory Bowel Disease	An umbrella term that includes ulcerative colitis and Crohn's disease. Both conditions are characterized by severe cramping, diarrhea, bleeding, and fever.
Intestinal Obstruction	Blockage of the intestinal contents. The blockage can occur at any location and can be caused by a number of abnormalities. Causes of obstruction include tumors, twisting of the intestines (volvulus), paralytic ileus (peristalsis stops), herniation (and trapping) of the bowel, and gangrene.
Pancreatitis	An inflammation of the pancreas. Pancreatitis causes severe pain and signs and symptoms that may end in death.

Summary Outline

I. Functions of the Digestive System
A. Ingestion (Eating)
B. Digestion
1. Mechanical digestion is the breakdown of large food particles into smaller pieces by physical means (chewing, mixing, mashing, and squishing).
2. Chemical digestion is the chemical alteration of food (by enzymes and hydrochloric acid).
3. Most digestion takes place in the small intestine.

C. Absorption
1. Absorption is the movement of digested food particles across the lining of the digestive tract into the blood.
2. Most absorption takes place in the duodenum.

D. Elimination

II. The Wall of the Digestive Tract and Membranes
A. Four Layers of the Digestive Tract
1. The mucosa is the innermost lining.
2. The submucosa contains glands, blood vessels, nerves, and lymphatic vessels.
3. The muscle layer is composed of two layers of smooth muscle, an inner circular layer and an outer longitudinal layer. The muscle layer is responsible for mixing/mashing movements and for peristalsis, a movement that moves the food in a forward direction.
4. The serosa is the outermost layer.

B. Peritoneal Membranes
1. The peritoneal membranes are extensions of the serosa.
2. The mesentery and the mesocolon are peritoneal membranes.
3. The greater and lesser omentum are peritoneal membranes located in front of the digestive organs.

III. Structures of the Digestive System
A. Mouth
1. The mouth is also called the oral cavity or the buccal cavity.
2. The mouth contains several accessory organs, such as the teeth, salivary glands, and tongue.

B. Teeth and Tongue
1. The teeth function in mechanical digestion (chewing).
2. The two sets of teeth are deciduous and permanent.
3. The three parts of a tooth are the crown, neck, and root.
4. The tongue is a muscular organ that facilitates chewing and swallowing of the bolus of food.

C. Salivary Glands
1. The three salivary glands are the parotid, submandibular, and sublingual.
2. The salivary glands secrete saliva and salivary amylase.

D. Pharynx (Throat)
1. There are three parts to the pharynx; only the oropharynx and the laryngopharynx are part of the digestive tract.
2. As food is swallowed, it moves from the pharynx to the esophagus.

E. Esophagus
1. The esophagus is a long tube that connects the pharynx to the stomach.
2. There are two sphincters: the upper (pharyngoesophageal) sphincter and the lower esophageal sphincter, or LES.

F. Stomach
1. The three parts of the stomach are the fundus, body, and pylorus.
2. The stomach functions in digestion, secretion of enzymes and hydrochloric acid (HCl), secretion of hormones and intrinsic factor, and regulation of the rate at which chyme is delivered to the small intestine.

G. Small Intestine
1. The three parts of the small intestine are the duodenum, jejunum, and ileum.
2. Most of the digestion and absorption occurs within the duodenum.
3. The inner lining of the small intestine, particularly the duodenum, looks like a velvety brush border.
4. The brush border cells are composed of villi and microvilli. Each villus has a lacteal (for fat absorption) and capillaries for the absorption of glucose and amino acids.

H. Large Intestine
1. The large intestine consists of the cecum, ascending colon, transverse colon, descending colon, sigmoid colon, rectum, and anus.
2. The large intestine functions in absorption of water and electrolytes, synthesis of vitamins, temporary storage of waste (feces), and elimination of waste from the body.

IV. Accessory Digestive Organs (Liver, Gallbladder, and Pancreas)
A. Liver
1. The liver functions in the synthesis of bile salts and bile, synthesis of plasma proteins, storage of glycogen and vitamins, detoxification of drugs and other harmful substances, excretion of cholesterol, bilirubin, and drugs, phagocytosis, and the metabolism of carbohydrates, proteins, and fats.
2. The liver receives arterial blood from the hepatic artery. It receives a large supply of venous blood from the hepatic portal system. Venous blood leaves the liver by the hepatic veins.

continued

Summary Outline *continued*

IV. Accessory Digestive Organs (Liver, Gall-bladder, and Pancreas), *continued*

  A. Liver, *continued*

    3. The liver lobule is the functional unit of the liver. The arrangement of the liver lobule allows the liver to remove selected substances from the blood.

    4. Bile is synthesized by the liver and flows through thousands of canaliculi into the hepatic ducts.

  B. Biliary Tree

    1. The biliary tree is composed of the bile ducts that connect the liver, gallbladder, and duodenum.

    2. The common bile duct empties into the duodenum.

  C. Gallbladder

    1. The gallbladder is connected to the biliary tree by the cystic duct.

    2. The gallbladder functions to store and concentrate bile.

    3. The gallbladder contracts and releases bile in response to the hormone cholecystokinin (CCK).

  D. Pancreas

    1. As an endocrine gland, the pancreas secretes two important hormones, insulin and glucagon. As an exocrine gland, the pancreas secretes the most important digestive enzymes and an important alkaline (bicarbonate-rich) secretion.

    2. The digestive enzymes are secreted by the acinar cells. The enzymes travel through pancreatic ducts and empty into the duodenum, near the base of the common bile duct.

V. Digestion and Absorption

  A. Carbohydrate Digestion

    1. To be absorbed, carbohydrates must be broken down to monosaccharides, primarily glucose.

    2. Carbohydrates are broken down by enzymes called amylases and disaccharidases.

  B. Protein Digestion

    1. To be absorbed, proteins must be broken down into amino acids.

    2. Proteins are broken down by proteolytic enzymes or proteases. Protein breakdown is aided by gastric HCl.

  C. Fat Digestion

    1. To be absorbed, fats must be broken down into fatty acids and glycerol.

    2. Fats are broken down by enzymes called lipases. Fats are first emulsified by bile before lipase can function efficiently.

VI. Nutrition and Body Energy

The body needs five categories of nutrients to function well. The food pyramid (see Fig. 19–13) defines a balanced diet.

  A. Carbohydrates

    1. Carbohydrates are either simple or complex.

    2. Glucose, the simplest carbohydrate, is the major fuel used by the body for energy.

  B. Protein

    1. The body needs essential amino acids, which it cannot synthesize, and nonessential amino acids, which it can synthesize.

    2. Dietary proteins are complete or incomplete. A complete protein is a food that contains all the essential amino acids.

  C. Fats (Lipids)

    1. Most dietary lipids are triglycerides.

    2. Fats are either saturated fats (like butter) or unsaturated fatty acids (like oils).

    3. For health reasons, the American Heart Association recommends limiting the dietary intake of fat.

  D. Vitamins

    1. Vitamins are small organic molecules that help regulate cell metabolism. Dietary vitamin deficiencies give rise to many diseases (see Table 19–2).

    2. Vitamins are either water soluble (vitamins B and C) or fat soluble (vitamins A, D, E, and K).

  E. Minerals

    1. Minerals are inorganic substances necessary for normal body function.

    2. Mineral deficiencies can cause serious health problems.

  F. Body Energy

    1. The body needs energy to do its work and maintain body temperature.

    2. Energy is measured in units called Calories. Carbohydrates and protein yield 4 Cal/gram; fats yield 9 Cal/gram.

    3. The basal metabolic rate (BMR) is the amount of energy the body requires per unit time to perform essential activities at rest.

    4. BMR is determined by many factors, including age, gender, surface area, emotional state, overall health status, and hormones (especially thyroxine).

Review Your Knowledge

1. What is the difference between digestion and absorption?

2. Describe mechanical and chemical digestion.

3. What are the four layers of the digestive tract, going from inside to outside?

4. Trace the pathway for food to travel from the mouth to the anus.

5. Name three pairs of salivary glands. What is the only enzyme found in saliva?

6. What structure closes the base of the esophagus, preventing reflux of stomach contents back into the esophagus?

7. List five functions of the stomach.

8. Describe the following clinical conditions: peptic ulcer, hiatal hernia, dumping syndrome, pyloric stenosis, and vagotomy.

9. Why is the duodenum considered the meeting point for digestion? From which organs does the duodenum receive secretions?

10. Describe the villus, the brush border, and the lacteal.

11. What are four functions of the large intestine?

12. List nine important functions of the liver.

13. Where is bile produced? Where is bile stored? What is the function of bile? If a person has gallbladder stones, the digestion of which food group will be disturbed?

14. Which secretions important to digestion are produced by the pancreas? Which food groups are digested by secretions from the pancreas?

15. Describe the following clinical conditions affecting the liver: jaundice, hepatitis, common bile duct obstruction, portal hypertension and hemorrhage, and ascites.

16. Where does the digestion of carbohydrates begin? Where are proteins digested? How are fats digested?

17. What is the difference between fat-soluble and water-soluble vitamins?

18. What are six factors that affect the basal metabolic rate?

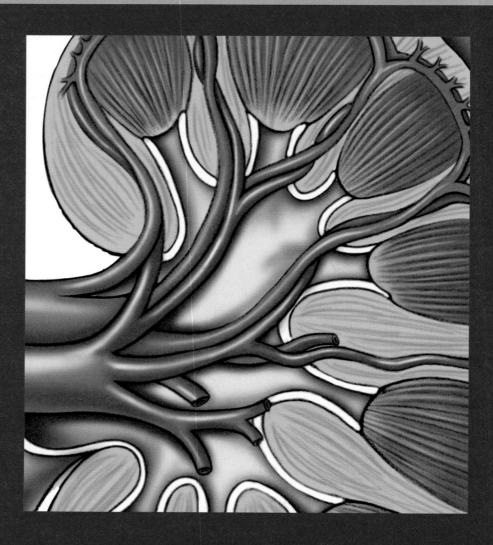

••• Key Terms

Aldosterone (ăl-dŏs′tə-rōn″)

Angiotensin (ăn″jē-ō-tĕn′sĭn)

Antidiuretic hormone (ADH)
(ăn′tē-dī″yə-rĕt′ĭk hôr′mōn)

Calyces (sing. calyx) (kā′lĭ-sēz)

Creatinine (krē-ăt′ĭ-nēn″)

Detrusor muscle (dē-trōō′zər mŭs′əl)

Dialysis (dī-ăl′ĭ-sĭs)

Diuresis (dī″yə-rē′sĭs)

Glomerular Filtration
(glō-mĕr′yə-lər fĭl-trā′shən)

Glomerulus (glō-mĕr′yə-ləs)

Kidney (kĭd′nē)

Nephron (nĕf′rŏn)

Oliguria (ŏl″ĭ-gyōō′rē-ə)

Renal tubule (rē′nəl tōō′byōol)

Renin (rĕn′ĭn)

Specific gravity (spĭ-sĭ′fĭk grăv′ĭ-tē)

Tubular reabsorption
(tōō′byə-lər rē-əb-sôrp′-shən)

Tubular secretion (tōō′byə-lər sĭ-krē′shən)

Ureter (yōō-rē′tər)

Urethra (yōō-rē′thrə)

••• Selected terms in bold type in this chapter are defined in the Glossary.

20 URINARY SYSTEM

Objectives

1. List four organs of excretion.

2. Describe the major organs of the urinary system.

3. Describe the location, structure, blood supply, and functions of the kidneys.

4. Explain the role of the nephron unit in the formation of urine.

5. Explain the three processes involved in the formation of urine: glomerular filtration, reabsorption, and secretion.

6. Describe control of water and electrolytes through aldosterone, antidiuretic hormone (ADH), atrial natriuretic factor (ANF), and parathyroid hormone.

7. Describe the role of erythropoietin.

8. List the normal constituents of urine.

9. Describe what happens when the kidneys shut down.

10. Describe the structure and function of the ureters, urinary bladder, and urethra.

Sammy with his soggy diaper is a friendly reminder of our hard-working urinary system. Indeed, Sammy may be a bundle of joy, but he is generally a wet bundle. What makes Sammy wet? Like a 'round-the-clock factory, Sammy's body burns fuel and produces waste products. To remain healthy, his body must remove waste and other unwanted materials. The kidneys play a crucial role in the excretion of waste. This process is what makes Sammy wet.

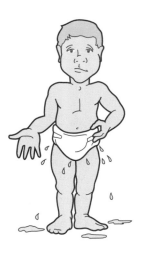

The kidneys are the most important excretory organs. They eliminate nitrogenous waste, water, electrolytes, toxins, and drugs. Other organs perform excretory functions. The sweat glands secrete small amounts of nitrogen compounds, water, and electrolytes. The lungs eliminate carbon dioxide and water, and the intestines excrete digestive wastes, bile pigments, and other minerals (Table 20–1). Note that while the skin, lungs, and intestines eliminate waste, only the kidneys can fine-tune the excretion of water and electrolytes to maintain the normal volume and composition of body fluids.

Table 20 • 1 — ORGANS OF EXCRETION

ORGAN	SUBSTANCE EXCRETED
Kidney	Water Electrolytes Nitrogenous waste Drugs
Skin (sweat glands)	Water Electrolytes Nitrogenous waste
Lungs	Carbon dioxide Water
Intestines	Digestive waste (feces) Bile pigments

The urinary system, shown in Figure 20–1, makes urine, temporarily stores it, and finally eliminates it from the body. The major organs of the urinary system are located extraperitoneally (outside of the peritoneum). They include the following:

- Two kidneys. The **kidneys** (kĭd′nēz) form urine from the blood.
- Two ureters. The **ureters** (yōō-rē′tərz) are tubes that conduct urine from the kidneys to the urinary bladder.
- One **urinary bladder.** The bladder acts as a temporary reservoir; it receives urine from the ureters and stores the urine until it can be eliminated.
- One **urethra** (yōō-rē′thrə). The urethra is a tube that conducts urine from the bladder to the outside for elimination. (Do not confuse the ureters with the urethra. They are different structures.)

KIDNEYS: REGULATION AND EXCRETION

Location of the Kidneys

The kidneys are located high on the posterior wall of the abdominal cavity, behind the parietal peritoneum (retroperitoneal space) (see Fig. 20–1A). A connective tissue membrane, called the renal fascia, holds the kidney in place. Masses of adipose tissue (fat) cushion the kidneys. The lower rib cage partially encloses and protects them.

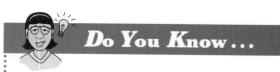

What is a floating kidney?

The kidney is normally held in its proper position by connective and adipose tissue. A very thin person has little adipose tissue. The kidney is more loosely attached to surrounding structures and may move about, or float. This in turn causes the ureters to kink and the flow of urine to be restricted.

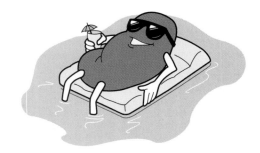

A

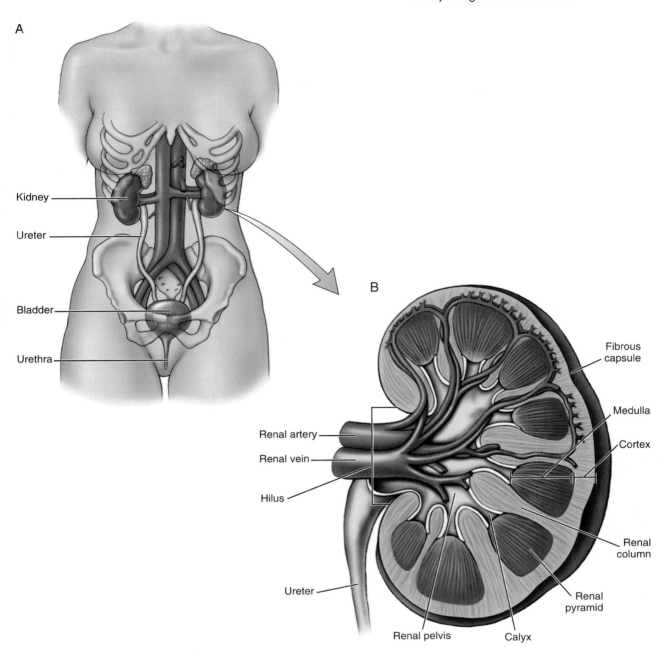

B

FIGURE 20–1 ● Organization of the urinary system. A, Organs of the urinary system. B, Internal structure of a kidney.

Structure of a Kidney

The kidney is a reddish-brown bean-like structure enclosed in a tough fibrous capsule. Each kidney is about 4 inches (10 cm) long, 2 inches (5 cm) wide, and 1 inch (2.5 cm) thick. The indentation of the bean-shaped kidney is called the **hilus.** It is the point where several structures (blood vessels, ureter, and nerves) enter or exit the kidney.

What do you see when you cut open a kidney? As Figure 20–1B shows, a kidney has three distinct regions: the renal cortex, the renal medulla, and the renal pelvis. The lighter, outer region is the **renal cortex** (*cortex* means bark). The darker triangular structure, the **renal medulla,** is located deeper within the kidney. The renal medulla forms striped, cone-shaped regions called **renal pyramids.** Each pyramid is separated by **renal columns.** These are extensions of the outer renal cortex. The lower ends of the pyramids point toward the **renal pelvis,** a basin that collects the urine made by the kidney and helps form the upper end of the ureter. The cup-like edges of the renal pelvis, closest to the pyramids, are calyces. **Calyces** (kă'lĭ-sēz) (singular, calyx) collect the urine formed in the kidney.

Blood Supply to the Kidney

Blood is brought to the kidney by the renal artery, which arises from the abdominal aorta (see Fig. 20–1B). The renal arteries deliver a large amount of blood to the kidneys. After entering the kidney, the renal artery branches into a series of smaller and smaller arteries, which make contact with the nephron units, the urine-making structures of the kidney. Blood leaves the kidneys through a series of veins that finally merge to form the renal vein. The renal vein empties into the inferior vena cava.

Functions of the Kidneys

In general, the kidneys cleanse the blood of waste products, help regulate the volume and composition of body fluids, and help regulate the pH of body fluids. Specifically, the kidneys

- Excrete nitrogenous waste such as urea, ammonia, and creatinine.
- Regulate blood volume by determining the amount of water excreted.
- Help regulate the electrolyte content of the blood.
- Play a major role in the regulation of acid-base balance (blood pH) by controlling the excretion of hydrogen ions (H^+). (See Chapter 21 for the renal regulation of acid-base balance.)
- Play a role in the regulation of blood pressure through the secretion of renin.
- Play a role in the regulation of red blood cell production through the secretion of a hormone called erythropoietin.

Urine Making: The Nephron Unit

The **nephron** (něf'rŏn) is the functional unit, or urine-making unit, of the kidney. Each kidney contains about 1 million nephron units. The number of nephron units does not increase after birth, and they cannot be replaced if damaged. The growth of the kidney is, therefore, due to enlargement of the original nephron units. Each nephron unit has two parts: a tubular component (**renal tubule** [rē'nəl too'byool]) and a vascular component (blood vessels).

RENAL TUBULES. The renal tubules consist of a number of tubular structures. The glomerular capsule, called **Bowman's capsule,** is a C-shaped structure that partially surrounds a cluster of capillaries called a **glomerulus** (glō-měr'yə-ləs). Note that Figure 20–2 shows two views of a

nephron unit: a realistic one and a schematic one. You should become familiar with both views.

Bowman's capsule extends from the glomerulus as a highly coiled tubule called the **proximal convoluted tubule.** The proximal convoluted tubule dips toward the renal pelvis to form a hairpin-like structure called the **loop of Henle.** The loop of Henle contains a descending and ascending limb. The ascending limb becomes the **distal convoluted tubule.** The distal convoluted tubules of several nephron units merge to form a **collecting duct.** The collecting ducts run through the renal medulla to the calyx of the renal pelvis. Urine is formed within these tubules.

Urine formation thus occurs in a sequence of tubular structures from Bowman's capsule to the proximal convoluted tubule to the descending limb to the ascending limb (of Henle) to the distal convoluted tubule to the collecting duct. The collecting duct empties the urine into the calyx (renal pelvis).

RENAL BLOOD VESSELS. The kidney receives blood from the renal artery. The renal artery branches into smaller blood vessels that form the afferent arteriole. The **afferent arteriole** branches into a cluster, or tuft, of capillaries called a glomerulus. The glomerulus sits in Bowman's capsule and exits from Bowman's capsule as the **efferent arteriole.** The efferent arteriole then forms a second capillary network called the **peritubular capillaries.** The peritubular capillaries converge into the venules, larger veins, and, finally, into the renal vein. The peritubular capillaries surround the renal tubule. (You need to understand the relationships of the vascular structures, the glomeruli, and the peritubular capillaries to the tubular structures. Become thoroughly familiar with Figure 20–2.)

Blood therefore flows into, through, and out of the kidney in a sequence of vascular structures: renal artery to smaller and smaller arteries to the afferent arteriole to the glomerulus to the efferent arteriole to the peritubular capillary to the renal venules to the larger veins to the renal vein to the inferior vena cava.

Urine Formation

Urine is formed in the nephron units as water and dissolved substances move between the vascular and tubular structures. Three processes are involved in the formation of urine: glomerular filtration, tubular reabsorption, and tubular secretion.

GLOMERULAR FILTRATION. Urine formation begins in the glomerulus and Bowman's capsule and then moves along the tubules. **Glomerular filtration** (glō-měr'yə-lər fĭl-trā'shən) causes water and dissolved substances to move from the glomerulus into Bowman's capsule. Understanding filtration means answering two questions: why does

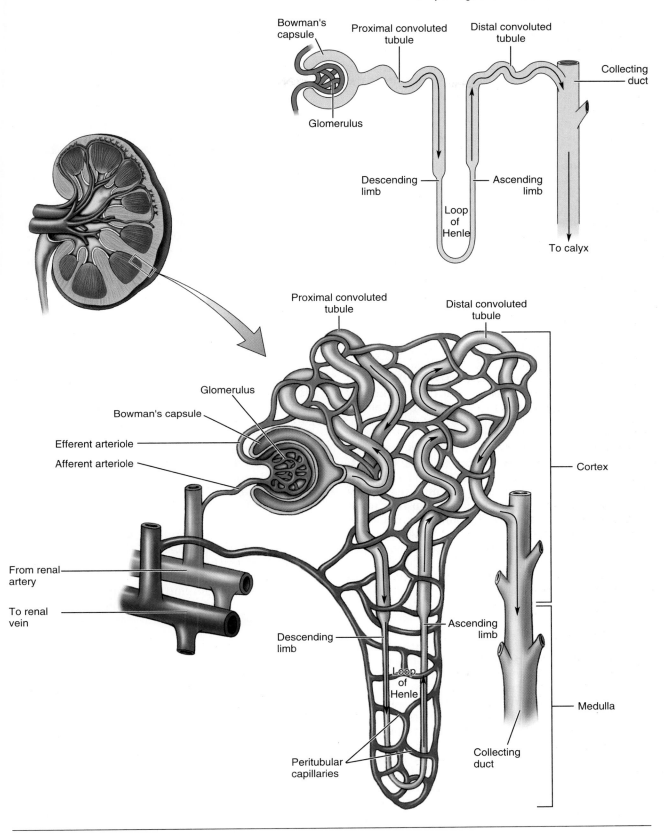

FIGURE 20–2 • The nephron unit: tubular and vascular structures.

filtration occur, and what substances are filtered across the glomerular membrane?

Why Filtration Occurs. Filtration occurs when the pressure on one side of a membrane is greater than the pressure on the opposite side. Blood pressure in the glomerulus is higher than the pressure within Bowman's capsule. It is this pressure gradient (pressure difference) that provides the driving force for filtration. (See Chapter 3 for a description of filtration.)

What Substances Are Filtered. The wall of the glomerulus contains pores and acts like a sieve, or a strainer. The size of the pores determines which substances can move across the wall from the glomerulus into Bowman's capsule. Small substances such as water, sodium, potassium, chloride, glucose, uric acid, and creatinine move through the pores very easily. These substances are filtered in proportion to their plasma concentration. In other words, if the concentration of a particular substance in the plasma is high, much of that substance is filtered. Large molecules such as red blood cells and large proteins cannot fit through the pores and therefore remain within the glomerulus. The water and the dissolved substances filtered into Bowman's capsule then form the **glomerular filtrate.** Note that the glomerular filtrate is protein-free; the presence of protein in the urine indicates abnormal nephron function, generally involving the glomerulus.

The rate at which glomerular filtration occurs is called the **glomerular filtration rate, or GFR.** Here is the amazing thing about GFR: The amount of filtrate formed is 125 mL per minute, or 180 liters (45 gallons) in 24 hours. Picture in your mind 180 liter bottles. This is the amount of filtrate formed by your kidneys in one day. Obviously, you do not excrete 180 liters of urine per day. Otherwise, you would do little more than drink and urinate. You excrete only about 1.5 liters per day. So the big question is this: What happens to the 178.5 liters that are filtered but not excreted?

TUBULAR REABSORPTION. Most of the filtrate, approximately 178.5 liters, is reabsorbed in the kidney and returned to the circulation. **Tubular reabsorption** (tōō′byə-lər rē-əb-sôrp′shən) is the process by which water and dissolved substances (glomerular filtrate) move from the tubules into the blood of the peritubular capillaries. Although reabsorption occurs throughout the entire length of the renal tubule, most occurs in the proximal convoluted tubule.

What is reabsorbed, and what is excreted? The kidney chooses the type and quantity of substances it reabsorbs. Some substances, such as glucose, are completely reabsorbed. For example, the amount of glucose filtered is the same as the amount reabsorbed, so that glucose normally does not appear in the urine. Some substances are incompletely reabsorbed. For instance, over 99% of water and sodium is reabsorbed, while only 50%

of urea is reabsorbed. Some waste products, such as creatinine, are not reabsorbed at all. Those substances not reabsorbed remain in the tubules, becoming part of the urine.

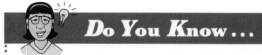

Do You Know...

Why is serum creatinine a measure of kidney function?

   Creatinine (krē-ăt′ĭ-nēn) is a waste product removed from the blood by the kidneys and eliminated in the urine. If kidney function declines, creatinine accumulates in the plasma. Thus, serum creatinine levels are used to monitor kidney function.

The reabsorption of substances by the kidney also varies with the mechanism of reabsorption. Absorption occurs through either active or passive transport. For instance, sodium is actively transported from the tubules into the peritubular capillaries. Water and chloride passively follow the movement of sodium. In general, when sodium is pumped from one location to another, water follows passively. This sequence is the basis for the action of most **diuretics,** drugs that increase the production of urine. The excess secretion of urine is **diuresis** (dī′yə-rē′sĭs). Most diuretics block the reabsorption of sodium and therefore also block the reabsorption of water. The excess sodium and water remain in the tubules and are eliminated as urine.

Hormones regulate the reabsorption of some substances. Sodium and potassium, for instance, are regulated in part by aldosterone.

TUBULAR SECRETION. While most of the water and dissolved substances enter the tubules because of filtration, a second process moves very small amounts of substances from the blood into the tubules. This is **tubular secretion** (tōō′byə-lər sĭ-krē′shən). It involves the active secretion of substances such as potassium ions (K^+), hydrogen ions (H^+), uric acid, ammonia, and drugs from the peritubular capillaries into the tubules.

Thus, urine is formed by three processes: filtration, reabsorption, and secretion. You must remember the structures involved in each process. Filtration causes water and dissolved substances to move from the capillaries (glomerulus) into the tubules. Reabsorption causes water and selected substances to move from the tubules into the peritubular capillaries. Secretion causes small amounts of specific substances to move from the peritubular capillaries into the tubules.

Table 20 • 2 — EFFECTS OF HORMONES ON THE KIDNEY

HORMONE	SECRETED BY	FUNCTION
Aldosterone	Adrenal cortex	Stimulates the reabsorption of sodium and water; stimulates the excretion of potassium; acts primarily on the distal tubule
Atrial natriuretic factor (ANF)	Atria of the heart	Decreases the reabsorption of sodium; causes greater excretion of sodium and water by the kidney
Antidiuretic hormone (ADH)	Neurohypophysis (posterior pituitary)	Stimulates the reabsorption of water
Parathyroid hormone (PTH)	Parathyroid gland	Stimulates the reabsorption of calcium and excretion of phosphate

HORMONAL CONTROL OF WATER AND ELECTROLYTES

Several hormones act on the kidney to regulate water and electrolyte excretion. Thus, these hormones play an important role in the regulation of blood volume, blood pressure, and electrolyte composition of body fluids. Hormones that affect blood volume and blood pressure include aldosterone, antidiuretic hormone (ADH), and atrial natriuretic factor (ANF). Aldosterone helps regulate sodium and potassium, while ANF affects sodium balance. ADH primarily affects the reabsorption of water. Parathyroid hormone (PTH) helps to regulate calcium and phosphate (Table 20–2).

Aldosterone

Aldosterone (ăl-dŏs′tə-rōn) is a hormone secreted by the adrenal cortex. Aldosterone acts primarily on the distal tubule. It stimulates the reabsorption of sodium and water and the excretion of potassium. Aldosterone expands or increases blood volume. Because aldosterone increases blood volume, it also increases blood pressure. A deficiency of aldosterone causes severely diminished blood volume, decline in blood pressure, and shock.

What causes the release of aldosterone? One of the most important stimuli for the release of aldosterone is renin. **Renin** (rĕn′ĭn) is a hormone that initiates a series of events called the **renin-angiotensin-aldosterone system.** Renin is secreted by a specialized collection of cells called the **juxtaglomerular apparatus,** located in the afferent arterioles. The renin-secreting cells are stimulated when either blood pressure or blood volume declines. As Figure 20–3 shows, renin sets off the following series of events:

• Renin activates **angiotensinogen** to form **angiotensin I** (ăn″jē-ō-tĕn′sĭn). Angiotensinogen

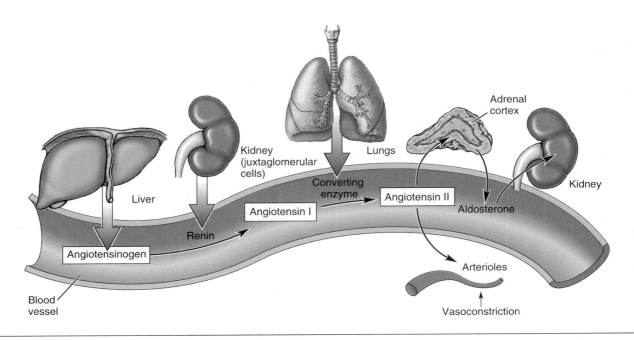

FIGURE 20–3 ● The renin-angiotensin-aldosterone system.

425

is secreted by the liver and circulates within the blood in its inactive form.

- An enzyme called **converting enzyme** acts in the pulmonary capillaries to change angiotensin I to **angiotensin II.**
- Angiotensin II stimulates the adrenal cortex to release aldosterone. The aldosterone, in turn, stimulates the distal tubule to reabsorb sodium and water and to excrete potassium.

In addition to stimulating aldosterone release, angiotensin II is also a potent vasopressor. Angiotensin II causes vasoconstriction and an elevation in blood pressure. Thus the activation of the renin-angiotensin-aldosterone system regulates blood volume and blood pressure.

A class of drugs called ACE inhibitors is used to lower blood pressure. (ACE stands for angiotensin-converting enzyme.) ACE inhibitors prevent the production of angiotensin II, which is a potent vasoconstrictor.

Antidiuretic Hormone

A second hormone exerting an important effect on water reabsorption is **antidiuretic hormone** (ăn′tē-dī″yə-rĕt′ĭk hôr′mōn) **(ADH).** The action of ADH allows the kidneys to concentrate urine. (Think of the name antidiuretic hormone. It literally means against diuresis, or urine production.) The posterior pituitary gland (neurohypophysis) secretes ADH.

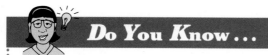

Why do both diabetes mellitus and diabetes insipidus cause polyuria?

Diabetes mellitus is a disease of insulin deficiency that results in hyperglycemia. The hyperglycemia, in turn, leads to excess filtration of glucose by the kidneys. Because all of the filtered glucose cannot be reabsorbed, glycosuria develops. The excess glucose in the tubules requires the excretion of large amounts of water. Thus, the person with diabetes mellitus experiences polyuria (*poly* means much; *uria* means urine). Diabetes insipidus is a disease of ADH deficiency. ADH is necessary for the reabsorption of water from the collecting duct. In the absence of ADH, the person may excrete up to 10 liters of a pale dilute urine. Note that both diabetes mellitus and diabetes insipidus are characterized by polyuria. The underlying causes of the polyuria, however, are different.

Antidiuretic hormone works primarily on the collecting duct by determining its permeability to water. In the presence of ADH, the collecting duct becomes permeable to water. Water is reabsorbed from the collecting duct into the peritubular capillaries. In other words, ADH decreases the excretion of water and causes excretion of a highly concentrated urine. In the absence of ADH, the membrane permeability of the collecting duct decreases, and water cannot be reabsorbed; the result is excretion of a very dilute urine. Because ADH affects the amount of water excreted by the kidneys, it plays an important role in the determination of blood volume and blood pressure. Excess ADH expands blood volume, while a deficiency of ADH diminishes blood volume.

What is the stimulus for the release of ADH? The two stimuli are a decrease in blood volume and an increase in the concentration of solutes in the plasma. Consider a person who becomes dehydrated by vomiting. The person loses large amounts of water and electrolytes. When the volume of blood decreases and the concentration of the blood increases, ADH is released. The ADH increases the reabsorption of water by the kidneys, expanding blood volume and diluting the blood. The increased blood volume eventually stops the stimulus for the release of ADH.

Atrial Natriuretic Factor

Atrial natriuretic factor (ANF) causes excretion of sodium (Na^+), a process called **natriuresis.** ANF is secreted by the walls of the atria of the heart in response to an increase in the volume of blood. ANF decreases the secretion of renin by the juxtaglomerular cells (kidney) and decreases the secretion of aldosterone by the adrenal cortex. The overall effect is to decrease sodium and water reabsorption. The effects of ANF are opposite to the effects of aldosterone and ADH.

Parathyroid Hormone

Parathyroid hormone (PTH) is secreted by the parathyroid glands. It does not affect water balance but plays an important role in the regulation of two electrolytes, calcium and phosphate. PTH elevates plasma calcium through its effects on three organs: bones, digestive tract, and kidneys. PTH stimulates the renal tubules to reabsorb calcium and excrete phosphate. The primary stimulus for the release of PTH is a low plasma level of calcium (see Chapter 12 for a detailed description of PTH).

Table 20•3 CHARACTERISTICS OF URINE

CHARACTERISTIC	DESCRIPTION
Amount (volume)	Average 1500 mL/24 hours
pH	Average 6.0
Specific gravity	Slightly heavier than water (1.001–1.035)
Color	Yellow (amber, straw colored, deep yellow in dehydration, pale yellow with overhydration)
Some Abnormal Constituents of Urine	
Albumin (protein)	Albuminuria: indicates an increased permeability of the glomerulus (eg, nephrotic syndrome, glomerulonephritis, hypertension); sometimes exercise or pregnancy will result in albuminuria
Glucose	Glycosuria: usually indicates diabetes mellitus
Red blood cells	Hematuria: bleeding in the urinary tract; indicates inflammation, trauma or disease
Hemoglobin	Hemoglobinuria: indicates hemolysis (transfusion reactions, hemolytic anemia)
White blood cells	Pyuria (pus): indicates infection within the kidney or urinary tract
Ketone bodies	Ketonuria: usually indicates uncontrolled diabetes mellitus (fats are rapidly and incompletely metabolized)
Bilirubin	Bilirubinuria: usually indicates disease involving the liver and/or biliary tree

COMPOSITION OF URINE

Finally, we can answer this question: What is in urine? Urine is a sterile fluid composed mostly of water (95%), nitrogen-containing waste, and electrolytes. Important nitrogenous waste includes urea, uric acid, ammonia, and creatinine. The light yellow color of urine is due to a pigment called urochrome formed from the breakdown of hemoglobin in the liver. Table 20–3 summarizes the composition of urine along with the significance of some abnormal constituents. Figure 20–4 summarizes the steps in urine formation.

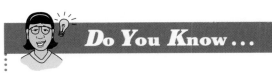

Do You Know ...

Why does urinary specific gravity increase in a dehydrated patient?

Specific gravity (spĭ-sĭ′fĭk grăv′ĭ-tē) is the ratio of the amount of solute to volume (solute/volume). The specific gravity of urine ranges from 1.001 to 1.035, depending on the amount of solute (substances such as glucose and creatinine) in the urine. The more solute, the higher the specific gravity. If a patient is dehydrated, less water is filtered by the kidneys; as a result, the volume of urine decreases. The ratio of solute to volume in the urine therefore increases. Thus, dehydration is characterized by an increase in urinary specific gravity.

✳ **SUM IT UP!** Water and dissolved solute (180 liters per 24 hours) are filtered across the glomerulus into Bowman's capsule. Reabsorption of water and solute occurs throughout the entire length of the tubule. Most of the reabsorption occurs in the proximal convoluted tubule. Water (178.5 liters in 24 hours) moves from the tubules into the blood (peritubular capillaries). Aldosterone affects primarily the distal tubule. Aldosterone stimulates the reabsorption of sodium (water follows sodium) and excretion of potassium. Atrial natriuretic factor (ANF) exerts an effect opposite to that of aldosterone. ADH determines the membrane permeability of the collecting duct, thereby regulating water reabsorption at this site. The peritubular capillaries secrete a small amount of solute into the tubules. Approximately 1.5 liters of urine is excreted from the body in 24 hours.

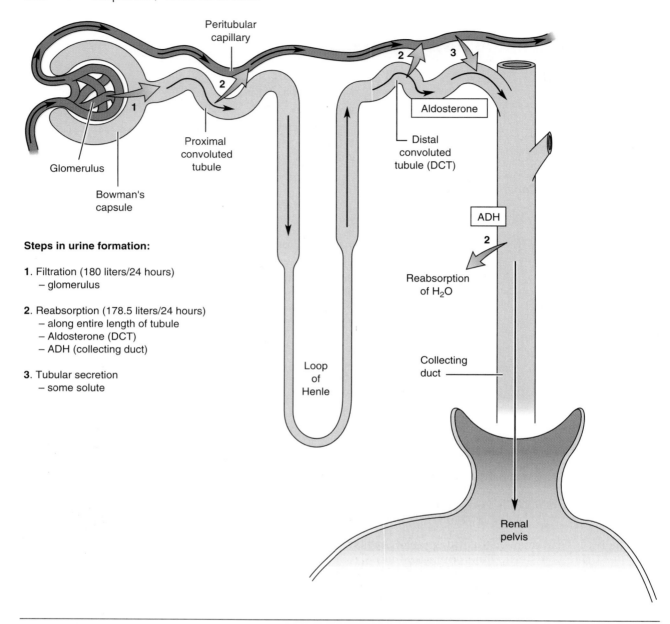

Steps in urine formation:

1. Filtration (180 liters/24 hours)
  – glomerulus

2. Reabsorption (178.5 liters/24 hours)
  – along entire length of tubule
  – Aldosterone (DCT)
  – ADH (collecting duct)

3. Tubular secretion
  – some solute

FIGURE 20–4 ● Steps in urine formation: filtration, reabsorption, and secretion. Note that the peritubular capillaries are shown here as long straight tubes. They actually surround the tubules, as in Figure 20–2.

WHEN THE KIDNEYS SHUT DOWN

Sometimes the kidneys stop working, or shut down. This condition is **renal failure** or **renal suppression.** The kidneys no longer make urine. The blood is not cleansed of its waste, and substances that should have been excreted in the urine remain in the blood. This condition is called **uremia,** which literally means urine in the blood.

Uremia may be prevented with an **artificial kidney,** a form of **dialysis** (dī-ăl′ĭ-sĭs) (Fig. 20–5). The artificial kidney consists of a cylinder filled

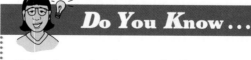

Why does circulatory shock cause oliguria?

In a state of circulatory shock, blood pressure is severely decreased. The low blood pressure, in turn, decreases glomerular filtration, thereby reducing urinary output. A low urinary output is called **oliguria** (ŏl′ĭ-gyōō′rē-ə) (*oligo* means scanty; *uria* means urine). Oliguria is a urinary output of less than 400 mL per 24 hours.

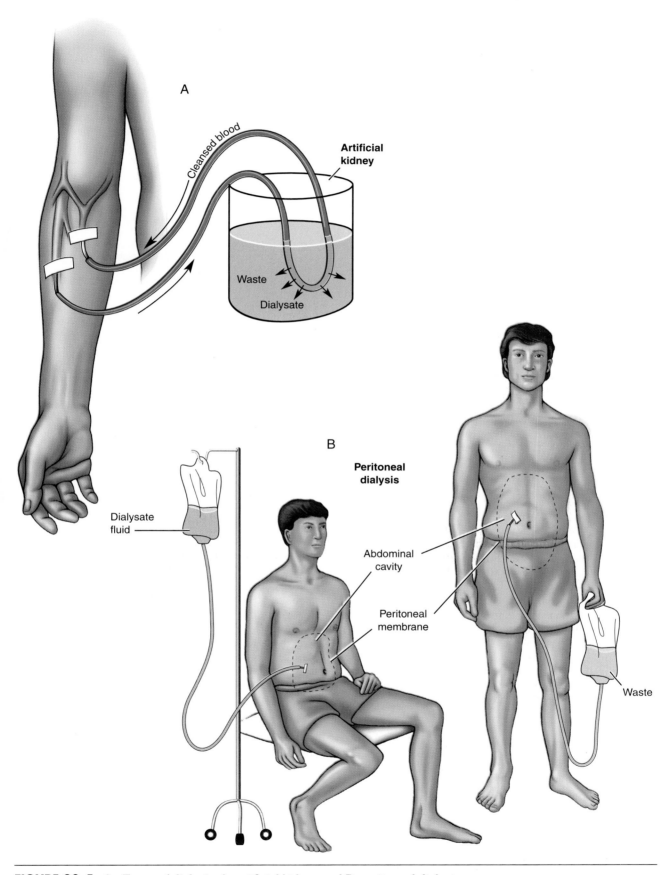

FIGURE 20–5 • Types of dialysis: A, artificial kidney and B, peritoneal dialysis.

with a plasma-like solution called the **dialysate.** The patient's blood is passed through a series of tiny tubes immersed in the dialysate. Waste products in the blood, such as potassium, creatinine, uric acid, and excess water, diffuse out of the tubes into the dialysate. The blood is thus cleansed of these waste products and returned to the patient. Because this procedure cleanses blood like a kidney, it is called an artificial kidney.

A second form of dialysis is **peritoneal dialysis.** With this procedure, the peritoneal cavity of the patient is used as the cylinder of an artificial kidney, and dialysate is infused into the peritoneal cavity. Waste products diffuse from the blood into the dialysate. The dialysate eventually drains out of the peritoneal cavity and is discarded.

YOUR PLUMBING: STRUCTURE AND FUNCTION

While the kidneys form urine, the remaining structures of the urinary system (ureters, bladder, and urethra) function as plumbing and form the **urinary tract** (Fig. 20–6). They do not alter the urine in any way; instead, they store and conduct urine from the kidney to the outside of the body. The urinary tract has an outer layer of connective tissue and a middle layer of smooth muscle. The tract is lined with mucous membrane.

Ureters

Two ureters connect the kidneys with the bladder. The ureters originate in the pelvis of the kidneys and terminate in the bladder. The ureters are long (10–13 inches or 25–33 cm), slender muscular tubes capable of rhythmic contractions called peristalsis. Urine moves along the ureters from the kidneys to the bladder in response to gravity and peristalsis.

Sometimes a kidney stone **(renal calculus)** lodges in the slender ureter, and the urine backs up behind the stone, causing severe pain and pressure known as **renal colic.** Unless the stone is washed out or removed, kidney damage may occur.

Urinary Bladder

The urinary bladder functions as a temporary reservoir for the storage of urine. When empty, the bladder is located below the peritoneal membrane and behind the symphysis pubis. When full, the bladder rises into the abdominal cavity. You can feel a distended bladder if you place your hand over the lower abdominal wall.

Four layers make up the wall of the bladder. The innermost layer is mucous membrane and contains several thicknesses of transitional epithelium. The mucous membrane is continuous with the mucous membrane of the ureters and urethra. The second layer is called the submucosa and consists of connective tissue and contains many elastic fibers. The third layer is composed of muscle. This involuntary smooth muscle is the **detrusor muscle** (dē-trōō′zər mus′əl). The outermost layer of the upper part of the bladder is the serosa. The lower portion of the bladder is covered by connective tissue.

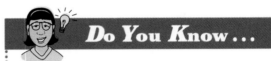

Do You Know...

Why can an ignored bladder infection cause a kidney infection?

The urinary bladder, especially in the female, is a frequent site of infection. An infection of the urinary bladder is called cystitis. If cystitis is not treated promptly, pathogens can travel from the bladder up the ureter into the kidney, causing a kidney infection (pyelonephritis). Because the pathogens travel to the kidney from the bladder, a kidney infection is often called an ascending infection.

How much can you hold? The bladder wall is arranged in folds called **rugae.** The rugae allow the bladder to stretch as it fills. The urge to urinate usually begins when it has accumulated about 200 mL of urine. As the volume of urine increases to 300 mL, the urge to urinate becomes more uncomfortable. A moderately full bladder contains about 500 mL, or 1 pint of urine. An overdistended bladder may contain more than 1 liter of urine. With overdistention, the urge to void may be lost.

One specific area of the floor of the bladder is the **trigone.** It is a triangular area formed by three points: the entrance points of the two ureters and the exit point of the urethra. The trigone is important clinically because infections tend to persist in this area. The exit of the urinary bladder contains a sphincter muscle, called the **internal sphincter.** The internal sphincter is composed of smooth muscle that contracts involuntarily to prevent emptying. Below the internal sphincter, surrounding the upper region of the urethra, is the **external sphincter.** This sphincter is composed of skeletal muscle and is voluntarily controlled. Contraction of the external sphincter allows you to resist the urge to urinate.

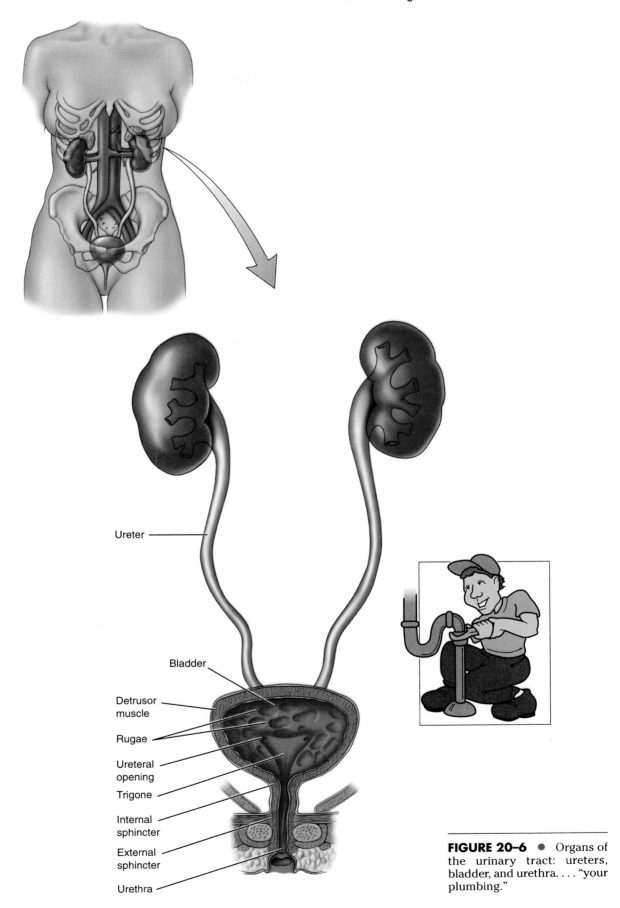

Ureter

Bladder

Detrusor muscle

Rugae

Ureteral opening

Trigone

Internal sphincter

External sphincter

Urethra

FIGURE 20–6 • Organs of the urinary tract: ureters, bladder, and urethra. . . . "your plumbing."

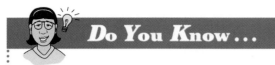

Do You Know...

Why does prolonged bedrest predispose the patient to a urinary tract infection?

Urine does not flow backward in a healthy person. The upright sitting and standing positions help prevent backflow of urine. Prolonged bedrest, however, slows the flow of urine toward the bladder, resulting in stagnation and infection.

Urination

Urination, also called **micturition** or **voiding,** is the process of expelling urine from the bladder. What causes micturition? As the bladder fills with urine, stimulated stretch receptors send nerve impulses through sensory nerves to the spinal cord. The spinal cord reflexively sends a motor nerve impulse back to the bladder, causing the bladder wall to contract rhythmically and the internal sphincter muscle to relax. This response is called the **micturition reflex.**

The micturition reflex gives rise to a sense of urgency. Contraction of the external sphincter prevents involuntary urination. In an infant, the micturition reflex causes the bladder to empty involuntarily. This is what causes baby Sammy to be a wet bundle of joy. As baby Sammy matures, he will learn to override this reflex by voluntarily controlling the external sphincter. Only then can Sammy move from diapers to training pants.

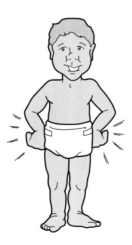

A patient may experience urinary retention, the inability to void or to empty the bladder. Urinary retention is usually due to the effects of drugs used during surgery. Note the difference between suppression and retention. Renal suppression means that the kidneys do not make urine. Urinary retention means that the bladder does not expel urine.

Urethra

The urethra is a tube that carries urine from the bladder to the outside. It is lined with mucous membrane that contains numerous mucus-secreting glands. The muscular layer of the urethra contracts and helps express urine during micturition.

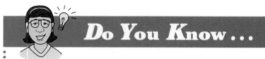

Do You Know...

Why does an enlarged prostate gland cause dysuria?

The male urethra is surrounded by the donut-shaped prostate gland. When the prostate gland enlarges, pressure is exerted on the outside of the urethra, closing the lumen of the urethra and impeding the flow of urine from the bladder. Urination becomes difficult (dysuria), and the incomplete emptying of the bladder sets the stage for repeated bladder infections. The incomplete emptying also causes nocturia (needing to urinate at night, thereby interfering with sleep), a bothersome symptom that may cause men to seek medical help.

The male and female urethras differ in several ways. In the female, the urethra is short (1.5 inches or 3.8 cm) and is part of the urinary system. The urethra opens to the outside at the **urethral meatus.** The female urethral meatus is located in front of the vagina and between the labia minora.

In the male, the urethra is part of both the urinary and the reproductive systems. The male urethra (8 inches or 20 cm) is much longer than the female urethra. As the male urethra leaves the bladder, it passes through the prostate gland and extends the length of the penis. Thus, the male urethra performs a dual purpose; it carries urine (its urinary function) and sperm (its reproductive function).

✳ **SUM IT UP!** The kidneys make urine. The urine is stored and transported by the structures that make up the urinary tract: ureters, bladder, and urethra. The accumulation of urine in the bladder is the stimulus for the micturition reflex and creates the urge to void. Voluntary control of the external sphincter allows you to void at a particular time. Urine exits the body through the urethral meatus.

As You Age

1. The number of nephron units progressively decreases so that, by the age of 70 to 80 years, there has been a 50% reduction. Clinically this decrease in nephron function causes a diminished ability to concentrate urine.

2. Glomerular filtration rate (GFR) declines with age. As a result, the elderly person excretes drugs more slowly and is at risk for drug overdose. The decrease in GFR also makes it difficult for the elderly person to excrete excess blood volume, so any intravenous fluids must be administered slowly and carefully. Overhydration is a common cause of heart failure in the elderly.

3. The aging urinary bladder shrinks and becomes less able to contract and relax. As a result, the elderly person must void more frequently. Because of less effective bladder contraction and residual urine, the incidence of bladder infection increases. The weakening of the external sphincter and a decreased ability to sense a distended bladder increase the incidence of bladder incontinence. Frequent urination in men may be caused by an enlarged prostate gland, a common age-related disorder.

Disorders of the Urinary System

Glomerulonephritis	Inflammation (antigen-antibody reaction) of the glomeruli that develops in response to streptococcal infection. The glomeruli are damaged in such a way that large amounts of albumin and other proteins are lost in the urine.
Inflammation of the lining of the urinary tract	Inflammation of the urinary tract, commonly caused by infection with *Escherichia coli*. Both urethritis and cystitis are lower urinary tract infections. Urethritis is an inflammation of the urethra. Cystitis is inflammation of the urinary bladder. Pyelitis is a form of upper urinary tract infection and refers to inflammation of the renal pelvis and calyces.
Polycystic kidney	A genetic disease characterized by the development of multiple fluid-filled sacs in the kidney. The sacs gradually cause destruction of kidney tissue and loss of kidney function.
Pyelonephritis	A bacterial infection of the pelvis of the kidney. Pyelonephritis is frequently caused by a neglected bladder infection that ascends through the ureters to the kidneys.
Renal calculi	Also called nephrolithiasis or kidney stones. Sharp stones (like those that form in the patient with gout) can damage the nephron units and cause gradual loss of renal function. Kidney stones typically get lodged in the ureter, blocking the flow of urine and causing accumulation of urine in the renal pelvis (hydronephrosis). The urine backs up in the kidney and may cause serious kidney damage and pain (renal colic).
Renal failure	Rapid kidney failure (acute renal failure) or gradual kidney failure (chronic renal failure). Renal failure has many causes: infections, acute hypotensive episodes, exposure to toxins, complications of diseases such as diabetes, genetic disorders such as polycystic kidney disease, and congenital defects. Unless dialyzed, the blood of a patient in renal failure accumulates waste products (uremia) and makes the person toxic.

Summary Outline

I. Urinary System and Urine Making

A. Kidney
1. The kidneys are the most important excretory organs. They eliminate nitrogenous waste, water, electrolytes, toxins, and drugs.
2. The kidney has three distinct regions: the renal cortex, the renal medulla, and the renal pelvis. The kidney is supplied by the renal artery and drained by the renal vein.
3. The kidney has six functions: it excretes nitrogenous waste, it regulates blood volume, electrolytes, pH, and blood pressure, and it helps red blood cell production.

B. Nephron Unit
1. The nephron unit is the functional (urine-making) unit of the kidney.
2. The nephron unit is composed of tubular structures and vascular structures.

C. Three Processes in Urine Formation
1. Glomerular filtration filters 180 liters of filtrate in 24 hours. It moves water and dissolved substances from the glomerulus into Bowman's capsule.
2. Tubular reabsorption causes the reabsorption of 178.5 liters of filtrate. It moves the filtrate from the tubules into the peritubular capillaries.
3. Tubular secretion causes the secretion of small amounts of specific substances from the peritubular capillaries into the tubules.

II. Hormonal Control of Water and Electrolytes

A. Aldosterone
1. Aldosterone stimulates the distal tubule to reabsorb Na^+ and water and to excrete K^+.
2. The secretion of aldosterone is regulated by the renin-angiotensin-aldosterone system.
3. The release of renin from the kidneys activates the renin-angiotensin-aldosterone system.

B. Antidiuretic Hormone (ADH)
1. ADH stimulates the collecting duct to reabsorb water.
2. ADH is released from the posterior pituitary gland in response to low blood volume and increased concentration of solute in the plasma.

C. Other Hormones
1. Atrial natriuretic factor inhibits the reabsorption of Na^+ and water, thereby causing natriuresis.
2. Parathyroid hormone stimulates the renal reabsorption of calcium and the excretion of phosphate.

III. Your Plumbing: Structure and Function
Your plumbing consists of two ureters, one bladder, and one urethra.

A. Ureters
1. The two ureters are long, slender tubes that carry urine from the renal pelvis to the bladder.
2. Urine moves in response to peristalsis.

B. Urinary Bladder and Urethra
1. The urinary bladder is a temporary reservoir that holds the urine.
2. The voluntary elimination of urine is called urination, micturition, or voiding.
3. The urethra is a tube that carries urine from the bladder to the outside of the body.

Review Your Knowledge

1. Trace the flow of urine from the kidneys to the outside of the body.

2. What are six functions of the kidneys?

3. What is the functional unit of the kidney?

4. Name the tubular structures that the urine flows through starting with Bowman's capsule and going to the calyx.

5. What substances are filtered across the glomerular membrane?

6. What are the differences between glomerular filtration, tubular reabsorption, and tubular secretion?

7. How much of the glomerular filtrate is excreted as urine?

8. What substances are reabsorbed by the kidneys? What substances are excreted by the kidneys?

9. How do diuretics increase the excretion of urine?

Review Your Knowledge *continued*

10. Explain how aldosterone, antidiuretic hormone (ADH), and atrial natriuretic factor (ANF) act on the kidney to regulate water and electrolyte excretion. Where is each hormone secreted?

11. What effect does aldosterone have on blood pressure? What causes the release of aldosterone?

12. Which hormone allows the kidneys to concentrate urine?

13. How is the parathyroid hormone (PTH) related to the kidneys?

14. What are the normal components of urine? What is blood in the urine called? What is glucose in the urine called? How much urine is excreted in 24 hours?

15. Describe the four layers of the wall of the bladder.

16. What causes micturition?

17. What is the difference between renal suppression and urinary retention?

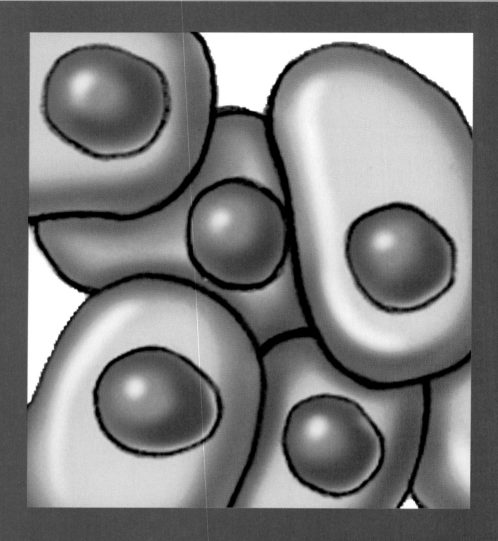

• • • Key Terms

Buffer (bŭf′ər)

Edema (ĭ-dē′mə)

Electrolyte balance (ĭ-lĕk′trə-līt″ băl′əns)

Extracellular fluid (ĕk″strə-sĕl′yə-lər flōo′ĭd)

Hyperkalemia (hī″pər-kə-lē′mē-ə)

Hyperventilation (hī″pər-vĕn″tĭl-ā′shən)

Hypokalemia (hī″pō-kə-lē′mē-ə)

Hypoventilation (hī″pō-vĕn″tĭl-ā′shən)

Intake (ĭn′tāk)

Interstitial fluid (ĭn″tər-stĭsh′əl flōo′ĭd)

Intracellular fluid (ĭn″trə-sĕl′yə-lər flōo′ĭd)

Kussmaul respirations
(kōos′môl rĕs″pə-rā′shənz)

Metabolic acidosis (mĕt″ə-bŏl′ĭk ăs″ĭ-dō′sĭs)

Metabolic alkalosis (mĕt″ə-bŏl′ĭk ăl″kə-lō′sĭs)

Output (out′pŏot)

Respiratory acidosis
(rĕs′pər-ə-tōr″ē ăs″ĭ-dō′sĭs)

Respiratory alkalosis
(rĕs′pər-ə-tōr″ē ăl″kə-lō′sĭs)

Skin turgor (skĭn tûr′gər)

Transcellular fluid (trăns″sĕl′yə-lər flōo′ĭd)

• • • Selected terms in bold type in this chapter are defined in the Glossary.

21

WATER, ELECTROLYTE, AND ACID-BASE BALANCE

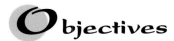

Objectives

1. Describe the two fluid compartments: intracellular and extracellular.

2. Describe the concept of intake and output.

3. List factors that affect electrolyte balance.

4. Describe the common ions: sodium, potassium, calcium, chloride, magnesium, and bicarbonate.

5. Describe factors that affect acid-base balance.

6. List three mechanisms that regulate pH in the body.

7. Discuss acid-base imbalances: acidosis and alkalosis.

The old saying "you're all wet" has some truth to it. Between 50% and 70% of a person's weight is water. In the average adult male, the water makes up 60% of the weight (about 40 liters), while in the female, water makes up about 50%. An infant is composed of even more water, up to 75%. Because adipose tissue contains less water than does muscle tissue, obese persons have less water than do thin persons.

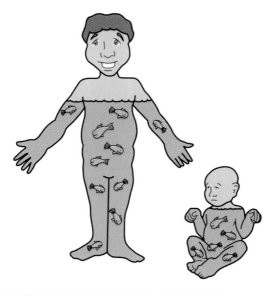

DISTRIBUTION OF BODY FLUIDS

Fluid Compartments

Water and its dissolved electrolytes are distributed into two major compartments: an intracellular compartment and an extracellular compartment (Fig. 21–1). The intracellular compartment includes the water located in all the cells of the body. Most water, about 63%, is located in the intracellular compartment.

The extracellular compartment includes the fluid located outside all the cells and represents about 37% of the total body water. The extracellular compartment includes the water located between cells (**interstitial fluid** [ĭn″tər-stĭsh′əl flōō′ĭd]), water within blood vessels (plasma), and water within lymphatic vessels (lymph). **Transcellular fluid** (trăns″sĕl′yə-lər flōō′ĭd) is extracellular fluid and includes cerebrospinal fluid (CSF), the aqueous and vitreous humors in the eyes, the synovial fluids of joints, the serous fluids in body cavities, and the glandular secretions. Interstitial fluid and plasma are the largest extracellular compartments.

Composition of Body Fluids

Intracellular and extracellular fluids vary in their concentrations of various electrolytes. **Extracellular fluids** (ĕk″strə-sĕl′yə-lər flōō′ĭdz) contain high concentrations of sodium (Na^+), chloride (Cl^-), and bicarbonate (HCO_3^-) ions. The plasma portion (extracellular) contains more protein than other extracellular fluids do. **Intracellular fluid** (ĭn″trə-sĕl′yə-lər flōō′ĭd) contains high concentrations of potassium (K^+), phosphate (PO_4^-) and magnesium (Mg^{++}) ions.

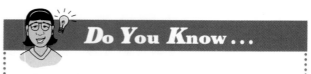

Why might a patient be given an intravenous infusion of normal saline or Ringer's lactate solution?

Some patients become deficient in body fluids. These may be surgical patients who are not permitted to drink, patients who have been vomiting, or those who are unconscious and unable to eat or drink. These patients frequently receive intravenous infusions of solutions that resemble plasma in ionic composition. Normal saline, for instance, contains 0.9% sodium chloride, a concentration equal to that of plasma. Ringer's lactate solution contains sodium, potassium, calcium, chloride, and lactate in concentrations that resemble plasma.

Smaller concentrations of other ions are present in both intracellular and extracellular flu-

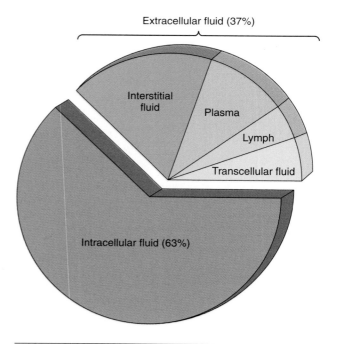

FIGURE 21–1 ● Fluid compartments. The two fluid compartments are the intracellular and the extracellular compartments. The extracellular compartment includes interstitial fluid, plasma, lymph, and transcellular fluid.

ids. While distributed across the fluid compartments, water and electrolytes can move from one compartment to another. The movement of fluid and electrolytes between compartments is well regulated (see Chapter 15).

WATER BALANCE

Normally, the quantity of water taken in (**intake** [ĭn′tāk]) equals the amount of water eliminated from the body (**output** [out′po͞ot]). Water balance exists when intake equals output (Fig. 21–2). As part of your clinical responsibilities, you will be measuring intake and output.

Water Intake

Although water intake can vary considerably, the average adult takes in about 2500 mL every 24 hours. About 60% comes from drinking liquids, and an additional 30% comes from water in foods. Ten percent comes from the breakdown of foods. This portion is called the water of metabolism.

Thirst is the primary regulator of water intake. The thirst center is in the hypothalamus of the brain. As the body loses water, the thirst center in the hypothalamus is stimulated. The stimulation causes you to drink. Drinking then restores the water content of the body. Both your thirst and your hypothalamus are satisfied.

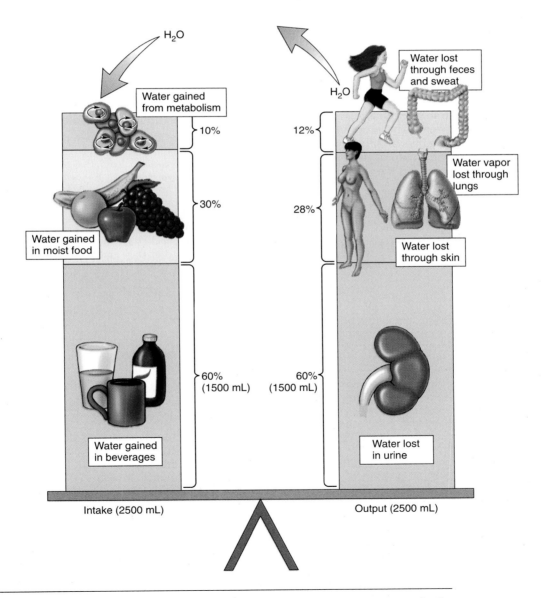

FIGURE 21–2   ●   Water balance: intake equals output. A person ingests most water in the form of beverages. Most water is lost as urine.

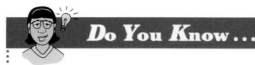

What is skin turgor?

Skin turgor (skĭn tûr′gər) is assessed by pinching the skin and then observing how quickly the skin flattens, or returns to its normal position. If a person is well hydrated, the pinched skin quickly flattens out. The skin of a dehydrated person, however, flattens out more slowly. The slower response is due to the depleted interstitial fluid, a condition characteristic of dehydration.

Water Output

In a healthy person, 24-hour intake and output are approximately equal. The individual who takes in 2500 mL of water should, therefore, eliminate 2500 mL. Water can leave the body through several routes: kidneys, skin, lungs, and digestive tract. The kidneys eliminate about 60% of the water as urine. About 28% is lost from the skin and lungs. Six percent is eliminated in the feces, and another 6% is lost as sweat. The amount lost by sweat can vary considerably, depending on the level of exercise and environmental temperatures. Water loss through the skin and lungs increases in a hot, dry environment.

What is edema?

Edema (ĭ-dē′mə) is the accumulation of excess fluid in the interstitial space. Depending on its location in the body, edema can cause a variety of symptoms. Edema of the ankles, for instance, causes the feet to swell, making it difficult to wear shoes. If edema occurs in the lungs, more life-threatening symptoms may develop. The excess fluid impairs the diffusion of oxygen into the pulmonary capillaries, making the patient hypoxic. The goal of therapy is to relieve symptoms (eg, hypoxia) and to eliminate the cause of the edema formation. Diuretics play a key role in eliminating excess fluid from the body.

The kidneys are the primary regulator of water output. Water regulation occurs primarily through the action of antidiuretic hormone (ADH) on the collecting duct. When body water content is low, the posterior pituitary gland releases ADH. It stimulates the collecting duct to reabsorb water, thereby decreasing water in the urine and increasing blood volume. When body water content is high, the secretion of ADH decreases. As a result, less water is reabsorbed from the collecting duct, and the excess water is eliminated in the urine.

ELECTROLYTE BALANCE

Electrolyte balance (ĭ-lĕk′trə-līt″ băl′əns) exists when the amounts of the various electrolytes gained by the body equal the amounts lost. **Electrolyte imbalances** are common, serious clinical challenges. Electrolytes are important components of the body fluids. The kidneys control the composition of body fluids by regulating the renal excretion of electrolytes. Table 21–1 includes the major electrolytes and their normal levels and functions.

What serious electrolyte imbalance is a common complication of diuretic therapy?

A diuretic agent increases the production of urine. Most diuretics work by blocking the reabsorption of sodium from the tubules. Generally, water follows sodium. If sodium is not reabsorbed, neither is the water. Hence, urinary output increases. This process is called **diuresis.** Unfortunately, diuresis also results in the elimination of potassium. The process of potassium loss by the kidney is called **kaliuresis.** Many diuretics are kaliuretic in that they cause the renal excretion of potassium. Prolonged therapy with diuretics frequently causes hypokalemia, a potentially life-threatening condition.

Quick Reference

Chapter 2 describes the chemical characteristics of electrolytes. You will want to review several terms listed here, for quick reference:

- **Ion:** an element or compound that carries an electrical charge. Common ions are Na^+, Cl^-, K^+, Ca^{++}, and Mg^{++}.
- **Cation:** a positively charged ion, such as Na^+, K^+, and Ca^{++}.
- **Anion:** a negatively charged ion, such as Cl^- and HCO_3^- (bicarbonate).
- **Electrolyte:** substances that form ions when they dissolve in water, such as NaCl (salt).

$$NaCl \rightarrow Na^+ \text{ (cation)} + Cl^- \text{ (anion)}$$

- **Ionization:** the chemical reaction caused when a salt splits into two ions.

Table 21 • 1 MAJOR IONS AND FUNCTIONS

ELECTROLYTE	PLASMA LEVELS	FUNCTION
Sodium (Na^+)	136–145 mEq/L	Chief extracellular cation Regulates extracellular volume Participates in nerve-muscle function
Potassium (K^+)	3.5–5.0 mEq/L	Chief intracellular cation Participates in nerve-muscle function
Calcium (Ca^{++})	4.5–5.8 mEg/L	Strengthens bone and teeth Participates in muscle contraction Helps in blood clotting
Magnesium (Mg^{++})	1.5–2.5 mEq/L	Strengthens bone Participates in nerve-muscle function
Chloride (Cl^-)	95–108 mEq/L	Chief extracellular anion Involved in extracellular volume control
Bicarbonate (HCO_3^-)	22–26 mEq/L	Part of bicarbonate buffer system Participates in acid-base balance
Phosphate (HPO_4^{--})	2.5–4.5 mEq/L	Strengthens bone Participates in acid-base balance

Most Important Ions

Sodium (Na^+)

Sodium is the chief *extra*cellular cation, accounting for nearly 90% of the positively charged ions in the extracellular fluid. Sodium is necessary for nerve impulse conduction, and it also helps maintain body fluid balance. The primary mechanism regulating sodium concentration is aldosterone (see Chapter 20). Aldosterone stimulates the distal tubule of the nephron unit to reabsorb sodium.

Potassium (K^+)

Potassium is the chief *intra*cellular cation. Like sodium, potassium plays an important role in nerve impulse conduction. The primary substance regulating potassium concentration is aldosterone. Aldosterone stimulates the distal tubule to excrete potassium.

The monitoring of serum potassium levels is an important clinical responsibility. Alterations in plasma levels of potassium can cause serious cardiac dysrhythmias. **Hyperkalemia** (hī″pər-kə-lē′mē-ə) refers to excess potassium (K^+) in the blood. **Hypokalemia** (hī″pō-kə-lē′mē-ə) refers to a lower-than-normal amount of potassium in the blood. (Do not confuse *hyperkalemia,* excess K^+, with **hypercalcemia,** excess calcium in the blood.)

Calcium (Ca^{++})

Calcium is necessary for bone and teeth formation, muscle contraction, nerve impulse transmission, and blood clotting. Ninety-nine percent of the body's calcium is in the bones and teeth. Parathyroid hormone is the primary regulator of plasma levels of calcium (see Chapter 12).

Magnesium (Mg^{++})

Next to potassium, magnesium is the most abundant cation in the intracellular fluid. Magnesium is important in the function of the heart, muscles, and nerves.

Chloride (Cl^-)

Chloride is the chief extracellular anion. Chloride usually follows sodium. That is, when sodium is actively pumped from the tubules into the peritubular capillaries (within the nephron unit), chloride follows the sodium passively.

Bicarbonate (HCO_3^-)

Bicarbonate is an important anion in acid-base balance. Bicarbonate is an alkaline (basic) substance that helps remove excess acid from the body. It is also the form in which carbon dioxide (CO_2) is transported in the blood. Bicarbonate excretion is controlled by the kidneys. Bicarbonate can be either reabsorbed or excreted, depending on the body's needs.

Other Ions

The plasma contains other ions, such as sulfate (SO_4^{--}) and phosphate (PO_4^-). The normal lab values for the major ions are summarized in Table 21–1.

✳ **SUM IT UP!** The volume (amount) and composition of body fluids are closely regulated. Body fluids are found in two main compartments. Most body fluid (63%) is in the intracellular compartment. The remaining 37% is in the extracellular compartment. The extracellular compartment contains interstitial fluid, plasma, lymph, and transcellular fluid. The electrolyte composition of the body fluids is important. The chief extracellular cation is sodium; the chief intracellular cation is potassium. Excesses and deficiencies of water and electrolytes cause serious problems.

ACID-BASE BALANCE

A normally functioning body requires a balance between acids and bases. Acid-base balance is described according to its regulation of pH. Why is the regulation of pH so important? All chemical reactions in the body occur at a particular pH level; any alteration in pH interferes with important chemical reactions. Chemical reactions that take place within extracellular fluids occur only when the pH is above 7. The neurons are particularly sensitive to changes in the pH of body fluids. For instance, if the plasma levels of hydrogen ion (H^+) decrease, the neurons become more excitable, and the person may experience a seizure. If the plasma H^+ concentration increases, however, neuronal activity decreases, and the person may become comatose.

Quick Reference

Chapter 2 describes acids, bases, and pH. You will want to review several terms listed here for quick reference:

- **Acid:** a substance that dissociates (splits) into H^+ and an anion like Cl^- (eg, $HCl \rightarrow H^+ + Cl^-$). An acid donates a hydrogen ion (H^+) during a chemical reaction.
- **Base:** a substance that combines with H^+ during a chemical reaction and removes H^+ from solution (eg, $OH^- + H^+ \rightarrow H_2O$). A base is an H^+ acceptor. The hydroxyl ion (OH^-), for example, combines with H^+ to create water. An example of a base is sodium hydroxide ($NaOH$). When added to an acidic solution, the $NaOH$ ionizes into Na^+ and OH^-; the OH^- then combines with H^+.
- **pH:** a unit of measurement that indicates the number of H^+ in solution. Remember: As the number of H^+ increases, the pH decreases. As the number of H^+ decreases, the pH increases. The normal plasma pH ranges from 7.35 to 7.45, with an average of 7.4. A plasma pH of less than 7.35 is called **acidosis**. A plasma pH of more than 7.45 is called **alkalosis** (Fig. 21–3).

Where the Acid (H^+) Comes From

Most of the hydrogen ions come from the body's chemical reactions during metabolism. For instance, when glucose is metabolized in the presence of oxygen, it produces carbon dioxide (CO_2), water, and energy. The CO_2 combines with water and forms carbonic acid. When glucose is metabolized in the absence of oxygen, it forms lactic acid. When fatty acids are metabolized very quickly, they yield ketoacids. Finally, when proteins are metabolized, some of them yield sulfuric acid. All these acids are produced by metabolizing cells. To maintain acid-base balance, the body must eliminate the acids.

How the Body Regulates pH

Three mechanisms work together to regulate pH: buffers, respirations, and kidney function (see Fig. 21–3B).

Buffers

The buffer system is the first line of defense in the regulation of pH. A **buffer** (bŭf′ər) is a chemical substance that prevents large changes in pH. There are two parts to a buffer, called a buffer pair. The **buffer pair** consists of a "taker" and a "giver" and works like this. If H^+ concentration in the blood increases, the "taker" part of the buffer removes H^+ from the blood. If the H^+ concentration decreases, the "giver" part of the buffer donates H^+ to the blood. By removing or adding H^+, the buffer pair can maintain a normal blood pH. The body has numerous buffer systems. The most important are the bicarbonate buffers, phosphate buffers, hemoglobin, and plasma proteins.

Respiration

The respiratory system is the second line of defense in the regulation of pH. What does breathing have to do with pH? To answer this question, you must understand the following chemical reaction:

$$CO_2 + H_2O \rightleftharpoons H_2CO_3 \rightleftharpoons H^+ + HCO_3^-$$

The reaction (reading from left to right) says this: carbon dioxide (CO_2) combines with water (H_2O) to form carbonic acid (H_2CO_3). Carbonic acid dissociates to form hydrogen ion (H^+) and bicarbonate (HCO_3^-). The important point is this: The reaction shows that carbon dioxide acts as an acid because it donates H^+. The respiratory system can control H^+ production because it regulates the plasma concentrations of carbon dioxide.

A

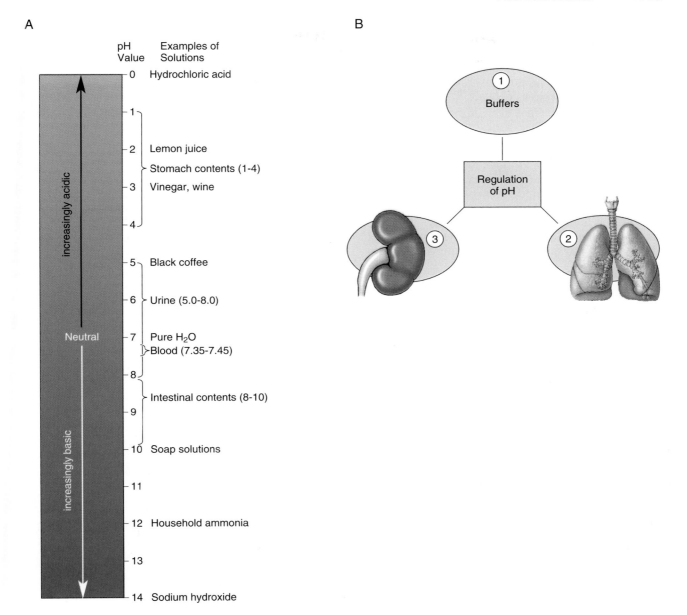

pH Value	Examples of Solutions
0	Hydrochloric acid
1	
2	Lemon juice
	Stomach contents (1-4)
3	Vinegar, wine
4	
5	Black coffee
6	Urine (5.0-8.0)
7	Pure H$_2$O
	Blood (7.35-7.45)
8	
	Intestinal contents (8-10)
9	
10	Soap solutions
11	
12	Household ammonia
13	
14	Sodium hydroxide

increasingly acidic

Neutral

increasingly basic

B

1 Buffers

Regulation of pH

3

2

FIGURE 21–3 ● Acid-base balance. A, pH scale showing the range of pH readings from acid (pH 0) to base (pH 14). B, Regulation of pH by buffers, respirations, and kidney function.

HOW INCREASING THE RESPIRATORY RATE INCREASES PH. By increasing respiratory rate, the body exhales, or blows off, carbon dioxide. The decrease in carbon dioxide causes the reaction (above) to move from right to left. (Read the reaction from right to left.) H$^+$ combines with HCO$_3^-$ to form H$_2$CO$_3$, which then forms CO$_2$ and H$_2$O. The CO$_2$ is then exhaled. What is accomplished by blowing off CO$_2$? The amount of H$^+$ decreases, and the pH increases.

HOW DECREASING THE RESPIRATORY RATE DECREASES PH. By decreasing the respiratory rate, the body retains carbon dioxide. (Read the reaction from left to right.) The CO$_2$ combines with H$_2$O to form H$_2$CO$_3$, which then forms H$^+$ and HCO$_3^-$. The increase in H$^+$ causes the pH to decrease. Note that CO$_2$ retention causes the formation of acid (H$^+$) and a decrease in pH.

HOW THE RESPIRATORY SYSTEM KNOWS. How does the respiratory system know that it should increase or decrease the respiratory rate? The medulla, the respiratory center in the brain, senses changes in H$^+$ concentration. As plasma H$^+$ concentration increases, the respiratory center is stimulated. The respiratory center then increases the rate and depth of breathing, thereby increasing the excretion of carbon dioxide by the lungs.

As plasma H^+ concentration decreases, the medullary respiratory center sends a slow-down signal, thereby decreasing the rate of breathing and the excretion of carbon dioxide by the lungs. As carbon dioxide accumulates in the plasma, it forms H^+ and decreases pH.

Kidneys

The kidneys are the third line of defense in the regulation of pH. The kidneys help regulate pH by reabsorbing or excreting H^+ as needed. The kidneys also help regulate bicarbonate (HCO_3^-), a major buffer. The kidneys can reabsorb bicarbonate when it is needed and can eliminate bicarbonate in the urine. Because the kidneys are major H^+ eliminators, patients in kidney failure are generally acidotic.

Acid-Base Imbalances

When the body is unable to regulate pH, acid-base imbalances result. The acid-base imbalances in the blood are called acidosis and alkalosis. These imbalances are common and often life-threatening (Table 21–2).

Acidosis

A decrease in plasma pH below 7.35 is acidosis. (Remember: An increase in the plasma H^+ concentration results in a decrease in pH.) The two types of acidosis are respiratory acidosis and metabolic acidosis. **Respiratory acidosis** (rĕs'pər-ə-tōr"ē ăs"ĭ-dō'sĭs) is caused by any condition that decreases the effectiveness of the respiratory system or causes prolonged **hypoventilation** (hī"pō-vĕn"tĭl-ā'shən) (inadequate air intake). For example, chronic lung disease (emphysema), high doses of narcotics, splinting of the chest, and injury to the medulla may all cause a decrease in respiratory activity. The hypoventilation, in turn, increases the plasma levels of CO_2 (Fig. 21–4).

To understand the effect of hypoventilation on pH, refer to the reaction below, reading the reaction from left to right.

$$CO_2 + H_2O \rightleftharpoons H_2CO_3 \rightleftharpoons H^+ + HCO_3^-$$

The CO_2 combines with H_2O to form $H_2CO_3^-$, which then forms H^+ and HCO_3^-. What has happened? The excess carbon dioxide has produced excess acid (H^+) and lowered the pH. In other words, CO_2 retention (hypoventilation) causes acidosis. Because the acidosis is caused by a respiratory dysfunction, it is classified as a respiratory acidosis.

How does the body try to correct respiratory acidosis? First, the buffer systems remove some of the excess H^+. Then the kidneys excrete some H^+. (The ability of the kidneys to correct respiratory

acidosis is called the renal compensation of respiratory acidosis. The respiratory system, however, cannot correct this pH imbalance, because it is the dysfunctional respiratory system that is causing the acidosis.)

Metabolic acidosis (mĕt"ə-bŏl'ĭk ăs"ĭ-dō'sĭs) is a decrease in pH due to nonrespiratory conditions. For instance, kidney disease, uncontrolled

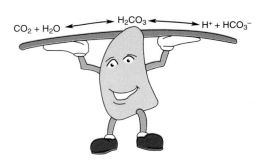

Normal lung maintains healthy acid–base balance.

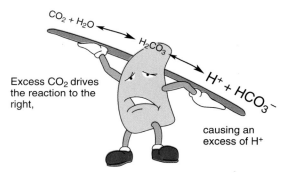

Excess CO_2 drives the reaction to the right, causing an excess of H^+

A lung that hypoventilates can cause respiratory acidosis

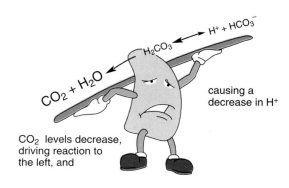

CO_2 levels decrease, driving reaction to the left, and causing a decrease in H^+

A lung that hyperventilates can cause respiratory alkalosis

FIGURE 21–4 • Acid-base balance. The lungs play an important role in acid-base balance. Hypoventilation causes respiratory acidosis. Hyperventilation causes respiratory alkalosis.

Table 21•2 pH IMBALANCES

IMBALANCE	CAUSES	COMPENSATIONS
Acidosis (pH < 7.35)		
Respiratory acidosis	Any condition that causes hypoventilation (chronic lung disease such as emphysema, asthma, splinting of the chest, high doses of narcotic drugs, myasthenia gravis)	Kidneys excrete H^+ and reabsorb HCO_3^- (renal compensation for respiratory acidosis)
Metabolic acidosis	Kidney disease, diarrhea, diabetic ketoacidosis, lactic acidosis, and vomiting of intestinal contents	Increased respiratory rate to blow off CO_2; Kussmaul respirations (respiratory compensation for metabolic acidosis)
Alkalosis (pH > 7.45)		
Respiratory alkalosis	Any condition that causes hyperventilation (anxiety)	Kidneys retain H^+ and excrete HCO_3^- (renal compensation for respiratory alkalosis)
Metabolic alkalosis	Persistent vomiting of stomach contents (loss of HCl), gastric suctioning, overingestion of antacids and bicarbonate-containing drugs	Decreased respiratory activity to retain CO_2 (respiratory compensation for metabolic alkalosis)

Do You Know...

Why does acidosis cause potassium (K^+) to move out of the cells into the blood?

As the amount of H^+ increases in the blood (acidosis), H^+ moves into the body cells. In exchange for the inward movement of H^+, the cell expels K^+ into the blood. The expulsion of K^+ can cause a dangerous hyperkalemia. In diabetic ketoacidosis, the acidosis causes the shift of the H^+ and K^+ across the cell membrane. The K^+ in the blood is gradually eliminated in the urine as the patient undergoes diuresis. When the patient is treated with insulin, the blood pH is gradually restored. As the acidosis gradually improves, the H^+ leaves the cell and enters the plasma in exchange for K^+. The movement of the K^+ back into the cell causes a decrease in blood K^+, and the patient becomes hypokalemic. Hypokalemia can cause life-threatening cardiac dysrhythmias. It is therefore important to closely monitor the patient's K^+ levels.

Do You Know...

Why does a person with diabetic ketoacidosis have breath with a fruity odor and Kussmaul respirations?

A person with uncontrolled diabetes rapidly and incompletely metabolizes fatty acids. This process results in the formation of ketone bodies. One of the ketone bodies is acetone; the other two are strong acids. The acetone has a fruity odor. Thus, when the diabetic patient exhales, you may detect a fruity odor on the patient's breath. The strong ketoacids cause an acidosis (here also called ketoacidosis). As the H^+ concentration increases, the acid stimulates the respiratory center in the brain to increase the rate and depth of respirations. This respiratory effect is called *Kussmaul respirations*. These are the body's attempt to correct and compensate for the acidosis by eliminating carbon dioxide.

diabetes mellitus, prolonged vomiting of intestinal contents (with loss of bicarbonate), and severe diarrhea (with loss of bicarbonate) are common causes of metabolic acidosis. A patient with poor kidney function is unable to excrete H^+ and becomes acidotic. A patient with uncontrolled diabetes mellitus produces excess ketoacids that overwhelm the buffer systems, accumulate in the plasma, and cause ketoacidosis.

How does the body try to correct metabolic acidosis? First, the buffer system removes some of the excess H^+. Second, the respiratory system helps remove excess H^+ through **hyperventilation** (hī″pər-ven″tĭl-ā′shən) or **Kussmaul respirations** (kōōs′mōl rĕs″pə-rā′shənz). Hyperventilation decreases plasma CO_2 and causes the reaction to move from right to left. To understand the effect of hyperventilation on pH, read the reaction from right to left.

$$CO_2 + H_2O \rightleftharpoons H_2CO_3 \rightleftharpoons H^+ + HCO_3^-$$

The H^+ combines with HCO_3^- to form H_2CO_3, which then forms CO_2 and H_2O. The CO_2 is then

445

exhaled. The hyperventilation decreases the amount of H^+ in the plasma, thereby increasing pH. (The increased respiratory activity is called the respiratory compensation for metabolic acidosis.)

Alkalosis

An increase in plasma pH above 7.45 is alkalosis. The two types of alkalosis are respiratory alkalosis and metabolic alkalosis. Respiratory alkalosis develops from hyperventilation and the resulting decrease in plasma CO_2. Common causes of respiratory alkalosis include anxiety and aspirin (salicylate) poisoning. Any condition that causes hyperventilation causes **respiratory alkalosis** (rĕs′pər-ə-tōr″ē ăl″kə-lō′sĭs).

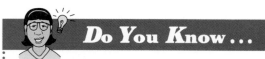

Do You Know...

Why might an overly anxious person feel numbness and tingling?

An anxious person often hyperventilates, causing a respiratory alkalosis. Calcium is less soluble in alkalotic blood. Consequently, the plasma levels of calcium decrease. Because calcium is necessary for normal nerve conduction, nerve function is impaired, and the person experiences numbness and tingling. If the person continues to hyperventilate, the plasma levels of calcium may decline so much that an episode of hypocalcemic tetany may occur.

The body tries to correct respiratory alkalosis by the buffers and the kidneys. The buffers donate H^+ to the plasma, thereby decreasing pH. The kidneys decrease the excretion of H^+; H^+ retention decreases pH. The kidneys also increase the excretion of bicarbonate, thereby excreting a basic or alkaline urine. The ability of the kidneys to correct respiratory alkalosis is called the renal compensation of respiratory alkalosis. The respiratory system cannot correct this pH disturbance because it is the overactivity, or hyperventilation, of the respiratory system that is causing the alkalosis.

Metabolic alkalosis (mĕt″ə-bŏl′ĭk ăl″kə-lō′sĭs) is an increase in pH caused by nonrespiratory disorders. Metabolic alkalosis can be caused by overuse of antacid and bicarbonate-containing drugs, persistent vomiting of stomach contents (loss of HCl), and frequent nasogastric suctioning (loss of HCl). The body tries to correct metabolic alkalosis through buffers, the kidneys, and the respiratory system. The buffers donate H^+, thereby decreasing pH. The kidneys decrease their excretion of H^+ and reabsorb base (bicarbonate). Finally, the respiratory system corrects the pH by

hypoventilation. Hypoventilation increases plasma CO_2 and causes the reaction to move from left to right. To understand the effect of hypoventilation on pH, refer to the reaction below, reading from left to right

$$CO_2 + H_2O \rightleftharpoons H_2CO_3 \rightleftharpoons H^+ + HCO_3^-$$

The CO_2 combines with H_2O to form H_2CO_3, which, in turn, forms $H^+ + HCO_3^-$. Hypoventilation increases CO_2, which in turn increases H^+ and decreases pH.

Note that the respiratory system can both cause a pH imbalance and help correct a nonrespiratory pH imbalance. Similarly, the kidneys can both cause and correct pH imbalances. The ability of the lungs and the kidneys to correct a pH imbalance is called its compensatory function.

✳ **SUM IT UP!** Plasma H^+ concentration is expressed as pH. The normal plasma pH is 7.4 (the range is 7.35 to 7.45). It is precisely regulated by three mechanisms: buffers, respirations, and kidney function. Acid-base balance is essential for the proper functioning of millions of chemical reactions in the body. Thus acid-base imbalances pose a serious threat to health. The imbalances are classified as either acidosis, a plasma pH less than 7.35 (respiratory and metabolic), or alkalosis, a plasma pH greater than 7.45 (respiratory and metabolic).

As You Age

1. As the kidneys age, the tubules become less responsive to antidiuretic hormone (ADH) and tend to lose too much water. The excess water loss is accompanied by a decrease in the thirst mechanism. As a result, the elderly person is prone to dehydration.

2. The ability to reabsorb glucose and sodium is also diminished. The presence of excess solute (sodium and glucose) in the urine contributes to excess urination and water loss. In addition, impaired reabsorption of glucose interferes with blood glucose monitoring in diabetes.

3. The kidney tubules are less efficient in the secretion of ions, including the hydrogen ion (H^+). As a result, the elderly person experiences difficulty in correcting acid-base imbalances.

4. With immobility and diminished exercise, calcium moves from the bones into the renal tubules. There the calcium precipitates, causing kidney stones.

Disorders Resulting From Fluid and Electrolyte Imbalance

Dehydration	A condition in which the water content of the body is decreased below normal. Dehydration develops when water output exceeds water intake and commonly occurs in conditions such as excessive sweating, vomiting, diarrhea, and overuse of diuretics.
Potassium imbalances	Common and often life-threatening imbalances. Hypokalemia is a decrease in the amount of potassium in the blood and is usually due to prolonged diarrhea and the overuse of diuretics. Hyperkalemia is an increase in the amount of potassium in the blood. Common causes include impaired renal function, tissue injury, and the use of drugs such as potassium-sparing diuretics.
Sodium imbalances	Increased or decreased plasma levels of sodium. Hypernatremia is an increase in plasma sodium. It is most often seen in patients with high fever and excessive water loss through evaporation. Hypernatremia also accompanies sustained decreased secretion of ADH. Hyponatremia is a decrease in plasma sodium and is commonly seen with excess sweating, vomiting, diarrhea, and some forms of renal disease. Excess ingestion of water can dilute the plasma, thereby decreasing tonicity (hyponatremia) and causing water intoxication.

Summary Outline

I. Distribution of Fluids and Electrolytes
Fluids and electrolytes must be distributed in the body compartments in the correct volumes and concentrations.

A. Major Fluid Compartments
1. The two major fluid compartments are the intracellular compartment (63% of the water) and the extracellular compartment (37% of the water).
2. The extracellular compartment includes interstitial fluid, intravascular fluid (plasma), lymph, and transcellular fluid.

B. Composition of Body Fluids
1. Intracellular fluid contains high concentrations of potassium (K^+), phosphate (PO_4), and magnesium (Mg^{++}).
2. Extracellular fluid contains a high concentration of sodium (Na^+), chloride (Cl^-), and bicarbonate (HCO_3^-).

II. Water Balance: Intake Equals Output
A. Intake
1. The average intake of water is 2500 mL per 24 hours.
2. The primary regulator of fluid intake is thirst.

B. Output
1. The average output of water is 2500 mL in 24 hours.
2. Water is excreted by the kidneys (60%), skin and lungs (28%), digestive tract (6%), and sweat (6%).

III. Electrolyte Balance
A. Sodium (Na^+)
1. Sodium is the chief extracellular cation.
2. Sodium is necessary for nerve-muscle conduction and helps maintain fluid balance.
3. Sodium is primarily regulated by aldosterone.

B. Potassium (K^+)
1. Potassium is the chief intracellular cation.
2. Potassium is necessary for nerve-muscle conduction.
3. Potassium is primarily regulated by aldosterone.

C. Calcium (Ca^{++})
1. Calcium is widely distributed throughout the body but is found primarily in teeth and bones.
2. Calcium strengthens bones and teeth and is necessary for muscle contraction, nerve-muscle conduction, and blood clotting.
3. Calcium is primarily regulated by parathyroid hormone.

D. Magnesium (Mg^{++}) and Chloride (Cl^-)
1. Magnesium performs important functions in heart, muscles, and nerves.
2. Chloride is the chief extracellular anion.
3. Chloride usually follows Na^+.

continued

Summary Outline *continued*

III. Electrolyte Balance, *continued*

E. Bicarbonate (HCO_3^-)

1. Bicarbonate is a major extracellular anion.
2. Bicarbonate plays three important roles: it is the major form in which CO_2 is transported, it acts as a base (alkaline substance), and it plays an important role in acid-base balance.

IV. Acid-Base Balance

A. pH

1. The pH refers to the concentration of H^+.
2. The normal blood pH is 7.35 to 7.45. If blood pH is less than 7.35, the person is in acidosis. If blood pH is greater than 7.45, the person is in alkalosis.

B. Regulation of Blood pH

1. Blood pH is regulated by three mechanisms: buffers, the respiratory system, and the kidneys.
2. Buffers (the buffer pair) can donate or remove H^+.
3. The respiratory system affects pH by regulating CO_2. By blowing off CO_2, the respiratory system lowers H^+ concentration (increases pH). By retaining CO_2, the respiratory system increases H^+ concentration (lowers pH).

4. The kidneys can vary their excretion of H^+. If the body has excess H^+, the kidneys excrete H^+. If the body does not have enough H^+, the kidneys retain H^+. The kidney can also vary its intake of bicarbonate, an important buffer.

V. Acid-Base Imbalances

A. Acidosis

1. Acidosis means that the blood pH is less than 7.35.
2. Respiratory acidosis is caused by hypoventilation (eg, emphysema, splinting of the chest, narcotics).
3. Metabolic acidosis is due to nonrespiratory causes, including kidney disease, uncontrolled diabetes mellitus, diarrhea, and lactic acid production.

B. Alkalosis

1. Alkalosis means that the blood pH is greater than 7.45.
2. Respiratory alkalosis is caused by hyperventilation (eg, anxiety).
3. Metabolic alkalosis is caused by nonrespiratory conditions, including overingestion of antacids and bicarbonate-containing drugs, severe vomiting of stomach contents, and prolonged gastric suctioning.

Review Your Knowledge

1. How much of an adult's body weight is water? Is there more water in the intracellular compartment or the extracellular compartment?

2. In what four locations is extracellular fluid found? Which portion of extracellular fluid contains the most protein?

3. What is the relationship of water intake and output? What is the average 24-hour intake and output?

4. List four routes through which water can leave the body. Which organ in the body is the primary regulator of water output?

5. What hormones regulate water balance in the body?

6. What is the main extracellular cation? What is the main intracellular cation? Which ion is necessary for bone and teeth formation? What is the main extracellular anion? What is an important anion in acid-base balance?

7. Which two ions play an important role in nerve impulse conduction? Which hormone regulates sodium and potassium concentration? What hormone regulates plasma levels of calcium? Which ion helps remove excess acid from the body?

8. Why is the regulation of pH so important to the body? What is the relationship of H^+ to seizures and comatose states?

9. How is acidosis different from alkalosis? Where does acid (H^+) in the body come from?

10. Name three mechanisms that work together to regulate pH.

11. List four important buffer systems in the body.

12. What is the relationship of carbon dioxide to acids? What happens to H^+ concentration and pH when carbon dioxide accumulates in the plasma?

13. How do the kidneys help regulate pH? Why are patients in kidney failure usually acidotic?

Review Your Knowledge *continued*

14. List two ways in which the body tries to correct respiratory acidosis. What are four causes of metabolic acidosis? What effect does hyperventilation have on pH?

15. How does the body try to correct respiratory alkalosis? What are three causes of respiratory alkalosis?

16. What is meant by the compensatory function of the lungs and kidneys?

17. If a person is dehydrated, what happens to skin turgor?

18. How do Kussmaul respirations help the body compensate for metabolic acidosis?

19. What types of intravenous infusions are given to persons deficient in body fluids?

20. How is hypokalemia related to the administration of diuretics? How can the administration of diuretics help relieve hypoxia?

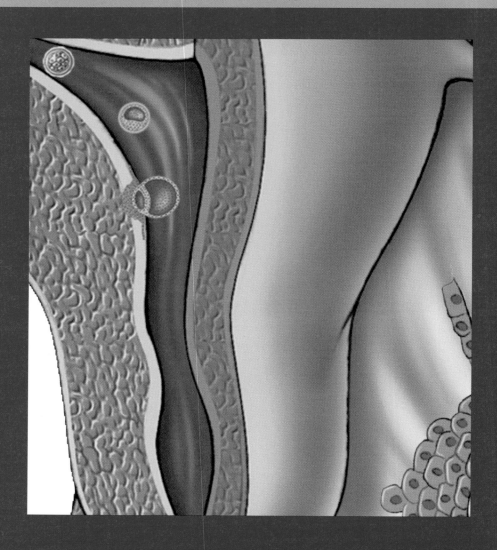

••• Key Terms

Cervix (sûr′vĭks)
Endometrium (ĕn″dō-mē′trē-əm)
Epididymis (ĕp″ĭ-dĭd′ə-mĭs)
Estrogen (ĕs′trō-jən)
Fallopian tube (fə-lō′pē-ən tōōb)
Gonad (gō′năd)
Gonadotropin (gō-năd′ə-trōp′ĭn)
Menopause (mĕn′ə-pôz)
Menses (mĕn′sēz)
Myometrium (mī″ō-mē′trē-əm)

Ovarian follicle (ō-vâr′ē-ən fŏl′ĭ-kəl)
Ovulation (ŏv″ū-lā′shən)
Progesterone (prō-jĕs′tə-rōn)
Prostate gland (prŏs′tāt glănd)
Scrotum (skrō′təm)
Semen (sē′mən)
Spermatogenesis (spûr″mə-tō-jĕn′ĭ-sĭs)
Testes (tĕs′tēz)
Testosterone (tĕs-tŏs′tə-rōn)
Vas deferens (văs′ dĕf′ər-ĕnz″)

••• Selected terms in bold type in this chapter are defined in the Glossary.

22

REPRODUCTIVE SYSTEM

Objectives

1. List the structures and function of the male and female reproductive systems.

2. Describe the structure and function of the testes.

3. Explain the process of sperm formation.

4. Describe the structure and function of the male genital ducts: epididymis, vas deferens, ejaculatory duct, and urethra.

5. Describe the accessory glands that add secretions to the semen: seminal vesicles, prostate gland, and bulbourethral glands.

6. Describe the male and female sexual response.

7. Describe the hormonal control of male reproduction, including the effects of testosterone.

8. Describe the structure and function of the ovaries, including the ovarian follicle, ovulation, and ovarian hormones.

9. Describe the structure and function of the female genital tract: fallopian tubes, uterus, and vagina.

10. Explain the hormonal control of the female reproductive cycle.

11. Describe common methods of birth control.

Few biologic drives are as strong as the urge to reproduce. As everyone knows and appreciates, human reproduction is **sexual,** meaning that both a female and a male partner are required. In contrast, reproduction in single-cell organisms is **asexual,** meaning that no partner is required. They simply divide by themselves. Think of how different your life would be in an asexual environment!

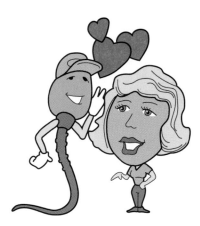

To carry out its role, the reproductive system performs two functions. It produces, nurtures, and transports ova and sperm, and it secretes hormones. The reproductive organs include the primary reproductive organs and the secondary reproductive organs. The **primary reproductive organs** are the **gonads** (gō′nădz). The female gonads are the ovaries. The male gonads are the testes.

The gonads perform two functions: they secrete hormones, and they produce the **gametes.** The gametes are the ova (eggs) and the sperm. All other organs, ducts, and glands in the reproductive system are **secondary,** or **accessory, reproductive organs.** The secondary reproductive structures nourish and transport the eggs and sperm. They also provide a safe and nourishing environment for the fertilized eggs.

MALE REPRODUCTIVE SYSTEM

The male reproductive system performs three roles. It produces, nourishes, and transports sperm. It deposits the sperm within the female reproductive tract, and it secretes hormones. Figure 22–1A shows the organs of the male reproductive tract.

Testes

The **testes** (tĕs′tēz), or **testicles,** are the male gonads. They perform two functions: the production of sperm and the secretion of the male hormone, **testosterone** (tĕs-tŏs′tə-rōn) (see Fig. 22–1A). The two oval testes are located outside the abdominal cavity and are suspended in a sac between the thighs called the **scrotum** (skrō′təm). Each testis (singular) is surrounded by a tough fibrous connective tissue capsule.

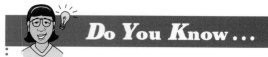

Why did Aristotle call the testicle the *orchis*?

The root of the orchid plant is olive shaped; in Greek the shape is called an *orchis.* Noticing the similarity between the shape of the orchid root and the testicles, Aristotle dubbed the testicle *orchis.* The word *orchis* is still used in medical terms. For example, orchitis refers to inflammation of the testicles, and orchiectomy refers to the surgical removal of the testicles. The word *testis* comes from the Latin and means to bear witness to. The word *testes* shares the same Latin root with the word *testify.* In ancient Rome, only men could bear witness, or testify, in a public forum. To show the importance of their testimony, they held their testicles as they spoke.

The testes begin their development within the abdominal cavity but usually descend into the scrotum during the last 2 months of fetal development. Failure of the testes to descend into the scrotum is called **cryptorchidism,** a condition that can result in sterility if it is left untreated. Why are undescended testicles associated with infertility? Sperm cannot live at body temperature (37°C [98.6°F]); instead, they prefer the cooler temperature of the scrotum, about 34°C (93.2°F). To avoid infertility, a surgeon will pull the undescended testicles into the scrotum.

The wearing of tight underwear and jeans can also elevate the temperature in the testes, thereby lowering sperm count. What happens when the outside, environmental temperature becomes excessively cold during the winter months? The scrotum, with the assistance of the cremaster muscle, pulls the testes close to the body, thereby keeping the sperm warm.

The testis is divided into about 250 smaller units called **lobules** (Fig. 22–2A). Each lobule contains seminiferous tubules and interstitial cells. The tightly coiled **seminiferous tubules** form sperm. The **interstitial cells** lie between the seminiferous tubules and produce the male hormones called **androgens.** The most important androgen is testosterone. Thus, the testes produce both sperm and testosterone.

A

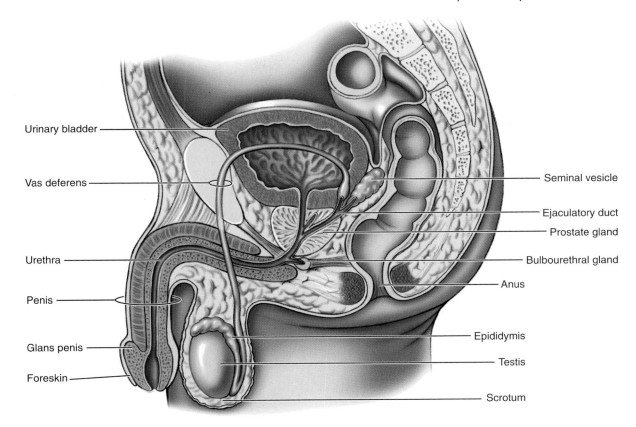

Urinary bladder

Vas deferens

Urethra

Penis

Glans penis

Foreskin

Seminal vesicle

Ejaculatory duct

Prostate gland

Bulbourethral gland

Anus

Epididymis

Testis

Scrotum

B

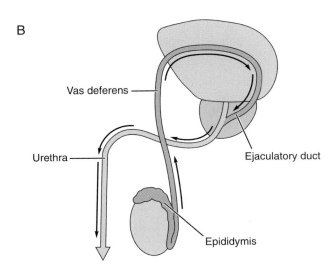

Vas deferens

Urethra

Ejaculatory duct

Epididymis

FIGURE 22-1 • A, Male reproductive organs. B, The pathway that sperm follow from the testes through the urethra.

Cells Involved in Sperm Formation

Each day a man makes millions of sperm. Sperm are formed by the epithelium of the seminiferous tubules. The seminiferous tubules contain two types of cells, spermatogenic cells and supporting cells. The spermatogenic cells are sperm-producing cells. The supporting cells have several names: sustentacular cells, Sertoli cells,

and "nurse" cells. The supporting cells support, nourish, and regulate the spermatogenic cells.

Spermatogenesis

Spermatogenesis (spŭr″mə-tō-jĕn′ĭ-sĭs) is the formation of sperm. The undifferentiated spermatogenic cells are called **spermatogonia.** Each spermatogonium contains 46 chromosomes, the

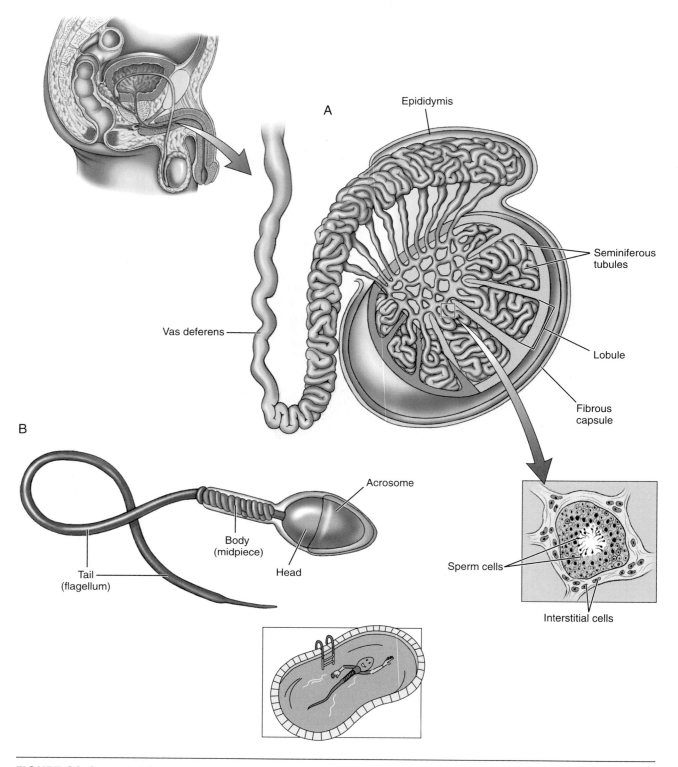

FIGURE 22–2 ● A, Male gonad. The testis consists of lobules containing seminiferous tubules surrounded by interstitial cells. Note the connection with the epididymis and vas deferens. B, Sperm showing the head, body, and tail. The long tail (flagellum) enables the sperm to swim.

normal number of chromosomes for human body cells. Under the influence of testosterone, the spermatogonia enlarge to become **primary spermatocytes.** The primary spermatocytes divide by a special type of cell division called **meiosis.** The important point about meiosis is this: Meiosis reduces the number of chromosomes by one half, from 46 to 23. Thus, a sperm has only 23 chromosomes. When the sperm unites with an egg, which also has only 23 chromosomes, the fertilized egg contains 46 chromosomes, the normal number for human body cells. Newly formed sperm are not functional and must undergo several maturational changes.

A sperm looks like a tadpole (Fig. 22–2B). The mature sperm has three parts: a head, a body, and a tail. The **head** is primarily a nucleus. The nucleus is important because it contains the genetic information. The front part of the head has a specialized structure called the **acrosome,** which contains enzymes that help the sperm penetrate the egg at the time of fertilization. The **body,** or midpiece, of the sperm is a spiral-shaped structure that contains many mitochondria and supplies the sperm with the energy needed for the "big swim." The tail of the sperm is a flagellum. Its whip-like movements enable the sperm to swim. Most sperm live only hours after being deposited in the female reproductive tract, but the hardier ones may survive for up to 3 days.

✳ **SUM IT UP!** The purpose of the reproductive system is to produce offspring. Human reproduction is achieved sexually through the union of an egg and a sperm. The primary reproductive organs are the gonads: the ovaries in the female, and the testes in the male. The gonads produce the gametes. The ovaries produce the female gametes (eggs). The testes produce the male gametes (sperm). The mature egg and sperm each contain 23 chromosomes. Upon union, the fertilized egg contains 46 chromosomes, the number of chromosomes that human cells contain.

Genital Ducts

As the sperm form, they gather in the seminiferous tubules and then move into a series of **genital ducts,** where they mature. They are then transported from the testes to the outside of the body. The ducts include two epididymides, two vas (ductus) deferens, two ejaculatory ducts, and one urethra.

Epididymis

The **epididymis** (ĕp″ĭ-dĭd′ə-mĭs) is the first part of the duct system. It is about 20 feet (6 meters) in length, is tightly coiled, and sits along the top and posterior side of the testis (see Fig. 22–1A). While in the epididymis, the sperm mature, becoming motile and fertile. The walls of the epididymis contract and push the sperm into the next structure, the vas deferens.

Vas Deferens and Ejaculatory Ducts

The **vas deferens** (văs′ dĕf′ər-ĕnz″) is continuous with the epididymis. It ascends as part of the **spermatic cord** through the **inguinal canal** in

the groin region into the abdominopelvic cavity. (There are two spermatic cords, one coming from the right and one from the left groin region.) In addition to the vas deferens, the spermatic cord includes blood vessels, lymphatic vessels, nerves, muscles, and connective tissue.

As the vas deferens courses through the pelvic cavity, it curves over the urinary bladder and joins with the duct of the seminal vesicle to form the **ejaculatory duct** (see Fig. 22–1A). The two ejaculatory ducts, from the right and left sides, pass through the prostate gland and join with the single urethra.

Urethra

The urethra extends from the base of the urinary bladder to the tip of the penis. The male urethra serves two organ systems, the reproductive system and the urinary system. The urethra carries urine from the urinary bladder to the outside. It also carries semen from the ejaculatory ducts to the outside. While serving two purposes, however, the urethra can only do one thing at a time. It passes either urine or semen, never both simultaneously.

Accessory Glands

Various secretions are added to the sperm as they travel through the genital ducts. The secretions come from three glands: the seminal vesicles, the prostate gland, and the bulbourethral glands (see Fig. 22–1A).

Seminal Vesicles

The seminal vesicles are located at the base of the bladder and secrete a thick yellowish material rich in substances such as fructose (sugar), vitamin C, and prostaglandins. These substances nourish and activate the sperm as they pass through the ducts.

Prostate Gland

The single doughnut-like **prostate gland** (prŏs′tāt glănd) encircles the prostatic urethra just below the bladder. The word *prostate* comes from the Greek, meaning one who stands before. The gland stands before the exit from the bladder into the urethra. The prostate gland secretes a milky alkaline substance that plays a role in increasing sperm motility. It also counteracts the acidic environment of the vagina and so helps protect the sperm as they enter the woman's body. During ejaculation, the smooth muscle of the prostate gland contracts and forces the secretions into the urethra.

Bulbourethral Glands

The bulbourethral glands, or Cowper glands, are tiny glands that secrete a thick mucus into the penile urethra. The mucus serves as a lubricant during sexual intercourse.

Semen

The mixture of sperm and the secretions of the accessory glands is called **semen** (sē′mən). About 60% of the volume of semen comes from the seminal vesicles. Most of the remainder of the volume comes from the prostate gland. Semen, or seminal fluid, is a milky-white liquid with an alkaline pH (7.2 to 7.6). The alkaline pH is important because sperm are sluggish in an acidic pH. Because the pH of the female vagina is acidic, the alkaline pH of semen neutralizes the acid in the vagina and therefore protects the sperm from the destructive effects of acid.

The secretions of the accessory glands perform several other functions: they nourish the sperm, aid in the transport of sperm, and lubricate the reproductive tract. The amount of semen per ejaculation is small, about 2 to 6 mL, or 1 teaspoon. The number of sperm per ejaculation, however, is impressive (50 to 100 million).

External Genitals

The external genitals (genitalia) of the male consist of the scrotum and the penis (see Fig. 22–1). The scrotum is a sac, or pouch of skin, that hangs loosely between the legs and contains the testes. This arrangement provides the testes with a temperature below body temperature.

The **penis** has two functions: it carries urine through the urethra to the outside of the body, and it acts as the organ of sexual intercourse (copulation). The penis deposits sperm in the female reproductive tract. The **shaft,** or **body,** of the penis contains three columns of erectile tissue and an enlarged tip called the **glans penis.** The opening of the urethra penetrates the glans penis.

The loose skin covering the penis extends downward and forms a cuff of skin around the glans called the **foreskin** or **prepuce.** Around puberty, small glands located in the foreskin and the glans secrete an oily substance. This secretion and the surrounding dead skin cells form a cheesy substance called **smegma.** As part of daily hygiene, a man should pull back the foreskin to remove the smegma. Occasionally, the foreskin is too tight and cannot be retracted. This condition is called **phimosis.**

The foreskin is often surgically removed after birth in a process called **circumcision.** While parents often have their sons circumcised to promote cleanliness, circumcision is also a religious ritual. In the United States, Jews and Muslims are the religious communities that typically perform circumcision.

Male Sexual Response: Erection, Emission, Ejaculation, and Orgasm

The urethra extends the length of the penis and is surrounded by three columns of erectile tissue. Erectile tissue is spongy. When a man is sexually stimulated, the parasympathetic nerves fire, the penile arteries dilate, and the erectile tissue fills with blood. The accumulation of blood in the erectile tissue causes the penis to enlarge and become rigid. This process is an **erection.** It enables the penis to penetrate the reproductive tract of the female. For a number of reasons, a man may be unable to achieve an erection and is said to have **erectile dysfunction.** (The older term is impotence.)

Orgasm refers to the pleasurable physiologic and psychologic sensations that occur at the height of sexual stimulation. Orgasm in the male is accompanied by emission and ejaculation. **Emission** is the movement of sperm and glandular secretions from the testes and genital ducts into the urethra, where they mix to form semen. Emission is caused by the influence of the sympathetic nervous system on the ducts, causing rhythmic peristaltic-type contractions.

Ejaculation is the expulsion of semen from the urethra to the outside. Ejaculation begins when the urethra fills with semen. Motor nerve impulses from the spinal cord stimulate the skeletal muscles at the base of the erectile columns in the penis to contract rhythmically. The rhythmic contraction provides the force necessary to expel the semen. The flow of semen during ejaculation is illustrated in Figure 22–1B. Immediately after ejaculation, sympathetic nerve impulses cause the penile arteries to constrict, thereby reducing blood flow into the penis. This process is accompanied by increased venous drainage of blood from the penis. As a consequence, the penis becomes flaccid and returns to its unstimulated size.

Male Sex Hormones

Effects of Testosterone

The male sex hormones are called androgens, the most important being testosterone. Most of the testosterone is secreted by the interstitial cells of the testes. A small amount is secreted by the adrenal cortex.

Secretion of testosterone begins during fetal development and continues at a very low level throughout childhood. When a boy reaches age 10 to 13, testosterone secretion increases rapidly, transforming the boy into a man. This phase in reproductive development is called **puberty.** After puberty, testosterone is secreted continuously throughout the life of the male.

Testosterone is necessary for the production of sperm and is responsible for the development of the male sex characteristics. The **primary sex characteristics** include the enlargement and development of the testes and the various accessory organs such as the penis. **Secondary sex characteristics** refer to special features of the male body and include the following:

- Increased growth of hair, particularly on the face (the beard), chest, axillary region, and pubic region
- Deepening of the voice due to enlargement of the larynx
- Thickening of the skin and increased activity of the oil and sweat glands; at puberty, the adolescent is faced with new challenges: acne and body odor
- Increased musculoskeletal growth and development of the male physique (broad shoulders and narrow waist)

Hormonal Control of Male Reproduction

The male reproductive system is controlled primarily by the hormones secreted by the hypothalamus, the anterior pituitary gland, and the testes. The hypothalamus secretes gonadotropin-releasing hormone (GnRH). This hormone, in turn, stimulates the anterior pituitary gland to secrete the **gonadotropins** (gō-năd″ə-trōp′ĭnz), **follicle-stimulating hormone (FSH),** and **luteinizing hormone (LH)** (Fig. 22–3). FSH promotes spermatogenesis by stimulating the spermatogenic cells to respond to testosterone. Note that spermatogenesis comes about through the combined action of FSH and testosterone. LH, also known as interstitial cell–stimulating hormone (ICSH) in the male, promotes the development of the interstitial cells of the testes and the secretion of testosterone.

After puberty, a negative feedback loop regulates testosterone production. When the level of testosterone in the blood increases, it causes the hypothalamus and the anterior pituitary gland to decrease their hormonal secretions, thereby decreasing the production of testosterone. As blood levels of testosterone decrease, the anterior pituitary gland increases its secretion of LH (ICSH), thereby stimulating the interstitial cells to secrete testosterone once again. The negative feedback mechanism maintains constant blood levels of testosterone.

✳ **SUM IT UP!** Four hormones—GnRH, FSH, LH, and testosterone—control the male reproductive system. GnRH stimulates the anterior pituitary gland to secrete FSH and LH (ICSH). FSH and testosterone stimulate spermatogenesis. LH stimulates the secretion of testosterone. Finally, testosterone stimulates the development of the male secondary sex characteristics. A male looks male because of testosterone.

FIGURE 22–3 ● Control of sperm production and testosterone secretion. GnRH stimulates the secretion of FSH and LH. FSH stimulates sperm production. LH stimulates the secretion of testosterone. The secretion of testosterone is controlled by negative feedback. The testosterone feeds back and shuts off GnRH and LH.

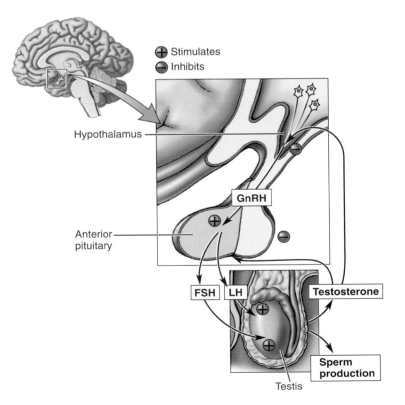

FEMALE REPRODUCTIVE SYSTEM

The female reproductive system produces eggs, secretes hormones, and nurtures and protects a developing baby during the 9 months of pregnancy. Figure 22–4A shows the organs of the female reproductive system.

Ovaries

The **ovaries** are the female gonads. Two almond-shaped ovaries, located on either side of the uterus in the pelvic cavity, are anchored in place by several ligaments, including the ovarian and the broad ligaments. The ovaries, while not attached directly to the fallopian tubes, are close to them.

Egg Development: The Ovarian Follicle

Within the ovary are many tiny sac-like structures called **ovarian follicles** (ō-vâr′ē-ən fŏl′ĭ-kəlz). A female is born with two million follicles. This number steadily declines with age, however, so that at puberty only about 400,000 follicles remain. Of these, only about 400 follicles ever fully mature, because a female usually produces only one egg per month throughout her reproductive years. The production of eggs begins at puberty and continues until menopause, at about 45 to 55 years of age. As with sperm, the supply of eggs far exceeds the actual need. This is nature's way of ensuring future generations.

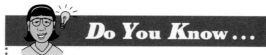

Do You Know...

What is in vitro fertilization?

In vitro fertilization refers to the fertilization of an egg that occurs in a test tube or a container other than the fallopian tube. The term *in vitro* literally means in glass. The fertilized egg is eventually implanted in the mother's uterus, where it will grow and develop for nine months.

Each ovarian follicle consists of an immature egg, called an **oocyte,** and cells surrounding the oocyte, called **follicular cells** (Fig. 22–4B). Beginning at puberty, several follicles mature, or ripen, every month, although usually only one fully matures. As the egg matures, it begins to undergo meiotic cell division, which will reduce the number of chromosomes by one-half, from 46 to 23. (Meiosis begins before fertilization and is completed after fertilization.)

At the same time, the follicle enlarges, a fluid-filled center is formed, and the follicular cells be-

Do You Know...

What do Plato, hysteria, and the concept of the wandering womb have in common?

Plato believed that the womb (uterus), if unused for a long period, became "indignant." This indignant womb then wandered around the body, inhibiting the body's spirit and causing disease. According to the male thinkers of the day, a woman was so thoroughly controlled by her wandering womb that she was considered irrational and prone to emotional outbursts and fits of hysteria. This belief was the reason that the womb was named the *hystera*. The term has persisted in medical terminology. For example, a hysterectomy refers to the surgical removal of the uterus.

gin to secrete estrogen. Lastly, the egg is surrounded by cells called the **zona pellucida** (inner) and **corona radiata** (outer). The mature ovarian follicle is known as the **graafian follicle.** The graafian follicle looks like a blister on the surface of the ovary that is ready to burst.

Ovulation

Once a month the ovarian follicle bursts. The ovary ejects a mature egg (ovum) with a surrounding layer of cells. This ejection phase is called **ovulation** (ŏv″ū-lā′shən). The egg travels from the surface of the ovary into the peritoneal cavity, where it is immediately swept into the fallopian tubes by the swishing motion of the **fimbriae** (finger-like projections at the ends of the fallopian tubes). The egg gradually travels through the fallopian tubes to the uterus. If the egg is fertilized, it implants in the uterine lining and grows into a baby. If the egg is not fertilized, the egg dies and is eliminated in the menstrual blood.

Once ovulation has occurred, the follicular cells that remain in the ovary develop into a glandular structure called the **corpus luteum** ("yellow body"). The corpus luteum secretes two hormones, large amounts of progesterone and smaller amounts of estrogen. If fertilization does not occur, the corpus luteum deteriorates in about 10 days and becomes known as the **corpus albicans** ("white body"). The dead corpus albicans is not capable of secreting hormones. If fertilization occurs, however, the corpus luteum does not deteriorate. It stays alive and continues to secrete its hormones until this role can be taken over by the placenta, a structure you will read about in Chapter 23.

Sometimes, after ovulation, the corpus luteum fills with fluid and forms an ovarian cyst. This condition usually resolves on its own, but it may become painful and require surgery.

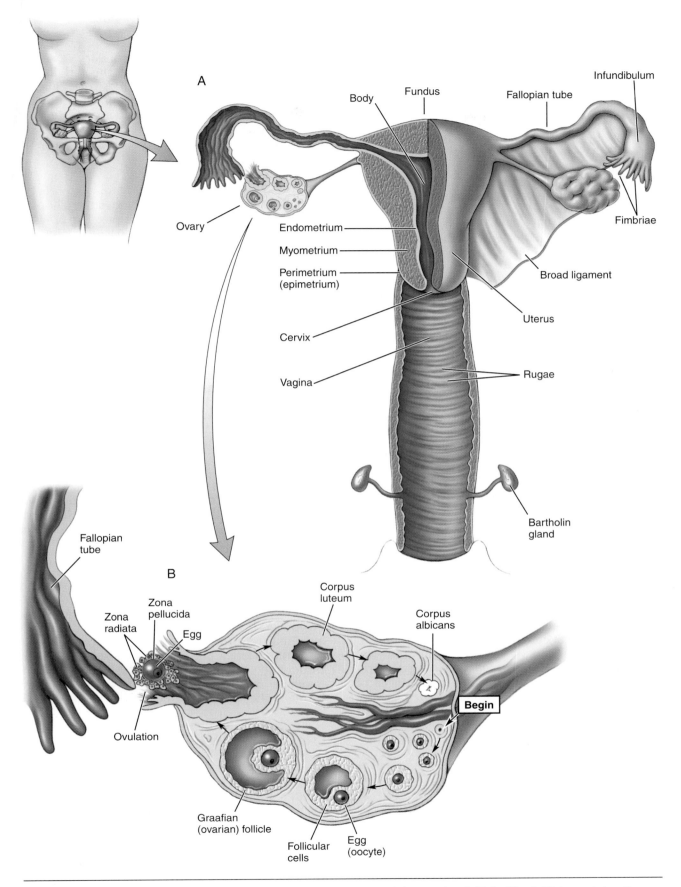

A

Fundus

Body

Fallopian tube

Infundibulum

Endometrium

Myometrium

Perimetrium
(epimetrium)

Cervix

Vagina

Ovary

Fimbriae

Broad ligament

Uterus

Rugae

Bartholin
gland

Fallopian
tube

B

Zona
radiata

Zona
pellucida

Egg

Ovulation

Corpus
luteum

Corpus
albicans

Begin

Graafian
(ovarian) follicle

Follicular
cells

Egg
(oocyte)

FIGURE 22–4 ● A, Female reproductive organs. B, Maturation of the ovarian follicle. The follicle contains the egg and follicular cells. The mature ovarian follicle is called the graafian follicle. At ovulation, the egg is expelled from the graafian follicle and is swept up into the fallopian tube. The follicular cells on the surface of the ovary form the corpus luteum. The corpus luteum deteriorates into the corpus albicans.

Ovarian Hormones

At puberty, the ovaries begin to secrete the sex hormones estrogen and progesterone. The follicular cells of the maturing follicles secrete estrogen, while the corpus luteum secretes large amounts of progesterone and smaller amounts of estrogen. These hormones transform the girl into a woman.

ESTROGEN. **Estrogen** (ĕs′trō-jən) is a term used for a group of similar hormones, the most important being estradiol. The correct term therefore is estrogens. We will use the conventional singular form, estrogen, however, understanding that it refers to the group of estrogen-related hormones.

Estrogen exerts two important effects: It promotes the maturation of the egg, and it helps develop the female secondary sex characteristics. Just as the male looks male because of testosterone, the female looks female because of estrogen. The feminizing effects of estrogen include

- Enlargement and development of the organs of the female reproductive system
- Enlargement and development of the breasts
- Deposition of fat beneath the skin, especially in the thighs, buttocks, and breasts
- Widening of the pelvis
- Onset of the menstrual cycle
- Closure of the epiphyseal discs in long bones, thereby stopping further growth in height.

PROGESTERONE. The corpus luteum secretes **progesterone** (prō-jĕs′tə-rōn). (Remember that the corpus luteum is the cluster of ovarian follicular cells that nourished the egg prior to ovulation.) Progesterone has three important effects: It works with estrogen in establishing the menstrual cycle, helps maintain pregnancy, and prepares the breasts for milk production during pregnancy, increasing their secretory capacity. Although the corpus luteum secretes enough progesterone to maintain pregnancy in the early months, the woman's body needs larger amounts of both estrogen and progesterone during the later stages of pregnancy. This role is performed by the placenta (see Chapter 23). Thus, most of the estrogen and progesterone secreted during pregnancy come from the placenta.

✻ **SUM IT UP!** The primary female reproductive organ is the ovary. Once a month, several ovarian follicles begin to ripen, or mature, although only one follicle usually fully matures. Each follicle contains an immature egg and estrogen-secreting follicular cells. Under the influence of LH, an egg is expelled from the mature graafian follicle. This event is ovulation. Following ovulation, follicular cells called the corpus luteum begin to secrete large amounts of progesterone. Thus, the ovary secretes both estrogen and progesterone. Estrogen helps mature the follicle and is primarily responsible for the secondary sex characteristics. Estrogen transforms the girl into a woman. Progesterone works with estrogen in controlling the menstrual cycle and plays an important role in preparing the reproductive system for pregnancy.

Genital Tract

The female genital tract includes the fallopian tubes, the uterus, and the vagina (see Fig. 22–4A).

Fallopian Tubes

The **fallopian tubes** (fə-lō′pē-ən tōōbz) are also called the **uterine tubes** or the **oviducts.** Each of the two fallopian tubes is about 10 cm (4 in) long. The tubes extend from either side of the uterus to the ovaries. The funnel-shaped end of the fallopian tube nearest the ovary is called the **infundibulum** and has finger-like projections called fimbriae. The fallopian tube does not attach directly to the ovary, but the fimbriae hang over the ovary, where their swishing motion sweeps the egg from the surface of the ovary into the fallopian tubes.

At ovulation, the fimbriae sweep the egg from the surface of the ovary into the fallopian tube. Once in the fallopian tube, the egg moves slowly toward the uterus. Because the egg cannot swim like sperm, peristaltic muscle contractions within the walls of the fallopian tubes move it forward. The swaying motion of the cilia of the cells lining the fallopian tubes also contribute to the egg's movement.

The fallopian tubes have two functions. First, the tube transports the egg from the ovary to the uterus. Second, the tube is the usual site of fertilization of the egg by the sperm. If fertilization does not occur, the egg deteriorates and is eventually excreted from the body in the menstrual flow. If fertilization does occur, the fertilized egg moves through the fallopian tube into the uterus, where it implants and grows into a baby. The journey through the fallopian tubes takes about 4 to 5 days.

Occasionally, the fertilized egg implants in the lining of the fallopian tube rather than in the uterus. This condition is an **ectopic pregnancy.** The word *ectopic* means in an abnormal site; a tubal pregnancy is therefore an ectopic pregnancy. An ectopic pregnancy usually results in a miscarriage. It causes maternal bleeding, possible hemorrhage, and even death.

Uterus

The **uterus,** or **womb,** is shaped like an upside-down pear and is located between the urinary bladder and the rectum. The **broad ligament** holds the uterus in place. The primary function of the uterus is to provide a safe and nurturing environment for the growing baby. It is the baby's cradle for 9 comfortable months. During pregnancy, the size of the uterus increases considerably. It must hold the growing baby and the placenta.

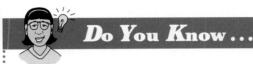

What are the spots on the outer surface of these organs?

These spots represent endometrial tissue adhering to the outer surface of the ovary, fallopian tube, rectum, and urinary bladder. How did the endometrial tissue get there? In some women, a portion of the menstrual discharge flows backward, into the fallopian tubes, and then into the pelvic cavity. The endometrial tissue adheres to the outer surface of the organs in the pelvic cavity. This condition is called **endometriosis.** The endometrial tissue acts as though it were still in the uterus. It responds to the ovarian hormones by thickening, becoming secretory, and then sloughing. A woman then feels the discomfort of menstruation throughout the pelvic cavity. In addition to causing severe pain, endometriosis causes scarring and the formation of adhesions.

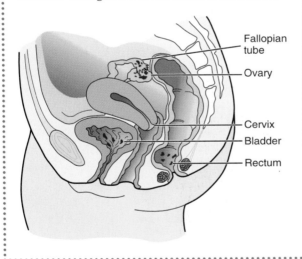

Fallopian tube

Ovary

Cervix

Bladder

Rectum

The uterus has three parts. The **fundus** is the upper dome-shaped region above the entrance of the fallopian tubes. The **body** is the central region. The **cervix** (sûr′vĭks) is the lower narrow region that opens into the vagina. The uterus has three layers: an outer serosal layer called the **epimetrium,** or **perimetrium,** a middle smooth muscular layer called the **myometrium** (mī″ō-mē′trē-əm), and an inner layer called the **endometrium** (ĕn″dō-mē′trē-əm). The endometrial uterine lining has two layers: the **basilar layer** and the **functional layer.** The basilar layer is thin and vascular and lies next to the myometrium. The functional layer responds to the ovarian hormones and thickens in preparation for the fertilized egg. It is also the layer that sloughs off during menstruation, when fertilization has not occurred.

Vagina

The **vagina** is a 4-inch muscular tube that extends from the cervix to the vaginal opening in the perineum. The vaginal opening is usually covered by a thin membrane called the **hymen.** The hymen may be ruptured in a number of ways, such as the first intercourse, use of tampons, or strenuous exercise. The upper portion of the vagina receives the cervix of the uterus. The cervix dips into the vagina so that pockets, or spaces, form around the cervix. The pockets are called **fornices.** The deepest is the **posterior fornix,** located behind the cervix.

What is a Pap smear?

The Pap smear is a diagnostic procedure used for detecting cancer of the cervix. The technique involves scraping some cells from the cervix and examining them for evidence of cancer. This simple and painless procedure has been used successfully to diagnose cancer in its early stages, when the cure rates are high. The technique is named for its developer, Dr. George Papanicolaou.

Why does a woman frequently develop a vaginal "yeast infection" after taking antibiotics?

Antibiotics are given to kill or injure pathogens. Unfortunately, they also destroy the microorganisms of the vagina (normal flora). These microorganisms normally keep the yeast population under control. With the alteration of the normal flora within the vagina, yeasts grow uncontrollably, causing itching and a thick vaginal discharge. Fortunately, over-the-counter medications allow a woman to treat this condition, once it has been determined that it is a fungal infection.

The mucosal lining of the vagina lies in folds (rugae) capable of expanding. The folding is important for childbearing because it permits the vagina to stretch and accommodate the baby. In addition to forming a part of the birth canal, the vagina is also the organ that receives the penis during intercourse and serves as an exit for menstrual blood. The bacterial population (normal flora) in the vagina creates an acidic environment that discourages the growth of pathogens.

✳ **SUM IT UP!** The genital tract consists of the fallopian tubes, the uterus, and the vagina. The fallopian tube, the usual site of fertilization, transports the egg from the ovary to the uterus. The uterus is the site where the fetus lives and grows for 9 months. The vagina receives the penis during intercourse and serves as part of the birth canal. A baby makes its entrance into the world through the vagina.

External Genitals

The female external genitals (genitalia) are together called the vulva (Fig. 22–5). The **vulva** includes the labia majora, the labia minora, the clitoris, and the vestibular glands.

The two **labia majora** are folds of hair-covered skin that lie external to the two smaller **labia minora.** The labia (the word literally means lips) are separated by a cleft containing the urethral and vaginal openings. The labia prevent drying of the mucous membranes. The labia majora merge anteriorly (in front) to form the rounded, hair-covered region over the symphysis called the **mons pubis.**

The **clitoris** is the structure that resembles the penis. Although small, the clitoris contains erectile tissue and is capped by a thin membrane called the **glans.** The labia minora extend forward and partially surround the clitoris to form a foreskin. Like the penis, the clitoris contains sensory receptors that allow the female to experience pleasurable sexual sensations.

The **vestibule** is a cleft between the labia minora. It contains the openings of the urethra and the vagina. A pair of **vestibular glands (Bartholin glands)** lie on either side of the vaginal opening and secrete a mucus-containing substance that moistens and lubricates the vestibule. Note that the female urinary system and the reproductive system are entirely separate. The female urethra carries only urine, whereas the male urethra carries both urine and semen.

The **perineum** refers to the entire pelvic floor. The common use of the word, however, is more limited. Most clinicians use the word *perineum* to

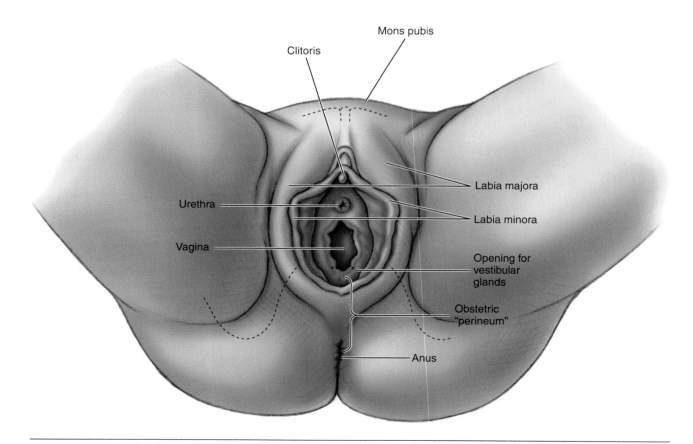

FIGURE 22–5 ● External genitals of the female.

mean the area between the vaginal opening and the anus.

Female Sexual Response

The female responds to sexual stimulation with erection and orgasm. Erectile tissue in the clitoris and the tissue surrounding the vaginal opening swell with blood in response to parasympathetically induced dilation of the arteries. Erectile tissue in the vaginal mucosa, breasts, and nipples also swell. Other responses include an enlargement of the vagina and secretion by the vestibular glands. At the height of sexual stimulation, a woman experiences orgasm, a pleasurable physiologic and psychologic sensation.

As it mediates pleasurable sensations, the orgasm also stimulates a number of reflexes. These reflexes cause muscle contractions in the perineum, uterine walls, and uterine tubes. The muscular activity associated with orgasm is thought to aid in directing and transporting the sperm through the genital tract.

Hormonal Control of the Reproductive Cycles

Let us review the female reproductive cycle. Each month, an egg is produced by the ovary in anticipation of producing a baby. As the egg develops in the ovary, the uterus prepares to receive the fertilized egg. Its preparation consists of the building up of a thick, lush endometrial lining. If the egg is not fertilized, the endometrial lining is no longer needed to nourish and house the fetus, and so it is shed in the menstrual flow. Then the

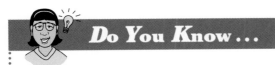

Do You Know...

Why do female athletes often experience menstrual irregularities?

Female athletes, especially those who train intensely, sometimes experience changes in their menstrual cycles. Some experience diminished menstrual flow, called **oligomenorrhea,** while others experience complete absence of menstrual flow (**amenorrhea**). The changes seem to be related to the amount of adipose tissue in the body. Adipose tissue normally stores and gradually releases a small amount of estrogen. As the amount of adipose tissue decreases with exercise, the amount of estrogen also decreases, causing changes in the menstrual cycle.

entire process begins again. A second egg ripens in the ovary, and the uterine lining starts the rebuilding process. This process repeats itself throughout the female reproductive years, all for the purpose of reproducing.

A number of hormones control the female reproductive cycle. Unlike male hormones, female hormonal secretion occurs in a monthly cycle with a regular pattern of increases and decreases in hormone levels. In fact, the word **menses** (měn'sēz) (menstrual) comes from the Greek word for month or moon. The hypothalamus, anterior pituitary gland, and ovaries secrete most of the hormones involved in the menstrual cycle. The hypothalamus secretes gonadotropin-releasing hormone (GnRH) into the hypothalamic portal vessels. GnRH then stimulates the anterior pituitary gland to secrete the gonadotropins FSH and LH. FSH and LH, in turn, stimulate the ovaries, causing them to secrete estrogen and progesterone. The hormones that regulate the female reproductive cycle are summarized in Table 22–1.

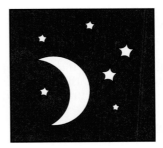

Two Reproductive Cycles

Two components of the female reproductive cycle are the ovarian cycle and the uterine cycle. These cycles begin at puberty and last about 40 years. Refer to Figure 22–6 as you read about the cyclic changes. Figure 22–6A illustrates the secretions of the anterior pituitary gland, FSH and LH, over a 28-day monthly cycle. (The 28-day cycle is an *average* length; a normal cycle may be shorter or longer than 28 days.) The hypothalamic-releasing hormone is not shown, but it is responsible for stimulating the anterior pituitary secretion of the gonadotropins FSH and LH.

For each day of the period, you should be able to identify the secretions of the anterior pituitary gland, the maturation of the ovarian follicle, the changes in the blood levels of ovarian hormones, and the growth of the endometrial lining of the uterus. Figure 22–6B illustrates the growth and maturation of the ovarian follicle, which causes ovulation and the development of the corpus luteum. Figure 22–6C shows the blood levels of the ovarian hormones estrogen and progesterone. Fig-

Table 22 • 1	**FEMALE HORMONES**		
HORMONE	**GLAND**	**TARGET ORGAN**	**EFFECTS**
Gonadotropin-releasing hormones (GnRH)	Hypothalamus	Anterior pituitary	Stimulate the secretion of the gonadotropins (FSH and LH)
Follicle-stimulating hormone (FSH)	Anterior pituitary	Ovary	Initiates development of the ovarian follicle Stimulates the secretion of estrogen by the follicular cells
Luteinizing hormone (LH)	Anterior pituitary	Ovary	Causes ovulation Stimulates the corpus luteum to secrete progesterone
Estrogen	Ovary (follicle)	Locally (ovary)	Stimulates maturation of the ovarian follicle
		Uterus (endometrium)	Stimulates the proliferative phase of endometrial development
		Other tissues and organs	Causes the development of the secondary sex characteristics
Progesterone	Ovary (corpus luteum)	Uterus (endometrium)	Stimulates the secretory phase of endometrial development
Human chorionic gonadotropin (hCG)	Trophoblast cells of the embryo	Corpus luteum	Maintains the corpus luteum during pregnancy

ure 22–6D illustrates the monthly changes in the uterine lining. Together, the parts of Figure 22–6 describe events that occur over a 28-day period.

Ovarian Cycle

The **ovarian cycle** consists of the changes that occur within the ovary over the 28-day monthly period (see Fig. 22–6B). The two phases of the ovarian cycle are the follicular phase and the luteal phase.

FOLLICULAR PHASE. The **follicular phase** begins with the hypothalamic secretion of GnRH. This hormone, in turn, stimulates the release of gonadotropins by the anterior pituitary gland. The FSH and small amounts of LH stimulate the growth and maturation of the ovarian follicle. The maturing ovarian follicle secretes large amounts of estrogen, causing the blood levels of estrogen to increase.

Estrogen dominates the follicular phase. Estrogen has an effect on both the ovary and the uterus. The estrogen helps the ovarian follicle to mature. The blood also carries the estrogen to the uterus, where it helps build up the uterine lining in the first half of the uterine cycle (days 1–14).

The follicular phase ends with ovulation, the expulsion of the egg from the surface of the ovary. A sharp rise (midcycle surge) of LH on day 14 causes ovulation. (See Figure 22–6A for the midcycle surge of LH and Figure 22–6B for ovulation.)

LUTEAL PHASE. The **luteal phase** immediately follows ovulation. The corpus luteum develops during the luteal phase. Follicular cells of the ruptured follicle on the surface of the ovary form the corpus luteum. LH then stimulates the corpus luteum to secrete progesterone and small amounts of estrogen. The progesterone and estrogen exert a negative feedback effect on the hypothalamus and anterior pituitary gland, thereby inhibiting further secretion of FSH and LH. Progesterone dominates the luteal phase.

When the corpus luteum dies, secretion of progesterone and estrogen declines. As a result of the decrease in estrogen and progesterone, FSH and small amounts of LH are once again secreted, and the cycle is repeated.

Uterine Cycle

The **uterine cycle,** also called the **menstrual cycle,** consists of the changes that occur in the endometrium over a 28-day period (see Fig. 22–6D). Estrogen and progesterone secreted by the ovaries cause the endometrial changes. Thus the ovarian cycle controls the uterine cycle. The uterine cycle has three phases: the menstrual phase, the proliferative phase, and the secretory phase.

MENSTRUAL PHASE. Bleeding characterizes the **menstrual phase.** It begins on the first day and continues for 3 to 5 days, varying from person to person. During the menstrual phase, the functional layer of the endometrial lining and blood leave the uterus through the vagina as menstrual flow. Women call this process "having your period."

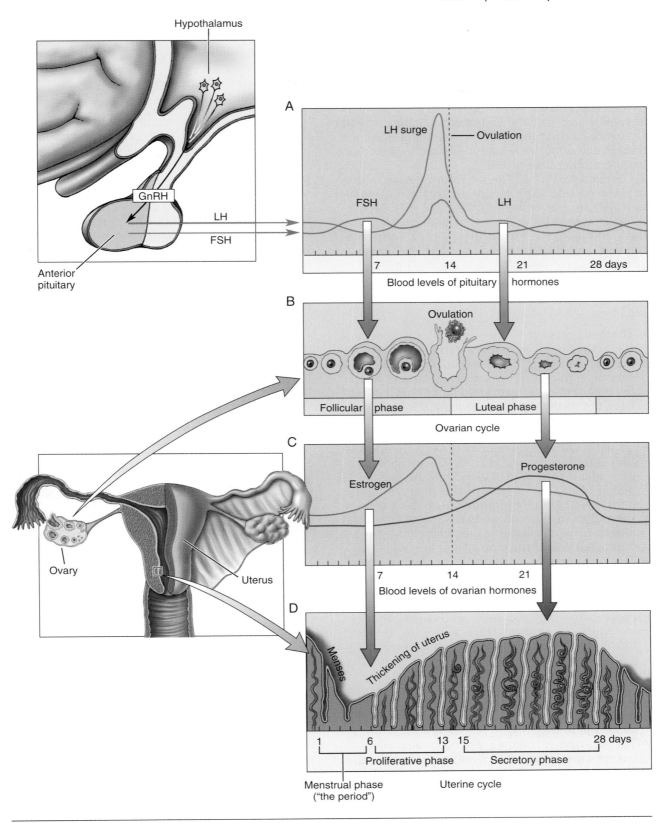

FIGURE 22–6 ● Hormonal control of the female reproductive cycle (28-day cycle). A, The anterior pituitary gland secretes the gonadotropins FSH and LH. B, Ovarian events: maturation of the ovarian follicle, ovulation at midcycle, and development of the corpus luteum. C, Blood levels of the ovarian hormones estrogen and progesterone. D, The uterine cycle.

PROLIFERATIVE PHASE. The **proliferative phase** begins with the end of the menstrual phase. Repair and growth of the inner endometrial lining characterize the proliferative phase. The lining grows primarily because of estrogen secreted by the ovaries (see Fig. 22–6B, 22–6C). The proliferative phase is so named because the cells proliferate and thus repair the endometrial lining. Note in Figure 22–6D that the endometrial lining becomes thicker and acquires additional blood vessels during the proliferative phase.

SECRETORY PHASE. The **secretory phase** is due to the secretion of progesterone by the corpus luteum of the ovary (see Fig. 22–6C, 22–6D). Progesterone causes the endometrial lining to become thick and lush, thereby forming a nutritious environment awaiting the arrival of a fertilized ovum.

✳ **SUM IT UP!** Let us highlight the events of the ovarian and uterine cycles. Refer again to Figure 22–6.

- The development of the ovarian follicle, during the follicular phase of the ovarian cycle, is due primarily to FSH. FSH stimulates the follicle to secrete estrogen. The estrogen, secreted by the follicular cells, performs two functions: It stimulates the growth of the follicle, and it is responsible for the proliferative phase of the uterine cycle.
- Ovulation is the expulsion of the egg at midcycle (day 14). A surge of LH from the anterior pituitary gland causes ovulation, and the egg is expelled from the surface of the ovary into the peritoneal cavity. The fimbriae at the edges of the fallopian tube immediately sweep the egg into the tube. A cluster of follicular cells remains on the surface of the ovary.
- The remaining follicular cells on the surface of the ovary form the corpus luteum. The corpus luteum secretes progesterone and some estrogen. Blood carries the hormones to the uterus.
- Progesterone in particular stimulates the uterine lining to become thick and lush, thereby forming a rich lining for the fertilized egg. Progesterone dominates the secretory phase of the uterine cycle.
- When blood levels of estrogen and progesterone decline, the endometrial lining sloughs off and causes bleeding. This process is the basis for menstruation.
- The ovarian hormones estrogen and progesterone exert a negative feedback effect on the hypothalamus and anterior pituitary gland. When blood levels of the ovarian hormones rise, secretions of FSH and LH are low. When the corpus luteum degenerates into the corpus albicans, however, the blood levels of estrogen and progesterone decrease. The decrease in the ovarian hormones in turn allows the anterior pituitary gland to secrete FSH and LH. Conse-

quently, FSH and LH are secreted in small amounts. The stimulated ovary then develops another follicle.

Implantation: Keeping the Corpus Luteum Alive

Note: The endometrial lining does not slough if blood levels of estrogen and progesterone are adequate. These levels are adequate if the corpus luteum does not deteriorate. How does the body prevent the deterioration of the corpus luteum?

If fertilization of the egg occurs, preserving the thick lush uterine lining is crucial. Menstruation must be prevented. The corpus luteum accomplishes this task. How? Soon after fertilization, the baby-to-be implants, or imbeds itself, in the uterine lining. Some of the cells at the site of implantation in the uterus secrete a hormone called **human chorionic gonadotropin (hCG).** Blood carries hCG from the uterus to the ovary, where it stimulates the corpus luteum. hCG prevents the deterioration of the corpus luteum, thereby ensuring the continued secretion of estrogen and progesterone. hCG prolongs the life of the corpus luteum for 11 to 12 weeks until the placenta can take over as the major estrogen/progesterone–secreting gland. (Chapter 23 takes the story from here.)

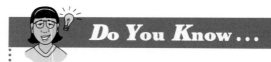

Do You Know...

What is gonorrhea ophthalmia?

Gonorrhea is a sexually transmitted disease caused by the bacterium *Neisseria gonorrhoeae.* Besides infecting the reproductive organs, the bacterium can also cause an eye infection (gonorrhea ophthalmia). A newborn can pick up gonorrhea ophthalmia by passing through the birth canal of an infected mother. This condition is called acquired ophthalmia neonatorum. To prevent ophthalmia neonatorum, an antibiotic is applied to the baby's eyes immediately after birth.

Menarche, Menses, and Menopause

In the female, puberty is marked by the first period of menstrual bleeding. This event is called **menarche.** Thereafter, the menstrual periods (menses) occur regularly until the woman reaches the late 40s or early 50s. At this time, the periods gradually become more irregular until they cease completely. This phase is called **menopause** (měn′ə-pōz). Menopause is also called the change of life, or the climacteric. Female reproductive function lasts from menarche to menopause.

Menopause is due to a decrease in the ovarian secretion of estrogen and progesterone. Without ovarian hormones, the uterine cycle ceases, and the woman stops menstruating. Other symptoms associated with menopause include hot flashes, sweating, depression, irritability, and insomnia. The symptoms are highly variable. Some women experience severe disturbances; others hardly notice any systemic effects.

METHODS OF BIRTH CONTROL

Birth control is the voluntary regulation of reproduction. Birth control can limit the number of offspring produced and help determine the timing of conception. Methods of **contraception** are forms of birth control that prevent the union of egg and sperm. Several methods of birth control are available. Most generally accepted methods are those that prevent fertilization of the egg after intercourse. Commonly used methods of birth control are summarized in Table 22–2.

Barrier Methods of Birth Control

Barriers prevent the sperm from entering the female: no union means no baby. Barrier methods are mechanical or chemical. The female and male

Table 22 • 2 COMMON BIRTH CONTROL METHODS

METHOD	DESCRIPTION	MECHANISM
Mechanical barrier		
Condom (male)	Latex sheath is placed over the erect penis	Blocks entrance of sperm
Condom (female)	Plastic lining is placed in the vagina	Blocks entrance of sperm
Diaphragm	Plastic cap fits over the cervical entrance	Blocks entrance of sperm
Chemical barrier		
Creams, foams, jellies	Possess spermicidal properties	Kills sperm
Sponge		
Hormonal contraceptives		
The pill	Hormone-containing pills taken daily (estrogen and progesterone)	Prevents ovulation by negative feedback
Implants	Progesterone-like hormone implanted under the skin	Prevent ovulation by negative feedback
Surgical		
Vasectomy	Both vas deferens cut and tied	No sperm in seminal fluid
Tubal ligation	Fallopian tubes cut and tied	No eggs in fallopian tubes
Intrauterine device	Solid object implanted in the uterine cavity	Prevents the implantation of the fertilized egg
Behavioral		
Abstinence	No intercourse	No sperm
Rhythm (natural family planning, timed coitus)	Avoidance of intercourse for several days prior to and following ovulation	No union of a sperm and egg
Coitus interruptus (withdrawal)	Penis withdrawn before ejaculation	Prevents sperm from entering the vagina
"Morning-after" pill (RU-486)	Pill taken the morning after intercourse	Prevents implantation

condoms and the diaphragm are mechanical barriers. For instance, the male condom is a thin latex sheath that covers the erect penis and prevents semen from entering the vagina during intercourse. The condom also protects against sexually transmitted diseases. Spermicidal creams, foams, and jellies are chemical barriers. The effectiveness of the chemical barriers is improved considerably when they are used with a mechanical barrier. For instance, many people use the spermicidal jelly and a diaphragm at the same time.

Hormonal Contraceptives

The birth control pill is a pharmacologic agent that contains estrogen and progesterone. As the blood levels of estrogen and progesterone increase, negative feedback inhibits the secretion of FSH by the anterior pituitary gland. This process, in turn, prevents ovulation: no egg means no baby.

Implants containing progesterone act in much the same way. Progesterone-containing capsules, or rods, can be surgically implanted under the skin of a woman's upper arm or scapular region. The progesterone is slowly but continuously released from the implant. As with the birth control pill, the elevated blood levels of progesterone prevent ovulation.

Surgical Methods of Birth Control

Surgical methods of contraception include a vasectomy in the male and a tubal ligation in the female (Fig. 22–7). A **vasectomy** involves removing a small section of each vas deferens and tying the cut ends. A vasectomy is contraceptive because the sperm cannot leave the epididymis: no sperm means no baby.

In the female, a tubal ligation involves removing a small section of each fallopian tube and tying the cut ends. After a **tubal ligation,** the egg cannot be transported from the ovary through the fallopian tubes, where fertilization normally takes place: no egg means no baby.

Intrauterine Devices

An **intrauterine device (IUD)** is a small solid object placed in the uterine cavity. The IUD prevents pregnancy because it stimulates the uterus to prevent implantation of the fertilized egg. Note that the IUD is not technically contraceptive. In

other words, it does not prevent conception; instead, it prevents implantation.

Behavioral Methods of Birth Control

Sexual partners can behave in ways to prevent pregnancy. Behavioral methods include abstinence, the rhythm method, and coitus interruptus. Abstinence, or the avoidance of sexual intercourse, is the most effective, though not the most popular, method of birth control.

The rhythm method, also called natural family planning or timed coitus, requires avoiding sexual intercourse at a time when the female is ovulating, generally at midcycle. Intercourse must be avoided a few days before and after ovulation. Because the menstrual cycle (and ovulation) are not always regular, the rhythm method is associated with a high pregnancy rate. Coitus interruptus involves the withdrawal of the penis from the vagina before ejaculation. It too is associated with a high pregnancy rate.

RU-486

RU-486 (mifepristone) is a pharmacologic agent used extensively outside the United States. It is sometimes called a morning-after form of birth control. RU-486 causes the loss of the implanted embryo by blocking progesterone receptors in the endometrium. The loss of progesterone receptors causes the endometrium to slough, carrying the implanted embryo with it. Note that RU-486, like the IUD, is not contraceptive. It does not prevent conception; instead, it prevents implantation.

Birth Control Choices

Each method of birth control has its advantages and disadvantages. Some methods are safer, more effective, or more convenient than others. Abstinence and the surgical methods (vasectomy and tubal ligation) are the most effective contraceptive practices. Unwanted pregnancy is most apt to occur in women who have unprotected sex and those who practice the rhythm method of birth control. The effectiveness of each method is summarized in Table 22–2.

✳ **SUM IT UP!** In the female, puberty is marked by the first period of menstrual bleeding. This event is called menarche. Thereafter, monthly menstrual periods (menses) occur regularly until menopause. Menopause, also called the climacteric or change of life, generally occurs when a

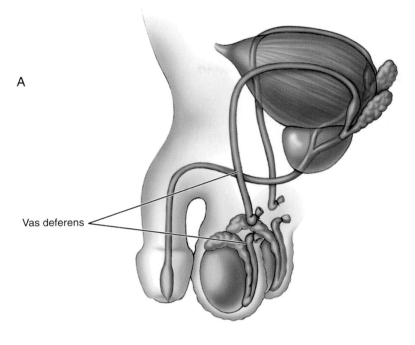

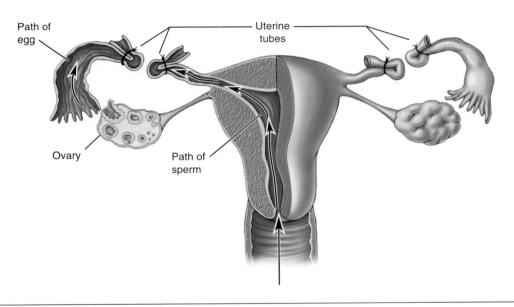

FIGURE 22–7 • Surgical methods of birth control. A, Vasectomy, the cutting and ligation (tying off) of the vas deferens. B, Tubal ligation, the cutting and ligation of the fallopian tubes.

woman is in her late 40s or early 50s. Menopause is caused by the decreased ovarian secretion of estrogen and progesterone.

Birth control is the voluntary regulation of reproduction. There are several methods of birth control: barrier methods (condoms, diaphragm),

hormonal contraceptives (the birth control pill and progesterone implants), surgical methods (vasectomy, tubal ligation), intrauterine devices, behavioral methods (abstinence, rhythm method, and coitus interruptus), and RU-486 (a morning-after pill).

As You Age

1. As a woman ages, her ovaries begin to atrophy, or shrink. Between the ages of 40 and 50, estrogen secretion decreases and symptoms of menopause appear; menstrual periods cease, signaling the end of her reproductive years.

2. The decrease in estrogen secretion causes a change in the accessory organs of reproduction. Tissues become thinner, with a decrease in secretions. The changes in these structures make the woman more prone to vaginal infections. Also, a decrease in vaginal secretions can make intercourse uncomfortable. The decrease in estrogen is also thought to cause weakening of bone, causing osteoporosis, and an increase in the incidence of cardiovascular diseases.

3. By the age of 50, the size of the uterus has decreased by 50%. The ligaments that anchor the uterus, urinary bladder, and rectum weaken, allowing these organs to drop down. Surgical correction is sometimes needed.

4. Breast tissue changes; the supporting ligaments weaken; fibrous cells replace glandular cells; and the amount of fat tissue decreases. These changes cause breast tissue to sag.

5. Around the age of 40, testicular function declines. This decline is accompanied by a decrease in the secretion of testosterone and a decreased sperm count (up to 50%). Despite these changes, a man continues to produce sperm and is capable of fathering children throughout most of his life span.

Disorders of the Reproductive Systems

Benign prostatic hyperplasia (BPH)	A noncancerous enlargement of the prostate gland. The enlarged prostate gland compresses the urethra, impeding urination and making the person prone to bladder infections.
Cancer of the reproductive organs	A number of cancers in both men and women. Cancer of the breast is a leading cause of death in women. Cervical cancer is a common form of cancer that is about 90% curable if diagnosed early. The routine use of the Pap smear as a screening test plays an important role in the high cure rate. Ovarian cancer is a particularly deadly form of cancer. Symptoms of ovarian cancer develop late in the course of the disease, thereby delaying diagnosis and treatment. Cancer of the prostate gland is a common cancer in men. A digital rectal examination is done routinely to detect any enlargement or changes in the prostate. The incidence of testicular cancer is increasing, particularly in athletes.
Dysmenorrhea	Painful or difficult menstruation.
Ovarian cyst	Fluid-filled bubbles of tissue that generally occur in the follicles or in the corpus luteum. Most cysts disappear spontaneously and require no treatment. Some cysts are painful; others may burst and require surgical intervention. All cysts must be evaluated to rule out cancer.
Pelvic inflammatory disease (PID)	A general term that includes inflammation of the uterus, uterine tubes (salpingitis), pelvic peritonitis, and abscess formation. PID is a serious complication of infection by *Neisseria gonorrhoeae (N. gonorrhoeae)* and *Chlamydia trachomatis (C. trachomatis)*.
Premenstrual tension	Also called premenstrual syndrome (PMS). Premenstrual tension is a syndrome characterized by abdominal bloating, fluid retention, and hyperirritability about 2 weeks before a menstrual period.

Disorders of the reproductive systems, *continued*

Sexually transmitted diseases (STDs)
Called venereal diseases, after Venus, the Roman goddess of love and beauty. STDs are infectious diseases transmitted from person to person mainly by sexual contact. Left untreated, most STDs cause sterility; some cause permanent disability and death. The most common STD is chlamydia, a nongonococcal urethritis, caused by a bacterium *(Chlamydia trachomatis)*. Genital herpes is caused by the herpes simplex virus and is characterized by painful blister-like sores on the external genitalia. The woman harbors the virus and may infect the fetus upon delivery. Pregnant women with genital herpes are encouraged to deliver their babies by cesarean section to prevent transmission of the virus to the baby. Other STDs include gonorrhea *(N. gonorrhoeae)*, syphilis *(Treponema pallidum)*, and trichomoniasis *(Trichomonas vaginalis)*.

Summary Outline

The reproductive system produces the cells and hormones necessary for reproduction.

I. Male Reproductive System

A. Testes
1. The testes, or testicles, are the male gonads.
2. The testis is composed of lobules with two types of cells: the seminiferous tubules, which produce sperm, and the interstitial cells, which secrete testosterone.

B. Genital Ducts and Glands
1. The sperm move through a series of genital ducts: the epididymis, the vas deferens, the ejaculatory ducts, and the urethra.
2. Three glands—the seminal vesicles, the prostate gland, and the bulbourethral glands—secrete into the genital ducts. The mixture of sperm and glandular secretions is called semen.

C. External Genitals
1. The male genitals consist of the scrotum and the penis.
2. The penis performs two functions: it is the organ of copulation (sexual intercourse), and it carries urine.

D. Male Sexual Response
1. Erection is due to the engorgement of the erectile tissue of the penis with blood. Erection causes the penis to enlarge and become rigid, thereby facilitating penetration.
2. Emission is the movement of sperm and glandular secretions from the testes into the urethra.
3. Ejaculation is the expulsion of the semen from the urethra to the outside.
4. Orgasm refers to the pleasurable physiologic and psychologic sensations that occur at the height of sexual stimulation.

E. Male Sex Hormones
1. The male sex hormones are called androgens, the most important being testosterone.
2. Testosterone determines the primary sex characteristics (eg, sperm production, growth of the penis) and the secondary sex characteristics (eg, growth of beard, deepening of the voice, musculoskeletal growth).
3. The male reproductive system is controlled by hormones from the hypothalamus (gonadotropin-releasing hormone) and from the anterior pituitary gland (FSH and LH).

II. Female Reproductive System
The female reproductive system produces eggs, secretes hormones, and nurtures and protects a developing baby during the 9 months of pregnancy.

A. Ovaries
1. The ovaries are the female gonads; the ovaries contain ovarian follicles.
2. Each ovarian follicle consists of an immature egg called an oocyte and cells surrounding the oocyte, called follicular cells.
3. On day 14 (of a 28-day cycle), the mature ovum bursts from the follicle in a process called ovulation. The ovum then enters the fallopian tubes.
4. The follicular cells on the surface of the ovary become the corpus luteum.
5. The ovaries secrete two hormones, estrogen and progesterone. The estrogen develops the secondary sex characteristics and makes a woman look like a woman. In general, the progesterone increases the secretory activities of the reproductive organs.

B. Genital Tract
1. The genital tract includes the fallopian tubes, the uterus, and the vagina.
2. The fallopian tubes, or uterine tubes, perform two roles. They transport the egg from the ovaries to the uterus, and they are the site where fertilization occurs.

continued

Summary Outline continued

II. Female Reproductive System, *continued*

B. Genital Tract, *continued*

3. The uterus, or womb, is the baby's cradle for the 9 months of pregnancy.
4. The uterus has three layers: epimetrium, myometrium, and endometrium. The myometrium is a muscle layer and expels the fetus from the uterus during labor. The endometrium responds cyclically to the female hormones.

C. External Genitals

1. The female external genitals are together called the vulva and include the labia majora, the labia minora, the clitoris, and the vestibular glands.
2. The perineum is a term commonly used to refer to the area between the vaginal opening and the anus.

D. Female Sexual Response

1. Erectile tissue (the clitoris and vaginal area) engorges with blood. This response is accompanied by an increase in secretions from the vestibular glands.
2. At the height of sexual stimulation the woman experiences orgasm.

E. Hormonal Control of the Female Reproductive Cycles

1. The two cycles are the ovarian cycle and the uterine cycle; the cycles are interrelated, and the average cycle lasts 28 days.
2. The ovarian cycle is divided into the follicular phase and the luteal phase.
3. During the follicular phase the ovarian follicle matures, primarily in response to FSH. The follicular phase ends with ovulation. The follicular phase is dominated by estrogen.
4. Ovulation is due primarily to a surge in the secretion of LH from the anterior pituitary gland.
5. The luteal phase of the ovarian cycle begins immediately after ovulation. This phase is dominated by the secretion of progesterone by the corpus luteum.
6. In the nonpregnant state, the corpus luteum deteriorates into the nonsecreting corpus albicans. In the pregnant state the corpus luteum stays alive because of the stimulatory effect of human chorionic gonadotropin, a hormone secreted by the cells of the baby-to-be as the fertilized egg implants into the uterus.
7. The uterine cycle is divided into the menstrual phase, the proliferative phase, and the secretory phase. The menstrual phase refers to the loss of a part of the endometrial lining and blood (women call this "having your period"). During the proliferative phase, the inner endometrial lining is thickening and becomes vascular, primarily in response to estrogen. During the secretory phase, the endometrial lining is becoming lush and moist from increased secretory activity; the secretory phase is dominated by progesterone.
8. See Figure 22–6 for a summary of the day-to-day hormonal relationships between the anterior pituitary gland, the ovaries, and the uterus.

III. Methods of Birth Control

The regulation of childbearing can be achieved with the use of barrier methods (eg, condoms), hormonal contraceptives (eg, the pill), surgical methods (tubal ligation, vasectomy), intrauterine devices (IUDs), behavioral methods (eg, rhythm), and the morning-after drugs such as RU-486.

Review Your Knowledge

1. How is human reproduction different from reproduction in single-cell organisms?

2. Name two functions of the reproductive system.

3. Name the male and female gonads. Name the male and female gametes.

4. What are three roles of the male reproductive system?

5. What happens to reproductive function when cryptorchidism, or failure of the testes to descend, occurs?

6. Where is testosterone produced? Where are sperm produced?

7. What is meiosis? How is it different from mitosis?

8. List the three parts of the sperm.

9. Trace the movement of sperm from the epididymis to the outside of the body.

10. What three glands contribute secretions to semen? What secretions are produced by each of these three glands?

Review Your Knowledge *continued*

11. Name the structures that make up the male external genitalia.

12. Which hormone stimulates spermatogenesis? Which hormone stimulates the secretion of testosterone? What are two functions of testosterone?

13. Where is the graafian follicle located? What is the corpus luteum? Which structures primarily secrete estrogen? What structure primarily secretes progesterone?

14. Which hormones stimulate the production of estrogen? Which hormones stimulate the production of progesterone?

15. Trace the movement of the ovum from the graafian follicle to the endometrium, when pregnancy occurs.

16. What are the three layers of the uterus? What are the names of the lower, central, and upper regions of the uterus?

17. Which structures make up the female external genitalia?

18. Describe the ovarian cycle and the uterine cycle. When does ovulation occur during the monthly cycle? What happens during the menstrual, proliferative, and secretory phases of the menstrual cycle?

19. Contrast *menarche, menses,* and *menopause.*

20. List commonly used methods of birth control.

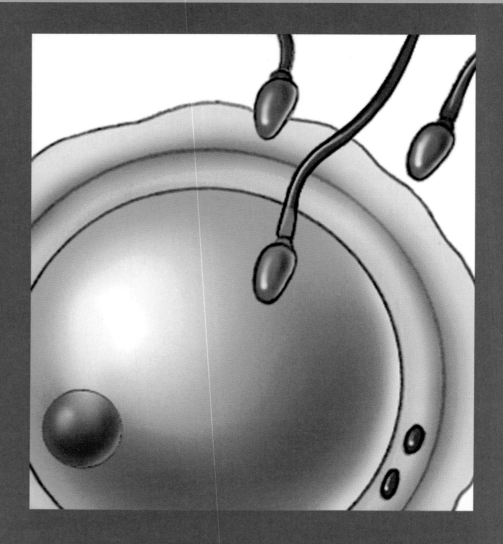

23 HUMAN DEVELOPMENT AND HEREDITY

Objectives

1. Describe the process of fertilization: when, where, and how it occurs.

2. Describe the process of development: cleavage, growth, morphogenesis, and differentiation.

3. Explain the three periods of prenatal development: early embryonic, embryonic, and fetal periods.

4. State two functions of the placenta.

5. Explain hormonal changes during pregnancy.

6. List six ways in which the mother's body changes during pregnancy.

7. Describe the process of labor, including the hormonal changes and the individual stages.

8. Describe the structure of the breast.

9. Describe the process of lactation.

10. Describe the relationships among DNA, chromosomes, and genes.

11. Explain dominant genes, recessive genes, and codominance.

12. Explain how the sex of the child is determined.

13. Define *meiosis*.

14. Describe sex-linked traits.

15. State the difference between congenital and hereditary diseases.

16. Define *karyotype*.

Nine months after conception, the reproductive process (Chapter 22) produces a baby. "Bundle of Joy" has arrived on the scene. Note that this term of endearment does not suggest "up, awake, and playing at 2 AM," gallons of the pink stuff (amoxicillin), and diapers-diapers-and-more-diapers. Nonetheless, Baby is cute, and the urge to reproduce is very strong. Let us follow Baby's start from fertilization through development and birth. Finally, we'll see what is meant by statements like "He's got his father's nose and his mother's smile." This is the genetic story.

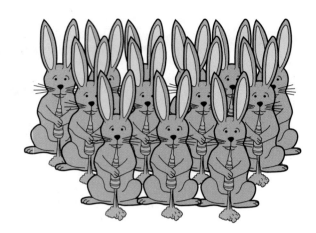

flex ovulators, and we all know about the rate of rabbit reproduction.

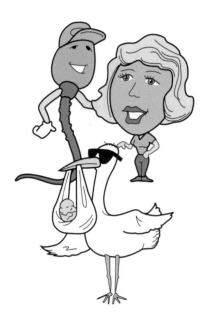

FERTILIZATION

Fertilization, also called **conception,** refers to the union of the nuclei of the egg and the sperm. When, where, and how does this union take place?

When Fertilization Occurs

Timing is everything. In the female, ovulation occurs at midcycle, around day 14 (see Chapter 22). The egg lives for about 24 hours after ovulation. Sperm usually live between 12 and 48 hours, with some surviving up to 72 hours. For fertilization to occur, sexual intercourse must take place around the time of ovulation, generally no earlier than 72 hours (3 days) before ovulation and no later than 24 hours (1 day) after ovulation. Alert: Evidence suggests that some women are reflex ovulators. These women ovulate in response to having intercourse. Think about it: The chance of pregnancy goes up. Remember that rabbits are re-

Where Fertilization Occurs

After ovulation, the egg enters the fallopian tube. Fertilization normally occurs in the first third of the fallopian tube, near the infundibulum (see Chapter 22).

How Fertilization Occurs

During intercourse, about 200 to 600 million sperm are deposited in the vagina, near the cervix of the uterus. Although many of the sperm are killed by the acidic environment of the vagina, about 100 thousand survive and swim through the uterus and into the fallopian tube, toward the egg. Within 1 to 2 hours after intercourse, thousands of sperm are gathered around the egg in the fallopian tube.

The acrosomes on the heads of the sperm rupture and release enzymes. The enzymes digest the linings of cells that surround the egg. Then, one and only one sperm penetrates the membrane of the egg. Upon penetration of the egg, the nuclei of the egg and sperm unite, thereby completing fertilization. The fertilized egg is called a **zygote** (zī'gōt''). The zygote is the first cell of a new individual.

The single-cell zygote has 46 chromosomes, 23 from the egg and 23 from the sperm. The zygote begins to divide, forming a cluster of cells that slowly makes its way through the fallopian tube toward the uterus. The zygote moves by peristalsis and by the swishing action of the cilia, which line the fallopian tubes. When this cluster of cells reaches the uterus, it implants itself into the plush endometrial lining, where it grows and develops into a human being with billions of cells.

PRENATAL DEVELOPMENT

Development is a process that begins with fertilization and ends with death. Human development is divided into two phases: prenatal development and postnatal development. Prenatal development begins with fertilization and is terminated at birth. The time of prenatal development is called **pregnancy, or gestation.** The normal gestation period lasts 38 weeks, or about 9 months. Pregnancy is divided into **trimesters** (3-month periods). The first trimester is the first 3 months of pregnancy. The second trimester is months 4, 5, and 6, and the third, or last, trimester is months 7, 8, and 9. Postnatal development begins with birth and terminates with death; it is what we are all doing now—it is called *life.*

What does prenatal development include? Prenatal development includes cleavage, growth, morphogenesis, and differentiation. **Cleavage** is cell division by mitosis. Mitosis produces two identical cells from a single cell. Thus, one cell splits into two cells. The two cells split into four cells, four cells split into eight cells, and so on. Each new cell is identical to the parent cell. Mitotic cell division increases the numbers of cells but not their actual size. The size of the cell increases through **growth.** Thus, as development progresses, both the number and the size of the cells increase.

Morphogenesis is the shaping of the cell cluster. Certain cells move, or migrate, to specific areas in the cell cluster. This process changes the shape of the cell mass. For instance, cells migrate to the side of the cell mass and take the appearance of tiny buds. These buds eventually become legs. Through morphogenesis, the round cluster of cells develops into an intricately and wonderously formed infant. Baby is shaping up!

Differentiation is the process whereby a cell becomes specialized. A cell differentiates to become a nerve cell, muscle cell, blood cell, or some other cell. The process of development is complex. It includes much more than a simple increase in the size and numbers of cells.

✳ **SUM IT UP!** Fertilization takes place in the fallopian tube, when the nuclei of a sperm and egg unite, producing a zygote. The zygote begins its early development in the fallopian tube. It gradually moves through the fallopian tube into the uterus, where it develops into an infant over a 9-month period. Prenatal development includes the processes of cleavage (mitosis), growth, morphogenesis, and differentiation.

Prenatal development is divided into three periods: the early embryonic period, the embryonic period, and the fetal period.

Early Embryonic Period

From Zygote to Blastocyst

The early embryonic period lasts for 2 weeks after fertilization. During this period, the zygote undergoes mitosis and other structural changes and travels from the fallopian tube into the uterus. Refer to Figure 23–1 as you follow these events. After fertilization (Fig. 23–1A), the zygote undergoes cleavage. Cleavage is accomplished by mitosis, cell division that increases the numbers of cells. The cells formed by mitotic cell division are **blastomeres** (Fig. 23–1B). Note the two-cell cluster, four-cell cluster, and eight-cell cluster.

When the number of cells increases to 16, the collection of cells is called a **morula** (Fig. 23–1C). The morula looks like a raspberry, so tiny that it is visible only through a microscope. Transformation from the zygote to a morula takes about 3 days. The morula enters the uterine cavity, where it floats around for 3 to 4 days and continues to undergo mitosis. By the end of the fifth day, the morula develops into a **blastocyst** (blăs′tə-sĭst).

Note the structure of the **early blastocyst** (Fig. 23–1D). The early blastocyst contains a hollow cavity surrounded by a single layer of flattened cells and a cluster of cells at one side. The single layer of flattened cells surrounding the cavity is called the **trophoblast.** These cells will help form the placenta and also secrete an important hormone. The cluster of cells within the blastocyst is called the **inner cell mass.** These cells will eventually form Baby.

The **late blastocyst** develops by day 7. The late blastocyst stage shows the beginnings of the amniotic cavity. The late blastocyst burrows into the endometrial lining of the uterus, where it is gradually covered over by cells of the endometrial lining. The burrowing process is called **implantation.** (Note that the zygote, blastomeres, morula, and early blastocyst are still surrounded by the zona pellucida and corona radiata. This layer disappears by the late blastocyst stage.)

During implantation the blastocyst also functions as a gland. The trophoblast, the flattened layer of cells that surrounds the cavity, secretes a hormone called **human chorionic gonadotropin** (hyōō′mən kôr″ē-ŏn′ĭk gō-năd″ə-trōp′ĭn) **(hCG).** hCG travels through the blood to the ovary, where it prevents the deterioration of the corpus luteum. In response to hCG, the corpus luteum continues to secrete estrogen and progesterone. The estrogen and progesterone stimulate the growth of the uterine wall and prevent menstruation.

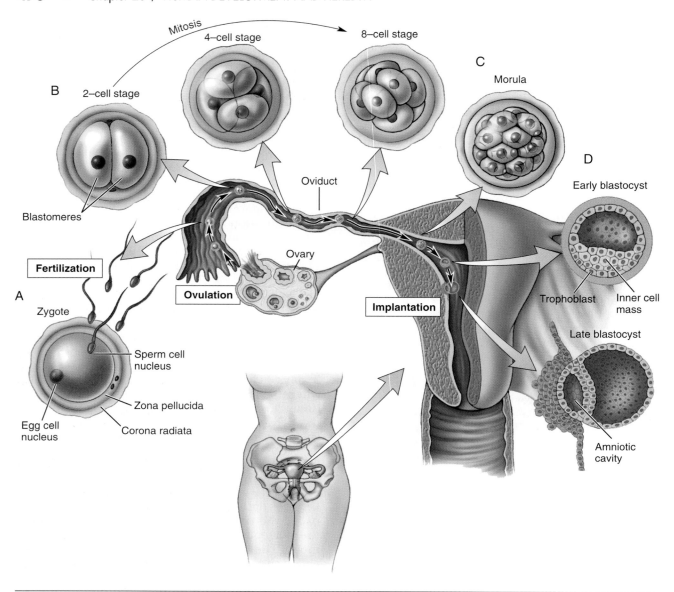

FIGURE 23–1 ● Stages of early embryonic development. A, Formation of the zygote during fertilization. B, Cleavage stage whereby the cells undergo mitosis and increase in number. C, Morula (16-cell cluster). D, Early blastocyst forms with an inner cell mass and trophoblast. The late blastocyst then implants itself into the uterine lining.

The secretion of hCG continues at a high level for about 2 months, then steadily declines as the placenta develops. The placenta eventually takes over the role of the corpus luteum by secreting large amounts of estrogen and progesterone. The blastocyst thus helps preserve its own survival through its secretion of hCG. With the implantation of the blastocyst and the organization of the inner cell mass, the early embryonic period comes to a close.

Seeing Double: How Twins Happen

Each cell within the morula or blastocyst can become a complete individual. Sometimes these cells split, and two embryos begin developing at the same time, thereby producing two offspring (twins) rather than one. These are **identical,** or **monozygotic, twins** because they develop from the same zygote and have identical genetic information. For monozygotic twins to develop, one sperm fertilizes one egg, and the zygote then splits.

Sometimes a mother ovulates two eggs, which are then fertilized by two different sperm. Because two babies are produced, they are called twins. These twins, however, are not identical. They do not develop from the same egg and do not have the same genetic information. They are called **fraternal,** or **dizygotic, twins** (meaning that they come from two different zygotes). Triplets, quadruplets, and other multiple births can develop in the same two ways.

Embryonic Period

Embryonic development lasts for 6 weeks, from week 3 through week 8. During this period, the baby-to-be is called an **embryo** (ĕm′brē-ō). The embryonic period involves the formation of extraembryonic membranes, the placenta, and all of the organ systems in the body.

Extraembryonic Membranes

The extraembryonic membranes form outside the embryo; hence the term *extra*embryonic. The membranes help to protect and nourish the embryo; they are also involved in the embryonic excretion of waste. At birth the membranes are expelled along with the placenta as the **afterbirth.** The four extraembryonic membranes are the amnion, the chorion, the yolk sac, and the allantois.

The **amnion** (ăm′nē-ŏn″) enlarges and forms a sac around the embryo (Fig. 23–2). The sac is called the **amniotic sac** and is filled with a fluid called the **amniotic fluid.** The amniotic fluid forms a protective cushion around the embryo and helps protect it from bumps and changes in temperature. The amniotic fluid also allows the baby-to-be to move around and exercise.

The embryo secretes waste and sheds cells into the amniotic fluid. This process is the basis for a diagnostic test called an **amniocentesis,** in which a sample of amniotic fluid is aspirated from the amniotic cavity and examined for evidence of fetal abnormalities (see Fig. 23–2B). The amniotic sac is often called the bag of waters. It breaks before delivery and generally signals the onset of labor.

A second extraembryonic membrane is the chorion. The **chorion** (kōr′ē-ŏn″) is the outer extraembryonic membrane. It develops many finger-like projections called chorionic villi. The **chorionic villi** penetrate the uterine wall and interact with the tissues of the mother's uterus to form the placenta. Sampling of the cells of the chorionic villi is another way to detect genetic defects (Fig. 23–3 and see Fig. 23–2C).

A third extraembryonic membrane is the **yolk sac.** The yolk sacs in birds and reptiles help nourish the offspring, but the yolk sac in humans serves different functions: it produces red blood cells and immature sex cells (which later become the egg and the sperm). After the sixth week, the yolk sac ceases to function. The embryonic liver then produces red blood cells, and by the seventh month, the bone marrow has assumed this function. By then the yolk sac has become part of the umbilical cord.

The **allantois** is the fourth extraembryonic membrane. The allantois contributes to the formation of several structures, including the urinary bladder. The blood vessels of the allantois also help form the umbilical blood vessels, which transport blood to and from the placenta. After the second month, the allantois deteriorates and becomes part of the umbilical cord.

Placenta

The **placenta** (plə-sĕn′tə) is a disc-shaped structure about 7 inches (15–20 cm) in diameter and 1 inch (2.5 cm) thick. Normally, the placenta is in the upper portion of the uterus. The placenta is a highly vascular structure formed from both embryonic and maternal tissue. By the end of the embryonic period (8 weeks), the placenta is functional. After the birth of the baby, the placenta is expelled as part of the afterbirth.

FORMATION OF THE PLACENTA. The placenta develops as the chorionic villi of the embryo burrow into the endometrial lining of the uterus (see Fig. 23–3). The chorionic villi contain blood vessels that are continuous with the umbilical arteries and vein of the embryo. The chorionic villi sit in blood-filled spaces (lacunae) in the mother's endometrium.

Pay special attention to the arrangement of the embryonic and maternal blood vessels. The chorionic villi contain blood that comes from the embryo. The endometrial spaces (lacunae) contain blood from the mother. The embryonic and maternal blood supplies, while intimately close, are separated by the **placental membrane.** The placental membrane is formed by the membranes of the chorionic villi and the walls of the embryonic capillaries in the chorionic villi. The placental membrane thus maintains two separate circulations: the embryonic and maternal circulations. The two circulations do not mix!

FUNCTIONS OF THE PLACENTA. The placenta plays two important roles. First, it is the site across which nutrients and waste are exchanged between mother and baby. Second, it functions as a gland for the mother. Nutrients and waste exchange at the placental membrane. Oxygen, food, and other nutrients diffuse from the mother's blood into the blood of the embryo. Carbon dioxide and other waste diffuse from the embryo's blood into the mother's blood. The mother then excretes the waste through her organs of excretion. Baby-to-be "breathes" and "eats" at the placenta. If the placenta is injured in any way, the oxygen supply to the embryo may be cut off, causing irreversible brain damage and possibly death.

In addition to its role in exchange, the placenta acts as a gland for the mother. It secretes hormones that help to maintain the pregnancy, prepare the body for the birthing process, and promote postnatal events such as breastfeeding. The placental hormones are listed and described in Table 23–1.

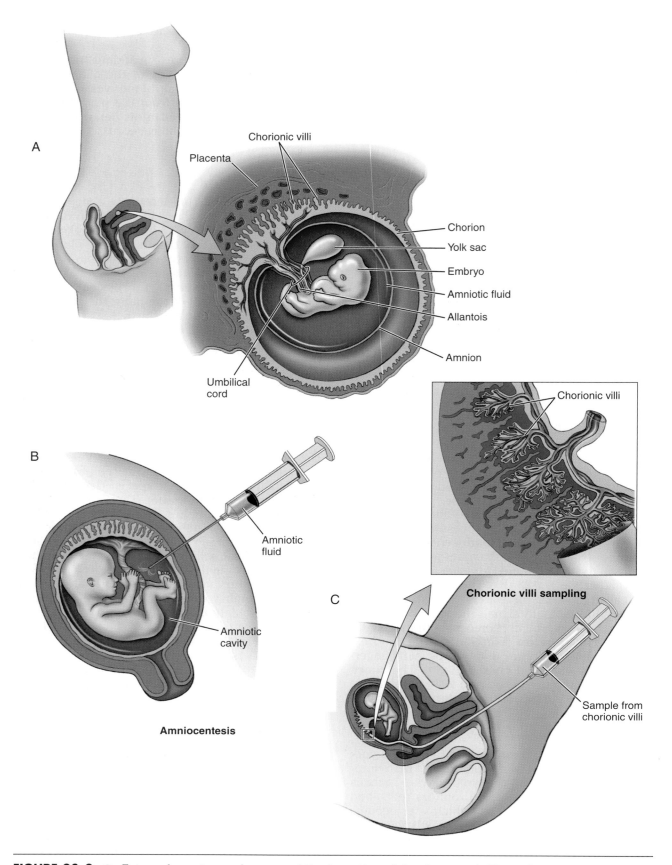

FIGURE 23–2 ● Extraembryonic membranes and the formation of the placenta. A, The embryo is surrounded by the amnion and the amniotic fluid in the amniotic cavity. The chorion forms the outer membrane. Chorionic villi containing blood vessels are projections extending into the uterine wall and helping to form the placenta. The third membrane is the yolk sac; the allantois is the fourth membrane. B, Amniocentesis: the insertion of a needle into the amniotic cavity and the aspiration of amniotic fluid. C, Chorionic villi sampling: the insertion of a tube into the area of the chorionic villi. A sample of fluid is aspirated and analyzed for the presence of fetal abnormalities.

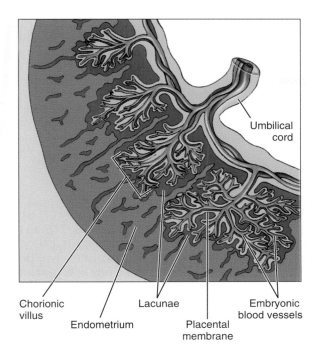

Chorionic villus
Endometrium
Lacunae
Placental membrane
Embryonic blood vessels

FIGURE 23–3 ● A cross-section of the chorionic villi. Note that the fetal circulation and the maternal circulation are separated by the placental membrane.

Hook Up: The Umbilical Cord

How does the embryo connect with the mother? The **umbilical cord** (ŭm-bĭl′ĭ-kəl kôrd) is the structure that connects embryo and mother at the placenta (see Fig. 23–2). The umbilical cord contains two umbilical arteries and one umbilical vein. Connective tissue strengthens the cord. Because the umbilical cord carries oxygen-rich blood to the developing infant, it is, literally, the baby's lifeline. Compression or injury to the umbilical cord can cause severe distress and possibly the death of the baby.

When the baby is delivered, the umbilical cord is cut, severing the infant from the placenta. The stump of the cord shrivels up, drops off, and leaves the **navel,** or belly button. The baby's organs, such as the lungs, kidneys, and digestive system must then take over the functions previously performed by the placenta.

Organogenesis

The embryonic period is a time of **organogenesis,** the formation of body organs and organ systems. The inner cell mass of the blastocyst forms a flattened structure called the **embryonic disc.** The embryonic disc, in turn, gives rise to three **primary germ layers,** the **ectoderm,** the **mesoderm,** and the **endoderm.**

All of the tissues and organs of the body develop from these germ layers. For instance, the ectoderm gives rise to the nervous system, portions of the special senses, and the skin. The skin is one of the earliest organs to develop and forms during the third week. The mesoderm gives rise to muscle, bone, blood, and many of the structures of the cardiovascular system. The endoderm gives rise to the epithelial lining of the digestive tract, respiratory tract, and parts of the urinary tract. By the end of the embryonic period (week 8) the main internal organs are established. The embryo weighs

Table 23•1	HORMONES OF PREGNANCY	
HORMONE	**SECRETED BY**	**EFFECTS**
Human chorionic gonadotropin (hCG)	Embryonic cells (trophoblasts) during implantation	Maintains the function of the corpus luteum; forms the basis of the pregnancy test.
Estrogen and progesterone	Corpus luteum during the first 2 months; placenta after 2 months	Both estrogen and progesterone stimulate the development of the uterine lining and mammary glands. Progesterone inhibits uterine contractions during pregnancy. Estrogen causes relaxation of the pelvic joints. At the beginning of labor, estrogen opposes the quieting effects of progesterone on uterine contractions and sensitizes the myometrium to oxytocin.
Prolactin	Anterior pituitary gland	Stimulates the breast to secrete milk.
Oxytocin	Posterior pituitary gland	Causes the release of milk from the breast (part of the milk let-down reflex initiated by suckling). Causes uterine contraction (participates in labor and postpartum uterine contractions to decrease bleeding).
Prostaglandins	Placenta	Stimulate uterine contractions.

about 1 gram, is about 1 inch (2.5 cm) in length, and has a human appearance (Fig. 23–4).

Be Careful: Teratogens

Because the organs of the body are being formed at this time, the embryonic period is most critical for development. Toxic substances such as alcohol, drugs, and certain pathogens can cross the placental membrane and interfere with embryonic development, causing severe birth defects. These toxic substances are called **teratogens** (tĕr′ə-tə-jənz), a word that means monster-producing and attests to the severity of teratogenic birth defects. Hazardous conditions such as exposure to radiation can also act as teratogens (Fig. 23–5).

Alcohol is a potent teratogen. Alcohol can cause a cluster of birth defects known as **fetal-alcohol syndrome.** In addition to causing facial deformities, alcohol interferes with neurologic and mental development. The tranquilizer thalidomide is another drug that produces teratogenic effects. The development of fin-like appendages instead of arms and legs has been correlated with the ingestion of thalidomide during pregnancy. Because of the sensitivity of the embryo to teratogenic agents, the mother must be extremely careful to protect her unborn child from toxic substances and hazardous conditions.

Fetal Period

The fetal period extends from week 9 to birth. At this time, the developing offspring is called a **fetus** (fē′təs). The fetal period is primarily a time of growth and maturation; only a few new parts appear. Body proportions, however, continue to

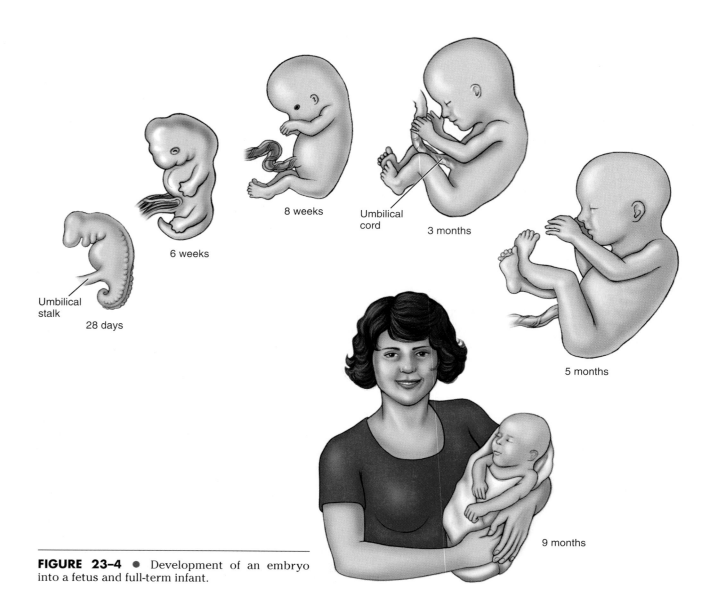

FIGURE 23–4 • Development of an embryo into a fetus and full-term infant.

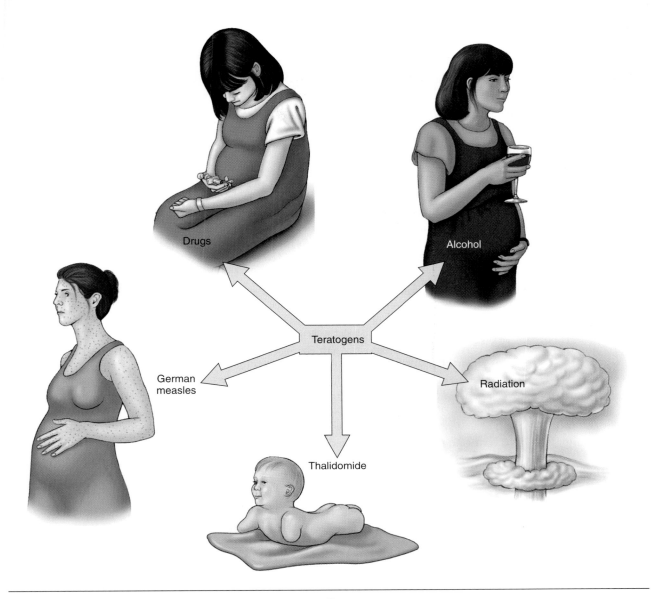

FIGURE 23–5 ● Teratogens: "monster-producing agents."

change. For instance, at 8 weeks the head is nearly as large as the body. At birth, the head is proportionately much smaller than the body. Note the change in body size and proportion in Figure 23–4.

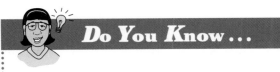

What is a sonogram?

A **sonogram** is an image produced by sound waves as they encounter different tissues and organs. During the procedure, sound waves are directed through the mother's abdomen. As the sound waves "hit" the fetus, an image appears on the scope showing an outline of the fetus. The sex of the fetus can be determined by sonography, as can certain fetal abnormalities.

Table 23–2 summarizes prenatal development. Note that a primitive nervous system begins to form in the third week. The heart and blood vessels originate during the second week. The heart is pumping blood to all the organs of the embryo by the second month, and a heartbeat can be detected during the third month, when the sex of the fetus can also be determined. Once the testes differentiate, they produce the male sex hormone testosterone. Testosterone stimulates the growth of the male external genitals. In the absence of testosterone, female genitals form.

The mother first feels the fetus move during the fifth month; this experience is called **quickening.** As the fetus grows, its skin becomes covered by a fine downy hair called **lanugo** (during the fifth month). The lanugo is covered by a white cheese-like substance called the **vernix caseosa.** The vernix is thought to protect the delicate fetal skin from the amniotic fluid. By the fifth month the fetus

Table 23 • 2	**HUMAN DEVELOPMENT**

TIME	DEVELOPMENTAL EVENT
Embryonic	
Second week	Implantation occurs. The inner cell mass is giving rise to the primary germ layers. Beginning of placental development.
Third week	Beginning of the nervous system.
Fourth week	Appearance of limb buds. Heart is beating. Embryo has tail. Other organ systems begin.
Fifth week	Enlarged head; nose, eyes, and ears are noticeable.
Sixth week	Fingers and toes are present; appearance of cartilage skeleton.
Second month	All organ systems are developing. Cartilaginous skeleton is being replaced by bone (ossification). Embryo is about 1.5 inches (3.8 cm) long.
Fetal	
Third month	Facial features present in crude form. Can determine gender (the external reproductive organs are distinguishable as male or female).
Fourth month	Sensory organs are present: eyes and ears attain shape and position. Eyes blink and the baby begins sucking movements. Skeleton is visible.
Fifth month	Vernix caseosa and a fine downy hair (lanugo) cover the skin. The proud parents first hear Baby's heartbeat during a prenatal visit. Quickening.
Sixth month	Continues to grow. Myelination of the spinal cord begins.
Seventh month	Eyes are open. Testes descend into scrotum. Weighs about 3 pounds (135 g). Bone marrow becomes the only site of blood cell formation.
Eighth month	Body is lean and well-proportioned. Subcutaneous fat begins to be deposited.
Ninth month	Full term and ready to be delivered. Average weight is 7.5 pounds (338 g). Average length is 21 inches (53.3 cm).

is in crowded quarters and is flexed anteriorly in fetal position. During the last 2 months the baby is gaining weight rapidly as fat is deposited in the subcutaneous tissue. As the time for birth approaches, the fetus rotates so that the head is pointed toward the cervix. At the end of 38 weeks, the fetus is full term. During this period the fetal weight has increased from less than ½ ounce (14 g) to 7.5 pounds (3.4 kg) (average weight of a full-term infant). The fetus has grown in length from about 1 inch (2.5 cm) to 21 inches (53 cm). Baby is ready to face the world!

Sometimes, the embryo or fetus is born too early, before the 9-month gestation period is completed. A number of terms are used to describe early birth. An **abortion** is the loss of an embryo or fetus before the twentieth week of development. A **spontaneous abortion** occurs naturally, with no artificial interference. Usually, a spontaneous abortion is caused by some fetal abnormality. A **miscarriage** is the layperson's term for a spontaneous abortion. An **induced abortion** is an abortion deliberately caused by some artificial or mechanical means. An unwanted pregnancy is a common cause of an induced abortion. A **therapeutic abortion** is performed by a physician as a form of treatment for the mother. For instance, a pregnancy that threatens the life of the mother may be terminated to save the mother's life or improve her medical condition.

A baby born before 38 weeks but capable of living outside the womb is a **premature** or **preterm infant.** A 20-week-old fetus is considered **viable,** that is, able to live outside the womb. A premature baby is small; but more importantly, it is immature and may require medical support. In particular, the hypothalamus is too immature to regulate body temperature well, and the surfactant produced by the fetal lungs is inadequate to maintain breathing. Premature infants frequently die from overexertion caused by respiratory distress associated with inadequate surfactants. Generally, the more premature the birth, the greater is the need for medical support.

✳ **SUM IT UP!** Prenatal development is divided into three periods: the early embryonic period, the embryonic period, and the fetal period. The early embryonic period lasts for 2 weeks and includes the development of the fertilized egg (zygote) to the blastocyst stage. Implantation of the blastocyst into the endometrium and the secretion of human chorionic gonadotropin (hCG) by the trophoblast are two important accomplishments of the early embryonic period. The period of embryonic development lasts for 6 weeks. The major accomplishments of the embryonic period include the formation of extraembryonic membranes and the development of the placenta and umbilical cord.

The embryonic period is also the period of organogenesis. Because all of the organ systems are developing at this time, the embryo is extremely sensitive to teratogenic, or monster-producing, effects. A teratogen is an agent (eg, drug) or force (eg, radiation) capable of interfering with organogenesis. Teratogens produce severe birth defects. The fetal period lasts from week 9 to birth and is primarily a period of rapid growth and maturation. Baby is shaping up, fattening up, and moving about. The mother can feel the fetus kick and stretch. Evidence suggests that babies even suck their thumbs at this time.

HORMONAL CHANGES DURING PREGNANCY

Pregnancy is characterized by complex hormonal changes. Several hormones are described in the text; a more complete list appears in Table 23–1.

Human Chorionic Gonadotropin (hCG)

After ovulation, the corpus luteum secretes estrogen and progesterone. In the nonpregnant condition, the corpus luteum deteriorates within 2 weeks, and the secretion of estrogen and progesterone declines. Deprived of its hormonal support, the endometrium sloughs, and menstruation begins. In the pregnant condition, secretion of hCG prevents the deterioration of the corpus luteum. Plasma levels of estrogen and progesterone are maintained, as is the endometrial lining. Menstruation is prevented. The trophoblast of the embryo secretes hCG. The secretion of hCG continues at a high level for the first 2 months of pregnancy and then declines to a low level by the end of 4 months. What happens to estrogen and progesterone after hCG levels decrease? By this time, the placenta is fully functional and secretes high levels of estrogen and progesterone. Thus, the placenta takes over the hormonal function of the corpus luteum.

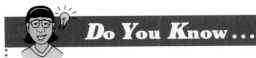

Do You Know...

What makes a pregnancy test positive?

Human chorionic gonadotropin (hCG) forms the basis of the pregnancy tests. hCG is secreted in early pregnancy and is eliminated by the mother's kidneys. Thus, hCG can be detected early in the mother's urine or blood. The pregnancy test may indicate positive results within about 8 to 10 days after fertilization.

Estrogen and Progesterone

The placenta secretes high levels of estrogen and progesterone throughout the second and third trimesters of pregnancy. Both hormones stimulate the continued development of the uterine lining. They also stimulate the development of the mammary glands, thereby preparing the mother for breastfeeding.

Estrogen causes an enlargement of the reproductive organs and relaxation of the ligaments of the pelvic joints. This process enlarges the pelvic cavity and facilitates the passage of the fetus through the birth canal at the time of delivery. Throughout early pregnancy, progesterone inhibits uterine contractions. The onset of labor, however, is associated with a decrease in the secretion of progesterone and an increase in the secretion of estrogen. This change in the concentration of estrogen and progesterone stimulates uterine contractions and contributes to the initiation of labor.

Other hormonal changes associated with pregnancy include increased secretion of aldosterone and parathyroid hormone. Aldosterone, secreted by the adrenal cortex, stimulates the kidney to reabsorb sodium and water. This increase in fluid, in turn, causes an increase in the maternal blood volume. Parathyroid hormone is secreted by the parathyroid gland and helps to maintain a high concentration of calcium in the maternal circulation. The fetus needs calcium for the development of the skeletal system. Other hormones are involved in the birthing process and lactation.

CHANGES IN THE MOTHER'S BODY DURING PREGNANCY

Throughout pregnancy the mother supplies all the food and oxygen for the fetus and eliminates all the waste. This added burden requires many changes in the mother's physiology:

- The rate of metabolism increases. For instance, the mother secretes greater amounts of the thyroid hormones triiodothyronine (T3) and thyroxine (T4). The increased metabolism, in turn, stimulates other organ systems. The mother's entire body responds to the demands of her unborn child.
- The mother's blood volume expands by as much as 40 to 50%. To pump the additional blood and meet the demands of an increased metabolism, the activity of the cardiovascular system increases. For instance, heart rate, stroke volume, and cardiac output increase.
- Respiratory activity increases to provide additional oxygen and to eliminate excess carbon dioxide.
- The kidneys work harder and produce more urine because they must eliminate waste for both the mother and the fetus.

- The size and weight of the uterus increase dramatically as the fetus grows to full term. To accommodate the growth of the uterus, the pelvic cavity expands as the sacroiliac joints and the symphysis pubis become more flexible. With growth, the uterus pushes, or displaces, the abdominal organs upward. In the later months of pregnancy especially, the upward displacement of abdominal organs exerts pressure on the diaphragm and hampers the mother's breathing.
- The mother's nutritional needs increase as the maternal organs (uterus and breasts) grow and she provides for the growing fetus.

Pregnancy brings some discomforts for some women. Nausea and vomiting, generally referred to as morning sickness, commonly occur in the first 3 months. Morning sickness may be due to hormonal changes, especially to the elevated levels of hCG. (Some women experience nausea and vomiting in the evening, not in the morning.) During the later months of pregnancy, the woman gains approximately 2 to 3 pounds per month. The added weight causes a shift in the mother's center of gravity, thereby affecting her balance and forcing her to adjust her walking style (eventually, many women appear to be waddling).

The added weight may also cause discomfort in the lower back and a multitude of other aches as the uterine ligaments and other supporting structures stretch. The expanding uterus stretches the abdominal skin, causing stretch marks, or **striae.** It also displaces the stomach upward, causing heartburn. Frequent urination results from increased urine formation and compression of the urinary bladder by the uterus. Lastly, the expanded uterus hampers the return of blood through the veins of the lower body region. This inhibited blood flow, in turn, may cause varicose veins and hemorrhoids. No wonder that the mother-to-be looks forward to giving birth!

While these discomforts of pregnancy are normal, several pregnancy-related conditions are not normal and are instead dangerous to both the mother and the child. For instance, the mother may develop a toxemia of pregnancy. This condition is characterized by an elevated blood pressure and progresses in severe cases to generalized seizures. The early stage is called **preeclampsia,** and the later seizure stage is called **eclampsia.**

✳ **SUM IT UP!** Pregnancy causes many changes in the mother. Hormonal changes are numerous and complex. Secretion of hCG, estrogen, and progesterone help maintain the pregnancy and prepare the organs of reproduction for 9 months of pregnancy. Other hormones, such as aldosterone, thyroid hormones, and parathyroid hormone, prepare the mother's body to nourish and sustain the growing unborn child. Almost every maternal organ responds to the presence of the fetus. The heart pumps more blood; the kidneys excrete more waste; and the increased metabolic rate indicates that every cell is working harder.

BIRTH OF THE BABY

Finally, Baby is ready to face the world. The birth process is called **parturition. Labor** is the process whereby forceful contractions expel the fetus from the uterus. Once labor starts, forceful and rhythmic contractions begin at the top of the uterus and travel down its length, forcing the fetus through the birth canal.

Labor

Hormonal Basis of Labor

The precise mechanism that starts labor is unknown. A number of hormonal stimuli do, however, play a role. For example, progesterone, which normally suppresses, or quiets, uterine contractions during pregnancy, is secreted in decreasing amounts after the seventh month. This decrease coincides with an increase in the secretion of estrogen. Estrogen has two effects on the uterus: it opposes the quieting effect of progesterone on uterine contractions, and it sensitizes the myometrium (uterine muscle) to the stimulatory effects of oxytocin.

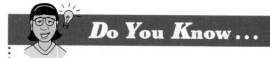

Why can aspirin and ibuprofen inhibit the onset of labor?

Aspirin and ibuprofen are antiprostaglandin drugs. Because prostaglandins stimulate uterine contractions, suppression of prostaglandin secretion by these drugs may inhibit uterine contractions, thereby inhibiting labor.

The secretion of prostaglandins by the placenta also plays a role in initiating labor. Prostaglandins stimulate uterine contractions. Finally, the stretching of the uterine and vaginal tissue in the late stage of pregnancy stimulates nerves, which send signals to the hypothalamus. The hypothalamus, in turn, stimulates the release of oxytocin from the posterior pituitary gland. Oxytocin exerts a powerful stimulating effect on the myometrium and is thought to play an important role in initiating labor.

Labor can, however, have a false start. Sometimes, a very pregnant and embarrassed mother is admitted to the hospital in false labor. What has happened? She has indeed felt uterine contractions. These contractions, however, are weak, irregular, and ineffectual. They are called **Braxton Hicks contractions,** and they normally occur during late pregnancy. These contractions are due to the increased responsiveness of the uterus to various hormones, particularly changing concentrations of estrogen and progesterone. The mother returns home to await the onset of true labor.

Stages of Labor

The three stages of true labor are the dilation stage, the expulsion stage, and the placental stage (Fig. 23–6). The **dilation stage** begins with the onset of labor and ends with full dilation of the cervix (10 cm). This stage is characterized by rhythmic and forceful contractions, rupture of the amniotic sac (the bag of waters), and cervical dilation. It is the longest stage of labor and generally lasts between 6 and 12 hours, although wide variation occurs from person to person. The **expulsion stage** extends from complete cervical dilation to the expulsion of the fetus through the vagina (birth canal). This stage generally lasts less than 1 hour. During this stage the mother has the urge to push, or to bear down, with abdominal muscles.

Do You Know...

What are placenta previa and abruptio placentae?

Sometimes the placenta forms too low in the uterus, near the cervix. When the cervix dilates during the later stages of pregnancy, the placenta detaches from the uterine wall, causing bleeding in the mother and depriving the fetus of an adequate supply of oxygen and nutrients. This condition is called **placenta previa. Abruptio placentae** refers to the premature separation of an implanted placentae at about 20 or more weeks of pregnancy. Without immediate treatment, abruptio placentae results in severe hemorrhage in the mother and death of the fetus.

In a normal delivery, the head is delivered first. A head-first delivery allows the baby to be suctioned free of mucus and to breathe even before the baby's body has fully exited from the birth canal. Because the vaginal orifice may not expand enough to deliver the baby, however, an episiotomy may be performed. An **episiotomy** is a surgical incision into the perineum, the tissue between the vaginal opening and the anus. The incision enlarges the vaginal opening and facilitates the delivery of the baby, thereby avoiding a lacerated perineum.

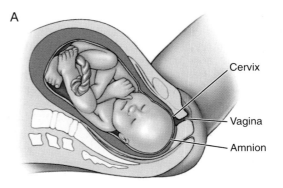

A

Cervix

Vagina

Amnion

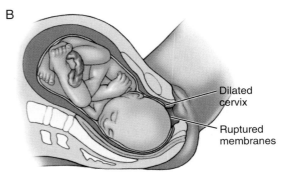

B

Dilated cervix

Ruptured membranes

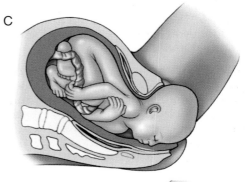

C

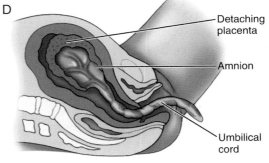

D

Detaching placenta

Amnion

Umbilical cord

FIGURE 23–6 ● Stages of labor. A, Before labor begins. B, Dilation stage. C, Expulsion stage. D, Placental stage.

The third stage is the **placental stage** and occurs 10 to 15 minutes after the birth of the baby. It involves the separation of the placenta from the uterine wall and expulsion of the placenta and attached membranes by forceful uterine contractions. The placenta and the attached membranes are collectively called the afterbirth. In addition to expelling the fetus and the placenta, the uterine contractions also cause vasoconstriction of the uterine blood vessels, thereby minimizing blood loss. Uterine contractions also help the uterus to return to its nonpregnant size and shape. About 500 mL of blood is lost during delivery.

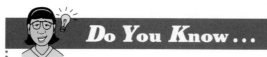

Do You Know...

What is a C-section?

A C-section, or cesarean section, refers to the delivery of the infant through a surgical incision in the abdominal and uterine walls. Rumor has it that Julius Caesar was born surgically; hence the name.

Sometimes, the fetus does not come out, or present, head first. Instead, another part of the body, such as the buttocks, is delivered first. This presentation is called a **breech birth.** A breech presentation makes delivery more difficult for both the mother and the infant.

✳ **SUM IT UP!** The birth process is called parturition. Labor is the forceful contractions that expel the baby and afterbirth from the uterus, through the birth canal. Labor begins in response to various hormones, particularly oxytocin. The three stages of labor are the dilation stage, the expulsion stage, and the placental stage.

FEMALE BREAST AND LACTATION

Structure of a Breast: The Mammary Glands

The anterior chest contains two elevations called breasts (Fig. 23–7A). The **breasts** are located anterior to the pectoralis major muscles and contain adipose tissue and mammary glands. **Mammary glands** (măm′əh-rē glăndz) are accessory organs of the female reproductive system. They secrete milk following the delivery of the baby. At the tip of each breast is a **nipple** surrounded by a circular area of pigmented skin called the **areola.** Each mammary gland contains 15 to 20 lobes. Each lobe contains many alveolar glands and a lactiferous duct. The **alveolar glands** secrete milk, which is carried toward the nipple by the **lactiferous duct.** Connective tissue, including the suspensory ligaments, helps support the breast.

Until a child reaches puberty, the mammary glands of male and female children are similar. At puberty, however, the female mammary glands are stimulated by estrogen and progesterone. The alveolar glands and ducts enlarge, and adipose tissue is deposited around these structures. The male breast does not develop because there is no hormonal stimulus to do so. If a male is given female hormones, however, he too develops breasts.

Hormones of Lactation

During pregnancy, the increased secretion of estrogen and progesterone have a profound effect on the breasts. The breasts may double in preparation for milk production, or **lactation,** following birth. Usually there is no milk production during pregnancy because lactation requires **prolactin,** a hormone secreted by the anterior pituitary gland (in response to a releasing hormone) (Fig. 23–7B). High plasma levels of estrogen and progesterone inhibit prolactin secretion during pregnancy. After delivery, however, plasma levels of estrogen and progesterone decrease, allowing the anterior pituitary gland to secrete prolactin. Milk production takes 2 to 3 days to begin. In the meantime, the mammary glands produce **colostrum,** a yellowish watery fluid rich in protein and antibodies.

While prolactin is necessary for milk production, a second hormone, **oxytocin,** is necessary for the *release* of milk from the breast. How does milk release happen? When the baby suckles, or nurses, at the breast, nerve impulses in the areola are stimulated. Nerve impulses then travel from the breast to the hypothalamus; the hypothalamus, in turn, stimulates the posterior pituitary gland to release oxytocin. The oxytocin travels through the blood to the breast, causing contraction of the lobules. This process squeezes milk into the ducts, where it can be drawn out of the nipple by the nursing infant.

The effect of suckling and oxytocin release is called the **milk let-down reflex** (mĭlk lĕt′doun rē′flĕks). Note that the stimulus for the milk let-down reflex is suckling at the breast. Thus, nursing mothers are encouraged to suckle their infants frequently. Breastfeeding encourages a good flow of milk. Note the distinction between the effects of prolactin and oxytocin. Prolactin stimulates milk production, or lactation. Oxytocin stimulates the milk let-down reflex and stimulates the flow of milk.

In addition to its effect on the flow of milk, oxytocin causes the uterus to contract. Uterine contraction helps minimize blood loss and more quickly returns the uterus to its nonpregnant state. A classification of drugs called **oxytocic agents** are sometimes administered to the mother after childbirth. Like oxytocin, these drugs cause uterine contractions and minimize postpartum bleeding.

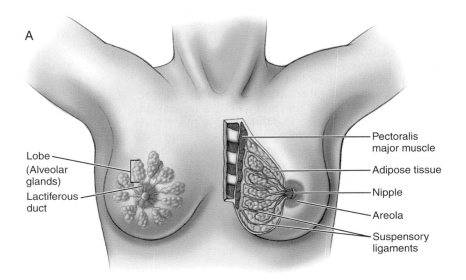

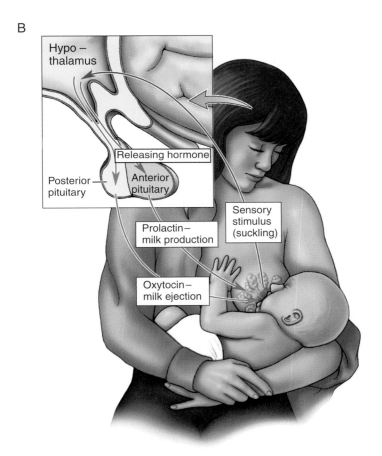

FIGURE 23–7 ● A, Breast and mammary glands. B, Hormones involved in breastfeeding. Prolactin stimulates milk production. Oxytocin is concerned with the flow of milk (milk let-down reflex).

Labels in figure A:
Lobe (Alveolar glands)
Lactiferous duct
Pectoralis major muscle
Adipose tissue
Nipple
Areola
Suspensory ligaments

Labels in figure B:
Hypo–thalamus
Releasing hormone
Posterior pituitary
Anterior pituitary
Prolactin–milk production
Oxytocin–milk ejection
Sensory stimulus (suckling)

POSTNATAL CHANGES AND DEVELOPMENTAL STAGES

Immediate Adjustments

Immediately after birth, the baby must make many important adjustments to survive. Most importantly, the baby must begin breathing. The first deep breaths, drawn as the baby cries, expand the lungs and provide the infant with life-giving oxygen. The cardiovascular system then makes a second major adjustment. These changes are summarized in Table 15–2. (Fetal circulation was described in Chapter 15.)

Just after birth, other organ systems also begin to function. For instance, the kidneys begin to make urine, and the digestive system begins a life-long career of eating, digesting, and excreting. The first stool produced by the newborn is soft and black; it is called **meconium.**

One minute after birth, the infant's physical condition may be rated according to the Apgar scale. A score of 0, 1, 2, and so on, with a maximum score of 10, is given for the following signs: heart rate, respirations, color, muscle tone, and response to stimuli. An Apgar evaluation is also made at 5 minutes. Infants with low Apgar scores require prompt medical treatment.

Development as a Lifelong Process

After the newborn makes the immediate adjustments, the infant continues to grow and develop. Throughout life, the person will pass through the following developmental stages:

- Neonatal period. The neonatal period begins at birth and lasts for 4 weeks. During this time, the baby is called a **neonate.**
- Infancy. The period of infancy lasts from the end of the first month to the end of the first year. Baby's first birthday marks the end of this stage.
- Childhood. The period of childhood lasts from the beginning of the second year to puberty.
- Adolescence. The period of adolescence lasts from puberty to adulthood. One word characterizes this stage: hormones. Now both young women and young men are physically capable of reproduction. The period of adolescence is a period of tremendous growth and upheaval. The teen moves toward adulthood, leaving behind childish ways and coming to grips with becoming an adult.
- Adulthood. Adulthood is the period from adolescence to old age. During this period, the person is usually concerned with family matters and career goals. Most of us are still trying to give up childish ways.
- Senescence. Senescence is the period of old age, ending in death. It is not only a time to reflect on a life well lived but also a time to pursue other goals and to pass on the collected wisdom of a lifetime.

✳ **SUM IT UP!** After the birth of the baby, both baby and mother make many physiologic adjustments. The mother's body returns to its nonpregnant state. For instance, cardiac output and blood volume decrease. She is physiologically prepared to breastfeed. Through the actions of prolactin and oxytocin, her mammary glands are producing milk (the process called lactation) and making it readily available to the suckling infant (through the milk let-down reflex). The baby has made an initial adjustment to life on the outside and is breathing, urinating, and eating. The newborn continues postnatal development as a neonate. From there, it is on to infancy, childhood, adolescence, adulthood, and senescence.

HEREDITY

"He has his father's nose and his mother's smile." How often have we made that kind of statement when we recognize the traits of a parent in a child? The transmission of characteristics from parent to child is called **heredity,** and the science that studies heredity is called **genetics.** It was the work of an Austrian monk, Gregor Mendel, in the early 19th century that paved the way for the modern science of genetics. Using garden peas, Mendel demonstrated a pattern of specific traits passed on from parent to child.

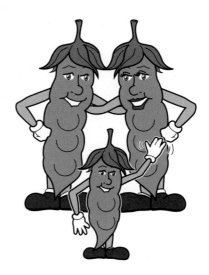

DNA, Genes, and Chromosomes

How are genetic structures related? Genetic information is located in the DNA molecule and more specifically in the DNA base-sequencing. (You may wish to review this topic in Chapter 4.) DNA is tightly wound into thread-like structures called **chromosomes** (krō′mə-sōmz), found in the nucleus of most cells in the body. **Genes** (jēnz) are segments of the DNA strand and carry information for a specific trait, such as skin color, freckles, and blood type. See Table 23–3 for other genetically determined characteristics. Some traits are determined by a single pair of genes, whereas other traits, such as height, require input from several genes. Each chromosome may carry thousands of genes, and each gene occupies a specific position on a chromosome.

Chromosomes exist in pairs. With the exception of the sex cells (egg and sperm) there are 23 pairs, or 46 chromosomes, in almost all human cells (red blood cells are the other exception). During fertilization, the egg from the female contributes 23 chromosomes to the zygote and the sperm from the male contributes 23 chromosomes to the zygote, for a total of 23 pairs, or 46 chromo-

Table 23•3 EXAMPLES OF GENETIC TRAITS

TRAIT	DOMINANT	RECESSIVE
Hairline	Widow's peak	Continuous hairline
Hair color	Dark	Light
Hair texture	Curly	Straight
Hair on back of hand	Present	Absent
Freckles	Present	Absent (few)
Dimples	Present	Absent
Eye color	Dark	Light
Color vision	Normal	Color blind
Ear lobes	Unattached	Attached
Cleft chin	Present	Absent
Rh factor	Present	Absent

somes. One member of each pair comes from the egg; the other comes from the sperm. Thus, for each trait, genetic instructions come from both the mother and the father. Forty-four chromosomes (22 pairs) are called **autosomes.** The autosomal gene pairs are numbered from 1 to 22. Two (one pair) of the 46 chromosomes are sex chromosomes; each is either an X or a Y chromosome.

Genetic Art: The Karyotype

It is possible to photograph the chromosomes in the cell. The photograph of the chromosomes is then cut apart, and the chromosomes are arranged in pairs by size and shape. The resulting display of the paired chromosomes is called a **karyotype** (kăr′ē-ə-tīp) (Fig. 23–8). This genetic art work displays 22 pairs of autosomes and one pair of sex chromosomes. The karyotype is a diagnostic tool. It can reveal structural abnormalities and errors in the numbers of chromosomes.

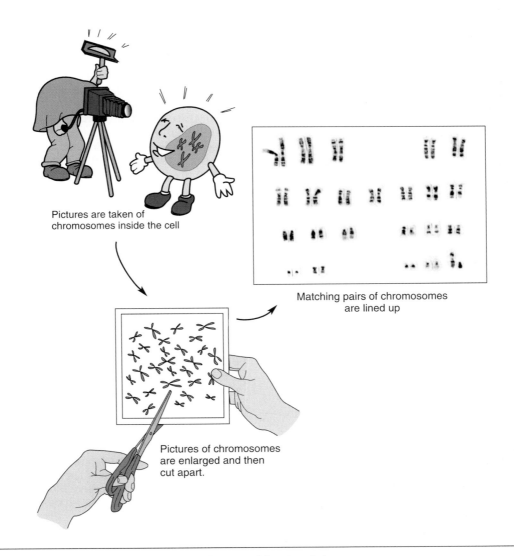

Pictures are taken of chromosomes inside the cell

Pictures of chromosomes are enlarged and then cut apart.

Matching pairs of chromosomes are lined up

FIGURE 23–8 ● Genetic art: the karyotype. There are 23 pairs of chromosomes.

Dominant, Recessive, and Codominant Genes

Remember: Each cell inherits two genes for each trait—tall/short, straight nose/curved nose, stubby fingers/long fingers, dark eyes/light eyes. Hence the choice: Will it be long or short, curved or straight? Genes can be dominant, recessive, or codominant. A **dominant gene** (dŏm′ə-nənt jēn) expresses itself; it gets noticed. The dominant gene overshadows the recessive gene, keeping it unnoticed, or unexpressed. Thus, a **recessive gene** (rĭ-sĕs′ĭv jēn) is not expressed if it is paired with a dominant gene. For instance, the genes for dark eyes are dominant, whereas the genes for light eyes are recessive. If the dominant genes (dark) and the recessive (light) genes are paired, the genes for dark eyes will be expressed (Fig. 23–9). The genes for light eyes will not be expressed. Gregor Mendel made the same observations about his peas—he found dominant and recessive traits in peas. **Codominant genes** express a trait equally. AB blood type is an example of codominance.

If recessive genes carry light eye coloring, how can an offspring develop blue eyes? Although blue eye coloring is recessive, a baby develops blue eyes because both the mother and the father are carrying the genes for blue eyes, a recessive trait (Fig. 23–9). If either the mother or the father had passed on a dominant gene for dark eyes, the child would have brown eyes.

The question put another way: If I have brown eyes, can any of my children have blue eyes? Yes! If I am carrying both a dominant (brown) and recessive (blue) gene for eye color, my child has a chance of having blue eyes. My recessive gene might pair with a recessive gene from my mate. If so, the pairing of two recessive genes produces a blue-eyed offspring. Brown-eyed-me is a **carrier,** one who shows no evidence of a trait (like blue eyes) but carries a recessive gene for that trait.

Too Many or Too Few Chromosomes

A person normally inherits 22 pairs of autosomal chromosomes (ie, the non-sex chromosomes). Sometimes, however, a person inherits too many or too few autosomal chromosomes. The most common autosomal abnormality is called **trisomy 21,** or **Down syndrome.** A child with trisomy 21 has three copies of chromosome 21 instead of two copies. Other types of trisomy occur very infre-

quently in live births. **Trisomy 18,** called **Edward syndrome,** is due to three copies of chromosome 18, while **trisomy 13,** called **Patau syndrome,** is due to three copies of chromosome 13. Autosomal abnormalities are usually due to nondisjunction.

Nondisjunction is the failure of the chromosomes (or chromatids) to separate during meiosis, thereby causing the formation of eggs or sperm with too many or too few chromosomes. If these eggs and sperm lead to pregnancy, the embryo may have one too many or too few chromosomes. Most pregnancies with an unbalanced number of chromosomes miscarry in the first trimester. Down syndrome is the most common chromosomal abnormality because the condition is least likely to cause the pregnancy to miscarry. Even so, an estimated 70% of pregnancies with Down syndrome spontaneously miscarry, usually in the first trimester.

Genetic Expression

Genetic expression determines what the offspring looks like. A person's genetic makeup, in turn, determines genetic expression. A person's genetic expression can be influenced by a number of factors, including the person's sex, the influence of other genes, and environmental conditions. For instance, certain types of baldness and color blindness may be inherited by both males and females, but these traits are more apt to appear in the male. A child may also have the genetic capability of growing very tall. If the child is deprived of adequate nutrition and exercise, however, that child may not grow as tall as genetic makeup predicted.

Genetic Mutations

Normally, DNA replicates all information with few mistakes. Because of this precision, information is passed along reliably and efficiently to the next generation. Sometimes, however, a change occurs in a gene, or a chromosome breaks in some unexpected way. The result may be a unique feature or a birth defect. This change in the genetic code is called a **mutation.** Some mutations occur spontaneously. Others are caused by **mutagenic agents.** Certain chemicals, drugs, and radiation are mutagenic. Mutations can be beneficial or harmful and may even cause the death of the offspring. For instance, a mutation in the cells of the immune system may render a child resistant to a

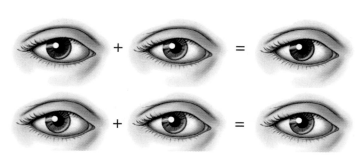

FIGURE 23–9 ● Eye color: dominant and recessive genes. A, The dominant brown-eye gene is expressed over the recessive blue-eye gene. B, Two recessive blue-eye genes produce a blue-eyed offspring.

particular disease, thereby enhancing health. Another mutation, however, may weaken the immune system, making it more susceptible to pathogens.

It's A Boy—It's A Girl: How the Sex of the Child Is Determined

Xs and Ys

Each human cell has 22 pairs of autosomal chromosomes and one pair of sex chromosomes (X and Y chromosomes). The female has two X chromosomes in her cells, a pair designated XX. A male has both an X and a Y chromosome in his cells, a pair designated XY (Fig. 23–10).

Sex Determination: A Male Thing

The **sex cells,** the egg and the sperm, divide by a special type of cell division called **meiosis** (mī-ō′sĭs). The important step in meiosis is the reduction (by one half) of the chromosomes. In other words, meiosis reduces the numbers of chromosomes from 46 to 23. The meiotic cell reduction also reduces the numbers of sex chromosomes by half. Consequently, each egg contains one X chromosome, and the sperm contains either an X chromosome or a Y chromosome. If a sperm containing an X chromosome fertilizes an egg, the child has an XX sex chromosome pair and is therefore female. If a sperm containing a Y chromosome fertilizes an egg, the child has an XY chromosome pair and is therefore male. Thus, the sperm (male) determines the sex of the child.

Sometimes a person inherits an abnormal number of sex chromosomes. For instance, a female with Turner syndrome inherits only one sex chromosome, an X chromosome. Turner syndrome is designated as XO. The X signifies the female chromosome; the O signifies the absence of the second sex chromosome. A child with Turner syndrome does not develop secondary sex characteristics, is shorter than average, and has a webbed neck. People with Turner syndrome have normal intelligence. Other genetic disorders involving extra sex chromosomes include Klinefelter syndrome (XXY) and the XYY male.

Sex-Linked Traits

The X and Y chromosomes differ structurally. The female X chromosome is larger than the Y chromosome and carries many genes for traits in addition to determining sex. The male Y chromosome is much smaller than the X chromosome and does not carry as much genetic information as the X chromosome does. Any trait that is carried on a sex chromosome is called a **sex-linked trait** (sĕks′lĭngkt″ trāt). Because the X chromosome has more genetic information than the Y chromosome, most sex-linked traits are carried on

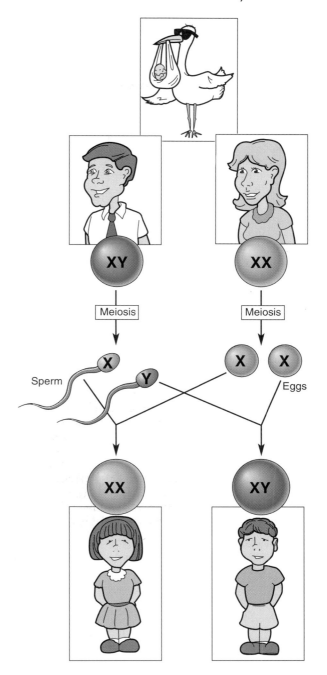

FIGURE 23–10 • Determination of sex: Xs and Ys. If an X chromosome from a male unites with an X chromosome of a female, the child is female. If a Y chromosome from a male unites with an X chromosome from a female, the child is male.

the female X chromosome. Sex-linked traits carried on the X chromosomes are also called **X-linked traits.**

While most sex-linked traits are carried on the X chromosome, they are expressed, or appear, in the male. Sex-linked diseases include hemophilia, Duchenne muscular dystrophy, and fragile X syndrome. Less serious sex-linked traits include baldness and red-green color-blindness.

Congenital and Hereditary Disease

You need to distinguish between congenital diseases and defects and hereditary diseases. **Congenital** (kən-jĕn′ĭ-tl) conditions are present at the time of birth. **Hereditary diseases** are genetically transmitted or transmissible. Any disease or defect present at birth is called congenital and includes both conditions that are inherited and those that are not. For instance, hemophilia is genetically transmitted and is therefore inherited. Because hemophilia is present at birth, it is also congenital.

A disease can, however, be congenital but not inherited. For instance, a mother may give birth to an infant who was exposed to the rubella virus (German measles) during her first trimester of pregnancy. This child may be born with cardiovascular defects, ocular defects, neural tube defects, and learning disabilities. These defects were not transmitted genetically from the parents to the child and are therefore not hereditary. The defects are congenital, however, because they were present at birth. Only 15% of congenital defects have a known genetic cause. Far fewer have a known environmental cause; for 70% of congenital birth defects, the cause is unknown.

Gene therapy offers hope for the treatment and eventual cure of genetic disorders. Gene therapy refers to the insertion of normal genes into cells that have abnormal genes. For instance, a person with congenitally high cholesterol levels might be successfully treated with genes that code for normal cholesterol production. Although in its early experimental stages, gene therapy provides hope for those with such genetic conditions as sickle cell disease, cystic fibrosis, and muscular dystrophy.

✳ **SUM IT UP!** A child resembles the parents because he or she inherits genetic information from each parent. Genetic information is stored in the DNA molecules, which are arranged in tightly woven strands called chromosomes. Almost every human cell contains 22 pairs of autosomal chromosomes and one pair of sex chromosomes. Egg and sperm cells each have only 23 chromosomes. Genes are segments of DNA that contain codes for specific traits such as eye color or blood type. The child receives two genes for each inherited trait, one from the mother and one from the father.

Genes are dominant, recessive, or codominant. The dominant gene expresses itself over a recessive gene. A recessive gene expresses itself only when it is paired with another recessive gene. Codominant genes express a trait equally (as with AB blood type). The sex chromosomes are designated X and Y. A female cell has two X chromosomes and is designated XX; a male cell has an X and a Y chromosome, designated XY. At fertilization, an XX combination produces a female child, while an XY combination produces a male. The father, with his Y chromosome, determines the sex of the child. Genetic information is passed along efficiently and reliably. Occasionally, incorrect or unhealthy information is passed along, thereby producing genetic diseases.

Disorders of Human Development

Cystic fibrosis	A disorder that results in the secretion of a thick mucus. The mucus obstructs the respiratory passages and the ducts of the pancreas. The child's main problem concerns inadequate respiratory function. Cystic fibrosis is the most common genetic disease within the white population.
Duchenne muscular dystrophy	A disorder caused by a defective protein and characterized by the replacement of muscle tissue with fat and scar tissue. There is a progressive decline in muscle function, so that the child is eventually confined to a wheelchair and dies because of poor muscle functioning of the heart and respiratory system.
Hemophilia	A disorder characterized by a deficiency of the antihemophilic factor (factor VIII). Hemophilia causes bleeding and immobility of the joints (see Chapter 13).
Huntington disease	A neurologic disorder characterized by uncontrollable muscle contractions and deterioration of the memory and personality. The onset of symptoms is delayed until 30 to 50 years of age, making genetic counseling difficult.
Neurofibromatosis	Also called elephant man disease. Neurofibromatosis is a disorder characterized by the growth of multiple masses along nerves throughout the body. The growths result in severe deformities. Many persons with this disorder become socially isolated and suffer more emotionally than physically.

Disorders of Human Development, *continued*

Osteogenesis imperfecta	Known as brittle bone disease and characterized by multiple fractures. Some bones may break in response to a simple change in posture.
Sickle cell disease	A genetic condition in which defective hemoglobin is synthesized (a single amino acid is out of place in the globin chain, causing a distortion of the hemoglobin molecule). The defective hemoglobin causes the red blood cells to sickle and then lyse, producing hemolytic anemia. The sickling also causes tissue hypoxia and severe pain.
Tay-Sachs disease	A disorder characterized by degeneration of the nervous system, resulting in death before the age of 2 years. Tay-Sachs disease is the most common genetic disease in persons of Jewish ancestry.

Summary Outline

The purpose of the reproductive system is to produce offspring whose genetic information is faithfully transmitted from generation to generation.

I. Fertilization to Birth

A. Fertilization
1. Fertilization is called conception and refers to the union of an egg and a sperm.
2. Fertilization takes place around the time of ovulation, usually at midcycle, and occurs in the fallopian tube.
3. The fertilized egg is called a zygote.

B. Human Development
1. Development is a process that begins with fertilization and ends with death; the two phases are prenatal development and postnatal development.
2. Prenatal development includes four processes: cleavage, growth, morphogenesis, and differentiation.

C. Prenatal Development
1. The prenatal period consists of the early embryonic period, the embryonic period, and the fetal period.
2. The early embryonic period lasts for 2 weeks after fertilization. Through the process of mitosis, the zygote evolves into a morula and then a blastocyst. The blastocyst implants into the uterine endometrial lining. The trophoblasts of the blastocyst secrete hCG (to maintain the secretion of the corpus luteum).
3. The two types of twins are monozygotic (identical) twins and dizygotic or fraternal (nonidentical) twins.
4. The embryonic period lasts for 6 weeks (from week 3 to week 8). The embryonic period involves the formation of the extraembryonic membranes, the placenta, and all of the organ systems.
5. The four extraembryonic membranes are the amnion, the chorion, the yolk sac, and the allantois. At birth the membranes are expelled with the placenta as the afterbirth.
6. The placenta develops as the chorionic villi of the embryo burrow into the endometrial lining of the uterus. The blood of the mother and embryo are very close but are still separate. The two blood circulations do not mix.

7. The placenta has two functions: it is the site of "exchange" of nutrients and waste, and it acts as a gland by secreting estrogen and progesterone throughout the pregnancy.
8. The embryo is hooked up to the placenta by the umbilical cord. The cord carries the large umbilical blood vessels.
9. The embryonic period is a period of organogenesis (the formation of the organs and organ systems). The organs arise from the primary germ layers: the ectoderm, the mesoderm, and the endoderm. During organogenesis, teratogens can exert very harmful effects.
10. The fetal period extends from week 9 to birth. It is a time of growth and maturation. See Table 23–2 for month-by-month growth.
11. The mother first feels the fetus moving during the fifth month. The experience is called quickening.
12. Hormonal changes during pregnancy include secretion of hCG, estrogen, and progesterone (and many others). See Table 23–1.
13. The mother-to-be experiences many physiologic changes during pregnancy. These include increased metabolism, increased cardiovascular function, increased blood volume, and increased kidney and respiratory function.

D. Birth (Parturition)
1. Labor is the forceful contractions that expel the fetus from the uterus.
2. Labor is caused by hormones (progesterone, estrogen, prostaglandins, and oxytocin).
3. The three stages of labor are the dilation stage, the expulsion stage, and the placental stage.

E. Breasts and Lactation
1. The breasts contain mammary (milk-secreting) glands and adipose tissue.
2. The mammary glands and surrounding structures are affected by two hormones, prolactin and oxytocin. Prolactin stimulates the

continued

I. Fertilization to Birth, *continued*

E. Breasts and Lactation, *continued*

mammary glands to increase the production of milk. Oxytocin stimulates the smooth muscle in the breast to release the milk (part of the milk let-down reflex).

II. Postnatal Development

A. Immediate Postnatal Changes

1. The baby takes a first breath and the cardiovascular system makes some major adjustments (changes from a fetal circulation to a postnatal circulation).
2. The baby's transition to "life on the outside" is monitored by the Apgar scale.

B. Developmental Periods

1. The neonatal period begins at birth and lasts for 4 weeks.
2. Infancy extends from the end of 1 month to 1 year.
3. Childhood lasts from year 2 to puberty.
4. Adolescence lasts from puberty to adulthood (there is no general agreement on the exact number of years).
5. Adulthood is the period from adolescence to old age.
6. Senescence is the period of old age ending in death.

III. Heredity

A. DNA, Genes, and Chromosomes

1. Genetic information is stored in the DNA of genes, which are arranged into chromosomes.
2. Chromosomes exist in pairs. With the exception of sex cells, most human cells have 23 pairs of chromosomes, or 46 chromosomes.
3. Genes are dominant, recessive, or codominant. A dominant gene expresses itself. A recessive gene does not express itself if it is paired with a dominant gene. Codominant genes express a trait equally.
4. A genetic mutation is due to a change in the genetic code. The code tells the cell to make a different protein; therefore the cell functions differently. Some mutations are helpful, most are harmless, and some are lethal.
5. The sex chromosomes are designated X and Y. A female has two X chromosomes, and a male has one X chromosome and one Y chromosome. Because only the male has the Y chromosome, the father determines the sex of the child.
6. Sex-linked traits are carried on the sex chromosomes. Most are carried on the X chromosome and are therefore also called X-linked traits.

B. Congenital and Hereditary Diseases

1. A congenital disorder is a condition present at birth. Congenital disorders include inherited and noninherited birth defects and diseases. A hereditary disease is transmitted genetically from parent to child.
2. Gene therapy is a form of treatment that attempts to replace an undesirable (disease-causing) gene with a more desirable gene.

Review Your Knowledge

1. When, where, and how does fertilization take place?

2. What is the difference between mitosis and meiosis?

3. Define *zygote, blastomere, morula,* and *blastocyst.*

4. What are the roles of hCG, estrogen, and progesterone in pregnancy?

5. Why is an amniocentesis done? When does the amniotic sac rupture?

6. What are two important functions of the placenta?

7. Define *embryo* and *fetus.* What are *teratogens?* How do teratogens affect the embryo and fetus?

8. What are the three stages of labor? Why is an episiotomy done? What is a *breech birth?*

9. How do oxytocin and prolactin affect lactation?

10. Define *DNA, genes,* and *chromosomes.*

11. How many chromosomes are in a zygote? How many are in a gamete?

12. What is the difference between a dominant gene and a recessive gene? What is a *carrier?*

13. What is an *autosomal abnormality?* What is *nondisjunction?*

14. What happens when a mutation occurs in a gene or a chromosome? What are some mutagenic agents?

15. How is the sex of a child determined? Which chromosomes are found in a male, and which ones are found in a female?

16. What is the difference between congenital disease and hereditary disease?

17. What accounts for variations in color of skin, hair, and eyes?

18. What is *gene therapy?*

Glossary

Abduction (ăb-dŭk'shən) Movement of a body part away from the midline.

Absorption (əb-sôrp'shən) Taking in of substances by cells or membranes; more specifically, referring to the movement of digested food from the digestive tract into the blood.

Accommodation (ə-kŏm"ə-dā'shən) The changes that take place in the eye, particularly the lens, that enable the person to focus on close or far-away objects.

Acetylcholine (ACh) (ăs"ə-tĭl-kō'lēn) A type of neurotransmitter that is secreted from the nerve terminals; ACh diffuses across the synapse and stimulates the postsynaptic membrane.

Acid (ăs'ĭd) A substance that donates or releases hydrogen ions when it ionizes in water.

Acidosis (ăs"ĭ-dō'sĭs) An imbalance in hydrogen ion (H^+) concentration. The increase in H^+ causes the blood pH to decrease to below 7.35. Acidosis can be classified as either respiratory or metabolic, depending on its cause.

Acrosome (ăk'rəo-sōm) Cap-like structure that covers the head of the sperm; it assists the sperm in penetrating the ovum.

ACTH See adrenocorticotropic hormone.

Actin (ăk'tĭn) One of the contractile proteins in muscle; also called the thin filaments. Actin in-

teracts with myosin to cause muscle contraction.

Action potential (ăk'shən pə-těn'shəl) Sequence of changes in the membrane potential that occur when a cell is stimulated to threshold; it includes depolarization and repolarization. Also called the nerve impulse.

Active transport (ăk'tĭv trănz'pôrt) A process that requires an input of energy (ATP) to move a substance from an area of low concentration to an area of high concentration.

Adaptation (ăd"ăp-tā'shən) Adjustment to a stimulus, such as the adaptation to odor.

Adduction (ə-dŭk'shən) Movement of a body part toward the midline of the body.

Adenohypophysis (ăd"ə-nō-hī-pŏf'ĭ-sĭs) Anterior pituitary gland.

Adenosine triphosphate (ATP) (ə-děn'ə-sēn trī-fŏs'fāt) An energy-storing and energy-transferring molecule found in all cells.

ADH See antidiuretic hormone.

Adipose tissue (ăd'ĭ-pōs tĭsh'ōō) A type of connective tissue that stores fat.

Adrenal gland (ə-drē'nəl glănd) An endocrine gland that consists of the adrenal cortex and the adrenal medulla. The cortex secretes steroids and the medulla secretes catecholamines.

Adrenalin (ə-drĕn′ə-lĭn) See epinephrine.

Adrenergic fiber (ăd″rə-nûr′jĭk fī′bər) A fiber that secretes norepinephrine at the axon terminal; postganglionic fibers of the sympathetic nervous system are adrenergic fibers.

Adrenocorticotropic hormone (ACTH) (ə-drē″no-kôr″tĭ-kō-trŏp′ĭk hōr′mōn) A hormone secreted by the anterior pituitary gland; it stimulates the adrenal cortex to secrete steroids, particularly cortisol.

Aerobic metabolism (âr-ō′bĭk mě-tăb′ə-lĭz-əm) Chemical reactions that require oxygen.

Afferent (ăf′ər-ənt) Carrying toward a center, such as afferent nerves carrying information toward the central nervous system.

Agglutination (ə-glōō″tĭ-nā′shən) Clumping of cells in response to an antigen-antibody reaction.

Albumin (ăl-byōō′mĭn) A plasma protein that helps regulate plasma osmotic pressure; it helps maintain blood volume by "holding" water within the blood vessels.

Albuminuria (ăl-byōō″mə-nōōr′ē-ə) The presence of albumin in the urine, usually due to a kidney disorder.

Aldosterone (ăl-dŏs′tərōn) A mineralocorticoid (steroid) secreted by the adrenal cortex. It stimulates the kidney to reabsorb sodium and water and to excrete potassium.

Alimentary canal (ăl″ə-měn′tə-rē kə-năl′) Tubular portion of the digestive tract that extends from the mouth to the anus.

Alkaline (ăl′kə-lĭn) A solution that contains more hydroxyl ions (OH$^-$) then hydrogen ions (H$^+$).

Alkalosis (ăl″kə-lō′sĭs) An imbalance in hydrogen ion (H$^+$) concentration. The decrease in H$^+$ increases blood pH to above 7.45. Alkalosis can be classified as either respiratory or metabolic, depending on its cause.

Allantois (ə-lăn′tō-ĭs) An extraembryonic membrane that forms the umbilical cord.

Allergen (ăl′ər-jən) Foreign substance or antigen that stimulates an allergic reaction.

Allergy (ăl′ər-jē) An overreaction to an antigen, causing a variety of symptoms; symptoms range from mild to severe life-threatening anaphylaxis; a hypersensitivity reaction.

Alopecia (ăl″ə-pē′shə) Loss of hair; baldness.

Alveolus (ăl-vē′ə-ləs) (pl. alveoli) Tiny grape-like sac in the lungs; it is the site of gas exchange (oxygen and carbon dioxide) between the air and the blood.

Amino acid (ə-mē′nō ăs′ĭd) A small organic compound that contains an amino group (NH$_2$) and an organic acid (COOH) group; the building block of protein.

Amniocentesis (ăm″nē-ō-sěn-tē′sĭs) The removal of amniotic fluid for analysis; a procedure used to detect birth defects.

Amniotic fluid (ăm″nē-ŏt′ĭk flōō′ĭd) Fluid in the amniotic sac that bathes and protects the fetus.

Amniotic sac (ăm″nē-ŏt′ĭk săk) Extraembryonic membrane that surrounds the fetus and contains amniotic fluid.

Amphiarthrosis (ăm″fē-är-thrō′sĭs) Slightly movable joint such as the joint between two vertebrae.

Amylase (ăm′ə-lās) Enzyme that digests carbohydrates. There is a salivary amylase (ptyalin) and a pancreatic amylase.

Anabolism (ə-năb′ə-lĭz-əm) Metabolic reactions that build complex substances from simpler substances.

Anaerobic metabolism (ăn″ə-rō′bĭk mě-tăb′ə-liz-əm) Chemical reactions that do not require oxygen.

Anaphylaxis (ăn′ə-fə-lăk′sys) A severe, life-threatening allergic reaction; characterized by difficulty in breathing and a hypotension-induced loss of consciousness.

Anastomosis (ə-năs″tə-mō′sĭs) An opening or communication between two tubular structures.

Anatomical position (ăn″ə-tŏm′y-kəl pə-zysh′ən) A position of the body; the body is standing in an erect position with the face forward and the arms at the side (palms and toes face in a forward direction).

Anatomy (ə-năt′ə-mē) Study of the structure of the body.

Androgen (ăn′drə-jěn) Male sex hormone; testosterone.

Anemia (ə-nē′mē-ə) A condition characterized by abnormally low amounts of hemoglobin or low numbers of red blood cells; results in decreased oxygen delivered to the body tissues.

Angina pectoris (ăn-jī′nə pěk′tôr-ĭs) Chest pain caused by inadequate oxygenation of the myocardium (heart muscle).

Angiotensin (ăn″jē-ō-těn′sĭn) A hormone produced by the action of renin on angiotensinogen. Angiotensin II causes vasoconstriction and stimulates the adrenal cortex to secrete aldosterone. These actions increase blood pressure.

Anion (ăn′ī-ŏn) A negatively charged ion.

Antagonist (ăn-tăg′ə-nĭst) A muscle that opposes another muscle.

Antecubital (ăn″tĭ-kyōō′bĭ-tl) Describing an area in front of the elbow joint.

Antibody (ăn′tĭ-bŏd″ē) A substance that reacts with a specific antigen.

Antidiuretic hormone (ADH) (ăn″tē-dī″yə-rět′ĭk hōr′mōn) A hormone released from the posterior pituitary gland; it increases the amount of water that the kidney reabsorbs, thereby increasing blood volume and decreasing urinary output.

Antigen (ăn′tĭ-jěn) A foreign substance that stimulates the production of antibodies.

Antitoxin (ăn″tē-tŏk′sĭn) A specific type of antibody produced by the body in response to a toxin.

Anus (ā′nəs) The terminal opening of the digestive tract for the elimination of feces.

Aorta (ā-ôr′tə) Large artery that conducts blood from the left ventricle of the heart.

Aortic valve (ā-ôr′tĭk vălv) Valve that prevents the backflow of blood from the aorta into the left ventricle.

Apocrine gland (ăp′ə-krĭn glănd) One of the sudoriferous glands; a type of sweat gland.

Aponeurosis (ăp″ə-nōō-rō′sĭs) Broad, flat sheet of fibrous connective tissue that connects muscle to another structure.

Appendicular skeleton (ăp″ən-dĭk′yə-lər skĕl′ĕ-tn) The part of the skeleton that includes the bones of the upper extremities, the lower extremities, the pelvic girdle, and the pectoral girdle.

Appendix (ə-pĕn′dĭks) The worm-shaped outpouching of the wall of the cecum; no known function.

Aqueous humor (ā′kwē-əs hyōō′mər) Watery fluid that fills the anterior cavity of the eye.

Arachnoid mater (ə-răk′noid mā′tər) Middle layer of the meninges.

Arachnoid villus (ə-răk′noid vĭl′əs) (pl. villi) A projection of the arachnoid mater into the dural sinus for the purpose of draining cerebrospinal fluid from the subarachnoid space and returning it to the general circulation.

Areolar tissue (ə-rē′ə-lər tĭsh′ōō) Loose connective tissue.

Arteriole (är-tîr′ē-ōl) Small artery that is composed largely of smooth muscle and is found between the larger artery and the capillaries; also called resistance vessel.

Artery (är′tə-rē) Blood vessel that carries blood away from the heart.

Arthritis (är-thrī′tĭs) Inflammation of the joints.

Articulation (är-tĭk″yə-lā′shən) Joining of structures at a joint.

Astigmatism (ə-stĭg′mə-tĭz′əm) A defect in the refracting function of the eye due to an abnormal curvature of the lens or cornea.

Astrocyte (ăs′trə-sīt) Type of neuroglia that helps form the blood-brain barrier.

Atom (ăt′əm) Fundamental unit of an element; the smallest part of the element that has the characteristics of that element.

ATP See adenosine triphosphate.

Atrioventricular node (AV node) (ā″trē-ō-vĕn-trĭk′yə-lər nōd) A part of the conduction system of the heart located in the septum separating the right atrium from the right ventricle; it conducts the electrical signal from the atrium to the ventricles.

Atrioventricular valve (AV valve) (ā″trē-ō-vĕn-trĭk′yə-lər vălv) Valve located between the septa separating the atrium from the ventricle. The tricuspid valve is located in the right heart, while the bicuspid (mitral) valve is located in the left heart.

Atrium (ā′trē-əm) (pl. atria) Upper chamber of the heart that receives blood from veins; there is a right and a left atrium.

Atrophy (ăt′rə-fē) A wasting or a decrease in the size of an organ or tissue, usually referring to a muscle.

Auditory tube (ô′dĭ-tôr″ē tōōb) Eustachian tube; the tube that connects the middle ear with the pharynx.

Autoimmune (ô″tō-ĭ-myōōn′) Immunity against one's own tissue.

Autonomic nervous system (ô″tə-nŏm′ĭk nûr′vəs sĭs′təm) The involuntary or automatic nervous system that controls the organs, glands, cardiac muscle, and smooth muscle. It has two divisions, the sympathetic nervous system and the parasympathetic nervous system.

Autosome (ô′tə-sōm) Any of the chromosomes except the sex chromosomes; for humans, there are 22 pairs of autosomes.

AV node (ā″vē″ nōd) See atrioventricular node.

AV valve (ā″vē″ vălv) See atrioventricular valve.

Axial skeleton (ăk′sē-əl skĕl′ə-tn) The part of the skeleton that includes the skull, vertebral column, ribs, and sternum.

Axillary (ăk′sə-lĕr″ē) Pertaining to the armpit.

Axon (ăk′sŏn) The elongated part of the neuron that conducts nerve impulses away from the cell body.

Baroreceptor (băr″ō-rĭ-sĕp′tər) Receptor that detects or senses changes in blood pressure; located in the carotid sinus and aortic arch.

Baroreceptor reflex (băr″ō-rĭ-sĕp′tər rē′flĕks) A nervous reflex that senses sudden changes in blood pressure and then stimulates the heart and blood vessels to return blood pressure to its normal range.

Basal ganglia (bā′səl găng′glē-ə) Masses of gray matter located in the cerebrum of the brain; helps control muscle coordination. Parkinson disease is a disorder of the basal ganglia.

Base (bās) A substance such as hydroxyl ion (OH^-) that combines with hydrogen ion.

Basement membrane (bās′mənt mĕm′brān) Layer that anchors epithelial tissue to an underlying connective tissue.

Base-pairing (bās′pâr-ĭng) The pairing of the bases of the nucleotides; adenine and thymine (DNA), guanine and cytosine (DNA and RNA), adenine and uracil (RNA).

Base-sequencing (bās″sē′kwən-sĭng) The sequence or arrangement of the bases in a strand of DNA or RNA. The sequence of bases contains the genetic code for protein synthesis; each sequence of three bases codes for an amino acid.

Basophil (bā′sə-fĭl) A granular white blood cell that absorbs a basic blue stain.

B cell (bē′ sĕl) B lymphocyte that produces and secretes antibodies.

Bicuspid valve (bī-kŭs′pĭd vălv) Atrioventricular valve located between the left atrium and the left ventricle; the mitral valve.

Bile (bīl) Fluid secreted by the liver and stored by the gallbladder; functions in fat digestion.

Bilirubin (bĭl′ĭ-roo′bĭn) Pigment produced from the breakdown of hemoglobin and secreted into the bile; an accumulation of bilirubin in the skin causes jaundice.

Biorhythm (bī′ō-rĭth″əm) Rhythmic or repeating pattern of secretion or activity that occurs within a living organism.

Blastocyst (blăs′tə-sĭst) An early preembryonic cluster of cells with a hollow interior. There is an early and a late blastocyst.

Bowman capsule (bō′mən kâp′səl) The C-shaped tubular structure that partially encloses the glomerulus. Water and dissolved substances are filtered from the glomerulus into the Bowman capsule.

Bradycardia (brăd″ĭ-kär′dē-ə) Abnormally slow heart rate, below 60 beats per minute.

Brain stem (brān′stĕm) Lower part of the brain that connects the brain with the spinal cord; consists of the midbrain, pons, and medulla.

Broca area (bro-kə′ â′rē-ə) A region in the frontal lobe that is concerned with motor speech.

Bronchiole (brŏng′kē-ōl″) Terminal end of the bronchus that carries air to and from the alveoli.

Bronchus (brŏng′kəs) (pl. bronchi) Large airway in the lungs that connects the trachea and the bronchioles; there is a right and left bronchus.

Buccal (bŭk′əl) Pertaining to the cheek.

Buffer (bŭf′ər) A substance that resists large changes in pH. A buffer can react with strong acids and bases, converting them to weaker acids and bases.

Bulbourethral glands (bŭl″bō-yoo-rē′thrəl glăndz) Glands that secrete fluid into the male urethra during sexual excitement; also called Cowper glands.

Bundle of His (bŭn′dl ŭv hĭz) Part of the conduction system that is located in the upper interventricular septum; splits into the right and left bundle branches.

Bursa (bûr′sə) (pl. bursae) Small, fluid-filled sac located near a joint.

Calcaneus (kăl-kā′nē-əs) The largest of the tarsals; the heel bone.

Calyx (kā′lĭks) Cup-like structure in the kidneys that collects urine from the nephron units.

Capillary (kăp′ə-lĕr″ē) The smallest and most numerous of the blood vessels; site of exchange of nutrients and waste between the blood and tissue fluid.

Carbohydrate (kär″bō-hī′drāt) Type of organic compounds including simple sugars, starch, and glycogen; primary source of energy.

Carbon dioxide (CO₂) (kär′bən dī-ŏk′sīd) The waste product of cellular metabolism.

Cardiac impulse (kär′dē-ăk ĭm′pŭls) An action potential that occurs in the cardiac conduction tissue.

Cardiac output (kär′dē-ăk out′poot) The amount of blood pumped by the heart in one minute; about 5000 mL per minute.

Cardiac tamponade (kär′dē-ăk tăm″pə-nād′) External compression or pressing on the heart, usually caused by a collection of fluid within the pericardial space; the pressure prevents the heart from filling with blood and causes a life-threatening decrease in cardiac output.

Cartilage (kär′tĭ-lĭj) Type of hard connective tissue formed from chondrocytes.

Catabolism (kə-tăb′ə-lĭz-əm) The metabolic breakdown of complex molecules into simpler molecules; the breakdown is accompanied by the release of energy.

Catalyst (kăt′ə-lĭst) Any substance that speeds up the rate of a chemical reaction.

Catecholamine (kăt″ĭ-kō′lə-mēn″) A classification of hormones that is secreted by the adrenal medulla; includes epinephrine (adrenalin) and norepinephrine.

Cation (kăt′ī-ŏn) A positively charged ion.

Cecum (sē′kəm) The part of the large intestine that connects the ileum of the small intestine and the ascending colon of the large intestine.

Cell (sĕl) The basic unit of life.

Cell life cycle (sĕl līf sī′kəl) The series of changes that a cell undergoes from the time it is formed until the time it divides; the two major periods are interphase and cell division.

Cell membrane (sĕl mĕm′brān) The membrane that surrounds the cell and regulates what enters and leaves the cell; also called the plasma membrane.

Central nervous system (CNS) (sĕn′trəl nûr′vəs sĭs′təm) The part of the nervous system that includes the brain and the spinal cord.

Centriole (sĕn′trē-ōl) Rod-shaped organelle that functions in cell division.

Cerebellum (sĕr″ə-bĕl′əm) Part of brain that is located under the cerebrum; it coordinates skeletal muscle activity.

Cerebrospinal fluid (CSF) (sĕr″ə-brō-spī′nəl floo′ĭd) Fluid secreted by the choroid plexus (capillaries and ependymal cells) into the ventricles of the brain. CSF circulates within the subarachnoid space around the brain and the spinal cord.

Cerebrum (ser′ə-brəm) The largest and uppermost part of the brain, which is divided into two cerebral hemispheres; most of the higher mental functioning is done by the cerebrum.

Cerumen (sə-roo′mən) Earwax found in the external ear.

Ceruminous gland (sə-roo′mə-nəs glănd) A modified sweat gland found in the external ear canal; it secretes cerumen, or earwax.

Cervix (sûr′vĭks) Constricted portion of an organ, usually referring to the lower portion of the uterus.

Chemoreceptor (kē″mō-rĭ-sĕp′tər) Receptor that detects changes in the chemical composition of a substance.

Chemotaxis (kē″mō-tăk′sĭs) Attraction of white blood cells, particularly the neutrophils and macrophages, to chemicals secreted by injured tissues.

Chordae tendineae (kôr′dē tĕn-dĭn′ē) Tough fibrous bands that attach the cuspid valves (bicuspid and tricuspid) to the walls of the ventricles of the heart.

Choroid (kôr′oid) The middle layer of the eye.

Choroid plexus (kôr′oid plĕk′səs) A tuft of capillaries and ependymal cells located in the ventricles of the brain. It secretes cerebrospinal fluid into the ventricles.

Chromosome (krō′mə-sōm) Coiled, thread-like structures that contain segments of DNA called genes.

Chyle (kīl) Milky-appearing substance that is absorbed into the lymphatics of the intestinal villi; the white appearance is due to fat.

Chyme (kīm) Paste-like mixture of partially digested food, water, and digestive enzymes that is formed in the stomach.

Cilia (sĭl′ē-ə) (sing. cilium) Hairs or hair-like processes on the surface of many cells.

Circumduction (sûr″kəm-dŭk′shən) Circular, "softball pitching" movement around a joint.

CNS See central nervous system.

Coagulation (kō-ăg″yə-lā′shən) Clotting of blood.

Cochlea (kŏk′lē-ə) Part of the inner ear that contains the organ of Corti, the receptors for hearing.

Collagen (kŏl′ə-jən) Flexible white protein found in bone and cartilage.

Colloidal suspension (kə-loi′dl səs-pĕn′shən) Mixture in which the particles do not dissolve but remain suspended in the solvent.

Colon (kō′lən) Major portion of the large intestine that extends from the cecum to the rectum.

Columnar epithelium (kə-lŭm′nər ĕp″ĭ-thēl′ē-əm) A type of epithelium that has column-shaped cells.

Complement (kŏm′plə-mənt) Group of blood proteins that helps antibodies destroy foreign cells.

Compound (kŏm′pound) Substance composed of two or more chemical elements, such as water (H_2O).

Conduction (kən-dŭk′shən) Loss of heat energy as it is transferred from the warm body to a cooler object, such as cooling blanket.

Cone (kōn) Photoreceptor that detects color.

Congenital (kən-jĕn′ĭ-tl) Present at birth.

Conjunctiva (kŏn″jŭngk-tĭ′və) Membrane that lines the eyelid and covers the anterior portion of the sclera.

Connective tissue (kə-nĕk′tĭv tĭsh′ōō) One of the four basic types of tissues that generally holds and supports body structures; includes bone, cartilage, and loose and dense fibrous connective tissue.

Contracture (kən-trăk′chər) An abnormal shortening of a muscle or the surrounding tissue, making the muscle resistant to stretching; often caused by immobility.

Convection (kən-vĕk′shən) Loss of heat energy to the surrounding cooler air. The layer of heated air next to the body is constantly being removed by a fan (or breeze) and replaced by cooler air.

Convolution (kŏn″və-lōō′shən) The surface folds, or bumps, of the cerebral cortex; a gyrus.

Cornea (kôr′nē-ə) Clear portion of the sclera that covers the anterior portion of the eye.

Coronary vessels (kôr′ə-nĕr-ē vĕs′əlz) The blood vessels that supply the heart muscle with blood. Include coronary arteries and veins.

Corpus callosum (kôr′pəs kə-lō′səm) The band of white matter that connects the right and left cerebral hemispheres.

Corpus luteum (kôr′pəs lōō′tē-əm) The yellow body formed from the ovarian follicle after ovulation; it secretes large amounts of progesterone and smaller amounts of estrogen.

Cortex (kôr′tĕks) Outer layer of an organ, such as the adrenal cortex and cerebral cortex.

Cortisol (kôr′tĭ-sōl) A steroid secreted by the adrenal cortex; considered one of the stress hormones.

Covalent bond (kō-vā′lənt bŏnd) A bond or attraction formed by the sharing of electrons between atoms.

Cranial nerves (krā′nē-əl nûrvz) The 12 pairs of nerves that emerge from the brain.

Cranium (krā′nē-əm) The bones of the skull that encase and protect the brain.

Creatinine (krē″ăt′ĭ-nēn) A waste product that is excreted by the kidney. Serum levels of creatinine are used to evaluate kidney function. A high serum creatinine level means that the kidneys are unable to excrete waste.

Cuboidal epithelium (kyōō-boĭd′l ĕp″ĭ-thēl′ē-əm) A type of epithelium that has cells shaped like cubes.

Cushing syndrome (kōōsh′ing sĭn′drōm) A group of symptoms that develop in response to increased plasma levels of cortisol. Symptoms include moon face, buffalo hump, poor wound healing, and fragile skin.

Cutaneous membrane (kyōō-tā′nē-əs mĕm′brān) Skin.

Cyanosis (sī″ə-nō′sĭs) Bluish coloring of the skin owing to insufficient oxygen in the blood.

Cystic duct (sĭs′tĭk dŭkt) Duct from the gallbladder; it joins the hepatic duct to form the common bile duct.

Cytoplasm (sī′tō-plă″zəm) Cellular material that surrounds the nucleus. The gel-like substance contains all of the organelles located outside of the nucleus.

Defecation (děf″ĭ-kā′shən) Act of eliminating undigested waste from the digestive tract; discharge of feces from the rectum.

Deglutition (děg″loo-tĭsh′ən) Act of swallowing.

Deltoid (děl′toid) Triangular muscle over the shoulder; refers to the shoulder region.

Dendrite (děn′drīt) Tree-like process of the neuron that receives the stimulus and carries it toward the cell body.

Dentin (děn′tĭn) The bone-like material that forms the body of the tooth.

Deoxyribonucleic acid (DNA) (dē-ŏk″sē-rī″bō-noo-klē′ĭk ăs′ĭd) A nucleotide that stores the genetic information of the organism; the sugar is deoxyribose and the bases are adenine, thymine, cytosine, and guanine.

Deoxyribose (dē-ŏk″sē-rī′bōs″) The five-carbon sugar that is found in DNA, deoxyribonucleic acid.

Depolarization (dē-pō″lər-ĭ-zā″shən) A change in the membrane potential across the cell membrane with the inside of the cell becoming less negative or less polarized.

Dermatome (dûr′mə-tōm″) A segment of the skin with sensory fibers from a single spinal nerve.

Dermis (dûr′mĭs) The thick layer of dense connective tissue that lies under the epidermis of the skin; called the true skin.

Diabetes insipidus (dī″ə-bē′tēz ĭn-sĭp′ĭdəs) A disorder characterized by the elimination of large amounts of urine because of a deficiency of antidiuretic hormone (ADH).

Diabetes mellitus (dī″ə-bē′tēz mə-lī′təs) A disease caused by an insufficient amount of insulin; it is characterized by hyperglycemia, polyuria, polyphagia, and polydipsia.

Dialysis (dī-ăl′ĭ-sĭs) A passive transport process that allows small particles to diffuse through a semipermeable membrane.

Diaphragm (dī′ə-frăm) Dome-shaped skeletal muscle that separates the thoracic and abdominal cavities; it is the chief muscle of inspiration (inhalation).

Diaphysis (dī-ăf′ĭ-sĭs) Shaft of a long bone.

Diarthrosis (dī″är-thrō′sĭs) Freely movable joint such as the knee joint; also called a synovial joint.

Diastole (dī-ăs′tə-lē) Relaxation phase of the cardiac cycle.

Diastolic pressure (dī″ə-stŏl′ĭk prĕsh′ər) The arterial pressure during the diastolic phase of the cardiac cycle; the "bottom number" of the blood pressure reading.

Diencephalon (dī″ĕn-sĕf′ə-lŏn) Part of the brain that consists primarily of the thalamus and the hypothalamus.

Differentiation (dĭf″ər-ĕn″shē-ā′shən) The process whereby a cell becomes specialized.

Diffusion (dĭ-fyoo′zhən) A passive transport process that causes movement of a substance from an area of high concentration to an area of low concentration.

Digestion (dĭ-jĕs′chən) The process of breaking down food into absorbable particles.

Disaccharide (dī-săk′ə-rīd) A carbohydrate that consists of two monosaccharides. Called a double sugar; includes sucrose, maltose, and lactose.

Distal (dĭs′təl) Farther from the midline or point of attachment to the trunk.

Diuresis (dī″yə-rē′sĭs) An increased excretion of urine. A drug that increases the excretion of urine is called a diuretic.

DNA. See deoxyribonucleic acid.

Dominant gene (dŏm′ə-nənt jēn) A gene that is always expressed.

Dorsal (dôr′səl) Toward the back; posterior.

Dorsal cavity (dôr′səl kăv′y-tē) The body cavity that is located toward the back part of the body; it is divided into the cranial cavity, which contains the brain, and the spinal cavity, which contains the spinal cord.

Dorsal root (dôr′səl root) Posterior region where the sensory branch of the spinal cord attaches to the spinal cord.

Ductus arteriosus (dŭk′təs är-tîr-ē-ō′sĭs) A fetal structure that allows blood to flow from the pulmonary artery into the aorta, thereby bypassing the lungs.

Duodenum (doo″ə-dē′nəm) The first part of the small intestine.

Dura mater (doo′rə mā′tər) The tough outer layer of the meninges; literally the "hard mother."

Dural sinus (doo′rəl sī′nəs) Space in the skull created by the dura mater and filled with blood; cerebrospinal fluid drains into the dural sinus and is returned to the general circulation.

Eccrine gland (ĕk′rĭn glănd) Type of sweat gland that secretes a watery substance; plays an important role in the regulation of body temperature.

Ectopic pregnancy (ĕk-tŏp′ĭk prĕg′nən-sē) A pregnancy that occurs outside the uterus.

Edema (ĭ-dē′mə) An abnormal collection of fluid, usually causing swelling.

Efferent (ĕf′ər-ənt) Movement away from a central point, such as a motor neuron that carries information away from the central nervous system.

Ejaculation (ĭ-jăk″yə-lā′shən) Expulsion of semen from the urethra.

Ejaculatory duct (ĭ-jăk′yə-lə-tō″rē dŭkt) The tube that transports sperm from the vas deferens to the urethra.

Electrocardiogram (ē-lĕk″trō-kär′dē-ə-grăm″) A graphic recording of the electrical events that occur during the cardiac cycle; called an ECG.

Electrolyte (ē-lĕk′trō-līt) A compound that dissociates into ions when dissolved in water.

Electrolyte balance (ĕ-lĕk′trō-līt băl′əns) The state in which the body contains the normal amounts of fluids and electrolytes.

Electron (ĕ-lĕk′trŏn) A negatively charged particle located in an orbital outside the nucleus of an atom.

Element (ĕl′ə-mĕnt) A substance composed of only one kind of atom.

Embolus (ĕm′bə-ləs) A detached clot or other foreign substance that eventually occludes or blocks a blood vessel.

Embryo (ĕm′brē-ō) The developing human between the gestational ages of 2 and 8 weeks.

Emulsification (ĭ-mŭl″sĭ-fĭ-kā′shən) The breaking down of large fat droplets into smaller droplets; accomplished by bile.

Endocardium (ĕn″dō-kär′dē-əm) The inner lining of the heart wall.

Endocrine gland (ĕn′də-krĭn glănd) A ductless gland that secretes hormones, usually into the blood.

Endocytosis (ĕn″dō-sī-tō′sĭs) Uptake of material through the cell membrane by forming a vesicle; pinocytosis and phagocytosis.

Endometriosis (ĕn″dō-mē″trē-ō′sĭs) A condition in which endometrial tissue occurs outside the uterus, usually in the pelvic cavity.

Endometrium (ĕn″dō-mē′trē-əm) The inner mucous membrane lining of the uterus.

Endoplasmic reticulum (ER) (ĕn″dō-plăz′mĭk rĕ-tĭk′yōō-lŭm) Intracellular membrane system that is concerned with the synthesis and transportation of protein; called the rough ER if ribosomes are attached; called the smooth ER if there are no ribosomes.

Endosteum (ĕn-dŏs′tē-əm) The inner lining of the marrow cavity of a long bone.

Energy (ĕn′ər-jē) The ability to perform work.

Enzyme (ĕn′zīm) Organic catalyst; it speeds up the rate of a chemical reaction.

Eosinophil (ē″ə-sĭn′ə-fĭl″) A granular leukocyte that stains red.

Epidermis (ĕp″ĭ-dûr′mĭs) Outer epithelial layer of the skin.

Epididymis (ĕp″ĭ-dĭd′ə-mĭs) A coiled tube that carries sperm from the testis to the vas deferens.

Epiglottis (ĕp″ĭ-glŏt′ĭs) Cartilage that guards the opening into the larynx; directs food and water into the esophagus.

Epinephrine (ĕp″ĭ-nĕf′rĭn) Hormone that is secreted by the adrenal medulla; its action is similar to stimulation of the sympathetic nervous system; also called adrenalin.

Epiphyseal disc (ĕp″ə-fĭz′ē-əl dĭsk) A band of cartilage that separates the epiphysis from the diaphysis in growing long bones. This is the site of longitudinal bone growth; also called the epiphyseal plate.

Epiphysis (ĕ-pĭf′ĭ-sĭs) End of a long bone. The two epiphyses are attached to the diaphysis.

Epithelial tissue (ĕp″ĭ-thē′lē-əl tĭsh′ōō) One of the four types of tissues. It is found on the surface of the body (skin) and lining the body cavities; it also forms glands.

Erection (ĭ-rĕk′shən) Engorgement of the erectile tissue by blood, causing the penis and clitoris to enlarge and become firm.

Erythroblastosis fetalis (ĕ-rĭth″rō-blăs-tō′sĭs fĭ-tăl-ĭs) A hemolytic disease of the newborn caused by an incompatibility between the maternal and fetal blood. It is characterized by anemia and jaundice.

Erythrocyte (ĕ-rĭth′rə-sīt) See red blood cell.

Erythropoiesis (ĕ-rĭth″rō-poi-ē′sĭs) The formation of red blood cells.

Erythropoietin (ĕ-rĭth″rō-poi′ə-tĭn) A hormone secreted primarily by the kidneys that stimulates the production of red blood cells.

Esophagus (ĕ-sŏf′ə-gəs) A hollow muscular tube that connects the pharynx (throat) with the stomach; the "food tube."

Estrogen (ĕs′trə-jən) The female sex hormone secreted by the developing ovarian follicle. Estrogen stimulates the growth of the reproductive organs, determines the secondary sex characteristics, and plays a crucial role in the menstrual cycle.

Eustachian tube (yōō-stā′kē-ən tōōb) See auditory tube.

Evaporation (ĭ-văp″ə-rā′shən) Loss of heat as water changes from the liquid to the vapor or gas state.

Exhalation (ĕks″hə-lā′shən) The process of moving air out of the lungs; the breathing out phase of ventilation; also called expiration.

Exocrine gland (ĕk′sə-krĭn glănd) A type of gland that secretes its products into ducts that open onto a surface.

Exocytosis (ĕk″sō-sī-tō′sĭs) Elimination of material from a cell through the formation of vesicles.

Expiration (ĕk″spə-rā′shən) See exhalation.

Extension (ĕk-stĕn′shən) An increase in the angle of a joint.

Extracellular (ek″strə-sĕl′yə-lər) Outside a cell.

Extracellular fluid (ĕk″strə-sĕl′yə-lər flōō′ĭd) The fluid that is located outside of the cell, such as the plasma and interstitial fluid.

Facial nerve (fā′shəl nûrv) Cranial nerve VII; a mixed nerve that supplies the face. Damage to this nerve causes Bell palsy.

Facilitated diffusion (fə-sĭl′ĭ-tāt-əd dĭ-fyōō′zhən) A process by which a substance moves with the assistance of a carrier molecule from an area of high concentration to an area of low concentration.

Fallopian tube (fə-lō′pē-ən tōōb) The passageway through which the egg or zygote moves from the ovary to the uterus; also called the oviduct or uterine tube.

Fascia (făsh′ē-ə) A fibrous connective tissue membrane that covers individual skeletal muscles or certain organs.

Fascicle (făs′ĭ-kəl) A small group or bundle of muscle fibers bound together by connective tissue.

Feces (fē′sēz) Waste material discharged from the rectum.

Femur (fē′mər) Large bone in the thigh.

Fertilization (fûr″tĭ-lĭ-zā′shən) Union of an ovum and a sperm to form a zygote.

Fetus (fē′təs) In prenatal development, the name given to the developing human at the end of the embryonic period; from the end of the eighth week of pregnancy to birth.

Fibrin (fī′brĭn) The protein strands formed by the action of thrombin on fibrinogen; the clot.

Fibrinogen (fī-brĭn′ə-jən) Protein clotting factor that is converted to fibrin when acted upon by thrombin.

Fibrinolysis (fī″brə-nŏl′ĭ-sĭs) Dissolving of a blood clot; occurs naturally by plasmin or by a class of drugs called thrombolytics.

Filtration (fĭl-trā′shən) The process by which water and dissolved substances move through a membrane in response to a pressure difference.

Fimbriae (fĭm′brē-ē″) Finger-like projections at the opening of the fallopian tube near the ovary.

Fissure (fĭsh′ər) A groove between parts of an organ, such as the longitudinal fissure of the brain.

Flagella (flə-jĕl′ə) Long whip-like organelles that serve to propel the organism, such as the tail of the sperm.

Flexion (flĕk′shən) A decrease in the angle of a joint; a bending movement.

Follicle-stimulating hormone (FSH) (fŏl′ĭ-kəl stĭm′yə-lāt-ĭng hōr′mōn) A gonadotropic hormone secreted by the anterior pituitary gland. FSH stimulates the gonads, the ovaries and testes, to produce ova and sperm.

Fontanel (fŏn″tə-nĕl′) A membraneous gap between the cranial bones of an infant's skull.

Foramen (fə-rā′mən) (pl. foramina) A hole or opening, usually in reference to a bone.

Foramen ovale (fə-rā′mən ō-văl′ē) An opening in the interatrial septum of the fetal heart; the opening allows blood to flow from the right atrium to the left atrium, thereby bypassing the lungs.

Foreskin (fôr′skĭn) The prepuce of the penis that is removed during circumcision.

Fovea centralis (fō′vē-ə sĕn-trā′lĭs) A depression in the retina (macula) of the eye that contains only cones and is the area of most acute vision.

Frontal lobe (frŭn′tl lōb) The anterior portion of the cerebrum that controls voluntary skeletal activity and plays an important role in emotions, critical thinking, and ethical decision-making.

Frontal plane (frŭn′tl plān) A vertical plane that divides the body into front (anterior) and back (posterior parts); also called the coronal plane.

Gallbladder (gôl′blăd-ər) A sac located on the undersurface of the liver that concentrates and stores bile.

Gamete (găm′ēt) An ovum or sperm.

Ganglion (găng′glē-ən) (pl. ganglia) One of a group of nerve cell bodies usually located in the peripheral nervous system.

Gastric juice (găs′trĭk jōōs) The secretions of the glands of the stomach that include mucus, hydrochloric acid, and pepsin.

Gastrin (găs′trĭn) A hormone that stimulates glands in the stomach to secrete hydrochloric acid.

Gene (jēn) A part of the chromosome that codes for a specific trait; the biologic unit of heredity.

Genetics (jə-nĕt′ĭks) The study of heredity.

Gestation (jĕs-tā′shən) The length of time from conception to birth; the human gestation period is approximately 9 months, or 40 weeks.

Gingiva (jĭn-jī′və) Gums.

Gland (glănd) A structure that secretes substances onto a surface, into a cavity, or into the blood; classified as exocrine or endocrine.

Glaucoma (glou-kō′mə) An eye disease characterized by increased intraocular pressure.

Glomerular filtration rate (GFR) (glŏ-mĕr′yə-lər fĭl-trā′shən rāt) The rate of filtration across the glomerular membrane.

Glomerulus (glŏ-mĕr′yə-ləs) Tuft of capillaries located within the Bowman capsule of the kidney. Water and dissolved solute are filtered across the glomerular membrane.

Glossopharyngeal nerve (glŏs″ō-fə-rĭn′jē-əl nŭrv) Cranial nerve IX; supplies the mouth and tongue and participates in the sensory part of the baroreceptor reflex.

Glottis (glŏt′ĭs) Opening between the vocal cords; an air passage for the respiratory tract.

Glucagon (glōō′kə-gŏn) A hormone secreted by the pancreas that raises the blood glucose level.

Glucocorticoid (glōō″kō-kôr′tĭ-koid) Steroid hormone that is secreted by the adrenal cortex; affects metabolism, especially carbohydrate metabolism. The principal glucocorticoid is cortisol.

Glucose (glōō′kōs) A monosaccharide, or simple sugar, that serves as the principal fuel for the cells of the body.

Glucosuria (glōō″kō-sōō′rē-ə) Condition characterized by glucose in the urine and often an indication of diabetes mellitus; also called glycosuria.

Glycogen (glī′kə-jən) Polysaccharide that is the storage form of glucose; stored primarily in skeletal muscles and the liver. Also called animal starch.

Glycolysis (glī-kŏl′ə-sĭs) The anaerobic catabolism of glucose into pyruvic acid.

Glycosuria (glī″kō-soo″rē-ə) See glucosuria.

Goblet cell (gŏb′lĭt sĕl) Mucus-secreting cell found in the respiratory and gastrointestinal tracts.

Goiter (goi′tər) Enlarged thyroid gland; may be toxic or nontoxic.

Golgi apparatus (gōl′jē ăp″ə-răt′təs) A membraneous organelle that is concerned with the final trimming and packaging of protein for exocytosis.

Gonad (gō′năd) Organ that produces gametes (ova or sperm); term for ovaries and testes.

Gonadotropic hormone (gō-năd″ə-trŏp′ĭk hōr′mōn) Hormone "aimed at" the gonads; includes follicle-stimulating hormone (FSH), luteinizing hormone (LH), and human chorionic gonadotropin (hCG).

Graafian follicle (gräf′ē-ən fŏl′ĭ-kəl) Mature ovarian follicle that releases an ovum.

Granulocyte (gran′yə-lō-sīt) White blood cell or leukocyte that is named for the staining characteristics of its granules; includes neutrophils, basophils, and eosinophils.

Graves disease (grāvz dĭ-zēz′) Hyperthyroidism.

Growth hormone (grōth hōr′mōn) Hormone secreted by the anterior pituitary gland. It primarily stimulates the muscle and skeletal systems, causing body growth. Also called somatotropin or somatotropic hormone.

Gustatory (gŭs′tə-tōr-ē) Pertaining to the sense of taste.

Gyrus (jī′rəs) (pl. gyri) A fold or "bump" on the surface of the brain; a convolution.

Hair follicle (hār fŏl′ĭ-kəl) The structure within the skin that produces the hair. The hair is formed by columns of dead, keratinized epithelial cells.

Hamstrings (hăm′strĭngz) Group of muscles in the posterior thigh; includes the biceps femoris, semimembranosus, and semitendinosus.

Hard palate (härd păl′ĭt) Anterior, hard portion of the roof of the mouth; formed by the fusion of parts of the maxilla and palatine bones.

Haversian system (hə-vûr′zhən sĭs′təm) The structural unit of compact bone; bone is layered in concentric circles around an osteonic canal. Also called an osteon.

Heart rate (härt rāt) The number of times the heart beats per minute.

Hematocrit (hĕ-măt′ə-krĭt) A laboratory test that expresses the percentage of red blood cells present in a volume of blood.

Hematopoiesis (hē″mə-tō-poi-ē′sĭs) Production of blood cells.

Hemoglobin (hē′mə-glō″bĭn) The iron-containing protein in the red blood cell that has the ability to take up and release oxygen; also transports carbon dioxide.

Hemolysis (hĕ-mŏl′ĭ-sĭs) Rupture of erythrocytes.

Hemostasis (hē″mə-stā′sĭs) Prevention of blood loss. Consists of three phases: vascular spasm, formation of a platelet plug, and blood coagulation.

Heparin (hĕp′ə-rĭn) An anticoagulant that prevents blood coagulation by removing thrombin.

Hepatic portal circulation or system (hĭ-păt′ĭk pōr′tl sûr-kyə-lā′shən) A system of veins, including the portal vein, that brings blood from the digestive organs and spleen to the liver.

Hereditary (hə-rĕd′ĭ-tĕr″ē) The transfer of genetic information from parent to child.

Hilus (hī′ləs) An indentation in an organ such as the kidney. The blood vessels, nerves, and other structures often enter and leave the organ at this indentation.

Histamine (hĭs′tə-mēn) A chemical released by the cells in response to injury; causes vasodilation (hypotension), bronchoconstriction (wheezing, dyspnea), and increased permeability of the blood vessels (edema).

Homeostasis (hō″mē-ō-stā′sĭs) The ability of the body to maintain a constant internal environment.

Hormone (hōr′mōn) A substance secreted by an endocrine gland. The hormone is carried by the blood to the target organs, where it stimulates a specific effect.

Human chorionic gonadotropin (hCG) (hyoo′mən kōr″ē-ŏn′ĭk gō-năd″ə-trŏp′ĭn) A hormone secreted by the trophoblastic cells; maintains the corpus luteum until the placenta can take over its glandular function.

Humerus (hyoo′mər-əs) Long bone of the upper arm.

Humoral immunity (hyoo′mər-əl) The type of immunity that involves antibodies.

Hydrogen bond (hī′drə-jən bŏnd) A weak intermolecular bond formed between hydrogen and a negatively charged atom such as oxygen or nitrogen.

Hymen (hī′mən) A membrane that partially covers the entrance to the vagina.

Hypercalcemia (hī″pər-kăl-sē′mē-ə) Abnormally high blood calcium level.

Hyperglycemia (hī″pər-glī-sē′mē-ə) Abnormally high blood glucose level, usually due to diabetes mellitus.

Hyperkalemia (hī″pər-kə-lē′mē-ə) Abnormally high blood potassium level.

Hypernatremia (hī″pər-nə-trē′mē-ə) Abnormally high blood sodium level.

Hypertension (hī″pər-tĕn′shən) Abnormally high blood pressure.

Hypertonic (hī″pər-tŏn′ĭk) Having a solute concentration greater than a reference solution.

Hypertrophy (hī-pûr′trə-fē) Increase in the size of a body part, usually referring to a muscle.

Hyperventilation (hī″pər-vĕn″tĭl-ā′shən) Abnormally rapid, deep breathing.

Hypoglossal nerve (hī″pə-glŏs′əl nŭrv) Cranial nerve XII that supplies the tongue with motor fibers.

Hypoglycemia (hī″pō-kə-lē′mē-ə) Abnormally low blood glucose.

Hypokalemia (hī″pō-kə-lē′mē-ə) A lower than normal amount of potassium in the blood.

Hyponatremia (hī″pō-nā-trē′mē-ə) A lower than normal amount of sodium in the blood.

Hypophysis (hī″pŏf′ĭ-sĭs) The pituitary gland.

Hypothalamic-hypophyseal portal system (hī″pə-thə-lă′mĭk hī″pə-fĭz′ē-əl pôr′tl sĭs′təm) The network of capillaries that connect the hypothalamus with the anterior pituitary gland. The capillaries carry the releasing hormones from the hypothalamus to the anterior pituitary.

Hypothalamus (hī″pō-thăl′ə-məs) A portion of the diencephalon that regulates the pituitary gland, the autonomic nervous system, water balance, appetite, temperature, and the emotions.

Hypothermia (hī″pə-thûr′mē-ə) A lower than normal body temperature.

Hypothyroidism (hī″pō-thī′roi-dĭz-əm) Decreased function of the thyroid gland causing a decrease in metabolism. Different forms cause cretinism in the unborn child and myxedema in the adult.

Hypotonic (hī″pō-tŏn′ĭk) Having a solute concentration less than a reference solution.

Hypoxia (hī″pŏk′sē-ə) Deficiency of oxygen.

Ileum (ĭl′ē-əm) The third part of the small intestine.

Ilium (ĭl′ē-əm) The upper flared part of the coxal (hip) bone.

Immunity (ĭ-myōō′nĭ-tē) The ability to resist and overcome injury by pathogens or antigenic substances.

Immunoglobulin (im″yōō-nō-glŏb′yə-lĭn) Antibodies produced by plasma cells in response to antigenic stimulation; includes IgG, IgM, IgA, IgD, and IgE.

Immunosuppression (im″yə-nō-sə-prĕsh′ən) Diminished ability of the immune system to defend the body against infection.

Implantation (ĭm″plăn-tā′shən) The embedding of the blastocyst into the uterine wall; occurs 7 to 8 days following fertilization.

Infection (ĭn-fĕk′shən) A disease process caused by microorganisms.

Inferior vena cava (ĭn-fĭr′ē-ər vē′nə kā′və) Large vein that returns blood from the lower parts of the body to the right atrium of the heart.

Inflammation (ĭn″flə-mā′shən) The body's response to infection or injury; characterized by redness, heat, swelling, and pain.

Inguinal canal (ĭng′gwə-nəl kə-năl′) The passageway through which the testis descends from the pelvic cavity into the scrotum.

Inhalation (in″hə-lā′shən) The process of moving air into the lungs; the breathing-in phase of ventilation. Also called inspiration.

Inner cell mass (ĭn′ər sĕl măs) The group of cells in the blastocyst that forms the embryo.

Inorganic (ĭn″ôr-găn′ĭk) Substances that do not contain carbon.

Inotropic effect (ĭn″ō-trŏp′ĭk ĭ-fĕkt′) A change in the strength or force of myocardial contraction that does not involve stretching the myocardial fibers. A positive inotropic effect is an increased force of contraction, whereas a negative inotropic effect is a decreased force of contraction.

Insertion (in-sûr′shən) The more movable attachment point of a muscle to a bone.

Inspiration (ĭn″spə-rā′shən) See inhalation.

Insulin (ĭn′sə-lĭn) A hormone secreted by the pancreas that lowers blood glucose; it facilitates the diffusion of glucose into the cells and stimulates the storage of excess glucose as glycogen.

Intake (ĭn′tāk) The amount of water taken into the body per day.

Integumentary system (ĭn-tĕg″yōō-mĕn′tə-rē sĭs′təm) The body system that consists of the skin and the accessory organs.

Intercellular (ĭn″tər-sĕl′yə-lər) Between the cells.

Interferon (ĭn″tər-fĭr′ŏn) Protein secreted by the cells that are infected with a virus; these proteins stimulate other cells to secrete antiviral proteins.

Interneuron (ĭn″tər-nōōr′ŏn) An association neuron; links the sensory and motor neurons in the central nervous system.

Interstitial cells (ĭn″tər-stĭsh′əl sĕlz) Cells located between the seminiferous tubules; they secrete testosterone. Also called the cells of Leydig.

Interstitial cell-stimulating hormone (ICSH) (ĭn″tər-stĭsh′əl sĕl stĭm′yə-lāt-ĭng hōr′mōn) In the male, luteinizing hormone is called ICSH. See luteinizing hormone.

Interstitial fluid (ĭn″tər-stĭsh′əl flōō′id) Fluid located between the cells; tissue fluid.

Interventricular septum (ĭn″tər-vĕn-trĭk′yə-lər sĕp′təm) The partition that separates the right and left ventricles.

Intervertebral disc (ĭn″tər-vûr′tə-brəl dĭsk) Cartilaginous disc located between two adjacent vertebrae.

Intracellular (ĭn″trə-sĕl′yə-lər) Refers to the inside of the cell.

Intrapleural pressure (ĭn″trə-plōōr′əl prĕsh′ər) The pressure in the pleural cavity between the visceral and the parietal pleurae; a negative intrapleural pressure is necessary for lung expansion.

Intrinsic factor (ĭn-trĭn′sĭk făk′tər) A protein secreted by the gastric cells that is necessary for the absorption of vitamin B_{12}; a deficiency causes pernicious anemia.

Ion (ī′ŏn) An electrically charged atom or group of atoms; either cations (positive charge) or anions (negative charge).

Ionic bond (ī-ŏn′ĭk bŏnd) A bond formed by the exchange of electrons between atoms.

Ionization (ī″ən-ĭ-zā′shən) The dissociation (breaking apart) of a substance into ions.

Iris (ī′rĭs) The part of the eye that describes a person as having brown, green, or blue eyes. It is a muscle that controls pupil size and regulates the amount of light that enters the eye.

Ischium (ĭs′kē-əm) The lower part of the coxal (hip) bone.

Islets of Langerhans (ī′lĭt ŭv läng′ər-hänz) The hormone-secreting cells of the pancreas. The alpha cells of the islets secrete glucagon; the beta cells secrete insulin.

Isotonic (ī″sə-tŏn′ĭk) Having the same concentration as the reference solution.

Isotope (ī′sə-tōp) An element that has the same number of protons and electrons, but a different number of neutrons.

Jaundice (jôn′dĭs) A yellow coloring of the skin and "whites" of the eyes caused by an increase in bilirubin in the blood.

Jejunum (jə-jōō′nəm) The second or middle part of the small intestine.

Joint (joint) The union of two or more bones; an articulation.

Karyotype (kăr′ē-ə-tīp) Arrangement of the chromosomes by pairs in a fixed order.

Keratin (kĕr′ə-tĭn) A hardening and "waterproofing" protein found in the skin, hair, and nails.

Ketone bodies (ke′tōn bod′ēz) Products of faulty fatty acid metabolism; includes acetone, acetoacetic acid, and beta hydroxybutyric acid.

Ketosis (kē-tō′sĭs) Abnormal condition caused by excessive fatty acid catabolism and characterized by elevated blood levels of ketone bodies; a complication of uncontrolled diabetes mellitus.

Kidney (kĭd′nē) The organ of the urinary system that produces the urine.

Korotkoff sound (kə-rŏt′kŏf sound) Sound heard over an artery through a stethoscope when a blood pressure reading is measured.

Kussmaul respirations (kōōs′mōl rĕs″pə-rā′shənz) An increase in respiratory activity that is stimulated by metabolic acidosis. The increased respiratory activity helps to "blow off" carbon dioxide, thereby decreasing the hydrogen ion concentration and correcting the acidosis; often seen in diabetic ketoacidosis.

Kyphosis (kī-fō′sĭs) Abnormal and exaggerated posterior curvature of the thoracic spine; hump-back.

Labia (lā′bē-ə) Lip-like folds of the female genitalia. The labia majora are the outer folds of skin and the labia minora are inner folds of mucous membrane.

Labor (lā′bər) The process by which the fetus is expelled from the uterus through the vagina.

Lacrimal gland (lăk′rĭ-məl) The gland of the eye that secretes tears.

Lactase (lăk′tās) A disaccharidase that breaks down lactose into glucose and galactose; a deficiency of this digestive enzyme causes lactose intolerance.

Lacteal (lăk′tēl) A lymph vessel in a villus of the small intestine.

Lactic acid (lăk′tĭk ăs′ĭd) A breakdown product of the anaerobic catabolism of glucose; thought to play a role in muscle soreness and fatigue.

Lactogenic hormone (LTH) (lăk″tə-jĕn′ĭk hōr′mōn) See prolactin.

Large intestine (lärj ĭn-tĕs′tĭn) The part of the intestine that extends from the small intestine to the anus.

Larynx (lăr′ĭngks) Structure that contains the vocal cords; voicebox.

Lens (lĕnz) Structure that refracts or bends light waves so as to focus them on the retina. A cloudy lens is called a cataract.

Leukocyte (lōō′kə-sīt) White blood cell; it functions primarily to defend the body against infection. Leukocytes include granulocytes (neutrophils, basophils, and eosinophils) and nongranulocytes (monocytes, lymphocytes).

Leukocytosis (lōō″kə-sī-tō′sĭs) A condition of having an abnormally large number of white blood cells; usually indicative of infection.

Leukopenia (lōō″kə-pē′nē-ə) An abnormally low number of white blood cells in the blood; usually due to myelosuppression.

Ligament (lĭg′ə-mĕnt) Strong band of connective tissue that joins bone to bone.

Limbic system (lĭm′bĭk sĭs′təm) Group of structures within the brain that produce emotional responses; the emotional brain.

Lipase (lī′pās) An enzyme that digests or breaks down fats into fatty acids and glycerol.

Lipid (lī′pĭd) Organic molecule that includes fats, oils, and steroids.

Loop of Henle (lōōp ŭv hĕn′lē) The U-shaped or "looped" part of the renal tubule that extends from the proximal tubule to the distal tubule.

Lordosis (lôr-dō′sĭs) Exaggerated lumbar curvature of the spine.

Lower esophageal sphincter (LES) (lō′ər ĕ-sŏf″ə-jē′əl sfĭngk′tər) Sphincter located at the base of the esophagus; prevents reflux of stomach contents and heartburn.

Lumbar puncture (lŭm′bär pŭngk′chər) A diagnostic procedure that involves the insertion of a needle into the subarachnoid space and the removal of cerebrospinal fluid for analysis.

Luteinizing hormone (LH) (lōō′tē-ə-nī″zĭng hōr′mōn) A gonadotropin secreted by the anterior pituitary gland. The target glands for LH are the gonads, the ovaries and testes. LH stimulates the corpus luteum in the ovaries and the interstitial cells in the testes. In the male, LH is also called interstitial cell-stimulating hormone (ICSH).

Lymph (lĭmf) Fluid that has the same composition as tissue fluid and is carried by the lymph vessels.

Lymphadenitis (lĭm-făd″n-ī′tĭs) Inflammation of the lymph nodes, whereby the lymph nodes become enlarged and tender; generally occurs when the lymph nodes are helping to fight an infection.

Lymphadenopathy (lĭm-făd″n-ŏp′ə-thē) Disease of the lymph nodes; includes human immunodeficiency virus infection, infectious mononucleosis, and Hodgkin disease.

Lymphatic duct (lĭm-făt′ĭk dŭkt) A lymphatic vessel or tube that carries lymph.

Lymph node (lĭmf nōd) A mass of lymphoid tissue located along the course of a lymphatic vessel; filters lymph and produces lymphocytes.

Lymphocyte (lĭm′fə-sīt) An agranular type of white blood cell. There are T lymphocytes and B lymphocytes.

Lymphokine (lim′fə-kīn) A group of chemicals secreted by T lymphocytes. The chemicals affect the functioning of other cells, especially the macrophages.

Lysosome (lī′sə-sōm) An organelle that contains powerful enzymes; engages in phagocytosis and does the "intracellular housecleaning."

Macrophage (măk′rə-fāj) An enlarged monocyte that eats foreign material; a "big eater."

Mammary gland (măm′ə-rē glănd) The gland of the female breast that secretes milk.

Mandible (măn′də-bəl) The lower jaw bone.

Manubrium (mə-noo′brē-əm) The upper part of the sternum.

Marrow (măr′ō) Connective tissue that occupies the spaces in bone; either the red marrow or the yellow marrow.

Matrix (mā′trĭks) Intercellular material of connective tissue.

Matter (măt′ər) Anything that occupies space; may occur as solid, liquid, or gas.

Maxilla (măk-sĭl′ə) The upper jaw bone.

Mechanoreceptor (měk″ə-nō-rĭ-sĕp′tər) Receptor that is stimulated by bending, pressing, or pushing; hearing receptors are bent and are therefore mechanoreceptors.

Mediastinum (mē″dē-ə-stī′nəm) Space between the lungs that contains the heart, trachea, thymus gland, esophagus, and large blood vessels.

Medulla (mĕ-dŭl′ə) The inner part of an organ, such as the adrenal medulla.

Medulla oblongata (mĕ-dŭl′ə ŏb″lŏng-gä′tə) A part of the brain stem that controls vital functions such as respiratory and cardiovascular function; the part of the brain that connects with the spinal cord.

Medullary cavity (mĕd′ə-lĕr″ē kăv′ĭ-tē) Cavity within the diaphysis of a long bone that is occupied by yellow marrow.

Megakaryocyte (mĕg″ə-kăr′ē-ō-sīt) Cell that fragments into platelets.

Meiosis (mī-ō′sĭs) A type of cell division used by the sex cells, the ovum and sperm, to reduce the number of chromosomes in each from 46 to 23.

Melanin (mĕl′ə-nĭn) A pigment that is responsible for the color of the skin and hair.

Melanocyte (mĕl′ə-nō-sīt) A melanin-producing cell.

Membrane (mĕm′brān) Sheet of tissue that may be made of epithelial or connective tissue.

Meninges (mə-nĭn′jēz) The membranes that cover the brain and spinal cord; include the dura mater, arachnoid mater, and pia mater.

Menopause (mĕn′ə-pōz) A normal developmental stage in women that marks the end of the ovarian and uterine cycles.

Menses (mĕn′sēz) Menstruation; the monthly discharge of blood from the uterus.

Menstruation (mĕn″stroo-ā′shən) Loss of blood and tissue from the uterus at the beginning of the uterine cycle; the "period."

Mesentery (mĕs′ən-tĕr″ē) The visceral peritoneum that covers the abdominal organs. A fold of peritoneal membrane attaches the small intestine to the posterior abdominal wall.

Metabolic acidosis (mĕt″ə-bŏl′ĭk ăs″ĭ-dō′sĭs) Acidosis caused by the accumulation of acids (with the exception of carbonic acid) or the loss of bases, including bicarbonate; see acidosis.

Metabolic alkalosis (mĕt″ə-bŏl′ĭk ăl″kə-lō′sĭs) An alkalosis caused by an excessive loss of hydrogen ions (H^+) or gain of bases; see alkalosis.

Metabolism (mĕ-tăb′ə-lĭz-əm) All the chemical reactions that occur within the cells; consists of anabolism and catabolism.

Micturition (mĭk″tə-rĭsh′ən) Act of eliminating urine from the bladder; urination or voiding.

Midbrain (mĭd′brān) The upper part of the brain stem; regulates visual, auditory, and equilibrium-related reflexes.

Mineral (mĭn′ər-əl) An inorganic substance such as sodium or potassium.

Miosis (mī-ō′sĭs) Constriction of the pupil of the eye.

Mitochondria (mī″tō-kŏn′drē-ə) Organelles that produce most of the ATP; the "powerplants" of the cell.

Mitosis (mī-tō′sĭs) Type of cell division that produces two identical daughter cells, each containing 46 chromosomes.

Mitral valve (mī′trəl vălv) See bicuspid valve.

Mixed nerve (mĭkst nŭrv) Nerve that contains both sensory and motor fibers.

Mixture (mĭks′chər) A combination of two or more substances that can be separated by ordinary physical means.

Molecule (mŏl′ĭ-kyool) A chemical combination of two or more atoms.

Monocyte (mŏn′ə-sīt) An agranular white blood cell that can become a macrophage; an important phagocyte.

Monosaccharide (mŏn″ō-săk′ə-rīd) A simple sugar consisting of hexoses (glucose, fructose, galactose) and pentoses (ribose, deoxyribose).

Morphogenesis (môr″fō-jĕn′ĭ-sĭs) The process by which an organism attains a shape; describes the "shaping-up" of Baby.

Morula (môr′yə-lə) A stage of preembryonic development characterized by a spherical solid mass of cells.

Motor nerve (mō′tər nûrv) A collection of motor neurons that carries information away from the central nervous system.

Motor neuron (mō′tər nōōr′ŏn) A neuron that takes information from the central nervous system to the effector organ; an efferent neuron.

Mucous membrane (myōō′kəs mĕm′brān) Type of membrane that lines the cavities and tubes that open to the outside.

Mutation (myōō-tā′shən) A change in the genetic code that may appear in the offspring.

Mydriasis (mĭ-drī′ə-sĭs) Dilation of the pupil of the eye.

Myelin (mī′ə-lĭn) White, fatty material that covers some nerve fibers; myelinated nerves conduct nerve impulses faster than nonmyelinated fibers.

Myelosuppression (mī″ĕ-lō-sə-presh′ən) Depressed activity of the bone marrow; results in diminished production of red blood cells, white blood cells, and platelets.

Myocardium (mī″ō-kăr′dē-əm) Heart muscle.

Myometrium (mī″ō-mē′trē-əm) The muscle layer of the uterus that contracts and causes the delivery of the infant.

Myosin (mī′ə-sĭn) A muscle protein that interacts with actin to cause muscle contraction; also called the thick filament.

Myxedema (mĭk″sĭ-dē′mə) Hypothyroidism in the adult.

Nares (nā′rēz) Openings into the nasal cavities; nostrils.

Nasal cavity (nā′zəl kăv′ĭ-tē) One of the two cavities through which air passes as it moves from the nostrils to the nasopharynx; separated by the nasal septum.

Nasal septum (nā′zəl sĕp′təm) The partition that separates the two nasal cavities.

Nasolacrimal duct (nā″zō-lăk′rĭ-məl dŭkt) A duct that carries tears from the lacrimal sac to the nasal cavities.

Neonate (nē′ō-nāt) A newborn infant from birth to 1 month; a baby.

Nephron (nĕf′rŏn) The structural and functional unit of the kidney that makes urine.

Nerve (nûrv) A bundle of nerve fibers that run toward and away from the central nervous system.

Nerve impulse (nûrv ĭm′pŭls) An action potential that occurs in nerves.

Nerve tract (nûrv trăkt) A group of neurons that share a common function within the central nervous system; may be ascending (sensory) or descending (motor).

Neurilemma (nōōr″ĭ-lĕm′ə) The sheath surrounding the axons of peripheral nerves; necessary for regeneration of damaged nerves.

Neuroglia (nōō-rŏg′lē-ə) Nerve cells that support, protect, and nourish the neurons; consist of astrocytes, ependymal cells, oligodendrocytes, and microglia.

Neurohypophysis (nōōr″ō-hī-pŏf′ĭ-sĭs) See posterior pituitary gland.

Neuromuscular junction (nōōr″ō-mŭs′kyə-lər jŭngk′shən) A junction or space that occurs between a motor neuron and a muscle fiber.

Neuron (nōōr′ŏn) Nerve cell that conducts the action potential (nerve impulse); composed of dendrites, a cell body, and an axon.

Neurotransmitter (nōōr″ō-trăns′mĭt-ər) A chemical made within the axon terminal that is responsible for transmission of the signal across the synapse or junction; common neurotransmitters include norepinephrine, acetylcholine, serotonin, dopamine, and epinephrine.

Neutrophil (nōō′trə-fĭl) A granular white blood cell that is motile and highly phagocytic; normally comprises about 60% to 70% of the total white blood cell count.

Node of Ranvier (nōd ŭv răn-vē-ā) A gap in the myelin sheath covering an axon; it is the exposed axonal membrane. The nerve impulse jumps from node to node as it moves toward the axon terminal.

Nondisjunction (nŏn″dĭs-jŭngk′shən) Failure of the chromosomes or chromatids to separate during meiosis.

Norepinephrine (nôr″ĕp-ə-nĕf′rĭn) Neurotransmitter released by adrenergic fibers (postganglionic fibers of the sympathetic nervous system) and by the adrenal medulla; causes the "fight or flight" response.

Nucleic acid (nōō-klē′ĭk ăs′ĭd) Composed of a series of nucleotides that store the genetic code and determine protein synthesis; DNA and RNA.

Nucleotide (nōō′klē-ō-tīd″) The building blocks of DNA and RNA; consists of a sugar (ribose or deoxyribose), a phosphate group, and a nitrogen-containing base (adenine, thymine, guanine, cytosine, or uracil).

Nucleus (nōō′klē-əs) (pl. nuclei) A large organelle separated from the cytoplasm by a nuclear membrane; stores the DNA in chromosomes and acts as the control center of the cell.

Occipital bone (ŏk-sĭp′ĭ-tl bōn) The flat bone that forms the back of the skull.

Occipital lobe (ŏk-sĭp′ĭ-tl lōb) The cerebral lobe located in the back of the head; concerned primarily with vision.

Oculomotor nerve (ŏk″yə-lō-mō″tər nûrv) Cranial nerve III; motor fibers to the extrinsic eye muscles, ciliary body, and pupil.

Olfactory nerve (ŏl-făk′tə-rē nûrv) Cranial nerve I; sensory for smell.

Olfactory receptor (ŏl-făk′tə-rē rĭ-sĕp′tər) Chemoreceptor located high in the nasal cavities; activation leads to the sense of smell.

Oliguria (ŏl″ĭ-gyoo′rē-ə) Scanty urine formation.

Oocyte (ō′ə-sīt) The developing female gamete; egg or ovum.

Oogenesis (ō″ə-jĕn′ĭ-sĭs) Production of eggs in the females; involves meiosis and maturation.

Optic chiasma (chiasm) (ŏp′tĭk kī-ăz′mə [kī′ăz-əm]) Site for the crossing of the medial fibers of the optic nerve to the opposite side of the brain; located in front of the anterior pituitary gland.

Optic nerve (ŏp′tĭk nûrv) Cranial nerve II; carries sensory information from the retina to the occipital lobe of the cerebrum for vision.

Oral cavity (ôr′əl kăv′ĭ-tē) Mouth.

Organ (ôr′gən) Group of tissues that performs a specialized function, such as the lungs.

Organelle (ôr″gə-nĕl′) A part of the cell that performs a specialized function, such as the energy-producing mitochondrion.

Organic (ôr-găn′ĭk) A carbon-containing substance.

Organ of Corti (ôr′gən ŭv kôr′tē) The cells in the cochlea of the inner ear that are the hearing receptors.

Organ system (ôr-gən sĭs″təm) A group of organs that perform a particular function, such as the organs of digestion.

Origin (ŏr′ə-jĭn) The part of the muscle that is attached to the more immovable structure.

Orthopnea (ôr-thŏp′nē-ə) Ability to breathe easily only in an upright position.

Osmosis (ŏz-mō′sĭs) The movement of water across a membrane from an area where there is more water to an area where there is less water.

Osseous tissue (ŏs′ē-əs tĭsh′oo) Bone tissue.

Ossicle (ŏs′ĭ-kəl) One of three tiny bones found in the middle ear; malleus (hammer), incus (anvil), stapes (stirrup).

Ossification (ŏs″ĭ-fĭ-kā′shən) The formation of bone.

Osteoblast (ŏs′tē-ə-blăst) A bone-building cell.

Osteoclast (ŏs′tē-ə-klăst″) A cell that causes the breakdown of bone; parathyroid hormone stimulates osteoclastic activity.

Osteocyte (ŏs′tē-ə-sīt″) A mature bone cell.

Osteoporosis (ŏs″tē-ō-pə-rō′sĭs) Weakened bones due to the loss of bone matrix.

Otitis media (ō-tī′tĭs mē′dē-ə) Middle ear infection.

Output (out′poot) The amount of water that the body eliminates per day.

Oval window (ō′vəl wĭn′dō) The membraneous oval structure in which the stapes sits.

Ovarian cycle (ō-vâr′ē-ən sī′kəl) Monthly changes in the secretion of the ovarian hormones, estrogen and progesterone.

Ovarian follicle (ō-vâr′ē-ən fŏl′ĭ-kəl) The ovarian structure that releases an egg at maturation; see graafian follicle.

Ovary (ō′və-rē) Female gonad that produces ova and the hormones estrogen and progesterone.

Ovulation (ŏv″yə-lā′shən) The discharge of the mature ovum from the graafian follicle.

Oxyhemoglobin (ŏk″sē-hē′mə-glō″bĭn) Hemoglobin that is loosely bound to oxygen.

Oxytocin (ŏk″sĭ-tō′sĭn) Hormone released from the posterior pituitary gland that causes contraction of the uterus during labor; literally means "swift birth."

Pacemaker (pās′māk″ər) The sinoatrial (SA) node located in the upper wall of the right atrium; sets the heart rate.

Pancreas (păn′krē-əs) An organ that has both endocrine and exocrine functions. The islets of Langerhans secrete the hormones insulin and glucagon. As an accessory organ of digestion, the pancreas secretes the most important of the digestive enzymes, amylase, lipase, and proteases.

Paranasal sinuses (păr″ə-nā′zəl sī′nəs-ĭz) Air-filled cavities in the skull; frontal, maxillary, sphenoidal, and ethmoidal sinuses.

Paraplegia (păr″ə-plē′jə) Paralysis of the lower extremities.

Parasympathetic nervous system (păr″ə-sĭm″pə-thĕt′ĭk nûr′vəs sĭs′təm) The division of the autonomic nervous system that is concerned with "feeding and breeding."

Parathyroid hormone (PTH) (păr″ə-thī′roid hōr′mōn) Hormone secreted by the parathyroid glands that regulates plasma levels of calcium. PTH raises the blood calcium level; a deficiency of PTH causes tetany.

Parietal (pə-rī′ĭ-təl) Pertaining to a wall of a cavity; the parietal peritoneum and the parietal pleura are membranes that hug the walls of their cavities.

Parietal lobe (pə-rī′ĭ-təl lōb) The cerebral lobe that is concerned primarily with generalized sensation.

Parkinson disease (pär′kĭn-sən dĭ-zēz′) A disease of the basal ganglia resulting in muscle weakness and rigidity, tremors, and a characteristic gait; caused by a deficiency of dopamine.

Parotid glands (pə-rŏt′ĭd glăndz) The largest of the three pairs of salivary glands. An inflammation of the parotid gland is called parotitis; a common viral inflammation of the parotids is called mumps.

Partial pressure (pär′shəl prĕsh′ər) The part of the total pressure exerted by a gas, such as the partial pressure of oxygen in room air.

Parturition (pär″tyoo-rĭsh′ən) The process of giving birth to a baby; the process includes the birth of the baby and the expulsion of the placenta.

Pectoral girdle (pĕk′tər-əl gûr′dl) Portion of the skeleton that supports and attaches to the upper extremities.

Pelvic cavity (pĕl′vĭk kăv′ĭ-tē) Lower or inferior portion of the abdominopelvic cavity; contains the urinary bladder, the sigmoid colon, the rectum, and the internal reproductive structures.

Pelvic girdle (pĕl′vĭk gûr′dl) Portion of the skeleton to which the lower extremities are attached.

Pelvis (pĕl′vĭs) Basin-like structure formed by the coxal (hip) bones, sacrum, and coccyx; also refers to a small cavity in the kidney that receives urine from the collecting ducts.

Penis (pē′nĭs) Male organ that functions in urination and copulation.

Pepsin (pĕp′sĭn) A protein-digesting enzyme found in gastric juice.

Peptide bond (pĕp′tīd bŏnd) Bond formed between two amino acids.

Pericardium (pĕr″ĭ-kär′dē-əm) A sling-like serous membrane that partially encloses the heart; supports the weight of the heart.

Perineum (pĕr″ə-nē′əm) The pelvic floor; extends from the anus to the vulva in the female and from the anus to the scrotum in the male.

Periosteum (pĕr″ē-ŏs′tē-əm) Fibrous connective tissue that covers the surface of a long bone.

Peripheral nervous system (pə-rĭf′ər-əl nûr′vəs sĭs′təm) The nerves and ganglia that lie outside the central nervous system.

Peristalsis (pĕr″ĭ-stŏl′sĭs) Rhythmic contraction of smooth muscle that propels a substance forward; peristalsis in the digestive tract moves food from the esophagus toward the anus.

Peritoneum (pĕr″ĭ-tə-nē′əm) A serous membrane located in the abdominal cavity. The parietal peritoneum lines the wall of the cavity; the visceral peritoneum surrounds the viscera.

Peritonitis (pĕr″ĭ-tə-nī′tĭs) Inflammation of the peritoneum.

Peritubular capillary (pĕr″ĭ-tōō′byə-lər kăp′ĭ-lĕr″ē) Capillary network that surrounds the renal tubules; water and dissolved solute are reabsorbed into the peritubular capillaries.

Pernicious anemia (pər-nĭsh′əs ə-nē′mē-ə) An anemic condition caused by a deficiency of vitamin B_{12} or intrinsic factor that is necessary for the absorption of vitamin B_{12}.

Peyer patches (pī′ər păch′əz) Lymph nodules in the walls of the small intestine, especially the ileum.

pH (pē″āch′) A measure of the hydrogen ion concentration. A blood pH greater than 7.45 is called alkalosis; a blood pH of less than 7.35 is called acidosis.

Phagocytosis (făg″ə-sī-tō′sĭs) The eating or engulfing of pathogens or cellular debris.

Phalanges (fā-lăn′jēz) Bones of the fingers, thumbs, and toes.

Pharynx (făr′ĭngks) A passageway for food, water, and air; also called the throat.

Photoreceptor (fō″tō-rĭ-sĕp′tər) Receptor that is stimulated by light such as the rods and cones of the retina.

Physiology (fĭz″ē-ŏl′ə-jē) The study of the functioning of the body.

Pia mater (pī′ə mā′tər) Soft innermost layer of meninges.

Pineal gland (pĭn′ē-əl glănd) Small gland located near the third ventricle of the brain; secretes melatonin and is involved in regulating biorhythms.

Pinocytosis (pĭn″ə-sī-tō′sĭs) Engulfing of water droplets by the cell membrane; cellular drinking.

Placenta (plə-sĕn′tə) Structure formed by the chorion and uterine tissue; the site of exchange of nutrients, oxygen, and waste for Baby-to-be. Also functions as a gland.

Plasma (plăz′mə) The yellow liquid portion of blood.

Plasma cell (plăz′mə sĕl) A cell that comes from a B lymphocyte and mass-produces antibodies.

Platelet (plāt′lĕt) Piece of a megakaryocyte that functions in hemostasis; also called thrombocyte.

Pleura (plōōr′ə) Serous membrane that surrounds the lungs; the two layers are the visceral pleura and the parietal pleura.

Plexus (plĕk′səs) A network of nerves such as the cervical plexus.

Polysaccharide (pŏl″ē-săk′ə-rīd″) A carbohydrate made of more than two simple sugars, such as glycogen.

Polyuria (pŏl″ē-yōō′rē-ə) Excessive excretion of urine as occurs in uncontrolled diabetes mellitus.

Pons (pŏnz) A portion of the brain stem located between the midbrain and the medulla oblongata; participates in breathing activity.

Portal vein (pôr′tl vān) See hepatic portal circulation.

Posterior pituitary gland (pŏs-tîr′ē-ər pĭ-tōō′ĭ-tĕr″ē glănd) An extension of the hypothalamus; releases antidiuretic hormone (ADH) and oxytocin; also called the neurohypophysis.

Prepuce (prē′pyōōs) Loose skin covering the glans of the penis or clitoris; removed during circumcision.

Presbyopia (prĕz″bē-ō′pē-ə) Condition of aging whereby the lens of the eye becomes less elastic, making it difficult to focus on near objects.

Prime mover (prīm mōō′vər) The muscle that is most responsible for a particular movement.

Progesterone (prō-jĕs′tə-rōn) A hormone secreted by the corpus luteum of the ovary. It stimulates the growth of the endometrium and helps maintain the pregnancy.

Projection (prə-jēk'shən) Process by which the brain causes a sensation to be felt at the point of stimulation.

Prolactin (prō-lăk'tĭn) A hormone secreted by the anterior pituitary gland that stimulates the breasts to make milk; also called lactogenic hormone.

Proprioception (prō'prē-ō-sĕp"shən) The sensation of movement and position of the body.

Prostaglandins (prŏs'tə-glăn'dĭnz) A group of compounds that are made from fatty acids in cell membranes; they exert powerful hormone-like effects.

Prostate gland (prŏs'tāt glănd) The gland that surrounds the upper portion of the urethra in the male; contributes to the formation of semen. An enlarged prostate gland impairs urination.

Protein (prō'tēn) A large, nitrogen-containing molecule that is composed of many amino acids.

Prothrombin (prō-thrŏm'bĭn) A plasma protein synthesized by the liver that plays a key role in blood coagulation. When activated it produces thrombin; requires vitamin K for its synthesis.

Proximal (prŏk'sə-məl) Closer to the midline or origin.

Proximal convoluted tubule (prŏk'sə-məl kŏn"və-lōōt'ĭd tōō'byōōl) Coiled region of the tubule that is close to the Bowman capsule.

PTH See parathyroid hormone.

Pulmonary (pŭl'mə-nĕr"ē) Pertaining to the lungs.

Pulmonary artery (pŭl'mə-nĕr"ē är'tə-rē) A large artery that transports unoxygenated blood from the right ventricle of the heart to the lungs.

Pulmonary circulation (pŭl'mə-nĕr"ē sūr-kyə-lā'shən) The path of blood through vessels that takes unoxygenated blood from the right ventricle to the lungs and oxygenated blood from the lungs to the left atrium.

Pulmonary edema (pŭl'mə-nĕr"ē ĭdē'mə) Accumulation of tissue fluid within the alveoli causing dyspnea, orthopnea, productive cough, and pink-tinged sputum.

Pulmonary vein (pŭl'mə-nĕr"ē vān) One of four pulmonary vessels that take oxygenated blood from the lungs to the left atrium.

Pulse (pŭls) Vibration of the arteries caused by rhythmic expansion and recoil of the large arteries following contraction of the ventricles. Pulse rate corresponds to heart rate.

Pulse pressure (pŭls prĕsh'ər) The difference between the systolic and diastolic blood pressure reading; average is 40 mm Hg.

Pupil (pyōō'pəl) An opening in the center of the iris through which light enters.

Purkinje fibers (pûr-kĭn'jē fī'bərz) Fast-conducting fibers located in the ventricular walls; conduct the electrical impulses from the bundle of His to the ventricular myocardium.

Pyloric sphincter (pī-lôr'ĭk sfĭngk'tər) A ring of smooth muscle that opens and closes the distal end of the pylorus.

Pylorus (pī-lôr'əs) Distal end of the stomach; exit is guarded by the pyloric sphincter.

Pyramidal tract (pĭ-răm'ĭ-dl trăkt) Major motor tract that descends from the precentral gyrus of the frontal lobe of the cerebrum to the spinal cord.

Pyrogen (pī'rə-jən) An agent that causes fever.

QRS complex (kyoo'är-ĕs" kŏm'plĕks) The ECG recording that represents ventricular depolarization.

Quadriplegia (kwŏd"rĭ-plē'jə) Paralysis of all four limbs, usually caused by an injury to the cervical spine.

Radiation (rā"dē-ā'shən) Loss of heat as it leaves a warm object, such as the body, to the surrounding cooler air.

Radius (rā'dē-əs) Long bone located on the thumb side of the forearm.

Receptor (rĭ-sĕp'tər) Sensory structure that responds to specific stimuli such as light, chemicals, or touch.

Recessive gene (rĭ-sĕs'ĭv jēn) Gene that only expresses itself when two copies are present; will not express itself in the offspring if it is paired with a dominant gene.

Red blood cell (rĕd blŭd sĕl) A blood cell that contains mostly hemoglobin; it functions in the transport of oxygen and carbon dioxide; also called an erythrocyte.

Red bone marrow (rĕd bōn măr'ō) Hematopoietic tissue located in certain bones, especially the flat bones; site of production of red blood cells, white blood cells, and platelets.

Referred pain (rĭ-fûrd'pān) Pain that feels that it originates in an area other than the part being stimulated.

Reflex (rē'flĕks) An automatic response to a stimulus; there are nervous reflexes and chemical reflexes.

Refraction (rĭ-frăk'shən) Bending of light waves; the chief refracting structures of the eye are the cornea and the lens.

Refractory period (rĭ-frăk'tə-re pĭr'ē-əd) Period of time during which nervous tissue cannot respond to a second stimulus.

Renal tubule (rē'nəl tōō'byōōl) Tubular part of the nephron unit that helps make and transport urine; consists of Bowman capsule, proximal convoluted tubule, loop of Henle, distal convoluted tubule, and collecting duct.

Renin (rē'nĭn) An enzyme secreted by the kidneys that causes the activation of angiotensin; helps regulate blood pressure.

Repolarization (rē"pō-lər-ĭ-zā'shən) Return of the membrane potential to its resting state after the nerve impulse.

Respiratory acidosis (rĕs′pər-ə-tôr″ē ăs″ĭ-dō′sĭs) An acidosis caused by hypoventilation; the cause of the acidosis is respiratory. See acidosis.

Respiratory alkalosis (rĕs′pər-ə-tôr″ē ăl″kə-lō′sĭs) An alkalosis caused by hyperventilation; the cause of the alkalosis is respiratory. See alkalosis.

Resting membrane potential (rĕst′ĭng mĕm′brān pə-tĕn′shəl) The membrane potential (electrical charge across the membrane) of an unstimulated or resting cell.

Reticular activating system (RAS) (rĭ-tĭk′yə-lər ăk′tə-vāt″ĭng sĭs′təm) The cells of the reticular formation that project to higher centers; concerned with wakefulness, alertness, and sleep.

Reticular formation (rĭ-tĭk′yə-lər fôr-mā′shən) A complex network of nerve fibers that arises within the brain stem and projects into the lower cerebrum; causes arousal of the cerebrum so that the person does not slip into a coma.

Reticulocyte (rĭ-tĭk′yə-lō-sīt″) An immature red blood cell that still has elements of an endoplasmic reticulum; an elevation of the reticulocyte count indicates bleeding.

Reticuloendothelial system (RES) (rĭ-tĭk″yə-lō-ĕn″də-thĕl′e-əl sĭs′təm) A group of phagocytic cells widely scattered throughout the body, especially in the lymph nodes, liver, lungs, and spleen; the RES destroys pathogens and foreign particles and removes tissue debris. (The newer term is the mononuclear phagocytic system.)

Retina (rĕt′ĭ-nə) The nervous inner layer of the eye; contains the photoreceptors, the rods and cones.

Rh factor (är″āch′ făk′tər) A type of antigen on the surface of the red blood cell.

Ribonucleic acid (RNA) (rī″bō-nōō-klē′ĭk ăs′ĭd) A nucleotide that copies or transcribes the genetic code from DNA; also involved in translation.

Ribose (rī′bōs) The five-carbon sugar that is found in RNA, ribonucleic acid.

Ribosome (rī′bə-sōm) An organelle that is concerned with the synthesis of protein; ribosomes either are bound to endoplasmic reticulum (rough ER) or are free in the cytoplasm.

Rickets (rĭk′ĭts) A vitamin D deficiency in children that causes bone softening and bowing of the legs.

Rod (rŏd) Photoreceptor that is stimulated by dim light; sees only black and white, not color.

Rugae (rōō′gē) Folds on the mucosal wall of an organ such as the stomach, urinary bladder, and vagina; permits expansion of the organ.

Sacrum (sā′krəm) The five fused sacral vertebrae at the base of the vertebral column.

Sagittal plane (săj′ĭ-tl plān) A vertical plane that divides the organ or body into right and left parts. A midsagittal plane divides the body into right and left halves.

Saliva (sə-lī′və) Secretions of the salivary glands; contains water, electrolytes, mucus, and an amylase (ptyalin).

Salivary glands (săl′ĭ-vĕr-ē glăndz) Three glands located in the mouth that secrete saliva; parotid, sublingual, submandibular glands.

Saltatory conduction (săl′-tə-tôr″ē kən-dŭk′shən) The rapid conduction of a nerve impulse as it jumps from node (of Ranvier) to node toward the axon terminal.

Sarcolemma (sär″kə-lĕm′ə) The plasma membrane of a muscle cell.

Sarcomere (sär′kə-mîr) The contractile unit of a muscle; extends from Z line to Z line and contains actin and myosin.

Schwann cell (shvän sĕl) Cell that surrounds a fiber of a peripheral nerve and forms the myelin and the neurilemma.

Sclera (sklē′rə) Outer layer of the eyeball; the white of the eye.

Scoliosis (skō′lē-ō′sĭs) Lateral curvature of the spine.

Scrotum (skrō′təm) A pouch of skin that encloses the testes.

Sebaceous gland (sĭ-bā′-shəs glănd) Gland located in the skin that secretes sebum.

Sebum (sē′bəm) The oily secretion of a sebaceous gland.

Semen (sē′mən) The sperm-containing secretion of the male.

Semicircular canal (sĕm″ē-sûr′kyə-lər kə-năl′) Structure in the inner ear that contains the receptors for balance.

Semilunar valve (sĕm″ē-lōō′nər vălv) A valve shaped like a half-moon located between the ventricles and their attached vessels; pulmonic valve and aortic valve.

Seminal vesicle (sĕm′ə-nəl vĕs′ĭ-kəl) Glands that produce about 60% of the volume of semen.

Seminiferous tubules (sĕm″ə-nĭf′ər-əs tōō′byōōlz) Highly coiled ducts within the testes that produce sperm.

Sensation (sĕn-sā′shən) A feeling or experience resulting from the brain's interpretation of sensory stimulation.

Sensory nerve (sĕn′sə-rē nûrv) A collection of sensory neurons that carries information toward the central nervous system.

Sensory neuron (sĕn′sə-rē nōōr′ŏn) A neuron that takes information toward the central nervous system; afferent neuron.

Serous membrane (sîr′əs mĕm′brān) Membranes that cover organs and line cavities that do not open to the outside.

Serum (sē′rəm) Blood plasma minus the clotting factors.

Sex chromosomes (sĕks krō′mə-sōm) Chromosomes that are responsible for the gender of the individual; XX for a female and XY for a male.

Sex-linked trait (sĕks′lĭngkt trāt) A trait whose genes are carried on the X or Y (sex) chromosome. Traits carried on the X chromosome are called X-linked traits.

Sickle cell disease (sĭk′əl sĕl dĭ-zēz) A genetic disorder involving abnormal synthesis of hemoglobin. The abnormal hemoglobin causes the red blood cells to sickle, thereby blocking the flow of blood to vital organs, and a type of anemia called sickle cell anemia.

Sigmoid (sĭg′moid) Distal S-shaped part of the colon; extends from the descending colon to the rectum.

Sinoatrial (SA) node (sī″nō-ā′trē-əl nōd) A small area of conducting tissue that initiates the heartbeat. Located in the upper wall of the right atrium; also called the pacemaker.

Sinus (sī′nəs) A cavity such as the paranasal sinuses in the head.

Sinusoid (sī′nyə-soid) Large, highly permeable capillary that permits free movement of proteins between the tissue fluid and the blood.

Skin turgor (skĭn tûr′gər) A condition of normal tension in the skin, effected by an adequate amount of fluid in the skin tissue. Poor skin turgor indicates dehydration.

Sliding-filament hypothesis (slīd′ĭng fĭl′ə-mənt hī-pŏth′ĭ-sĭs) Theory that a series of events causes actin and myosin to slide past one another, causing muscle contraction.

Small intestine (smōl ĭn-tĕs′tĭn) The portion of the digestive tract that extends from the stomach to the large intestine; duodenum, jejunum, ileum.

Soft palate (sôft păl′ĭt) The "soft" posterior portion of the roof of the mouth.

Solute (sŏl′yōōt) A substance that is dissolved in another substance (solvent).

Solution (sə-lōō′shən) A mixture in which the particles that are mixed together remain evenly distributed.

Solvent (sŏl′vənt) A substance in which the solute is dissolved or mixed.

Somatic nervous system (sō-măt″ĭk nûr′vəs sĭs″təm) The part of the peripheral nervous system that stimulates the skeletal muscles.

Somatotropin (sō″mə-tə-trō′pĭn) See growth hormone.

Specific gravity (spĭ-sĭ′fĭk grăv′ĭ-tē) The weight of urine compared to the weight of an equal volume of water.

Spermatogenesis (spûr″mə-tə-jĕn′ĭ-sĭs) Production of sperm in the male; involves meiosis and maturation.

Spermatozoon (spûr″mə-tə-zō′ŏn) A developing sperm.

Sphincter (sfĭngk′tər) A circular muscle that opens and closes a tube, such as the anal sphincter.

Spinal cord (spī′nəl kôrd) The part of the central nervous system located in the vertebral canal; transmits information to and from the brain.

Spinal nerve (spī′nəl nûrv) A nerve that arises from the spinal cord.

Spleen (splēn) A large organ located in the left upper quadrant of the abdominal cavity; phagocytoses red blood cells and platelets and produces lymphocytes.

Splenomegaly (splē″nō-mĕg′ə-lē) Enlarged spleen.

Spongy bone (spŭn′jē bōn) Soft or cancellous bone.

Stapes (stā′pēz) Middle ear ossicle, also called the stirrup; tiny bone that articulates with the incus and sits in the oval window.

Starling's law of the heart (stär′lĭngz lô uv thə härt) Refers to the relationship between myocardial stretch and the strength of myocardial contraction; the greater the stretch of the myocardial fibers, the greater the number of crossbridges formed, and the greater the force of contraction.

Stem cell (stĕm sĕl) Immature and undifferentiated cell found in the red bone marrow. It is the precursor of other blood cells such as the red blood cell, white blood cell, and platelet.

Stenosis (stə-nō′sĭs) An abnormal constriction or narrowing of an opening, as in mitral valve stenosis.

Sternum (stûr′nəm) The breastbone; parts are the manubrium, body, xiphoid process.

Steroid (stĕr′oid) Lipid-soluble hormone such as estrogen, testosterone, and cortisol; cholesterol is the precursor for steroid synthesis.

Stomach (stŭm′ək) The expandable digestive organ that receives food from the esophagus and delivers a partially digested chyme to the duodenum.

Strabismus (strə-bĭz′məs) A deviation of either eye so that the eyes are unable to focus on the same object at the same time; the medial deviation of the eye is called cross-eye.

Stratified (străt″ə-fīd) Layered, as in stratified epithelium.

Stratum corneum (strā′təm kôr′nē-əm) Outermost layer of the epidermis.

Stratum germinativum (strā′təm jûr″mĭ-nə-tĭv′əm) Innermost layer of the epidermis where cell division takes place.

Striated (strī′āt-əd) Banded or striped, such as striated muscle.

Stroke volume (strōk vŏl′yōōm) The amount of blood that the ventricle pumps in one beat; 60 to 80 mL per beat.

Subarachnoid space (sŭb″ə-răk′noid spās) The space between the arachnoid mater and the pia mater; the space through which cerebrospinal fluid circulates.

Subcutaneous (sŭb″kyōō-tā′nē-əs) Tissue beneath the dermis that contains fat cells.

Sudoriferous gland (soo″də-rĭf′ər-əs glănd) A sweat gland.

Superior vena cava (sŏŏ-pē′rē-ər vē′nə kā′və) The large vein that takes unoxygenated blood from the head, shoulders, and upper extremities to the right atrium.

Surfactant (sər-făk′tənt) Chemical substance that reduces surface tension; pulmonary surfactants prevent the collapse of alveoli.

Suspension (sə-spĕn′shən) A mixture in which the large particles gradually settle to the bottom unless continuously shaken or agitated (eg, a sand and water suspension).

Suture (soo′chər) A type of immovable joint (synarthrosis) found between the bones of the skull.

Sympathetic nervous system (sĭm″pə-thĕt′ĭk nûr′vəs sĭs′təm) A division of the autonomic nervous system that causes the "fight-or-flight" response.

Symphysis (sĭm′fĭ-sĭs) A slightly movable joint between bones separated by cartilage such as the symphysis pubis.

Synapse (sĭn′ăps) The area between two nerves, usually referring to the area between an axon and a dendrite; consists of a presynaptic membrane, synaptic cleft, and a postsynaptic membrane.

Synaptic cleft (sĭ-năp′tĭk klĕft) The small space between the presynaptic membrane and the postsynaptic membrane of a synapse.

Synarthrosis (sĭn″är-thrō′sĭs) An immovable joint such as a suture.

Synergist (sĭn′ər-jĭst) A muscle that assists or works with another muscle.

Synovial fluid (sĭ-nō′vē-əl floo′id) Fluid secreted by the synovial membrane into a synovial joint to decrease friction.

Synovial joint (sĭ-nō′vē-əl joint) A freely movable joint; a diarthrosis.

Synovial membrane (sĭ-nō′vē-əl mĕm′brān) Membrane that lines synovial or diarthrotic joints.

Systemic circulation (sĭs-tĕm′ĭk sûr-kyə-lā′shən) The part of the circulatory system that serves all parts of the body except the blood vessels that supply the gas-exchanging portions of the lungs.

Systole (sĭs′tə-lē) Contraction of the myocardium; there is atrial and ventricular systole.

Systolic pressure (sĭs-tŏl′ĭk prĕsh′ər) The arterial pressure during the systolic phase of the cardiac cycle; the "top number" of a blood pressure reading.

Tachycardia (tăk″ĭ-kär′dē-ə) An abnormally fast heart rate in excess of 100 beats per minute.

Target tissue (tär′gĭt tĭsh′oo) The tissue at which a hormone is aimed; adrenocorticotropic hormone (ACTH) is aimed at its target tissue (or organ), the adrenal cortex.

T cell (tē′ sĕl) A type of lymphocyte that engages in cell-mediated immunity; helper T cells stimulate other immune cells. Also called T lymphocyte.

Temporal lobe (tĕm′pə-rəl lōb) A lobe of the cerebrum that is responsible for hearing, smelling, speech, and memory.

Tendon (tĕn′dən) A strong band of connective tissue that anchors muscle to bone.

Teratogen (tĕr′ə-tə-jən) Means "monster-producing"; anything that causes developmental abnormalities in the embryo, such as the rubella virus or alcohol.

Testes (tĕs′tēz) (sing. testis) Male gonads that produce sperm and testosterone.

Testosterone (tĕs-tŏs′tə-rōn) The most important male hormone; androgen.

Tetanus (tĕt′ə-nəs) Sustained muscle contraction; also a disease caused by the *Clostridium tetani* pathogen.

Tetany (tĕt′ə-nē) Sustained muscle contraction caused by a deficiency of calcium.

Thalamus (thăl′ə-məs) Part of the diencephalon that acts primarily as a relay station for nerve tracts; passes information between the spinal cord and the cerebrum.

Thermoreceptor (thûr″mō-rĭ-sĕp′tər) Receptors that detect changes in temperature.

Thoracic duct (thə-răs′ĭk dŭkt) A large lymphatic vessel that receives lymph and empties it into the left subclavian vein.

Thrombin (thrŏm′bĭn) The enzyme produced when prothrombin is activated; it causes the conversion of fibrinogen into fibrin threads during blood coagulation.

Thrombocyte (thrŏm′bə-sīt) See platelet.

Thrombus (thrŏm′bəs) A blood clot formed within a blood vessel or a heart chamber.

Thymosin (thī′mə-sĭn) A hormone secreted by the thymus gland.

Thymus gland (thī′məs glănd) A lymphatic organ that lies in the upper chest region and plays an important role in immunity.

Thyroid gland (thī′roid glănd) A gland located in the anterior neck; secretes T_3, T_4 (thyroxine), and calcitonin.

Thyroid-stimulating hormone (TSH) (thī′roid stĭm′yə-lāt-ĭng hōr′mōn) Hormone secreted by the anterior pituitary gland that stimulates the thyroid gland to secrete T_3 and T_4.

Thyroxine (thī-rŏk′sĭn) A hormone secreted by the thyroid gland that regulates metabolic rate; called T_4 or tetraiodothyronine.

Tibia (tĭb′ē-ə) The shin bone found in the lower leg.

Tidal volume (tīd′l vŏl′yoom) Amount of air that is inhaled and exhaled during normal, quiet breathing.

Tissue (tĭsh′oo) A group of cells that perform a specialized function.

T lymphocyte (tē″lĭm′fə-sīt) See T cell.

Tonsil (tŏn′səl) Patches of lymphoid tissue embedded in the throat region; palatine, lingual, and pharyngeal tonsils.

Tonus (tō′nəs) The continuous contraction of a muscle.

Toxoid (tŏk′soid″) A toxin that is treated with heat or a chemical so that its disease-producing ability is destroyed while maintaining its antigenic properties; the toxoid can still stimulate the production of antitoxin.

Trachea (trā′kē-ə) Large airway located between the larynx and the bronchus; windpipe.

Tract (trăkt) Bundle of nerve fibers located in the central nervous system.

Transcellular fluid (trăns″sĕl′yə-lər flōō′ĭd) Extracellular fluid that includes cerebrospinal fluid, aqueous and vitreous humor, synovial fluid of the joints, serous fluid within body cavities, and exocrine gland secretions (eg, gastric juice).

Transverse plane (trăns′vŭrs plān) A plane that divides the body into a top (superior) and bottom (inferior) part.

Tricuspid valve (trī-kŭs′pĭd vălv) Atrioventricular valve found between the right atrium and the right ventricle.

Trigeminal nerve (trī-jĕm′ə-nəl nŭrv) Cranial nerve V; sensory to the face and teeth and motor to the chewing muscles.

Triglyceride (trī-glĭs′ə-rīd) A lipid molecule composed of three fatty acid molecules joined to glycerol.

Trigone (trī′gōn) Triangular area on the floor of the bladder formed by the openings for the two ureters and the urethra.

Triiodothyronine (trī″ī-ō″dō-thī′rə-nēn) A hormone secreted by the thyroid gland that regulates metabolic rate and is essential for normal growth and development; called T_3.

Trisomy (trī′sō-mē) Having three chromosomes instead of the normal pair of two.

Trochlear nerve (trŏk′lē-ər nŭrv) Cranial nerve IV; motor to an extrinsic eye muscle.

Trophoblast (trŏf′ə-blăst) The outermost layer of the blastocyst that becomes the chorion.

Tropic hormone (trō″pĭk hōr′mōn) A hormone that is "aimed at" another gland and helps to regulate that gland.

Trypsin (trĭp′sĭn) A proteolytic digestive enzyme produced by the pancreas.

Tubular reabsorption (tōō′byə-lər rē″əb-sôrp′shən) The movement of water and dissolved substances from the tubules into the peritubular capillaries; can be active or passive transport processes.

Tubular secretion (tōō′byə-lər sĭ-krē′shən) The movement of substances from the peritubular capillaries into the tubules.

Tunica (tōō′nĭ-kə) A layer or coat.

Twitch (twĭch) A single muscle contraction and relaxation.

Tympanic membrane (tĭm-păn′ĭk mĕm′brăn) Membrane that separates the external and middle ears; called the eardrum.

Ulna (ŭl′nə) The long bone located on the "little finger" side of the lower arm.

Umbilical arteries (ŭm-bĭl′ĭ-kəl är′tə-rēz) The fetal blood vessels that carry unoxygenated blood from the fetus to the placenta.

Umbilical cord (ŭm-bĭl′ĭ-kəl kôrd) The long structure that connects the fetus to the placenta; contains the umbilical arteries and umbilical vein.

Umbilical vein (ŭm-bĭl′ĭ-kəl vān) The fetal blood vessel that carries oxygenated blood from the placenta to the fetus.

Urea (yōō-rē′ə) A nitrogenous waste product formed by the liver and excreted by the kidneys.

Uremia (yōō-rē′mē-ə) Condition in which there are nitrogenous waste products in the blood; literally means "urine in the blood" and indicates that impaired kidney function is responsible for this syndrome.

Ureter (yōō-rē′tər) The tube that conducts urine from the kidney to the urinary bladder.

Urethra (yōō-rē′thrə) The tube that conducts urine from the bladder to the exterior of the body.

Urinalysis (yōōr″ĭ-năl′ĭ-sĭs) Examination of a urine sample for evidence of disease.

Urinary bladder (yōōr′ĭ-nĕr″ē blăd′ər) A muscular sac in the pelvic cavity that temporarily stores urine.

Urine (yōōr′ĭn) The fluid formed by the kidneys from the blood plasma; contains water, waste, and ions.

Urticaria (ûr″tĭ-kā′rē-ə) See hives.

Uterine tube (yōō′ter-in, u′ter-īn toob) See fallopian tube.

Uterus (yōō′tər-əs) The organ that houses "Baby-to-be" during development; the womb.

Vaccine (văk′sēn) Antigens that have been altered so as to produce active immunity without causing the disease.

Vagina (və-jī′nə) Long, muscular tube in the female that can receive the penis during intercourse and serves as the birth canal.

Vagus nerve (vā′gəs nŭrv) Cranial nerve X; called "the wanderer" because of its wide distribution to the thoracic and abdominal organs.

Valve (vălv) A structure that ensures a one-way flow of a liquid.

Varicose veins (văr′ĭ-kōs vānz) Distended and tortuous veins usually located in the legs.

Vascular (văs′kyə-lər) Pertaining to the blood vessels.

Vascular resistance (văs′kyə-lər rĭ-zĭs′təns) The amount of resistance that the blood vessels offer to the flow of blood; most resistance is caused by the arterioles.

Vas deferens (văs dĕf′ər-ĕns) The tube that carries sperm from the epididymis to the ejaculatory duct. Also called the ductus deferens.

Vasectomy (və-sĕk′tə-mē) A sterilization procedure in which a portion of each vas deferens is removed or severed.

Vasoconstriction (văs″ō-kən-strĭk′shən) The narrowing of blood vessels; usually refers to arterioles.

Vasodilation (văs″ō-dī-lā′shən) The widening of blood vessels; usually refers to arterioles.

Vein (vān) A blood vessel that takes blood toward the heart.

Vena cava (vē′nə kă′və) The large vein that takes unoxygenated blood to the right atrium; there is a superior and inferior vena cava.

Ventilation (věn″tĭ-lā′shən) Moving air into and out of the lungs. There are two phases: inhalation (breathing in) and exhalation (breathing out).

Ventral cavity (věn′trəl kăv′ĭ-tē) The cavity that is located toward the front part of the body. It is divided by the diaphragm into the upper thoracic cavity and the lower abdominopelvic cavity.

Ventral root (věn′trəl rōōt) Anterior region where the motor branch of the spinal nerve attaches to the spinal cord.

Ventricle (věn′trĭ-kəl) A cavity in an organ, such as the ventricles in the heart and brain.

Venule (věn′yōōl) A tiny vein.

Vermiform appendix (věrm′ĭ-fôrm ə-pěn′dĭks) See appendix.

Vernix caseosa (vûr′nĭks kā″sē-ō′sə) Cheese-like substance covering the skin of the fetus.

Vertebral column (vûr′tə-brəl kŏl′əm) The long chain of vertebrae that forms the spine and houses the spinal cord; also called the backbone.

Vesicle (věs′ĭ-kəl) A small membraneous sac that stores substances within a cell.

Vestibule (věs′tə-byōōl) A part of the inner ear that is concerned with balance.

Vestibulocochlear nerve (věs-tĭb″yə-lō-kŏk′lē-ər nûrv) Cranial nerve VIII. The cochlear branch is concerned with hearing; the vestibular branch is concerned with balance.

Villi (vĭl′īs) (sing. villus) Finger-like projections such as the villi that line the intestine; function in absorption.

Viscera (vĭs′ə-rə) The internal organs of the body.

Viscosity (vĭ-skŏs′ĭ-tē) Refers to the tendency of fluids to resist flowing; for instance, molasses is more viscous than water.

Vital capacity (vī′tl kə-păs′ĭ-tē) The greatest amount of air that can be exhaled following maximal inhalation.

Vitreous humor (vĭt′rē-əs hyōō′mər) The gel-like substance that occupies the posterior cavity of the eye.

Vocal cords (vō′kəl kôrdz) The folds of mucous membrane in the larynx that make sound when they vibrate; there are true and false vocal cords.

Vulva (vŭl′və) The external genitalia of the female.

White blood cell (WBC) (wīt blŭd sěl) See leukocyte.

White matter (wīt măt′ər) Nervous tissue in the central nervous system that is primarily composed of myelinated fibers.

Xiphoid process (zĭf′oid prŏs′ěs) The tip or lower end of the sternum.

Yellow marrow (yěl′ō măr′ō) Substance composed of fatty material and found primarily in the medullary cavity of the long bones of an adult.

Zygote (zī′gōt) Fertilized ovum; the cell resulting from the union of the egg and the sperm.

Appendix A
Microbiology Basics

OVERVIEW

A leading cause of disease in humans is the invasion of the body by **pathogens,** or disease-producing microorganisms. Although most microorganisms are harmless or even beneficial to the body, some are harmful, causing disease and sometimes death. Indeed, the history of the world has been shaped by great plagues and infectious diseases caused by pathogens.

The invasion of the body by a pathogen and the symptoms that develop in response to this invasion are called an **infection.** A **localized infection** is restricted to a small area, whereas a **systemic infection** is generalized, or more widespread. A systemic infection is usually spread by the blood; it affects the entire body and generally makes you feel sick. An **opportunistic infection** develops when the person is in a weakened state. For instance, the person with acquired immunodeficiency syndrome (AIDS) has a weakened immune system. As a result, organisms that are usually harmless and live amicably in or on the body are unchecked by immune defenses. As a result, their numbers increase and they cause infections. A **nosocomial infection** is a hospital-acquired infection. As health care professionals, we must protect our patients from becoming infected while in the hospital. With regard to nosocomial infections, the single most important preventive measure is frequent HANDWASHING. You will be unpleasantly surprised by the numbers of health professionals who do not wash their hands as they move from one patient to the next. As a result, pathogens are carried from patient to patient by contaminated hands and equipment.

The study of tiny living organisms is called **microbiology.** There is a vast amount of information about microbiology. We will limit this review to the microorganisms that cause the most common infectious diseases. See Table A–1 for key microbiologic terms and definitions.

TYPES OF MICROORGANISMS

Bacteria

Bacteria are single-cell organisms that are found everywhere. Most bacteria experience living conditions within the human body as ideal, so they move right in. The good news is that many bacteria perform useful roles. For instance, the **normal flora** (organisms that normally live in or on the human body) prevent the overgrowth of other organisms, keeping them under control. The bad news is that bacteria can cause disease. In fact, bacteria make up the largest group of pathogens.

Most bacteria are classified into three groups based on shape: coccus (round), bacillus (rod-shaped), and curved rod. Rickettsiae and chlamydiae are also classified as bacteria, although they differ in several important ways from the cocci, bacilli, and curved rods.

The **cocci** are round cells and are arranged in patterns. Cocci that are arranged in pairs are called **diplococci. Streptococci** are arranged in chains, like a chain of beads. **Staphylococci** look like bunches of grapes and are arranged in clusters. The cocci cause many diseases, including gonorrhea, meningitis, pneumonia, and rheumatic fever. The **bacilli** are long and slender and are shaped like a cigar. Diseases caused by bacilli include tetanus, diphtheria, and tuberculosis. The **curved rods** include the vibrio, the spirillum, and the spirochete. The **vibrio** has a slight curve and resembles a comma. Cholera is caused by a vibrio *(Vibrio cholerae).* The **spirillum** is a long cell that curves or coils and resembles a corkscrew. Highly coiled spirilla that are capable of waving and twisting motions are called **spirochetes.** The most famous spirochete *(Treponema pallidum)* causes syphilis. Bacterial infections are treated with antibiotics.

Rickettsiae and Chlamydiae

Rickettsiae and chlamydiae are classified as bacteria. However, they are smaller than most bacteria and must reproduce within the living cells of

Table A • 1   KEY MICROBIOLOGIC TERMS

TERM	DEFINITION
Anthelmintics	Chemicals that are harmful to worms (helminths).
Antibiotics	Chemicals that are used to treat bacterial infections. A broad-spectrum antibiotic destroys many different types of bacteria, whereas a narrow-spectrum antibiotic destroys only a few types.
Arthropods	Members of an animal phylum that have an exoskeleton (external skeleton) and jointed legs (name means jointed legs); include insects and ticks.
Carrier	A person who harbors a pathogen but does not display any symptoms of illness.
Communicable disease	Any disease that can be spread from one host to another.
Contagious disease	A disease that is easily spread from one person to another. Measles and chicken-pox are contagious diseases because they are easily spread. Although AIDS is an infectious disease, it is not considered contagious because it is not easily spread.
Culture	A population of microorganisms grown in an artificial medium.
Endemic disease	A disease that is always present in a population.
Epidemic disease	A disease acquired by many people in a given area over a short period of time.
Epidemiology	The study of the patterns and spread of disease.
Fecal-oral route	Transfer of a pathogen from contaminated feces (usually by the hands or contaminated linens) to the mouth.
Fomite	A nonliving object, such as eating utensils, that can spread an infection.
Host	An organism that is infected by a pathogen.
Host resistance	The defenses that the body uses to prevent infection by a pathogen.
Incubation period	The time interval between the invasion of the body by a pathogen and the appearance of the first symptoms of disease.
Infectious disease	A disease caused by pathogens or their toxins.
Noncommunicable disease	An infectious disease that cannot be transmitted directly or indirectly from host to host. For instance, a bladder infection due to *E. coli* cannot be spread from the infected person to another person.
Normal flora	A group of microorganisms that colonize a host without causing disease. There are normal flora that colonize the mouth, intestinal tract, vagina, nasal cavities, and other areas of the body. Microorganisms that are not pathogenic in one area may become pathogenic when transferred to another area. For instance, when the *Escherichia coli (E. coli)* bacteria that is part of the normal flora of the large intestine is unintentionally transferred to the urinary bladder, it causes a bladder infection.
Nosocomial infection	An infection that develops during the course of hospitalization and was not present on admission to the hospital; a hospital-acquired infection.
Opportunistic pathogen	An organism that is ordinarily not pathogenic but can become pathogenic under special conditions. See *normal flora.*
Pandemic disease	A worldwide epidemic.
Parasite	An organism that derives its nutrition from a living host.
Pasteurization	The process of heating a substance, such as milk or beer, at a specific temperature for a specific period of time. Milk is pasteurized by being heated to 62.8°C (145°F) for 30 minutes.
Portals of entry	The route or avenue by which a pathogen enters the body (breaks in the skin, inhalation, ingestion of contaminated water and food, introduction of the pathogen into the blood by biting insects).
Portals of exit	The route by which a pathogen leaves the body (excretion in the feces and urine, other body secretions such as semen, respiratory droplets, drainage from lesions [cutaneous, mucous membrane]).
Reservoir of infection	A continual source of infection.
Spore	A dormant or inactive stage of a bacterium characterized by an inner shell, called an endospore, that is resistant to harsh environmental changes (heat or drying). The ability of a bacterium to form spores increases its chances of survival.
Sterilization	A process that destroys all living organisms.
Toxin	A chemical produced by the pathogen that poisons the host.
Vector	A carrier of pathogens from host to host. The mosquito is the animal vector carrying the *Plasmodium* bacteria (malaria) to humans.

a host. Because they require a living host, they are called **parasites.** The rickettsiae are often carried by arthropod vectors such as fleas, ticks, and body lice. For instance, the rickettsia that causes Rocky Mountain spotted fever is carried by a tick. Body lice carry the rickettsia responsible for epidemic typhus. The chlamydiae are smaller than rickettsiae and cause several important human diseases. One of the most prevalent sexually transmitted diseases in the United States today is caused by *Chlamydia trachomatis* bacteria. Chlamydia infection is also responsible for trachoma, a serious eye infection that is the leading cause of blindness in the world. Like other bacterial infections, rickettsial and chlamydial infections are treated with antibiotics (see Table A–2).

Viruses

Viruses are the smallest of the infectious agents. They are not cells and consist of either RNA or DNA surrounded by a protein shell. Since viruses can only reproduce within the living cells of a host, they are parasites. Viruses cause many human diseases and generally do not respond to antibiotics. Examples of viral diseases are measles, mumps, influenza, poliomyelitis, and AIDS. Because of the intimacy of the virus-host relationship, the development of nontoxic antiviral agents has been slow and difficult. This point is well illustrated by the drug zidovudine (AZT), used in the treatment of AIDS. While exerting antiviral effects, the drug also causes widespread damage to the host cells (see Table A–2).

Fungi

Fungi are plant-like organisms, such as mushrooms, that grow best in dark, damp places. Yeasts and molds (as in bread mold) are types of fungi. A few fungi are pathogenic, causing **mycotic infections** (*myco* means fungus). Mycotic infections are usually localized and include athlete's foot, ringworm, thrush (mouth), and vaginitis. *Candida albicans* is a yeast-like fungus that normally inhabits the mouth, digestive tract, and vagina. When *Candida* overgrows, it causes an infection in the mouth (thrush), intestinal symptoms, and vaginitis. Systemic fungal infections are rare but, when they do occur, are life-threatening and difficult to cure (see Table A–2).

Protozoa

Protozoa are single-cell, animal-like microbes. There are four main types of protozoa: amebas, ciliates, flagellates, and sporozoa. Protozoa are found in the soil and in most bodies of water. Amebic dysentery and giardiasis are caused by protozoan parasites. The parasites are ingested in contaminated water and food and cause severe diarrhea. Malaria is caused by a sporozoon called a *plasmodium. Plasmodium malariae* is carried by a mosquito. The mosquito is capable of spreading malaria over a wide region. Indeed, malaria still causes over 3 million deaths per year in the more tropical regions of the world. Two other members of the sporozoa group pose a serious health threat to those persons with compromised immune systems. *Pneumocystis carinii* and *Cryptosporidium* cause opportunistic infections in persons with AIDS. *Pneumocystis carinii* causes pneumonia, and *Cryptosporidium* causes severe diarrhea (see Table A–2).

Parasitic Worms

Worms, called **helminths,** are multicellular animals that are parasitic and pathogenic to humans. The identification of most worm infestations requires microscopic examination of body samples (usually stool), which reveals the presence of the adult worms or the larval forms. The worms are classified as roundworms or flatworms. **Roundworms** include ascarides, pinworms, hookworms, trichinae, and the tiny worms that cause filariasis (elephantiasis). Infestation by pinworms is common in children and is very hard to control. The pinworms live in the intestinal tract but lay their eggs on the outer perianal area. The deposition of the eggs causes itching. The child then scratches the anal area and transfers the eggs to his mouth and to his friends. The eggs are swallowed and the newly hatched pinworms grow into adulthood in the intestine. Most worm infestations are transmitted by the fecal-oral route. (Hands contaminated by feces introduce the worms/eggs/larvae into the mouth.) Trichinosis is transmitted by ingestion of undercooked contaminated pork, and filariasis is transmitted by biting insects (see Table A–2).

The **flatworms** include the tapeworms and the flukes. Tapeworms that live in the intestines may grow from 5 to 50 feet in length. Flukes are flat, leaf-shaped worms that invade the blood and organs such as the liver, lungs, and intestines. Because these large flatworms feed from the host (human), infestation causes weight loss, anemia, and generalized debilitation. Infestation by worms is treated with drugs called anthelmintics (meaning against worms) (see Table A–2).

Arthropods

Arthropods are creatures with jointed legs and include insects and ticks. They are of concern for two reasons. Arthropods such as mites and lice are **ectoparasites,** meaning that they live on the surface of the body (skin and mucous membranes). Ectoparasites cause itching and discomfort but are not life-threatening. More seriously, arthropods such as mosquitoes, biting flies, fleas, and ticks act

PATHOPHYSIOLOGY: PATHOGENS AND THE DISEASES THEY CAUSE

PATHOGEN	DISEASE AND DESCRIPTION
Bacteria	
Cocci	
Neisseria gonorrhoeae	Gonorrhea. Inflammation of the mucous membrane of the reproductive and urinary tracts. May cause scarring of the fallopian tubes, leading to sterility. May also cause pelvic inflammatory disease (PID). Infants of infected mothers may develop ophthalmia neonatorum. [gram-negative gonococcus, no vaccine]
Neisseria meningitidis	Meningitis. Inflammation of the meninges, the membranes covering the brain and the spinal cord. [gram-negative meningococcus, vaccine available]
Staphylococcus aureus (other staphylococcal infections)	Skin infections such as boils and impetigo, pneumonia, kidney and bladder infections, osteomyelitis, septicemia, and food poisoning. *S. aureus* is a leading cause of nosocomial (hospital-acquired) infections. [gram-positive coccus, no vaccine]
Streptococcus pneumoniae	Pneumonia, middle ear infection, meningitis. [gram-positive diplococcus, vaccine available]
Streptococcus pyogenes	Septicemia, strep throat, middle ear infection, scarlet fever, pneumonia, endocarditis, and puerperal sepsis. Immunologic response to this organism can cause rheumatic fever with permanent damage to the heart valves, and glomerulonephritis. [gram-positive coccus, no vaccine]
Bacilli	
Bordetella pertussis	Pertussis (whooping cough). A severe infection of the trachea and bronchi characterized by episodes of violent coughing. The "whoop" is an effort to inhale after the coughing bouts. [gram-negative bacillus, vaccine available]
Clostridium botulinum	Botulism. A potentially fatal form of food poisoning. Associated with improper processing of foods. The toxin causes respiratory paralysis and death. [gram-positive, spore-forming, no vaccine]
Clostridium perfringens	Gas gangrene. Causes an acute wound infection. Death of the tissue is accompanied by the production of a gas. The dead tissue provides a favorable environment for further growth of this anaerobe. [gram-positive, spore-forming, no vaccine]
Clostridium tetani	Tetanus, or "lockjaw." Causes intense muscle spasms, leading to respiratory paralysis and death. The idea that you can get tetanus by stepping on a rusty nail is related to the fact that the organism is normally found in the soil and that it grows best under anaerobic conditions (conditions established by a deep puncture wound). [gram-positive, spore-forming, vaccine available]
Corynebacterium diphtheriae	Diphtheria. Inflammation of the throat with the formation of a thick, leathery membrane that may cause respiratory obstruction and death by asphyxiation. The toxin also causes heart damage and paralysis. [gram-positive, vaccine available]
Escherichia coli	Normal flora of the intestines. Causes local and systemic infections, food poisoning, diarrhea, septicemia, and septic shock. *E. coli* and related bacilli are the leading cause of nosocomial infections. [gram-negative, no vaccine]
Francisella tularensis	Tularemia, deer fly fever, or rabbit fever. Contracted by the bite of an insect (tick or fly), by ingestion of infected meat, or by inhalation. [gram-negative, no vaccine]
Haemophilus aegyptius	Conjunctivitis. Inflammation of the conjunctiva. The infection is spread by direct contact or by fomites. Often occurs in areas where there are many young children. [gram-negative, no vaccine]
Haemophilus influenzae	Meningitis (in children, especially those less than 2 years of age) and upper respiratory infection in older adults; also causes pneumonia, septicemia, pericarditis, and septic arthritis. [gram-negative, vaccine available]
Helicobacter pylori	Gastritis and ulceration of the stomach and duodenum.
Legionella pneumophila	Legionnaires' disease or legionellosis. A type of pneumonia seen in localized epidemics. The organism contaminates water supplies, including air-conditioning units. A milder, self-limiting form is called Pontiac fever. Has become a common cause of nosocomial pneumonia. [gram-negative, no vaccine]

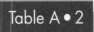
PATHOGEN	DISEASE AND DESCRIPTION
Mycobacterium tuberculosis	Tuberculosis (TB). The organism, also called the tubercle bacillus, causes primary lesions called tubercles. The tubercle bacillus can affect all parts of the body, but the lungs are the most commonly affected organs. The incidence of TB is increasing in the homeless population, in persons with AIDS, and in closed populations, such as in prisons. Generally, overcrowding and substandard living conditions favor the spread of TB. The development of drug resistance makes the treatment and control of TB difficult. Because of its staining characteristics, the organism is also called the acid-fast bacillus. [gram-positive, vaccine available, but generally not used in the United States]
Pseudomonas aeruginosa	Common cause of wound and urinary infections in debilitated patients (such as patients with severe burns, cancer, and other chronic conditions). [gram-negative, no vaccine]
Salmonella enteritidis (and others)	Salmonellosis. A common cause of food poisoning, characterized by severe diarrhea and generally due to the ingestion of contaminated poultry or eggs. [gram-negative, no vaccine]
Salmonella typhi	Typhoid fever. An intestinal infection and ulceration; the infection causes widespread involvement, including septicemia, and infection of the liver, gallbladder, or kidneys. Typhoid fever is rare in the United States because of the chlorination of the water supply. Flooding increases the probability of an outbreak of typhoid fever. [gram-negative, vaccine available]
Shigella dysenteriae	Dysentery. An acute intestinal infection characterized by severe diarrhea. Most often seen where sanitary conditions are poor. [gram-negative, no vaccine]
Yersinia pestis	Bubonic plague; in earlier times, called the "Black Death." The disease is contracted through the bite of fleas that have fed on infected rodents. The most common form of the disease is characterized by swollen, infected lymph nodes called buboes. Another form of the disease causes a fatal pneumonia. [gram-negative, vaccine not reliable]
Curved Rods	
Borrelia burgdorferi	Lyme disease. Characterized by a rash, palsy, and joint inflammation. The spirochete is transmitted by a small deer tick. [vaccine recently developed]
Treponema pallidum	Syphilis. The spirochete is transmitted primarily by sexual intercourse. There are three stages. The primary stage is characterized by the appearance of a lesion (chancre). The secondary stage is characterized by a rash on the skin and mucous membranes. After an extended period of time (5 to 40 years), a tertiary stage develops, characterized by the development of necrotic lesions (gummas) in the central nervous system, heart, aorta, and other organs. [no vaccine]
Vibrio cholerae	Cholera. Characterized by vomiting and profuse, watery diarrhea. Usually spread by water that has been contaminated by human feces. [gram-negative, vaccine is not reliable]
Rickettsiae and Chlamydiae	
Rickettsia prowazekii	Epidemic typhus. Characterized by high fever, delirium, a red rash, and hypotension. Transmitted to humans by lice and found primarily in places where sanitary conditions are poor.
Rickettsia rickettsii	Rocky Mountain spotted fever (RMSF). Characterized by high fever, rash, and pneumonia. Transmitted by ticks that have fed on contaminated wild rodents and dogs. Despite its name, RMSF is not confined to the Rocky Mountain region; it occurs throughout the United States.
Rickettsia typhi	Endemic typhus or murine typhus. A condition that is rarely found in the United States. The symptoms are milder, but similar to those of epidemic typhus. Transmitted by fleas that have fed on contaminated rats and wild rodents.
Chlamydia trachomatis (serogroups A–C)	Trachoma. Characterized by conjunctivitis and corneal scarring and blindness. Leading cause of blindness in the world.
Chlamydia trachomatis (serogroups D–K)	Nongonococcal urethritis. This is currently the most prevalent sexually transmitted disease in the United States. Causes inflammation of the reproductive tract. May lead to pelvic inflammatory disease, ectopic pregnancy, and miscarriage. Newborn infants of infected mothers may develop conjunctivitis or pneumonia. [no vaccine]

Table continued on following page

Table A • 2	PATHOPHYSIOLOGY: PATHOGENS AND THE DISEASES THEY CAUSE *Continued*

PATHOGEN	DISEASE AND DESCRIPTION
Viruses	
Cytomegalovirus (CMV)	Common mild infection of the salivary glands. Causes serious infections in immunosuppressed patients; these infections involve the retina (causing blindness), brain, lungs, liver, and digestive tract. [no vaccine]
Encephalitis viruses	Encephalitis. Inflammation of the brain characterized by confusion, lethargy, or coma. Wild animals and mosquitoes spread the disease. [vaccines available]
Hepatitis A (HAV)	Inflammation of the liver accompanied by nausea, vomiting, fatigue, and jaundice. Spread by fecal-oral route. Full recovery with no carrier state. [vaccine available]
Hepatitis B (HBV)	Inflammation of the liver. Spread by sexual activity or contact with contaminated blood and body fluids. Can develop into a chronic disease, a carrier state, or a fatal disease such as cirrhosis or cancer of the liver. [vaccine available]
Hepatitis C (HCV)	Inflammation of the liver. Known as post-transfusion hepatitis because it is caused by contaminated blood. Can become chronic, develop into a carrier state, or deteriorate to hepatic failure.
Herpes simplex virus	Type 1: cold sores or fever blisters. Appear on the lip, in the oral cavity, or in the nose. The virus lies dormant in the nerves between attacks. Spread in the saliva and causes eye infection through self-inoculation.
	Type 2: genital herpes. A common sexually transmitted disease characterized by painful lesions in the genitalia. [no vaccine]
Herpes varicella-zoster	Chickenpox (varicella). A mild infection, usually in children, and characterized by generalized skin lesions. Upon remission of the infection, the virus becomes dormant and may reactivate in later years as shingles (herpes zoster). Herpes zoster is characterized by painful skin lesions that form on the skin, tracing the path of the infected nerves. [vaccine available]
Human immunodeficiency virus (HIV)	Acquired immunodeficiency disease (AIDS). Characterized by destruction of the helper T cells, suppression of the immune system, and the development of life-threatening opportunistic infections. Spread by sexual contact or contact with contaminated blood and body fluids; placental transmission also occurs. [no vaccine]
Human papillomavirus (HPV)	Genital warts. Transmitted sexually. [no vaccine]
Influenza viruses	Influenza. Caused by different strains of the influenza viruses. A serious complication of the "flu" (muscle aches, fever, chills, malaise) is a secondary bacterial pneumonia. These are mutating viruses, each of which requires a new vaccine.
Measles virus	Measles (rubeola). An acute respiratory inflammation characterized by fever, sore throat, skin rash, and Koplik spots (white spots in the mouth). Many dangerous complications are possible, including measles encephalitis. [vaccine available]
Mumps virus	Mumps (epidemic parotitis). An acute inflammation of the parotid glands. Many complications are possible, including orchitis and sterility in males. [vaccine available]
Polio viruses	Poliomyelitis (infantile paralysis). Acute infection that may destroy nerve cells in the spinal cord, causing paralysis. [vaccine available]
Rhabdovirus	Rabies. A fatal disease characterized by headache, fever, seizures, and spasm of the throat muscles while swallowing (called hydrophobia). Spread by the saliva of infected animals such as dogs and other wild animals. [human rabies immune globulin (post-exposure prevention) and vaccine available]
Rhinoviruses	Common cold (coryza). A self-limiting upper respiratory infection characterized by runny nose, sore throat, and malaise. [no vaccine]
Rubella virus	German measles. A milder form of measles that is characterized by upper respiratory symptoms. The teratogenic birth defects, occurring during the first trimester, are severe and include blindness, deafness, brain damage, and heart defects. [vaccine available]

PATHOPHYSIOLOGY: PATHOGENS AND THE DISEASES THEY CAUSE *Continued*

PATHOGEN	DISEASE AND DESCRIPTION
Fungi	
Candida albicans	Candidiasis. An infection that involves the skin and mucous membranes. Infection of the mucous membranes of the oral cavity is called thrush. Causes important opportunistic infections.
Coccidioides immitis	Coccidioidomycosis. Called San Joaquin fever. A systemic fungal disease that attacks the lungs and produces symptoms similar to those of tuberculosis.
Cryptococcus neoformans	Cryptococcosis. A pulmonary infection that can progress to meningitis and infection of the brain. The most frequent fungal infection of the central nervous system. The incidence of the disease has recently increased because of opportunistic infections in persons with AIDS.
Histoplasma capsulatum	Histoplasmosis. Symptoms range from mild respiratory symptoms (usually self-limiting) to tuberculosis-like symptoms, including cavitation (often fatal). Other forms of the infection involve the liver, spleen, and lymph nodes.
Tinea	Ringworm. A highly contagious fungal infection of the skin. One form of ringworm (tinea pedis) is found on the foot and is called athlete's foot. Other forms of ringworm are found on the scalp (tinea capitis), and on the bearded areas of the face and neck (tinea barbae). Each form is caused by an organism belonging to a group of fungi called dermatophytes. (Ringworm is not caused by a worm, nor is the lesion always ring-shaped.)
Protozoa	
Balantidium coli	Balantidiasis. Gastrointestinal discomfort and diarrhea; often mild.
Entamoeba histolytica	Amebic dysentery. Ulceration of the wall of the large intestine often accompanied by severe diarrhea. The organism may invade the liver, lungs, and brain, causing abscesses in these areas.
Giardia lamblia	Giardiasis. Gastrointestinal discomfort and diarrhea; a common problem in day-care centers.
Plasmodium malariae (various forms)	Malaria. The plasmodium is carried by the mosquito (vector) and invades the red blood cells of the host. The plasmodium matures within the red blood cell, causing it to burst and making the host anemic.
Pneumocystis carinii	Pneumonia. Develops only in debilitated and immunosuppressed persons. A common cause of death in persons with AIDS.
Toxoplasma gondii	Toxoplasmosis. An asymptomatic infection in healthy people. Causes teratogenic effects such as mental retardation, blindness, and death. Causes a fatal encephalitis in immunosuppressed persons. Reservoirs are cats and raw meat.
Trichomonas vaginalis	Trichomoniasis. A sexually transmitted disease. The female experiences cervicitis and vaginitis; the male may be asymptomatic or experience painful urination.
Worms	
Ascaris	Twelve-inch-long worms that live in the small intestine. Large infestations may cause intestinal obstruction.
Clonorchis (Chinese liver fluke)	Acquired by eating contaminated raw fish. The worms live in the bile ducts and invade the liver, eventually causing cirrhosis if not treated.
Hookworm *(Necator)*	Larval worms burrow their way through the skin of a bare foot, migrate to the intestine, and hook onto the intestinal wall. The worms feed on the blood of the host, causing anemia and fatigue.
Pinworm *(Enterobius)*	The most common worm infestation in the United States. The adult worms live in the colon but lay their eggs on the perianal skin area, causing itching. Spread by fecal-oral route.
Tapeworms *(Taenia,* others)	Acquired by eating poorly cooked contaminated food such as beef, fish, and pork.
Trichinella spiralis	Trichinosis. Acquired by eating contaminated, poorly cooked pork. The worms migrate to muscles, forming cysts that become calcified. The calcified cysts cause severe muscle pain.

Table continued on following page

as vectors of disease. The bite of these arthropods introduces pathogens into the host, causing infection. For instance, the mosquito can carry the pathogens for malaria, encephalitis, and yellow fever. The tick can carry the pathogens for Lyme disease and Rocky Mountain spotted fever.

LABORATORY IDENTIFICATION

Many laboratory procedures and techniques are used to identify pathogens. One of these techniques is called staining and involves the use of various dyes.

Many bacteria are identified (and classified) according to staining characteristics using the Gram stain (a dye). A **gram-positive** bacterium is one that stains purple or blue. Streptococcus is an example of a gram-positive bacterium. A **gram-negative** bacterium, such as *Escherichia coli,* does not absorb the purple Gram stain. Instead, a gram-negative bacterium picks up a pink or red stain. Since most bacteria are either gram-positive or gram-negative, Gram staining is an important first step in the identification of the causative organism of an infection.

Another stain is called the **acid-fast stain.** The bacterium is first stained with a red dye and then washed with an acid. Most bacteria lose the red stain when washed with acid. However, several bacteria retain the red stain and therefore are called acid-fast. The most well known of the acid-fast bacteria is *Mycobacterium tuberculosis,* the causative organism of tuberculosis (TB). This organism is commonly called the acid-fast bacillus.

A few organisms do not stain with any of the commonly used dyes. Thus, the spirochetes and rickettsiae must be stained with special dyes and techniques.

You will frequently be asked to collect samples for laboratory analysis. There are specific rules that must be followed for each specimen. For instance, in collecting a urine specimen that will be analyzed for the presence of pathogens, you must be careful not to contaminate the urine with microorganisms from your hands or unsterile containers. The proper diagnosis depends on the correct technique.

Appendix B

Medical Terminology and Eponymous Terms

MEDICAL TERMINOLOGY

Anatomy and physiology has its own vocabulary. You must learn this vocabulary to understand the scientific concepts and to communicate effectively with other medical professionals. This special vocabulary consists of prefixes, word roots, and suffixes arranged in various combinations. By recognizing the meanings of the various prefixes, word roots, and suffixes, you can understand most words.

The **word root** is the main part of the word; it provides the central meaning of the word. For instance, *cardi-* refers to heart, while *cerebr-* refers to brain. Sometimes, two word roots are combined. For instance, *cardio-* (heart) and *pulmon-* (lungs) are combined in cardiopulmonary, a reference to both the heart and the lungs. Refer to the list in Table B–1 for other common word roots.

The **prefix** is the part of the word placed before the word root. The prefix alters the meaning of the word root. For instance, the prefix *mal-*, when placed before nutrition *(malnutrition)*, modifies or alters the meaning of nutrition; it means bad or poor nutrition. The prefix *hyper-*, as in *hypersecretion*, means that there is excessive secretion, while the prefix *hypo-*, as in *hyposecretion*, means that secretion is insufficient. Refer to the list in Table B–1 for commonly used prefixes.

The **suffix** is the part of the word that follows the word root; it is a word ending that may modify or alter the meaning of the word root. For instance, the suffix *-cide,* as in *germicide,* refers to a substance that kills germs. Refer to the list in Table B–1 for commonly used suffixes.

EPONYMOUS TERMS

As you study anatomy and physiology, you will notice that some terms incorporate the name of a person. For instance, the Krebs cycle is named after Hans Krebs, the famous biochemist who worked out and described the chemical reactions of this cycle. The person for whom something is named is an **eponym;** the descriptive term is an **eponymous term.**

Because eponymous terms do not provide much useful information, they are being replaced with more informative terms. For instance, the Krebs cycle has been renamed the citric acid cycle because citric acid is an important part of the cycle.

The following list provides some of the commonly used eponymous terms and the newer, more descriptive terms.

Eponymous Term	Newer Term
Achilles tendon	calcaneal tendon
Adam's apple	thyroid cartilage
ampulla of Vater	hepatopancreatic ampulla
Bowman capsule	glomerular capsule
bundle of His	atrioventricular bundle
canal of Schlemm	scleral venous sinus
cells of Leydig	interstitial cells
circle of Willis	cerebral arterial circle
Cowper glands	bulbourethral glands
eustachian tube	auditory tube
fallopian tube	uterine tube, oviduct
fissure of Rolando	central sulcus
graafian follicle	vesicular ovarian follicle
haversian canal	central canal
haversian system	osteon
islets of Langerhans	pancreatic islet cells
Krebs cycle	citric acid cycle
Sertoli cells	sustentacular cells
sphincter of Oddi	sphincter of the hepatopancreatic ampulla
Wernicke area	posterior speech area

Table B • 1   PREFIXES, SUFFIXES, AND WORD ROOTS

	MEANING	EXAMPLE
Prefixes		
a-, an-	lack of, without	anoxia (without oxygen)
ab-	away from	abduction (movement away from the midline)
ad- (af-)	to, toward	adduction (movement toward the midline), afferent (toward a center)
ante-	forward, before	antenatal (before birth)
anti-	against	antibiotic (against life), anticoagulant (against blood clotting)
bi-	two	biceps (two heads of a muscle)
bio-	life	biology (study of life)
brady-	slow	bradycardia (abnormally slow heart rate)
co-, com-, con-	with, together	congenital (born with)
contra-	against, opposite	contralateral (opposite side), contraception (against conception)
cyan-	blue	cyanotic (having a blue coloring)
de-	away from	dehydration (loss of water)
dextro-	right	dextrocardia (heart abnormally shifted to the right)
di-	two	disaccharide (double sugar)
dys-	difficult	dysphagia (difficulty in eating)
ect-, exo-, extra-	outside	extracellular (outside the cell)
epi-	on, upon	epidermis (upon the dermis)
erythr-	red	erythrocyte (red blood cell)
eu-	good, well	euphoria (sense of well-being), eupnea (normal breathing)
hemi-, semi-	one half	hemiplegia (paralysis of one half or one side of the body), semilunar valve (valve that resembles a half-moon)
hyper-	over, above normal	hypersecretion (excessive secretion)
hypo-	under, below normal	hyposecretion (insufficient secretion)
inter-	between	intercellular (between the cells)
intra-	within	intracellular (within the cells)
leuk(o)-	white	leukocyte (white blood cell)
macro-	large	macrophage (large phagocytic cell)
mal-	bad	malnutrition (bad or inadequate nutrition), malfunction (bad or inadequate function)
micro-	small	microbiology (study of small life such as bacteria)
melan-	black	melena (darkening of the stool by blood pigments)
necr-	dead	necrosis (death, as of tissue)
neo-	new	neonate (newborn infant), neoplasm (new growth)
noct-	night	nocturia (excessive urination at night)
olig-	scanty	oliguria (scanty urine)
orth-	straight	orthopnea (ability to breathe easily only in an upright, or straight, position)
peri-	around	pericardium (membrane surrounding the heart)
pleur-	rib, side	pleural membranes (membranes that enclose the lungs)
poly-	much, many	polyuria (much urine); polysaccharide (many sugars)
post-	after	postnatal (after birth)
pre-	before	prenatal (before birth)
presby-	elder, old	presbyopia (diminished vision due to aging)
pseudo-	false	pseudopod (false foot)
retro-	behind, backward	retroperitoneal (behind the peritoneum)

Table B • 1	**PREFIXES, SUFFIXES, AND WORD ROOTS** *Continued*

	MEANING	**EXAMPLE**
sten-	narrow	mitral valve stenosis (narrowing of the mitral valve)
sub-	underneath	subcutaneous (underneath the skin)
super-, supra-	above	suprarenal glands (glands located above the kidneys)
syn-	with, together	synergistic muscle (a muscle that works with another muscle)
tachy-	rapid	tachycardia (abnormally rapid heart rate)
trans-	across	transcapillary exchange (movement across the capillary membrane)

Suffixes

-algia	pain	neuralgia (nerve pain)
-cele	hernia	omphalocele (umbilical hernia)
-centesis	puncture to remove fluid	thoracentesis (aspiration of fluid from the chest)
-cide	to kill	germicide (kills germs)
-cyte	cell	leukocyte (white blood cell)
-ectomy	removal of	hysterectomy (removal of the uterus)
-emia	blood	hypoglycemia (decreased glucose in the blood)
-gram	record	mammogram (x-ray or record of the breasts)
-iasis	condition of	cholelithiasis (condition of having gallstones)
-itis	inflammation of	appendicitis (inflammation of the appendix)
-logy	study of	physiology (study of the function of the body)
-lysis, lytic	breakdown	hemolysis (breakdown of blood)
-malacia	softening	osteomalacia (softening of the bones)
-megaly	enlargement	hepatomegaly (enlarged liver)
-oma	tumor	adenoma (tumor containing glandular tissue)
-osis	abnormal condition	leukocytosis (abnormal condition of white blood cells)
-ostomy	to create an abnormal opening	colostomy (an opening into the colon)
-pathy	disease	nephropathy (disease of the kidney)
-penia	deficiency, poor	thrombocytopenia (a deficiency of platelets)
-plasty	to shape	pyloroplasty (to surgically shape the pylorus)
-rrhaphy	to suture or sew	herniorrhaphy (to repair or sew a hernia)
-rrhea	discharge from	rhinorrhea (discharge from the nose, a runny nose)
-scopy	visualization	colonoscopy (insertion of a scope to see the inside of the colon)
-stasis	to stand still, stop	hemostasis (stop the flow of blood)
-uria	urine	glucosuria (glucose in the urine)

Word Roots

aden	gland	adenoma (tumor of glandular tissue)
angi	vessel	angioma (tumor of a vessel)
arthr	joint	arthritis (inflammation of the joints)
blast	immature cell	osteoblast (immature bone cell)
brachi	arm	brachialgia (pain in the arm)
cardi	heart	cardioactive (having an effect on the heart)
cephal	head	cephalad (toward the head)
cervic	neck	cervicodynia (pain in the neck)
chondr	cartilage	chondroma (tumor of the cartilage)

Table continued on following page

Table B • 1	PREFIXES, SUFFIXES, AND WORD ROOTS *Continued*	
	MEANING	**EXAMPLE**
crani	skull	craniometry (measurement of the skull)
derm(at)	skin	dermatitis (inflammation of the skin)
gastr	stomach	gastritis (inflammation of the lining of the stomach)
gingiv	gums	gingivitis (inflammation of the gums)
gloss	tongue	glossitis (inflammation of the tongue)
glyc(y), gluc	sugar, glucose	hyperglycemia (high blood sugar)
hem(at)	blood	hematuria (blood in the urine)
hepat	liver	hepatitis (inflammation of the liver)
hyster	uterus	hysterectomy (removal of the uterus)
lact, galact	milk	lactogenic hormone (milk-producing hormone)
lith	stone	cholelithiasis (condition of gallstones)
mast, mamm	breast	mastitis (inflammation of the breast)
my	muscle	myocardium (heart muscle)
myel	marrow, spinal cord	myelosuppression (depression of the bone marrow)
nephr	kidney	nephritis (inflammation of the kidney)
neur	nerve	neuritis (inflammation of a nerve)
oo	egg	oocyte (egg cell)
oophor	ovary	oophorectomy (removal of the ovary)
ophthalm	eye	ophthalmoscope (an instrument used to view the eye)
path	disease	pathology (study of disease)
ped, pedia	child	pediatrics (branch of medicine dealing with the child)
phag	eat, swallow	dysphagia (difficulty swallowing)
pharyng	throat	pharyngitis (sore throat)
phleb	vein	phlebitis (inflammation of the vein)
pneum	air, breath	pneumothorax (air in the chest)
pneumon, pulmo(n)	lung	pneumonectomy (removal of the lung)
psych	mind	psychology (study of the mind)
rhin	nose	rhinorrhea (discharge from the nose; runny nose)
therm	heat	hyperthermia (higher than normal temperature)
thorac	chest	thoracotomy (incision into the chest)
thromb	clot	thrombolytic (an agent that dissolves a clot)
trache	windpipe	tracheostomy (incision into the trachea)

Appendix C

Laboratory Values

TEST	NORMAL VALUES*	CLINICAL SIGNIFICANCE
Blood Tests		
Blood Counts (Formed Elements)		
Platelet count	150,000–350,000/mm^3	Increases in heart disease, cirrhosis, and cancer; decreases in myelosuppression
Red blood cell count	Men: 4.5–6.0 million/mm^3 Women: 4.2–5.4 million/mm^3	Decreases in anemia; increases in polycythemia, dehydration
Reticulocyte count	0.5–1.5% of RBCs/mm^3	Increases in anemia following hemorrhage
White blood cell count	5000–10,000/mm^3	Increases in infection, inflammation, and dehydration; decreases in myelosuppression
White blood cell count (differential)		See Table 13–1
Other Counts		
Clotting time	5–10 minutes	Increases in severe liver disease and deficiencies of coagulation factors
Hematocrit	Men: 40–50% Women: 37–47%	Increases in dehydration and polycythemia; decreases in anemia and hemorrhage
Hemoglobin	Men: 13.5–17.5 g/dL Women: 12–16 g/dL	Increases in polycythemia and dehydration; decreases in anemia, bleeding, and hemolysis
Prothrombin time	11–15 seconds	Increases in liver disease, vitamin K deficiency, and oral anticoagulation
Blood Electrolytes and Metabolites		
Albumin	3.5–5.5 g/dL	Decreases in kidney disease, liver disease, and burns
Bicarbonate	22–26 mEq/L	Increases in chronic lung disease; decreases in metabolic acidosis (uncontrolled diabetes mellitus) and diarrhea
Bilirubin (total)	0.3–1.4 mg/dL	Increases in hepatobiliary disease and hemolytic reactions
Calcium	9.0–11 mg/dL	Increases in hyperparathyroidism and cancer; decreases in alkalosis and hyperphosphatemia

*Values vary from laboratory to laboratory.

Chloride	95–108 mEq/L	Increases in dehydration and heart failure; decreases when body fluids are lost, as in vomiting, diarrhea, and diuresis
Cholesterol	120–220 mg/dL	Increases in coronary artery disease
Creatinine	0.6–1.5 mg/dL	Increases in kidney disease
Glucose	70–110 mg/dL (affected by meals)	Increases in diabetes mellitus, severe illness, pregnancy; decreases in insulin overdose
pH	7.35–7.45	Increases in hyperventilation and metabolic alkalosis; decreases in diabetes mellitus and hypoventilation
Potassium	3.5–5.0 mEq/L	Increases in kidney failure, cell destruction, and acidosis; decreases in loss of body fluid (vomiting, diarrhea, diuretic-induced polyuria)
Sodium	136–145 mEq/L	Increases in dehydration; decreases when body fluids are lost (burns, diuresis, vomiting, diarrhea)
Urea nitrogen (BUN)	8–25 mg/dL	Increases in kidney disease and high protein diet
Uric acid	3.0–7.0 mg/dL	Increases in gout, leukemia, and kidney disease

Urinalysis

General Characteristics

Color	Amber, straw	Affected by hydration; dehydration causes a deeper yellow color, overhydration causes a pale color; hepatobiliary disease causes a deeper yellow color; color changes in response to drugs
Clarity	Clear, slightly hazy	Becomes cloudy on refrigeration or in the presence of urinary tract infection (bacteria clouds urine)
Odor	Aromatic	Foul-smelling with a urinary tract infection; fruity odor in ketoacidosis (diabetes mellitus)
Specific gravity (SG)	1.003–1.030	Affected by hydration. In dehydration, the SG increases; in overhydration the SG decreases. Polyuria (diabetes) causes a low specific gravity; also decreases in kidney damage.
pH	4.6–8.0	Decreases in acidosis and high protein diet; increases in alkalosis and vegetarian diet

Metabolites

Ammonia	20–70 mEq/L	Increases in diabetes mellitus and liver disease
Bilirubin	negative	Increases in liver disease and biliary obstruction
Creatinine	1–2.5 mg/24 hrs	Increases in infection; decreases in kidney disease
Glucose	negative	Increases in diabetes mellitus
Ketone bodies	negative	Increases in ketoacidosis (diabetes mellitus and starvation)

Protein	negative	Increases in kidney disease
Uric acid	0.4–1.0 g/24 hrs	Increases in gout and liver disease; decreases in kidney disease
Urobilinogen	0–4 mg/24 hrs	Increases in liver disease and hemolytic anemia

Formed Elements, Other Large Substances

Red blood cells	few	Increases in inflammation and trauma to the urinary tract
White blood cells	few	Increases in urinary tract infection
Bacteria	few	Increases in urinary tract infection

Index

Note: Page numbers in italics refer to illustrations; page numbers followed by the letter t refer to tables.